TEXTBOOK OF REMEDIAL
Massage

TEXTBOOK OF REMEDIAL
Massage

Sandra Grace PhD, MSc, Grad Cert Sports Chiro, Cert Clinical Chiro Paediatrics, Dip Acup, DBM, DO, DC, Dip Ed, BA

Professor of Osteopathy, Southern Cross University

Jane Graves MChiro, BSc, DRM, Cert IV TAE

Chiropractor, Massage Therapist and Educator
Associate Lecturer in Medical Education, Western Sydney University

ELSEVIER

ELSEVIER

Elsevier Australia. ACN 001 002 357
(a division of Reed International Books Australia Pty Ltd)
Tower 1, 475 Victoria Avenue, Chatswood, NSW 2067

ISBN: 978-0-7295-4334-7

National Library of Australia Cataloguing-in-Publication Data

A catalogue record for this
book is available from the
National Library of Australia

Content Strategist: Larissa Norrie
Content Project Manager: Sukanthi Sukumar
Edited by Annabel Adair
Cover by Natalie Bowra
Index by Innodata Indexing
Typeset by Toppan Best-set Premedia Limited
Printed in China by 1010 Printing International Limited

Last digit is the print number: 9 8 7 6 5 4 3 2 1

Contents

CONTENTS

CONTENTS

Preface

The second edition of this book maintains the focus of safe and evidence-based healthcare that was a key feature of the previous edition. It reflects evolving understandings of conditions that are frequently treated by remedial massage therapists, including low back pain, osteoarthritis, acute inflammation and tendinopathy. Extensive searches of academic databases were conducted to locate high quality research evidence to inform clinical practice. This edition also contains many traditional remedial massage treatments, many of which await rigorous scientific assessment. These treatments are presented with a focus on critical appraisal and lifelong learning, both of which are served by remaining conversant with current research.

The aim of this book is to present a comprehensive practical guide for students, practitioners and educators of remedial massage. It assumes mastery of the knowledge and skills required for therapeutic relaxation massage (Certificate IV level). Remedial massage practitioners treat a broad range of conditions, often as first contact practitioners. Safe practice requires a sound knowledge of clinical (red) and psychosocial (yellow) flags and a willingness to collaborate with other healthcare practitioners to provide client-centred care.

STRUCTURE OF THE BOOK

The book is presented in three sections. The first discusses the scope of practice of remedial massage, its place in the Australian healthcare system, and its potential role in the key field of integrative health. It presents a comprehensive and evidence-based approach to assessment and principles of treatment. The approach to short- and long-term treatment planning prioritises client safety and the use of current research, and highlights the important role of client education.

The second section deals with some of the most important and widely used techniques of remedial massage. The exposition of each technique is accompanied by a rationale based on current supporting evidence and an explanation of contraindications and precautions. Applications of techniques are illustrated by photographs and drawings. A demonstration of integrated techniques is also presented on the DVD accompanying the book.

The final section of the book is divided into regions of the body. Each chapter contains a description of common conditions of the region, relevant assessment procedures and a range of remedial massage techniques that can safely be applied in treatment. A distinctive feature of this book is its approach to treatment: it presents techniques as they are often integrated in practice and clearly articulates the clinical reasoning that supports treatment choices. Summary tables illustrating a range of remedial massage techniques for specific muscles are included in each chapter. The final chapter of the book focuses on remedial massage assessment and treatment considerations for specific population groups.

The content of this book aligns with the competencies for remedial massage practice that were developed by educators, curriculum designers and professional association representatives in Australia. This content is also highly applicable to other jurisdictions where remedial massage is practised. This book clarifies what constitutes remedial massage and what separates it from other manual therapies like relaxation massage, osteopathy and physiotherapy. Such clarification is necessary if the benefits of remedial massage are to be recognised in their own right and the safety and competence of its practitioners are to be assured. Remedial massage would then be assured of its rightful place within the healthcare system.

Acknowledgements

We are indebted to our colleagues Catrin Jonsson and Mark Deal whose expertise was indispensable to the relevance and currency of content. Thanks are also due to Larissa Norrie and Sukanthi Sukumar from Elsevier who guided our second edition and to Greg Gaul and Alan Laver who drew the high quality illustrations. Thanks also to our photographers Dianne and Veronique from Diverze Photography, and to Dragan Dimitrovski from Mak Video who shot the videos. Jane, Catrin and Mark were outstanding demonstrators. I am also deeply indebted to our models Aynur Aksu, Umit Aksu, Yavus Aksu, Hannah Temby, Eleanor Nurse, Michael Boyley and Pierce Boyley.

Thanks to our editor Stephen Clarke, who brought his formidable skills to imposing precision and clarity wherever they were needed, and to Annabel Adair who copy-edited the manuscript. Many skilled and experienced therapists and teachers contributed their expert knowledge and time to reviewing sections of the book. We are extremely grateful for their insights, which contributed so much to the final form of the book. Thanks also to Sasha Chaitow for her kind endorsement of this book. This also gives us an opportunity to acknowledge the inspiration we have had over thirty years of practice and pedagogy from the teachings of many leading lights in the field of manual therapies, none more cherished than Leon Chaitow and such pioneers as Janet Travell and Vladimir Janda.

Foreword

The rapid expansion of research providing a scientific underpinning for bodywork modalities has led to much progress in the acceptance and integration of massage as an adjunct to medical treatment for a variety of conditions. Distinct from other professions in a number of ways, in recent years therapeutic massage has constructively evolved towards a much-needed standardisation of vocabulary, training, and techniques supported by the latest evidence. The *Textbook of Remedial Massage* makes a significant contribution to this effort, and this new edition ensures a balance between the most recent research and the value of clinical experience.

For this new edition, the authors of this excellent textbook have diligently distilled a vast amount of new research to provide solid foundations for well-established techniques, while offering readers a robust understanding of assessment procedures and the dysfunctions they are treating. This edition takes account of changes in understanding of a variety of conditions and best practices, providing up-to-date information complete with the necessary guidelines for real-world use in the practice. They also highlight the continuing need for trials of higher methodological quality to produce rigorous, useful evidence for remedial massage, and the significance of research literacy and application among massage professionals.

As noted in the foreword to the first edition a clinician must make numerous complex decisions together with their patient when selecting the most appropriate techniques and approaches. This requires both a sound understanding of physiological and biopsychosocial factors, as well as a finely tuned critical ability to support clinical reasoning that can interpret and incorporate the evidence alongside tried-and-tested experience, while taking into account the contraindications depending on the multiple variables present. The structure and presentation of this book offers students and practitioners a solid and well-supported framework within which to do so.

In line with their stated aim of focusing on critical appraisal and lifelong learning, they have provided the best possible development of translational research, through clear, succinct tables of evidence regarding the management of a wide variety of conditions that incorporate the most recent findings and changes in approaches to acute and chronic conditions. These are accompanied with self-test review sections to further assist the proactive practitioner. This makes the book an essential guide for all involved in remedial massage as well as related professions utilising similar techniques, moving from definitions and key techniques, to focus on the body according to region and associated conditions. The clearly stated objectives, careful, comprehensive, evidence-based explanations of rationale, immediately useful illustrations, and provision of all the possible tools needed for safe and effective practice will benefit students and veteran therapists alike.

These features mark a significant contribution to the massage profession and the authors' stated aim of supporting a deeper integration of remedial massage into mainstream healthcare. While this has been conducted with reference to Australia, it possesses rich potential as an example to follow in other locales where such streamlining in education, training and practice is not yet standard, and it is to be hoped that this will indeed be achieved.

Sasha Chaitow MA, MA, PhD
Managing Editor, Journal of Bodywork and
Movement Therapies
London, UK

Contributor

Mark Deal, BSc, DC, DO, Dip Ed
(Technical)
Chiropractor, Osteopath, Acupuncturist and
Educator, Independent Contractor to Noosa
Parade Medical Centre

Remedial massage in Australian healthcare

Learning Outcomes

- Define remedial massage and describe the difference between remedial massage and other levels of massage training including relaxation massage.
- Demonstrate an understanding of the context of remedial massage practice including the extent of public use of remedial massage and attitudes of other healthcare practitioners towards remedial massage.
- Demonstrate an understanding of the evidence base for remedial massage.

DEFINING REMEDIAL MASSAGE

Many authors writing about massage therapy fail to distinguish between different types of massage, differences in training requirements for practitioners and varying levels of recognition by professional associations, medical benefit funds and WorkCover authorities.[1, 2] In particular, there is confusion between what constitutes relaxation or Swedish massage and remedial massage, the terms often being used interchangeably.[3] The Australian and New Zealand Standard Classification of Occupations (ANZSCO)[4] described only one massage occupation, that of massage therapist, who 'performs therapeutic massage and administers body treatments for health, fitness and remedial purposes'. Moreover, Australian professional associations often use definitions of massage and set levels of practice that they develop independently.[5-7]

Most Australian training institutions refer to two levels of massage therapy: a basic level (Certificate IV) for relaxation massage; and a more advanced level (Diploma) for diagnosing and treating musculoskeletal and other conditions. Myotherapy is now established as a third level with a more advanced approach, usually involving neurological assessment.

The national vocational education and Health Training Package recognises two levels of massage practice: Certificate IV in Massage Therapy Practice[8] and Diploma of Remedial Massage[9] that align with the Australian Qualifications Framework (Table 1.1).[10] The consensus among practitioners and educators of massage therapy is that remedial massage therapists assess and treat musculoskeletal and other system disorders.

Diploma-qualified therapists are expected to demonstrate a level of analysis, judgment, problem-solving skills, responsibility for their own work and the work of others, and self-evaluation capabilities in practice. (A diploma is the minimum qualification required for most Australian medical benefit funds.) Massage therapists with more basic levels of training, on the other hand, require sufficient knowledge and skills to determine the suitability of their clients for treatment using a contraindications checklist, and to perform a massage therapy routine with a limited range of variations. Any definition of remedial massage must reflect not only the level of technical skills required for this qualification, but also the level of analysis, evaluation and responsibility required for assessing and treating musculoskeletal and other conditions amenable to massage therapy. A common practice of training institutions is to interpret curriculum purely in terms of the range of content to be included. Such an interpretation is not only prone to misuse of the graduate capabilities outlined in Table 1.1, but also runs the risk of ignoring other important aspects of curriculum, including hidden or implicit ones (e.g. acculturation that occurs in student training clinics).

In this book we define remedial massage as:
i) the application of a range of diagnostic techniques[a] to identify clients and their conditions as suitable for remedial massage therapy and to enable adaptation of remedial massage therapy techniques to suit the needs of individual clients;

and
ii) the use of a range of basic and advanced massage techniques (e.g. trigger points, myofascial release and lymphatic drainage) to treat a variety of musculoskeletal and other system conditions.

THE CONTEXT OF REMEDIAL MASSAGE: USE OF COMPLEMENTARY AND ALTERNATIVE MEDICINE IN AUSTRALIAN HEALTHCARE

Remedial massage is one of the many modalities that are encompassed by the term *complementary and alternative medicine* (CAM). One study estimated that the number of Australians using CAM was high as 70% at an annual cost of about $4 billion.[11] A systematic review of the prevalence of CAM in six countries (Australia, Canada, Singapore, South Korea, UK, US) found that those surveyed were more likely

---

[a]The terms diagnosis/diagnostic techniques refer to assessment practices accepted as falling within the scope of remedial massage. They are to be understood solely as remedial massage diagnosis/diagnostic techniques whenever they are used in this book.

Table 1.1 Comparison between certificate IV and diploma qualifications

	Certificate IV	Diploma
Purpose	Graduates at this level will have theoretical and practical knowledge and skills for specialised and/or skilled work and/or further learning.	Graduates at this level will have specialised knowledge and skills for skilled/paraprofessional work and/or further learning.
Knowledge	Graduates of a Certificate IV will have broad factual, technical and some theoretical knowledge of a specific area or a broad field of work and learning.	Graduates at this level will have technical and theoretical knowledge in a specific area or a broad field of work and learning.
Skills	Graduates at this level will have a broad range of cognitive, technical and communication skills to select and apply a range of methods, tools, materials and information to: • complete routine and non-routine activities • provide and transmit solutions to a variety of predictable and sometimes unpredictable problems	Graduates at this level have a broad range of cognitive, technical and communication skills to select and apply methods and technologies to: • analyse information to complete a range of activities • provide and transmit solutions to sometimes complex problems • transmit information and skills to others
Application of knowledge and skills	Graduates at this level will apply knowledge and skills to demonstrate autonomy, judgement and limited responsibility in known or changing contexts and within established parameters.	Graduates at this level will apply knowledge and skills to demonstrate autonomy, judgement and defined responsibility in known or changing contexts and within broad but established parameters.
Volume of learning	The volume of learning of a Certificate IV is typically 0.5–2 years. There may be variations between short duration specialist qualifications that build on knowledge and skills already acquired and longer duration qualifications that are designed as entry level requirements for work.	The volume of learning of a Diploma is typically 1–2 years.

(Qualification descriptors reproduced with permission of the Australian Qualifications Framework Council[10])

to visit a massage therapist than an acupuncturist, homeopath, osteopath or medical herbalists. Only chiropractors were visited more frequently and this was thought to be due to their popularity in Australia, Canada and the US.[12] Massage therapy is particularly popular with people with musculoskeletal problems. For example, massage therapy consultations were reported by up to 81.5% by people with ankylosing spondylitis.[13]

THE REMEDIAL MASSAGE WORKFORCE IN AUSTRALIA

There have been few attempts to collect data on the number of remedial massage therapists working in Australia. Such a task is confounded by the lack of a central register or government registration and because many remedial massage therapists work part-time or casually and may not report remedial massage as their occupation. Most graduates of colleges and courses accredited with professional associations seek membership with their respective associations. Practitioners who have trained overseas, trained with a non-accredited college, who have not undertaken any formal training or who have not sought professional association membership may also be in practice. It is possible that the number of remedial massage therapists in Australia is considerably higher than the official professional association figures. An estimate based on 2009 information from professional massage associations put the number of massage therapists working in Australia at that time at just over 22,000.[14]

Three national surveys of CAM practitioners, funded by the Department of Health and Ageing, were conducted in Australia in 2000.[15, 16, 17] At the time the remedial massage workforce was predominantly female, part time and sole practice (see Table 1.2).

More recent surveys have demonstrated that the profession remains female dominated and that nearly three-quarters are over 36 years of age. The majority continue to work part time and about 40% of the profession have been in practice for more than 10 years (see Table 1.2).[18, 19]

ATTITUDES TOWARDS CAM BY MEDICAL AND OTHER HEALTHCARE PRACTITIONERS

Attitudes towards CAM among members of the medical profession and other non-CAM healthcare providers has fluctuated over time, with those CAM products and services that are evidence-based being more readily accepted. The Australian Medical Association's position statement on complementary medicine recognised that evidence-based aspects of complementary medicine can be part of patient care by a medical practitioner.[20] In Australia, members of the medical profession are also more likely to refer to, and to share practices with, practitioners of CAM occupations that have wider acceptance, such as acupuncture, chiropractic and massage, and less likely to do so with lower-profile CAM occupations such as Reiki and flower essences. Apart from clinical efficacy, they also consider potential risk and alignment with medical principles.[21] Medical practitioners can also be willing to explore new approaches, including CAM, when mainstream medical approaches are failing to bring improved health outcomes for their patients.[22]

Table 1.2 A comparison of surveys of the Australian massage therapy workforce

Massage workforce survey	Hale (2002)[15] (n = 2192)	Grace et al (2013)[18] (n = 3177)	Wardle et al (2015)[19] (n = 301)
Gender	Male: 25.2% Female: 74.8%	Male: 18.8% Female: 81.2%	Male: 32.8% Female: 67.2%
Age (years)	Age range: 26–55	< 25: 7.0% 25–35: 9.4% 36–45: 23.9% 46–55: 25.1% 56–65: 25.1% > 65: 6.1%	-
Number of consultations per week	Average: 12	< 5: 33.1 6–10: 24.3 11–20: 27 21–30: 10.5 31–40: 3.0 41–50: 1.6 > 50: 0.6	< 5: 21.6 6–10: 25.2 11–20: 26.9 > 20: 26.2
Type of practice	Solo practice: 64% Group practice: 18%	Solo practice: 61.8% Group practice: 26.7%	-
Years in clinical practice	1–5 years: 64%	1–5: 32% 6–10: 29.5% 11–15: 19.8% 16–20: 10.3% > 20: 8.3%	-

EVIDENCE FOR REMEDIAL MASSAGE PRACTICE

The evidence for the effectiveness of massage therapy is conflicting. Systematic reviews are regarded as the strongest form of evidence because they bring together all relevant studies on a specific topic and research question. They assess the risk of bias and critically appraise the quality of the studies to draw conclusions. These conclusions are invariably limited by the low quality of the available trials.

Several systematic reviews have reported short-term benefits of massage therapy compared to placebo or no treatment. For example, Kumar et al[23] reviewed nine systematic reviews of the effectiveness of massage therapy in the treatment of non-specific low back pain and concluded that 'massage may be an effective treatment option when compared to placebo and some active treatment options (such as relaxation), especially in the short term. There is conflicting and contradictory findings for the effectiveness of massage therapy for the treatment of non-specific low back pain when compared against other manual therapies (such as mobilization), standard medical care, and acupuncture'.

In another example, a systematic review of 26 randomised controlled trials found that massage therapy had short-term benefits for people with common musculoskeletal disorders compared to no treatment. Massage therapy, as a stand-alone treatment, was found to reduce pain and improve function compared to no treatment in some musculoskeletal conditions. When massage was compared to another active treatment, no clear benefit was evident.[24]

Another systematic review of seven randomised controlled trials reporting the effects of massage therapy on people with osteoarthritis or rheumatoid arthritis found that the risk of bias ranged from 4–7 on the PEDro scale (scores of 6 or above are considered high-quality trials and scores lower than 6 are considered low quality)[25] and low- to moderate-quality evidence that massage therapy was 'superior to non-active therapies in reducing pain and improving certain functional outcomes. It is unclear whether massage therapy is more effective than other forms of treatment'.[26]

Appendix 1.1 provides further examples of systematic reviews on the effectiveness of massage therapy. They have been sourced from the Cochrane Library (https://www.cochranelibrary.com/).

The message for massage research is clear. There is an urgent need to improve the quality of the trials that are conducted so that therapeutic interventions can be informed by the highest quality evidence. There are particular challenges for massage therapy that need to be overcome, including the lack of consensus on what massage therapy is, managing risk of bias, reliance on small sample sizes and other methodological flaws. Boyd[27] suggested the following be taken into consideration when designing massage therapy trials:

- Using appropriate controls
  - Comparing massage therapy to controls that are 'equally credible, acceptable and seemingly identical to massage'. Trials often compare massage therapy to another active therapy (i.e. usual care, exercise therapy, relaxation therapy). Complications can arise when assigning people to usual care if they have already found it unsuccessful. Wait list controls do not control for placebo effects.
  - Comparing massage therapy to no treatment (most massage therapy trials typically use no treatment controls but this does not rule out the possibility of effects being

'non-specific', that is, effects that result from attention and touch.

- Comparing massage therapy to sham therapy (e.g. sham massage, light touch). Some people argue that any touch control will have non-specific physiological effects and is therefore not a true placebo. Even patient expectation can contribute to a placebo effect. Boyd[27] suggested including questions about patient and practitioner expectation during the trial period so that the influence of expectation on trial outcomes can be considered.
- Using standardised patient-reported outcomes that have been found to be valid, sensitive and reliable. For example, the Patient Reported Outcomes Measurement Information System (PROMIS®), developed as a reliable and valid tool for evaluating medical interventions for people with chronic diseases, may be a useful outcome measure for massage therapy trials (see Appendix 1.2).

Comparative effectiveness research, incorporating cost benefit analyses on the use of massage therapy in a range of population groups, also needs to be conducted.

FUTURE DIRECTIONS

The escalating costs associated with the healthcare needs of ageing populations have focused attention on the role of healthcare strategies for chronic health conditions and for preventive healthcare.[28] Remedial massage has relevance for many Australians, including those with chronic non-life-threatening conditions. An increasing number of clients will rely on remedial massage, along with exercise and other therapies, to minimise or eliminate pain and other symptoms that assist their return to optimal function. Remedial massage therapists can also make an important contribution to preventive healthcare through their capacity for identifying sub-clinical indicators of musculoskeletal problems.

Given the increasing use of CAM in modern Western societies, it is reasonable to expect an increasing acceptance of remedial massage as a legitimate part of Australian healthcare by the public and other healthcare workers. From the perspectives of medical and other healthcare workers, acceptance will inevitably be linked to an increasing evidence base for CAM. High-quality research in remedial massage therapy depends on both available funding and training for those interested in CAM research. Increasing research literacy of remedial massage students and practising therapists is likely to influence the effectiveness of clinical practice as they draw on research results to inform their practice choices. More consistent and clearly defined levels in massage therapy training and graduate attributes linked to those levels, and stronger links between private colleges, TAFEs and university courses, will secure pathways and support for students and practitioners who are interested in remedial massage research projects. As research into remedial massage continues to emerge, some of the claims about its efficacy will be confirmed and some will be refuted. A robust remedial massage profession will want to be involved in, or at least kept abreast of, current research findings. It will be able to critique those findings, adjust education programs and inform its practitioners to ensure safe and competent remedial massage practice.

APPENDIX 1.1

Systematic reviews for massage therapy from the Cochrane Library

Title	Author, Year	Author's conclusions
Massage for mechanical neck pain	Patel KC, Gross A, Graham N, Goldsmith CH, Ezzo J, Morien A, Peloso PMJ, 2012[29]	No recommendations for practice can be made at this time because the effectiveness of massage for neck pain remains uncertain. As a stand-alone treatment, massage for mechanical neck pain was found to provide immediate or short-term effectiveness or both in pain and tenderness. Additionally, future research is needed in order to assess the long-term effects of treatment and treatments provided on more than one occasion.
Massage therapy for preventing pressure ulcers	Zhang Q, Sun Z, Yue J, 2015[30]	There are currently no studies eligible for inclusion in this review. It is, therefore, unclear whether massage therapy can prevent pressure ulcers.
Massage for low back pain	Furlan AD, Giraldo M, Baskwill A, Irvin E, Imamura M, 2015[31]	We have very little confidence that massage is an effective treatment for LBP. Acute, sub-acute and chronic LBP had improvements in pain outcomes with massage only in the short-term follow-up. Functional improvement was observed in participants with sub-acute and chronic LBP when compared with inactive controls, but only for the short-term follow-up. There were only minor adverse effects with massage.
Massage with or without aromatherapy for symptom relief in people with cancer	Shin E, Seo K, Lee S, Jang J, Jung Y, Kim M, Yeon J, 2016[32]	There was a lack of evidence on the clinical effectiveness of massage for symptom relief in people with cancer. Most studies were too small to be reliable and key outcomes were not reported. Any further studies of aromatherapy and massage will need to address these concerns.

Title	Author, Year	Author's conclusions
Deep transverse friction massage for treating lateral elbow or lateral knee tendinitis	Loew LM, Brosseau L, Tugwell P, Wells GA, Welch V, Shea B, Poitras S, De Angelis G, Rahman P, 2014[33]	We do not have sufficient evidence to determine the effects of deep transverse friction on pain, improvement in grip strength, and functional status for patients with lateral elbow tendinitis or knee tendinitis, as no evidence of clinically important benefits was found. The confidence intervals of the estimate of effects overlapped the null value for deep transverse friction massage in combination with physical therapy compared with physical therapy alone in the treatment of lateral elbow tendinitis and knee tendinitis. These conclusions are limited by the small sample size of the included randomised controlled trials. Future trials, utilising specific methods and adequate sample sizes, are needed before conclusions can be drawn regarding the specific effects of deep transverse friction massage on lateral elbow tendinitis.
Massage, reflexology and other manual methods for pain management in labour	Smith CA, Levett KM, Collins CT, Dahlen HG, Ee CC, Suganuma M, 2018[34]	Massage, warm pack and thermal manual methods may have a role in reducing pain, reducing length of labour and improving women's sense of control and emotional experience of labour, although the quality of evidence varies from low to very low and few trials reported on the key GRADE outcomes. Few trials reported on safety as an outcome. There is a need for further research to address these outcomes and to examine the effectiveness and efficacy of these manual methods for pain management.
Massage for promoting mental and physical health in typically developing infants under the age of six months	Bennett C, Underdown A, Barlow J, 2014[35]	These findings do not currently support the use of infant massage with low-risk groups of parents and infants. Available evidence is of poor quality, and many studies do not address the biological plausibility of the outcomes being measured, or the mechanisms by which change might be achieved. Future research should focus on the impact of infant massage in higher-risk groups (e.g. demographically and socially deprived parent–infant dyads), where there may be more potential for change.
Manual lymphatic drainage for lymphoedema following breast cancer treatment	Ezzo J, Manheimer E, McNeely ML, Howell DM, Weiss R, Johansson KI, Bao T, Bily L, Tuppo CM, Williams AF, Karadibak D[36]	Manual lymphatic drainage (MLD) is safe and may offer additional benefit to compression bandaging for swelling reduction. Compared to individuals with moderate-to-severe breast cancer related lymphoedema, those with mild-to-moderate breast cancer-related lymphoedema may be the ones who benefit from adding MLD to an intensive course of treatment with compression bandaging. This finding, however, needs to be confirmed by randomised data. In trials where MLD and sleeve were compared with a non-MLD treatment and sleeve, volumetric outcomes were inconsistent within the same trial. Research is needed to identify the most clinically meaningful volumetric measurement, to incorporate newer technologies in LE assessment, and to assess other clinically relevant outcomes such as fibrotic tissue formation. Findings were contradictory for function (range of motion), and inconclusive for quality of life. For symptoms such as pain and heaviness, 60% to 80% of participants reported feeling better regardless of which treatment they received. One-year follow-up suggests that once swelling had been reduced, participants were likely to keep their swelling down if they continued to use a custom-made sleeve.
Muscle energy technique for non-specific low back pain	Franke H, Fryer G, Ostelo RWJG, Kamper SJ, 2015[37]	The quality of research related to testing the effectiveness of muscle-energy technique (MET) is poor. Studies are generally small and at high risk of bias due to methodological deficiencies. Studies conducted to date generally provide low-quality evidence that MET is not effective for patients with LBP. There is not sufficient evidence to reliably determine whether MET is likely to be effective in practice. Large, methodologically-sound studies are necessary to investigate this question.
Manual therapy and exercise for adhesive capsulitis (frozen shoulder)	Page MJ, Green S, Kramer S, Johnston RV, McBain B, Chau M, Buchbinder R, 2014[38]	The best available data show that a combination of manual therapy and exercise may not be as effective as glucocorticoid injection in the short term. It is unclear whether a combination of manual therapy, exercise and electrotherapy is an effective adjunct to glucocorticoid injection or oral NSAID. Following arthrographic joint distension with glucocorticoid and saline, manual therapy and exercise may confer effects similar to those of sham ultrasound in terms of overall pain, function and quality of life, but may provide greater patient-reported treatment success and active range of motion. High-quality RCTs are needed to establish the benefits and harms of manual therapy and exercise interventions that reflect actual practice, compared with placebo, no intervention and active interventions with evidence of benefit (e.g. glucocorticoid injection).

Continued

Title	Author, Year	Author's conclusions
Manipulation and mobilisation for neck pain contrasted against an inactive control or another active treatment	Gross A, Langevin P, Burnie SJ, Bédard-Brochu M, Empey B, Dugas E, Faber-Dobrescu M, Andres C, Graham N, Goldsmith CH, Brønfort G, Hoving JL, LeBlanc F, 2015[39]	Although support can be found for use of thoracic manipulation versus control for neck pain, function and quality of life, results for cervical manipulation and mobilisation versus control are few and diverse. Publication bias cannot be ruled out. Research designed to protect against various biases is needed. Findings suggest that manipulation and mobilisation present similar results for every outcome at immediate/short/intermediate-term follow-up. Multiple cervical manipulation sessions may provide better pain relief and functional improvement than certain medications at immediate/intermediate/long-term follow-up. Since the risk of rare but serious adverse events for manipulation exists, further high-quality research focusing on mobilisation and comparing mobilisation or manipulation versus other treatment options is needed to guide clinicians in their optimal treatment choices.

(https://www.cochranelibrary.com/, accessed on 14/12/2018)

APPENDIX 1.2
PROMIS Scale v1.2 – Global Health[40]

Please respond to each question or statement by marking one box per row.

		Excellent	Very good	Good	Fair	Poor
Global01	In general, would you say your health is:	☐ 5	☐ 4	☐ 3	☐ 2	☐ 1
Global02	In general, would you say your quality of life is:	☐ 5	☐ 4	☐ 3	☐ 2	☐ 1
Global03	In general, how would you rate your physical health?	☐ 5	☐ 4	☐ 3	☐ 2	☐ 1
Global04	In general, how would you rate your mental health, including your mood and your ability to think?	☐ 5	☐ 4	☐ 3	☐ 2	☐ 1
Global05	In general, how would you rate your satisfaction with your social activities and relationships?	☐ 5	☐ 4	☐ 3	☐ 2	☐ 1
Global09r	In general, please rate how well you carry out your usual social activities and roles. (This includes activities at home, at work and in your community, and responsibilities as a parent, child, spouse, employee, friend, etc.)	☐ 5	☐ 4	☐ 3	☐ 2	☐ 1
		Completely	**Mostly**	**Moderately**	**A little**	**Not at all**
Global06	To what extent are you able to carry out your everyday physical activities such as walking, climbing stairs, carrying groceries, or moving a chair?	☐ 5	☐ 4	☐ 3	☐ 2	☐ 1

In the past 7 days …

		Never	Rarely	Sometimes	Often	Always
Global10r	How often have you been bothered by emotional problems such as feeling anxious, depressed or irritable?	☐ 5	☐ 4	☐ 3	☐ 2	☐ 1

		None	Mild	Moderate	Severe	Very severe
Global08r	How would you rate your fatigue on average?	☐ 5	☐ 4	☐ 3	☐ 2	☐ 1

Global07r	How would you rate your pain on average?	☐ 0 No pain	☐ 1	☐ 2	☐ 3	☐ 4	☐ 5	☐ 6	☐ 7	☐ 8	☐ 9	☐ 10 Worst pain imaginable

REFERENCES

1. Posadzki P, Ernst E. The safety of massage therapy: an update of a systematic review. Foc Altern Complement Ther 2013;18. Doi 10.1111/fct.12007
2. Bervoets D, Luijsterburg P, Alessie J, et al. Massage therapy has short-term benefits for people with common musculoskeletal disorders compared to no treatment: a systematic review. J Physiothe 2015; 61(3):106–16.
3. Cash M. Sports and remedial massage Therapy. London: Ebury Press; 2012.
4. Australian and New Zealand Standard Classification of Occupations, Version 1.2. Online. Available: http://www.abs.gov.au/ausstats/abs@.nsf/Product+Lookup/1220.0~2013,+Version+1.2~Chapter~UNIT+GROUP+4116+Massage+Therapists; 2013.
5. Massage & Myotherapy Australia. What is massage and myotherapy? Online. Available: https://www.massagemyotherapy.com.au/ccms.r?pageid=10034&TenID=AAMT; 2019.
6. Australian Natural Therapists' Association. Remedial massage therapy. Online. Available: https://www.australiannaturaltherapistsassociation.com.au/Public/ANTA_Therapies/RemedialTherapy.aspx; 2019.
7. Australian Traditional Medicine Society. Remedial massage. Online. Available: https://www.atms.com.au/remedial-massage; 2019.
8. training.gove.au. Qualification details Certificate IV in Massage Therapy Practice. Online. Available: https://training.gov.au/Training/Details/HLT40312; 2019.
9. training.gov.au. Qualification details HLT52015 – Diploma of Remedial Massage. Online. Available: https://training.gov.au/Training/Details/HLT52015; 2019.
10. Australian Qualifications Framework Council. AQF Qualifications. 2nd edn. Online. Available: http://www.aqf.edu.au/AbouttheAQF/AQFQualifications/tabid/98/Default.aspx; 2013.
11. Xue C, Zhang A, Lin V, et al. Complementary and alternative medicine use in Australia: a national population-based survey. J Altern Complement Med 2007;13(6):643–50.
12. Harris P, Cooper K, Relton C, et al. Prevalence of visits to massage therapists by the general population: a systematic review. Complement Ther Clin 2014;20:16–20.
13. Chatfield SM, Dharmage SC, Boers A, et al. Complementary and alternative medicines in ankylosing spondylitis: a cross-sectional study. Clin Rheumatol 2009;28:213–17. doi 10.1007/s10067-008-1029-3.
14. Grace S. Integrative medicine in Australian health care. Rotterdam: Sense; 2009.
15. Hale A. 2002 National survey of remedial therapists. J Aust Tradit Med Soc 2003;9(3):119–24.
16. Bensoussan A, Myers S, Wu SM, et al. A profile of naturopathic and western herbal medicine practitioners in Australia. Sydney: CompleMED, University of Western Sydney; 2003.
17. Hale A. 2002 Survey of ATMS: acupuncturists, herbalists and naturopaths. J Aust Trad Med Soc 2002;8(4):143–9.
18. Grace S, Rogers S, Eddey S. The natural medicine workforce in Australia: part 1. J Aust Trad Med Soc 2013;19:113–18.
19. Wardle JL, Barnett R, Adams J. Practice and research in Australian massage therapy: a national workforce survey. Int J Ther Massage Bodywork 2015;8(2):1–11.
20. Australian Medical Association. Position Statement: Complementary Medicine. Online. Available: https://ama.com.au/position-statement/ama-position-statement-complementary-medicine-2018; 2018.
21. Wardle JL, Sibbritt DW, Adams J. Primary care practitioner perceptions and attitudes of complementary medicine: a content analysis of free-text responses from a survey of non-metropolitan Australian general practitioners. Prim Health Care Res 2018;19(3):246–55.
22. Grace S, Higgs J. Integrative medicine: enhancing quality in primary health care. J Altern Complem Med 2010;16(9):945–50.
23. Kumar S, Beaton K, Hughes T. The effectiveness of massage therapy for the treatment of nonspecific low back pain: a systematic review of systematic reviews. Int J General Med 2013;6:733–41.
24. Bervoets D, Luijsterburg P, Alessie J, et al. Massage therapy has short-term benefits for people with common musculoskeletal disorders compared to no treatment: a systematic review. J Physiother 2015;61(3):106–16.
25. PEDro Physiotherapy Evidence Database. PEDro scale. Online. Available: https://www.pedro.org.au/english/downloads/pedro-scale/; 2018.
26. Nelson NL, Churilla JR. Massage therapy for pain and function in patients with arthritis: a systematic review of randomized controlled trials. Am J Phys Med Rehabil 2017;96(9):665–72.
27. Boyd C, Crawford C, Paat C, et al. The impact of massage therapy on function in pain populations—a systematic review and meta-analysis of randomized controlled trials: part II, Cancer pain populations. Pain Med 2016;17(8):1553–68.
28. Australian Government Department of Health and Ageing. Health workforce. Online. Available: http://www.health.gov.au/internet/main/publishing.nsf/Content/Health%20Workforce-2; 2019.
29. Patel K, Gross A, Graham N, et al. Massage for mechanical neck disorders. Cochrane Database Syst Rev 2012;Issue 9:Art. No.: CD004871.
30. Zhang Q, Sun Z, Yue J. Massage therapy for preventing pressure ulcers. Cochrane Database Syst Rev 2015;Issue 6:Art. No.: CD010518.
31. Furlan A, Giraldo M, Baskwill A, et al. Massage for low-back pain. Cochrane Database Syst Rev 2015;Issue 9:Art. No.: CD001929.
32. Shin E, Seo K, Lee S, et al. Massage with or without aromatherapy for symptom relief in people with cancer. Cochrane Database Syst Rev 2016;Issue 6:Art. No.: CD009873.
33. Loew LM, Brosseau L, Tugwell P, et al. Deep transverse friction massage for treating lateral elbow or lateral knee tendinitis. Cochrane Database Syst Rev 2014(11):CD003528.
34. Smith C, Levett K, Collins C, et al. Massage, reflexology and other manual methods for pain management in labour. Cochrane Database Syst Rev 2018;Issue 3:Art. No.: CD009290.
35. Bennett C, Underdown A, Barlow J. Massage for promoting mental and physical health in typically developing infants under the age of six months. Cochrane Database Syst Rev 2013;Issue 4: Art. No.: CD005038.
36. Ezzo E, Manheimer M, McNeely D, et al. Manual lymphatic drainage for lymphedema following breast cancer treatment. Cochrane Database Syst Rev 2015;21(5):CD003475.
37. Franke H, Fryer G, Ostelo R, et al. Muscle energy technique for non-specific low-back pain. Cochrane Database Syst Rev 2015;Issue 2:Art. No.: CD009852.
38. Page M, Green S, Kramer S, et al. Manual therapy and exercise for adhesive capsulitis (frozen shoulder). Cochrane Database Syst Rev 2014;Issue 8:Art. No.: CD011275.
39. Gross A, Langevin P, Burnie S, et al. Manipulation and mobilisation for neck pain contrasted against an inactive control or another active treatment. Cochrane Database Syst Rev 2015;Issue 9:Art. No.: CD004249.
40. Northwestern University. HealthMeasures. Online. Available: http://www.healthmeasures.net/explore-measurement-systems/promis/obtain-administer-measures; 2019.

2

Assessment procedures for remedial massage: an evidence-based approach

Learning Outcomes

- Demonstrate an understanding of the role of assessment in remedial massage practice.
- Demonstrate an understanding of the current evidence-based approach to musculoskeletal assessment.
- Identify red and yellow flags when conducting remedial massage assessment.
- Perform appropriate remedial massage assessments (case histories, outcome measures, postural observation, gait analysis, functional assessments and palpation) on a range of clients.
- Analyse and interpret assessment findings to guide the assessment process.

INTRODUCTION

As primary care practitioners, remedial massage therapists are required to make clinical judgments including identifying those clients whose treatment lies outside their scope of practice. It is estimated that between 34% and 40% of clients who visit complementary medicine practitioners have not been previously assessed by a general medical or other health practitioner.[1,2] It is, therefore, a key safety requirement of remedial massage training to adequately prepare practitioners for their primary contact role. Moreover, remedial massage is not entirely risk free, even though adverse events appear to be rare.[3,4] Competent performance and analysis of appropriate remedial massage assessments, including the selection of appropriate assessment procedures for individual clients, is essential for safe and effective remedial massage practice.

PRINCIPLES OF ASSESSMENT IN REMEDIAL MASSAGE PRACTICE

- Remedial massage should always be performed in conjunction with appropriate and ongoing assessment.[a]

- A definitive assessment is not always possible or necessary for many musculoskeletal problems. It is essential, however, that clients requiring referral to other healthcare practitioners are identified (red and yellow flags).
- A holistic approach to assessment considers all aspects of a client's biopsychosocial health.
- Remedial massage assessments are conducted in a logical order, usually beginning with a case history. Interpretations of assessment findings progressively guide the need for further assessments.
- Findings of individual assessments should always be interpreted cautiously and correlated with findings from other assessments. Evidence confirms the importance of case history and limited and conflicting support for physical assessments.
- Assessment findings guide remedial massage practice: negotiating treatment plans with clients, monitoring responses to treatment, adjusting treatments and reviewing plans as required.
- Strategies for assessing remedial massage clients may change with emerging evidence about the efficacy of individual assessments.

PURPOSE OF ASSESSMENTS

The purpose of remedial massage assessment is to:

- identify indicators of serious conditions (red flags)
- identify the presence of psychosocial factors that may influence presenting symptoms and response to treatment (yellow flags)
- assess clients' functional limitations
- guide treatment and management options
- monitor clients' responses to treatment so that treatment plans can be adjusted if required
- assess treatment effectiveness.

DEMONSTRATING TREATMENT EFFECTIVENESS

To monitor clients' responses to treatment, remedial massage therapists must first collect suitable baseline data, including information collected from case histories and observed or measured by practitioners. The pain scale is commonly used for this purpose. Repeated collection of pain scale data enables changes in clients' perceptions of pain to be recorded and may demonstrate the perceived effectiveness of treatment. The amount of medication that clients require to manage

---

[a]This is the current view of educators and professional associations of remedial massage in Australia. However, remedial massage, particularly seated massage, corporate massage and post-event sports massage are frequently performed without full assessment of clients.

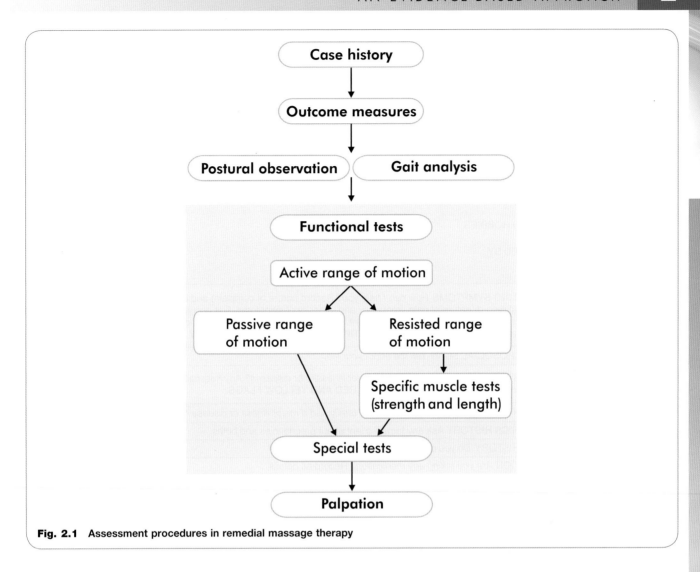

Fig. 2.1 Assessment procedures in remedial massage therapy

symptoms can also be used in this way. Recording details of medication at the initial consultation and changes in medication use over the ensuing period of treatment provides evidence of progress towards treatment goals.

ASSESSMENT PROCEDURES

The most commonly used assessment tools in remedial massage therapy are presented below in the order in which they are usually applied and easiest to learn. In reality, assessments are overlapping and ongoing throughout the consultation from first encounters with clients in waiting rooms to the continual assessments and adjustments that are required when applying any technique (e.g. for pain tolerance, for age, to meet clients' expectation). A flowchart of remedial massage assessments is illustrated in Figure 2.1.

CLIENT HISTORY

Taking a comprehensive client history is one of the most important assessment tools of healthcare practitioners. It is an important opportunity to establish relationships with clients that enhance positive outcomes of treatment.[4] It also enables the practitioner to learn about the biopsychosocial influences

Table 2.1   Red and yellow flags

Red flags	Yellow flags
Clinical features that may be associated with the presence of a serious physical condition.	Psychosocial and occupational factors that may influence presenting symptoms, treatment approach and outcomes.

on the client's health. The first responsibility of remedial massage therapists is to determine clients' suitability for remedial massage or for referral to another healthcare practitioner. The term *red flag* refers to clinical features (signs or symptoms) that may indicate the presence of serious underlying medical conditions requiring further investigation. Such conditions include cancers, fractures and infections (see Table 2.1). Although individual red flags have low specificity for a particular condition, they do prompt thinking about whether the overall clinical picture could indicate a serious cause of pain.[5] Clients who choose to complement medical treatment of serious conditions with remedial massage therapy require supervision by their medical practitioner and liaison between practitioners (or at the very least their practitioners need to be

NAME .... DATE OF BIRTH ....

ADDRESS ....

.... POSTCODE ....

PHONE B/H _____ A/H_____ Mobile _____

EMAIL _____

OCCUPATION

SPORTS / HOBBIES

REFERRED BY

PRESENTING SYMPTOMS *How can I help you?* Record nature of complaint and duration. Inquire and record: nature of pain, frequency and intensity of symptoms, first occurrence, mode of onset. If recurrent, previous treatment. Associated symptoms. Aggravating and relieving factors. Any other symptoms. IDENTIFY POSSIBLE RED AND YELLOW FLAGS.
BIOPSYCHOSOCIAL SCAN *Tell me about your life.*
PAST HISTORY *Have you ever had any major illnesses or diseases? Any hospitalisations? Any major accidents?* IDENTIFY POSSIBLE RED AND YELLOW FLAGS.
FAMILY HISTORY *Has any member of your family had a major illness or disease?*
OBSTETRICS HISTORY Ask any female client about pregnancies and births.
SOCIAL HISTORY *Do you drink or smoke? Recreational drugs?*
MEDICATION *Are you taking any medication?* Record all details.
ALLERGIES *Do you have any allergies?* Record all details.
SYSTEMS REVIEW Either by questionnaire or orally, ask a few questions relating to each system as required. (Central nervous: headaches, dizziness, numbness. Cardiovascular: chest pain, shortness of breath. Respiratory system: shortness of breath, wheezing, cough. Alimentary: nausea, vomiting, indigestion, abdominal pain, change in bowel habit. Urogenital: pain on urination, frequency of urination. Endocrine: Heat or cold intolerance, change in sweating, excessive thirst.)

Fig. 2.2 A typical case history form for remedial massage

aware of the entirety of their clients' treatments). Clients should always be encouraged to disclose their remedial massage treatment to their doctor.[6] However, many remedial massage clients do not have serious medical conditions. If there are no signs or symptoms associated with specific diseases or serious conditions, further investigations (such as X-rays, MRIs or blood tests) are generally not indicated.[7]

Once practitioners have dismissed the likelihood of serious conditions, they gather information to guide further assessments: identifying likely contributing factors, types of tissues that could be involved, clients' responses to previous treatments, aggravating and relieving factors and psychosocial factors that could affect clients' responses to treatment (yellow flags). Questions should proceed logically and presenting conditions prioritised. A sound grounding in physiology, pathology and symptomatology is required for analysing the health information collected and for recognising deviations from normal findings and signs and symptoms of common pathophysiologies. Practitioners are not required to read X-rays,

MRIs or other diagnostic imaging but they are expected to interpret their reports. Figure 2.2 is a typical remedial massage case history.

Assessing the well client

Remedial massage has long played a role in health maintenance and preventive medicine. Assessment of the well client is based on lifestyle history, postural and gait observations, functional tests, particularly those for muscle and joint function, and palpation. Clients who present for massage therapy without symptoms are sometimes surprised when massage elicits pain or tenderness or when they feel the ropiness of fibrotic tissues or the tightness of a muscle being stretched. They are being made aware of potential musculoskeletal stresses that could lead to future problems (sub-clinical indicators). Early interventions (e.g. advising patients to avoid prolonged awkward postures that could lead to musculoskeletal injury, improving manual handling techniques, or modifying an exercise program) may prevent many potential problems.

THE NATURE OF PAIN

Pain is a common presenting symptom of remedial massage clients. Perceptions of pain are complicated by its multidimensional nature and its changing nature over time. Questioning clients about pain helps determine their suitability for remedial massage and possible sources of pain. Ask clients about:

- the location of the pain
- the character of the pain, e.g. sharp shooting pain in a relatively narrow band (radicular pain), a dull ache that is hard to localise (referred pain), burning pain (from trauma to sympathetic and somatic sensory nerves)
- the severity of the pain
    - A number of pain intensity measures are available although the validity and reliability of such measures continues to be debated.[8] A simple procedure is to ask clients to rate their pain on a pain scale from 0 to 10, where 0 is no pain and 10 is extreme pain. Alternatively, practitioners can use a Visual Analogue Scale of Pain Intensity (VAS), a 10 cm line on which clients are asked to put a mark to show their current pain level.
- the onset of the pain
- the duration of the pain
- the course of the pain, e.g. intermittent, constant, episodic
- aggravating and relieving factors.

Questions designed to distinguish between pain of local origin and pain referred from a distant site (in particular, from a spinal segment) are useful in directing treatment to the source of pain. As a guide for determining the nature of pain, consider the following:

- local pain
    - usually sharp
    - well localised
- referred pain
    - dull
    - poorly localised
    - often refers in a predetermined pattern (e.g. nerve impingement at the spinal segment will refer pain in dermatomal patterns, trigger points refer in predictable patterns).

If a client reports numbness in an area of skin, the nerves supplying that dermatome[b] could be involved. Similarly, if a client reports weak muscles in a particular myotome, the motor neuron in that spinal segment may be involved. Knowing the spinal cord segment which supplies each dermatome and myotome can help locate the source of pain (see Figure 2.3).

Table 2.2 (p 13) is designed to assist practitioners identify red flags associated with pain of the lumbar, thoracic and cervical regions.

Identifying yellow flags

Yellow flags are indicators of psychosocial and occupational factors that may affect clients' presenting symptoms and responses to treatment. Identifying the presence of yellow flags may prompt early interventions and better outcomes for clients. For example, clients with high stress levels may benefit from referral to a counsellor; clients with concern about job security after extended absences from work may benefit from reassurance from their employer. The presence of yellow flags is not a contraindication for remedial massage. Rather, yellow flags alert the practitioner to possible complicating factors which may prompt referral to other health practitioners or delay the normal recovery process.

Yellow flags include:[9]

- belief that pain and activity are harmful
- sickness behaviours (e.g. extended rest)
- low or negative moods, social withdrawal
- problems with claims and compensation
- overprotective or unsupportive family
- apportioning blame
- overt anxiety or depression
- non-compliance with rehabilitation program
- long time between injury and referral.

Informed consent

As part of the initial interview clients need to have proposed assessments and treatments and any associated risks fully explained. Informed consent must be obtained for all assessment and treatment procedures.

Clients are entitled to make their own decisions about their healthcare. To be able to do this they require adequate information about the nature of the proposed treatment or management, its benefits, side effects, risks or possible complications, the expected duration of the treatment or management and alternatives to the proposed treatment or management, including costs. Remedial massage may occasionally lead to moderately severe adverse effects, most commonly associated with massage techniques applied to the neck region.[10]

Informed consent is only valid if the client has the capacity to understand and authorise the proposed healthcare. This means using words that the client can understand, allowing time for questions, and using an interpreter if needed. The client must be free to accept or reject the advice provided by the practitioner and to change their decision at any stage.[11] If an adult is unable to consent to a treatment, consent is dependent on a third party for their ongoing care (e.g. people with an intellectual disability under a guardianship order). Clients under 18 years are required to have informed consent provided by a parent or guardian. In some circumstances a person under 18 years may be deemed competent to provide informed consent. Check local requirements as the legislation relating to consent by a person under 18 years of age varies across jurisdictions. While it may not be necessary to ask the patient to sign a consent form for the proposed treatment in some jurisdictions, it is important that the practitioner document in the client's notes that informed consent has been provided, together with a summary of the information that was provided to the client to obtain that consent.

Consent remains valid until it is withdrawn by the client or if there is a change in their circumstances. Consent is required to be reaffirmed with the client at regular intervals during the treatment and management of the condition and if they bring a new presenting condition to the clinic.

---

[b]Every spinal nerve contains both sensory and motor neurons. Somatic sensory neurons carry impulses from the skin to the spinal cord and brain stem. A dermatome is the area of skin that provides sensory input to one pair of spinal nerves. Somatic motor neurons carry impulses from the spinal cord to skeletal muscles. All muscles innervated by the motor neurons in a single spinal segment constitute a myotome. In general, dermatomes overlie corresponding myotomes.

Fig. 2.3 Dermatomes: anterior and posterior view

OUTCOME MEASURES

Outcome measures are standardised questionnaires in which clients record perceived changes to their health status. They are used to assess clients' perceived health status and also to demonstrate the benefits of treatment. Three common outcome measures for musculoskeletal pain and disability are the Oswestry Disability Index, the Vernon Mior Neck Disability Questionnaire, and the Patient Specific Functional Scale which can be used for disability in any region of the body. Research into the use of outcome measures demonstrates high validity[c] and reliability[d] for some questionnaires which may account for their increasing use in clinical trials and in clinical practice.

The Patient-Reported Outcomes Measurement Information System (PROMIS) was funded by the National Institutes of Health in the US to provide item banks which offer 'efficient, flexible, and precise measurement' of commonly studied patient reported outcomes.[12] These freely available questionnaires provide health practitioners with reliable, valid, and flexible measures of clients' physical, mental and social wellbeing (see Appendix 1.2).

They are simple to administer and their standardised scoring systems allow comparisons of clients' responses over time. They are also readily interpreted by healthcare practitioners from other disciplines.

Completing questionnaires takes time and clients with low levels of English literacy will need assistance. Appointment times may need to be adjusted accordingly or clients invited to come to the clinic a few minutes before their scheduled appointment to complete the questionnaires. Outcome measures should be used at every opportunity by remedial massage therapists to demonstrate perceived effectiveness of their treatments.

[c]Validity is the extent to which a measure estimates the true nature of what it purports to measure.
[d]Reliability is the consistency of repeated applications of a measurement.

Table 2.2 Red flags of serious conditions associated with acute low back, thoracic and neck pain

Red flags	Possible condition
For acute low back pain	
Symptoms and signs of infection (e.g. fever) Risk factors for infection (e.g. underlying disease, immunosuppression, penetrating wound)	Infection
History of trauma Minor trauma (if >50 years, history of osteoporosis, taking corticosteroids)	Fracture
Past history of malignancy Age >50 years Failure to improve with treatment Unexplained weight loss Pain at multiple sites Pain at rest	Cancer
Absence of aggravating factors	Aortic aneurysm Other serious condition
Widespread neurological symptoms and signs in the lower limb (e.g. gait abnormality, saddle area numbness) ± urinary retention, faecal incontinence	Cauda equina syndrome (a medical emergency and requires urgent hospital referral)
For acute thoracic pain	
Minor trauma (if >50 years, history of osteoporosis, taking corticosteroids) Major trauma	Fracture
Symptoms and signs of infection (e.g. fever, night sweats) Risk factors for infection (e.g. underlying disease, immunosuppression, penetrating wound)	Infection
Past history of malignancy Age >50 years Failure to improve with treatment Unexplained weight loss Pain at multiple sites Pain at rest Night pain	Cancer
Chest pain or heaviness Movement/change in posture has no effect on pain Abdominal pain Shortness of breath, cough	Other serious condition
For acute neck pain	
Symptoms and signs of infection (e.g. fever, night sweats) Risk factors for infection (e.g. underlying disease, immunosuppression, penetrating wound)	Infection
History of trauma Minor trauma (if taking corticosteroids)	Fracture
Past history of malignancy Age >50 years Failure to improve with treatment Unexplained weight loss Dysphagia, headache, vomiting	Cancer
Neurological symptoms in the limbs	Neurological condition
Cerebrovascular symptoms or signs, anticoagulant use	Cerebral or spinal haemorrhage
Cardiovascular risk factors; transient ischaemic attack	Vertebral or carotid aneurysm

Note that acute pain in this context refers to pain of less than three months' duration.
Adapted from the New Zealand Guidelines Group[9].

POSTURAL ANALYSIS

Postural observation involves observing clients standing erect to assess structural and habitual postures and their associated musculature. Observing the whole client, regardless of the complaint, is consistent with the holistic approach of complementary medicine. Postural observation along with case history and other assessment findings, may contribute useful information to the development of treatment plans. However, static postural alignment is likely to be less important than the ability to change positions to avoid postural stresses that might occur. Postural analysis helps therapists to identify potential structural contributions to presenting symptoms.

By observing erect postures from the posterior and lateral aspects, practitioners can compare one side of the body with the other, the upper half with the lower half, the left foot with the right foot and so on to identify postural patterns and/or factors that could contribute to presenting conditions or predispose to future symptoms. Postural observation can provide information about the effects on the musculoskeletal system of right or left dominance, of regular sports and hobbies, of work-related activities and of adaptations to diseases and traumas. For example, cervicogenic headaches may be perpetuated by a scoliosis and without postural observation this connection could remain undetected. Failing to take such predisposing factors into account could result in short-lived treatment effects. Moreover, identifying postural tendencies (sometimes incidentally) can prompt appropriate advice from therapists. For example, advising a client with bilateral pes planus about appropriate footwear, or a client who works at a computer all day about the importance of regular pectoralis major stretches, may prevent compensatory movement patterns and reduce susceptibility to injury.

Identifying anatomical landmarks

To accurately describe and record postural observations, practitioners should be familiar with the following anatomical landmarks (see Figure 2.4):

ANTERIOR AND LATERAL

- The nipple line is approximately level with the 5th rib or 4th intercostal space.
- The umbilicus is approximately level with the L3/4 disc.
- The iliac crests are approximately level with L4.

POSTERIOR

- The spine of the scapula is approximately level with T2 spinous process.
- The inferior angle of the scapula is approximately level with T7.
- T12 is usually the lowest level of the attachment of the trapezius muscle.
- The PSISs are approximately level with S2.

Performing postural observation

Clothing that does not obscure posture is required for accurate postural assessments. Swimwear or sportswear are suitable. Alternatively, clients may disrobe to their underwear and wear a gown that opens at the back. Stand two or three metres behind the client. Ask the client to walk up and down on the spot a few times with their eyes closed and then to open their eyes, and stand comfortably, hands by their sides.

A plumb line (either real or imaginary) is used to project a centre of gravity line onto the external surface of the body. Postural analysis, particularly using this visual method, is not an exact science. It is not intended to identify deviations from 'good' posture. However, by observing static upright posture therapists can learn about their client's whole physical structure and potential effects that habitual postural stresses (e.g. from work) may have had on musculoskeletal function. In the erect posture, the plumb line passes as follows (see Figure 2.5).

In the posterior view:

- equidistant through the heels, ankles, calves, knees and thighs

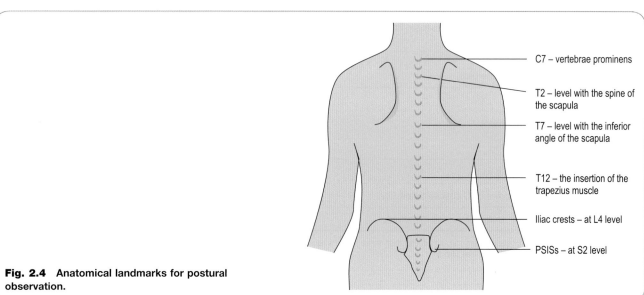

C7 – vertebrae prominens

T2 – level with the spine of the scapula

T7 – level with the inferior angle of the scapula

T12 – the insertion of the trapezius muscle

Iliac crests – at L4 level

PSISs – at S2 level

Fig. 2.4 Anatomical landmarks for postural observation.

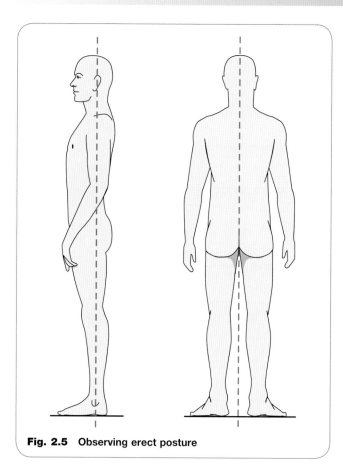

Fig. 2.5 Observing erect posture

- through the midline of the trunk
- through the midline of the neck and head.

In the lateral view:

- anterior to the lateral malleolus[e]
- anterior to the axis of the knee joint
- posterior to the hip joint
- through the bodies of L1 and L5
- bisecting the shoulder joint
- bisecting the ear.

General observations

A common reason that remedial massage therapists find postural observation difficult is that they look for detail before making general observations. Always begin by asking, 'What stands out? Are there any regions of the body that appear to be over-developed, under stress or very different from normal?' Next, focus on pelvic alignment which is useful for identifying common posture deviations like hyperlordosis or scoliosis. Learning to observe details like colour changes (e.g. the pallor of poor circulation, butterfly rash across the cheeks in rheumatoid conditions, a hairy tuft in the lumbosacral area in spondylolisthesis[f]), and unusual skin markings (e.g. petechiae, surgical scars, stretch marks, moles[g]) can be developed after the basics of postural observation have been mastered. Remember that postural observations are one of a number of assessments that contribute to understanding the overall clinical presentation of clients.

In the posterior view, observe:

1. The level of the pelvis. One of the most important findings of postural observation is the level of the pelvis, as many treatment plans address musculoskeletal adaptations to pelvic tilt. The pelvis comprises two ilia which articulate with each other at the symphysis pubis anteriorly and with the sacrum at the sacroiliac joints. Observe the level of the gluteal folds, PSISs, iliac crests, deviation of the gluteal cleft, the waist curvature and the distance between arms and trunk. To assist your determination of the level of the pelvis, the following describes the pattern of postural adaptations most often observed when the pelvis tilts. In this example, the client's pelvis is lower on the left than the right when observed posteriorly (see Figure 2.6). (For a client whose pelvis tilts lower on the right, the reverse would follow.) For a client whose pelvis is lower on the left than the right:
   - the PSIS is usually lower on the left
   - the gluteal fold is usually lower on the left
   - the gluteal cleft usually deviates to the left
   - the iliac crest is usually lower on the left
   - the waist curve usually flattens on the left
   - the lumbar scoliosis is usually convex on the left
   - the left foot is usually anterior and everted.

   If the level of the pelvis is not easily determined by observation, palpate the pelvis by placing your thumbs on the PSISs and fingers (held horizontally) on the iliac crests. Use your palpatory findings to confirm the presence (or absence) of a pelvic tilt.
2. The level of the shoulders
   Look at the contour of the trapezius muscle between the neck and the acromion and compare both sides.
3. Determine the nature of the scoliosis.
   Estimates of the shape of the curve can be ascertained from the presence of pelvic or shoulder tilt. Figure 2.7 illustrates common C-shaped and S-shaped spinal curvatures. Most thoracic scolioses are convex to the right (see Chapter 11).
4. Any other features of the back, neck or head that stand out (e.g. hypertonic muscles mid thoracic area, asymmetrical development from sports, work, or right or left dominance, muscle wasting).
5. Any lower limb features (e.g. ankle pronation, genu valgus or varus, oedema, feet everted) (see Figure 2.8).

In the lateral view, note:

1. the relation of the body to the centre of gravity line: assess the alignment of the ear, shoulder, hips and lateral malleoli
2. the level of the pelvis (e.g. hyperlordosis, hypolordosis)
3. the shape of the kyphosis (e.g. hyperkyphosis, flattened thoracic curvature)

---

[e]Some controversy exists among authors about the location of the centre of gravity line in the lateral view. It is sometimes said to bisect the lateral malleolus, rather than pass anteriorly to it.

[f]Spondylolisthesis is the anterior displacement of a vertebra in relation to the vertebra below (see Chapter 10).

[g]Massage therapists can play an important role in the detection of skin cancers among their clients. See Appendix 2.1 for a useful checklist.

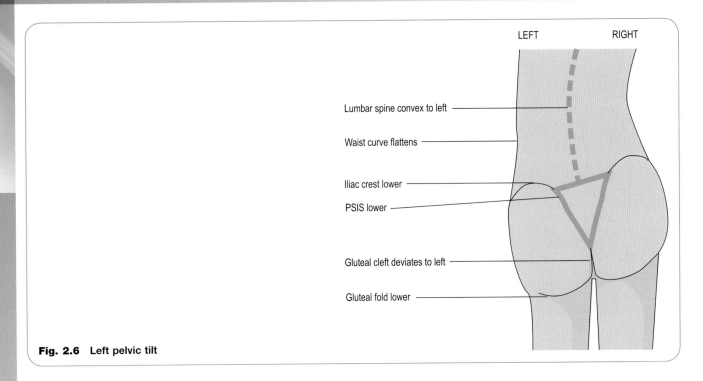

Fig. 2.6 Left pelvic tilt

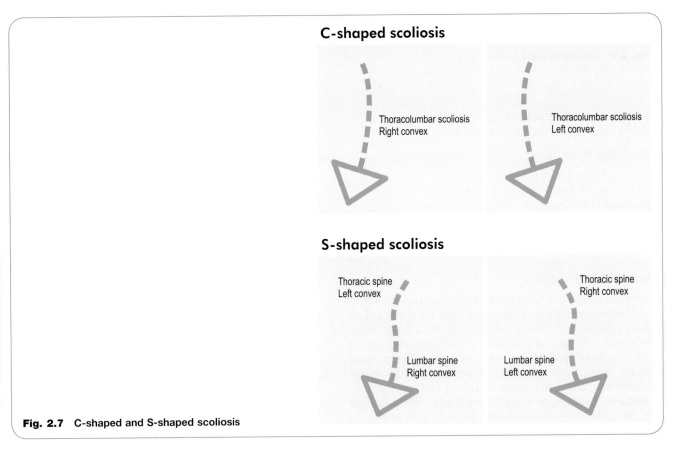

Fig. 2.7 C-shaped and S-shaped scoliosis

4. the position of the head (ear position in relation to shoulder, cervical hyper or hypolordosis)
5. the position of shoulders (e.g. rounded), arms and hands
6. any lower limb features (e.g. genu recurvatum, pes planus, pes cavus, hallux valgus, claw and hammer toes).

Method of recording

Postural observations are most easily recorded by marking diagrams of the posterior and lateral aspects of the erect body. Only the most obvious and important findings need be recorded. These include the level of the pelvis, any

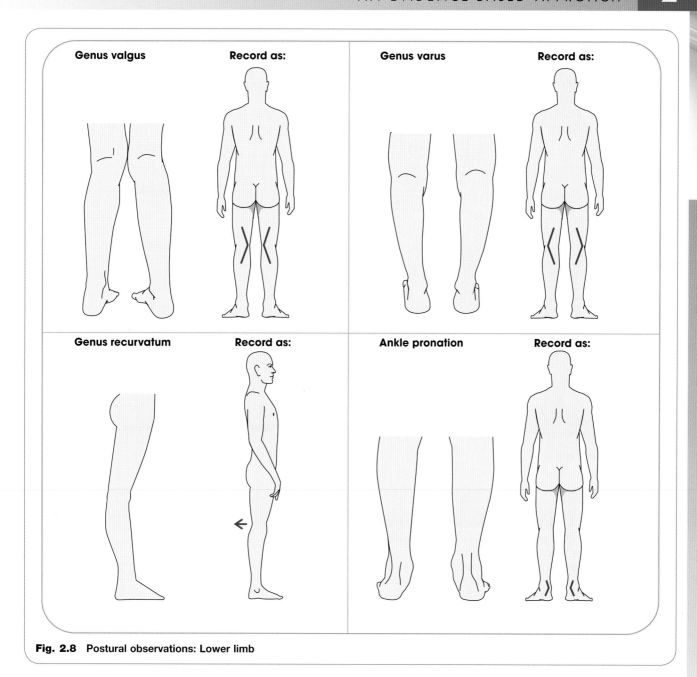

Fig. 2.8 Postural observations: Lower limb

major postural observations (e.g. scoliosis, hyperlordosis), and any possible factors that could predispose to current or future symptoms. In the following section ways of recording common posture observations are presented. Figure 2.8 shows how common posture observations of the lower limb can be recorded.

COMMON POSTURAL OBSERVATIONS

In the posterior view:

Scoliosis

Scoliosis refers to a lateral curvature of the spine, observed when the client is viewed anteriorly or posteriorly. Diagnostic imaging is required to determine the exact nature and

degree of spinal curvature. Postural observation enables practitioners to estimate large changes in spinal curvature and to suggest postural factors that may contribute or predispose to symptoms.

There are two major types of scoliosis:

- **Structural (idiopathic) scoliosis.** This is a curvature of the spine of unknown cause. It is relatively fixed and does not straighten on forward bending of the trunk (Adam's test) (see Figure 2.9 on p 18). It is often associated with vertebral and rib abnormalities and in severe cases can require bracing and surgery. Scoliosis screening tests in schools are designed to detect severe idiopathic scolioses that require such medical interventions. As a general rule, refer any child under 16 with a moderate or severe rib hump on

Fig. 2.9 Adam's test

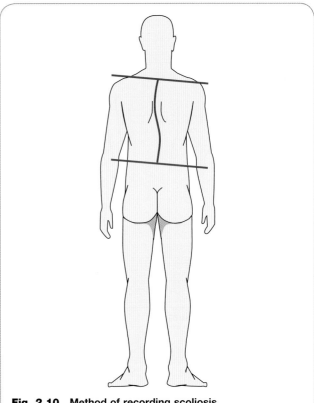

Fig. 2.10 Method of recording scoliosis

forward flexion (Adam's test) who has not been previously screened by a medical practitioner, chiropractor, osteopath, physiotherapist or in a school screening program.

- **Functional scoliosis.** This is a compensatory curvature that may be associated with pelvic tilt and mechanical overload due to work and sport activities. This type of scoliosis usually straightens on forward bending of the trunk (i.e. Adam's test is negative). It is usually correctable with such interventions as exercise programs, remedial massage and spinal manipulation.

Scoliosis is recorded on a posterior posture diagram by drawing three lines: i) a straight line at the level of the iliac crests angled to indicate the pelvic tilt. Try to make the angle of the straight line indicate the degree of pelvic tilt: an almost horizontal line would represent a small degree of pelvic tilt; a more diagonal line would represent a greater degree of pelvic tilt; ii) a straight line indicating the level of the shoulders; and iii) a curved line estimating the scoliosis (see Figure 2.10).

In the lateral view:

Lumbar hyperlordosis

This is a commonly observed posture (see Figure 2.11). Its causes include an anteriorly tilted pelvis, weak abdominal muscles relative to tight erector spinae muscles, and/or weak hamstring muscles relative to tight hip flexor muscles. Hyperlordosis is commonly associated with lower crossed syndrome (see Chapter 10).

Fig. 2.11 Method of recording hyperlordosis

Standing hyperlordosis test

Another quick test for hyperlordosis: The client removes their shoes and stands with their shoulders, buttocks and heels against a wall. Without adjusting the position, the client places one hand into the space between their waist and the wall. One flat palm in the space between the back and the wall is usual. Any more than this could indicate lumbar hyperlordosis. (Some clients can fit two fists placed one on top of the other.)

(Note: There could be other reasons for excessive space between the wall and the client's body, such as overdeveloped gluteus maximus muscles.)

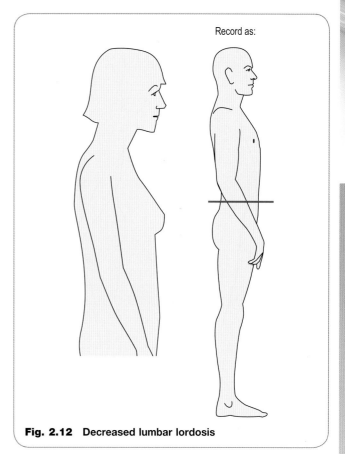

Fig. 2.12 Decreased lumbar lordosis

Hyperlordosis is recorded on a lateral posture diagram by a straight line indicating the level of the sacral base. Try to indicate the degree of anterior pelvic tilt with the angle of the line.

Decreased lumbar curvature

Spinal curvatures that appear to flatten or reverse may indicate a serious underlying condition.[h] For example, decreased lumbar lordosis is sometimes observed in clients with acute lumbar disc herniation. The symptoms may be severe and the client may be unable to stand upright, adopting an antalgic lean to reduce their level of pain (see Chapter 10 and Figure 2.12). Such clients require referral to a medical practitioner, chiropractor, osteopath or physiotherapist.

Hypolordosis is recorded on a lateral posture diagram by a straight line indicating the level of the sacral base. Try to indicate the degree of pelvic tilt with the angle of the line.

Increased thoracic kyphosis

Increased thoracic kyphosis is commonly observed in people with sedentary jobs as a result of prolonged sitting and is associated with upper crossed syndrome (see Chapter 12 and Figure 2.13). Another important cause is Scheuermann's disease which produces a fixed kyphosis, often in the thoracolumbar area. It occurs in 3–8% of the population and in males more than females. Clients may become round shouldered and find it difficult, if not impossible, to stand with shoulders held back. Early intervention (ideally before late teens or early twenties) with massage and exercise may help reduce the hypomobility associated with this condition (see Chapter 11).

Hyperkyphosis and hypokyphosis are recorded on a lateral posture diagram by drawing a curve to represent the position and degree of curvature of the thoracic spine.

Decreased thoracic kyphosis

A flattened thoracic kyphosis, also called 'dishing' or 'saucering', may be observed in the thoracic spine, particularly between the level of T2 and T7 (between the shoulder blades) (see Figure 2.14 on p 20).

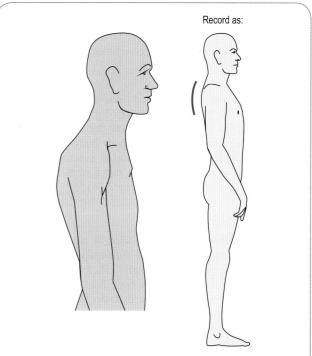

Fig. 2.13 Increased thoracic kyphosis

[h]An exception is the adaptation that sometimes occurs in pregnancy when the centre of gravity shifts posteriorly to accommodate the growing foetus.

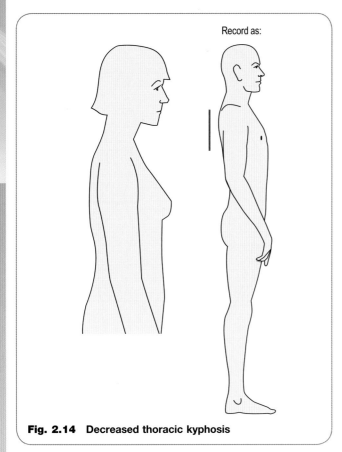

Record as:

Fig. 2.14   Decreased thoracic kyphosis

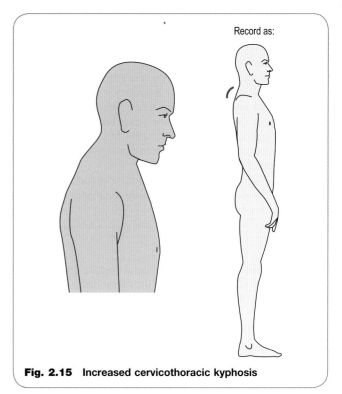

Record as:

Fig. 2.15   Increased cervicothoracic kyphosis

Record as:

Fig. 2.16   Sway back

Increased cervicothoracic curvature

This kyphotic curve of the cervicothoracic spine (C7 to T3), also called a 'dowager's hump', is most commonly observed in postmenopausal women and is associated with osteoporotic compression fractures and low levels of oestrogen (see Chapter 12 and Figure 2.15).

Cervicothoracic hyperkyphosis is recorded on a lateral posture diagram by drawing a curve to represent the position and degree of curvature of the cervicothoracic spine.

Sway back

Sway back has been distinguished from hyperlordosis by the relationship of the body to the centre of gravity line. In sway back the pelvis is tilted posteriorly but the pelvis is anterior to the centre of gravity line. The upper body extends backwards as a counterbalance. The lumbar erector spinae and hamstrings are short and tight; the hip flexors and thoracic erector spinae are lengthened (Figure 2.16).

GAIT ANALYSIS

Gait analysis, although not widely used by remedial massage therapists, can contribute useful information to treatment plans and can be performed simply, efficiently and without recourse to expensive equipment. Gait disturbances can arise from upper motor neuron lesions, disorders of the cerebellar, vestibular and proprioceptive systems, and dysfunctions of the musculoskeletal system. Many gait and other movement abnormalities are easily observed as clients enter the clinic. Remedial massage therapists will recognise the festinating gait of Parkinson's disease (short, shuffling steps with knees,

trunk and neck held in flexion), the hemiplegic gait that results from upper motor neuron lesions (leg abducted in a semicircle with each step, shoulder adducted, elbow flexed, wrist flexed and pronated), and the staggering ataxic gait of cerebellar disease or diminished sensation in the extremities (wide base of support and exaggerated movements).

Less pronounced disturbances in the symmetry, rhythm and speed of gait are also easily detected. Of particular interest to remedial massage therapists is the influence of joint and muscle function on normal gait. Common musculoskeletal causes of gait disturbance include functional short leg, sore feet, muscle shortness and weakness, and hypomobility or hypermobility of joints.[13] A range of remedial massage techniques can be used to release muscle contractures, increase the mobility of hypomobile joints and, in some cases, to normalise muscle firing patterns and gait reflex patterns through muscle energy techniques.[13]

Normal gait has two phases:

- stance phase which accounts for 60% of the cycle
- swing phase which takes up the remaining 40%.

These two phases can be further subdivided (see Table 2.3):

Stance phase

HEEL STRIKE

When the heel first strikes the ground the foot is approximately 90° to the leg. The knee is extended but not locked.

FOOT FLAT

In this phase the ankle plantarflexes under the control of anterior and posterior leg muscles, especially the eccentric contraction of tibialis anterior. The foot arch flattens slightly as it takes the load of the body and the foot pronates to absorb shock. The quadriceps and gluteal muscles stabilise the hip and knee.

MIDSTANCE

As the body moves over the foot the centre of gravity shifts to the weight-bearing limb. Gluteus medius and minimus control the hip as it internally rotates, adducts slightly and the pelvis drops on the opposite side. The pronated foot moves to slight supination and body weight is transferred to the lateral aspect of the foot. The ankle dorsiflexes.

PUSH-OFF

Weight is transferred to the ball of the foot and the gastrocnemius strongly contracts to plantarflex the ankle to about 20°. Tibialis posterior inverts the heel and the foot supinates. The metatarsophalangeal joints passively extend and the knee flexes to about 35°. Continued toe extension is controlled by the plantar fascia and eccentrically contracting toe flexors. The hip and knee extend and externally rotate.

Swing phase

ACCELERATION

In the acceleration phase, the knee flexes and the ankle dorsiflexes to shorten the limb to clear the ground. The forward swing of the leg is initiated by the quadriceps muscle.

MIDSWING

The hip flexors and knee extensors move the limb forward. The ankle is slightly dorsiflexed and the toes extended to clear the ground. Next, the hip extensors (especially gluteus maximus) and knee flexors (hamstrings) eccentrically contract to slow the forward motion. The hip internally rotates.

DECELERATION

The hamstrings contracting eccentrically and the quadriceps contracting concentrically stop the forward motion of the limb.[14]

Gait assessment: the procedure

Observe the client walking without shoes at their normal walking pace from the front, from the side and from behind. As with static postural observation, begin with general observations, this time about the symmetry, rhythm and speed of gait.

1. GENERAL OBSERVATIONS

Note any changes in the smooth coordinated pattern of normal gait.

- Step length is the distance between the point of first contact of one foot to the point of first contact of the other foot. In a study by Latt et al[15] involving 10 healthy adults (four male and six female) with ages ranging from 17 to 31 years, the average step length was 73 ± 3 cm. Step length decreases with age, fatigue, pain and pathology in the lower limb. (Note: Stride length is the distance between the first point of contact of one foot to the first point of contact with the same foot, i.e. two steps.)
- Adults walk at an average cadence of 90–120 steps per minute.[15, 16] The rate decreases with age, fatigue, pain and if footing is uncertain (e.g. if the surface is slippery or uneven).
- The width of the base (i.e. the distance between the feet) is usually 5–10 cm in adults.[17] Clients widen their base if they have cerebellar problems, decreased sensation in the soles of their feet, or if they feel dizzy or unsteady on their feet.
- In normal gait the body oscillates vertically usually no more than 5 cm with each step.[16]
- The pelvis makes a figure-eight movement, alternately shifting laterally over the weight-bearing limb in stance phase and then rotating forward approximately 40° in swing phase.[13]

2. IDENTIFY THE PHASE OF GAIT THAT IS DISRUPTED AND THE PARTS AFFECTED

A useful strategy for identifying gait disturbances that arise from local musculoskeletal problems is to locate the phase of gait that is affected. Common problems arising in each phase and possible causes are listed in Table 2.4 on p 23.

Stance phase

Most gait problems are apparent in stance phase. Clients who experience pain in stance phase when the single weight-bearing limb is loaded with the entire body weight may shorten the normal duration of the phase or adopt an antalgic gait (e.g. walking on the ball of the foot). Footwear as a source of pain should always be considered when symptoms occur in stance phase.

Heel strike

Pain from a heel spur, bruise or retrocalcaneal bursitis may cause the client to hop onto the foot to avoid heel strike. Normal knee extension may be prevented by a joint fused in flexion or weak quadriceps muscles. In the latter case, the client may push their knee into extension with their hand. If the hip extensors are weak, the client may increase their lumbar lordosis to compensate. Weak hip adductors may result in abnormal rotation of the pelvis and lower limb.

Table 2.3 Phases of gait

Phases of gait

	Stance phase				Swing phase		
	Heel strike	**Foot flat**	**Midstance**	**Push off**	**Acceleration**	**Mid swing**	**Deceleration**
	The foot makes first contact with the ground and the limb decelerates. A closed kinetic chain for the lower limb is initiated.	Foot adapts to surface and takes the weight of the body. The pelvis is stabilised. Trunk is carried forward by momentum.	The knee remains stabilised. Momentum continues to carry the body forward.	The body is accelerated into forward motion.	The lower limb is shortened and swung forward. The innominate moves anteriorly.	The foot clears the ground. On the weight-bearing side the innominate moves posteriorly; the sacrum tilts laterally towards the side of loading.	Decelerate the limb, and prepare for first contact with the ground.
Major muscle groups	*Concentric* Ankle dorsiflexors *Eccentric* Hip extensors Tibialis anterior	*Concentric* Knee extensors Ankle plantar flexors Isometric Hip abductors *Eccentric* Hip extensors Quadriceps Tibialis anterior	*Isometric* Ankle plantar flexors Hip abductors *Eccentric* Plantar flexors	*Concentric* Ankle plantar flexors *Eccentric* Toe flexors	*Concentric* Hip flexors Knee flexors Ankle dorsiflexors	*Concentric* Hip flexors Ankle dorsiflexors *Eccentric* Hip extensors	*Concentric* Quadriceps Ankle dorsiflexors *Eccentric* Knee flexors Hip extensors

Table 2.4 Common gait problems

Stance phase

Antalgic gait (often minimising the duration of stance phase)	Any condition causing pain, especially in the weight-bearing limb or lower back (e.g. shoe problems, osteoarthritis of the ankle, knee, hip, lumbar disc herniation)
Avoiding heel strike (e.g. hopping onto flat foot)	Heel spurs, bruise, bursitis
Drop foot gait	Weak tibialis anterior
Trendelenburg gait The pelvis drops and the trunk lurches to the unaffected side to maintain balance	Weak gluteus medius
Hip extensor gait Immediately after heel strike, the hip is thrust forward and the trunk thrown into extension	Weak gluteus maximus
Back knee gait to lock the knees into extension, pushing knee into extension with hand	Weak quadriceps
Unstable knee which may suddenly buckle into flexion	Dislocating knee cap, torn menisci, torn collateral ligaments
Walking on the balls of the feet	Gastrocnemius/soleus shortening or tear; heel or foot pain (antalgic gait)
Flat foot gait, no forceful toe-off	Weak gastrocnemius/soleus; hallux rigidus

Swing phase

Steppage gait (lifting knee high)	Weak dorsiflexors
Abnormal hip rotation in acceleration	Weak quadriceps
Heavy heel strike	Weak hamstrings

Foot flat

Weak or non-functioning dorsiflexors (tibialis anterior, extensor digitorum longus, extensor hallucis longus) may cause the foot to slap down after heel strike. If the ankle joint is fused, the client may not reach foot flat until midstance.

Midstance

The foot supports the entire body weight and the hip and knee move into extension. Osteoarthritis, pes planus or plantar fasciitis may cause pain in the weight-bearing ankle or foot. Painful calluses may develop over the metatarsal heads, often as a result of fallen transverse arches of the foot. If gluteus medius is weak, the pelvis drops on the non-weight-bearing side (gluteus medius or Trendelenburg or abductor gait). Weak quadriceps may cause excessive knee flexion.

Push off

If gluteus maximus is weak the client may thrust their trunk backwards to maintain hip extension (gluteus maximus or hip extensor gait). If the knee extensors are weak the knee may buckle. Weak gastrocnemius, soleus or flexor hallucis longus may lead to flat-footed (calcaneal) gait. Osteoarthritis or hallux rigidus may interrupt normal push off which requires extension of the metatarsophalangeal joint. Clients with hallux rigidus push off from the lateral aspect of their foot. Calluses on the metatarsal heads and corns can also cause pain during push off.

Swing phase

Acceleration

In the acceleration phase the ankle dorsiflexors help shorten the lower limb so it can clear the ground. Weak ankle dorsiflexors may cause foot drop. The hip flexes and medially rotates as the knee flexes to a maximum of 65° to shorten the leg. If the quadriceps muscles are weak the leg is swung forward with an exaggerated anterior pelvic rotation.

Midswing

If ankle dorsiflexors are weak in mid swing, the client may flex the hip excessively to bend the knee to avoid scraping the toe on the ground (steppage gait).

Deceleration

If the hamstrings are weak heel strike can be excessively hard and the knee may hyperextend (back knee gait).

Findings from gait analysis should be correlated with findings from other assessments, particularly length and strength tests for specific muscles which are detailed in Chapters 10–20 and assessment of the sacroiliac joints, and hip, knee, ankle and foot regions (Chapters 10, 18, 19 and 20 respectively). Further assessments such as muscle firing patterns (see Fritz et al[13]) and neuromuscular treatments like muscle energy techniques (see Chaitow[18]) are beyond the scope of this book but will be of interest to remedial massage therapists who use advanced soft tissue techniques.

FUNCTIONAL TESTS

As part of their assessment procedures, remedial massage therapists use a range of functional tests. These include active and passive range of motion, resisted muscle tests and other tests of functional limitation (e.g. tests for the strength of specific muscles, muscle length tests and other special tests including straight leg raising, Valsalva, Adam's test), and less commonly vital signs (blood pressure, temperature, pulse rate). Active, passive and resisted tests are usually performed before more specific tests.

Although functional tests are widely used by physical therapists including physiotherapists, chiropractors and osteopaths, several studies have found that many tests lack validity and reliability. Practitioners are urged to interpret clinical signs elicited during physical assessment cautiously.[7] 'Eyeballing' a client's active range of motion (i.e. measuring by eye without the use of a goniometer or other measuring tool) is particularly unreliable in clinical practice. Many functional tests have not been fully researched; however, increasingly, information about their diagnostic accuracy is becoming available. Measures of sensitivity (the probability of a positive test among clients with the condition) and specificity (the probability of a negative test among clients who don't have the condition) are available for some tests, however such measures are really only useful when they are very high (≥95%) to help rule a condition in or out.[19]

Likelihood ratios (LRs) are another measure of the usefulness of diagnostic tests. LRs greater than 1 indicate an increased probability that a condition is present. LRs of 10 or more usually rule in a condition. LRs less than 1 indicate a decreased probability that a condition is present. LRs of 0.1 or less usually rule out a condition. Figure 2.17 summarises common measures used to rate the diagnostic accuracy of functional tests.

The decision to perform diagnostic tests is based on client history and other findings that indicate the likelihood of a condition and also whether it is important to have a definitive diagnosis. Remember that in many cases it is not possible or necessary to have a definitive diagnosis of the cause of acute musculoskeletal pain to have effective management of the condition. Where diagnostic tests are appropriate, tests with the highest diagnostic accuracy are preferred. However, even results of functional tests with good ratings for diagnostic accuracy are best interpreted as indicators of possible conditions, such as hamstring strain, tennis elbow or osteoarthritis and used to guide treatment planning (see Table 2.6 on p 25). Physical testing demonstrates clients' functional limitations and suggests the types of tissues involved, the range of treatment options likely to benefit clients, and guides the application of techniques (e.g. depth and duration). However, the evidence for the validity and reliability of many physical assessments is preliminary at best.[20]

Active range of motion (AROM) tests

LOCATING THE REGION

Active tests require the client to move the body through ranges of motion. Muscles are activated and joints move so active movements are not specific to the types of tissues involved. They are useful in locating regions of the body that are likely sources of symptoms. For example, active range of motion tests of a client with posterior thigh pain will help determine if the lumbar spine, hip or knee regions are likely sources of pain and guide the choice of further assessments and treatment options.

SAFE PRACTICE

Safe practice is based on assessing functional limitations and making realistic interpretations of verbal and non-verbal information from clients. AROM testing has an important safety function. It precedes all other functional assessments. Observing clients' active movements helps practitioners determine appropriate pressure, speed and range for passive range of motion (PROM) and other tests. For example, if a client reports pain at 30° active lumbar flexion, all further assessment and treatment procedures must take this into account. In this case, bilateral knee to chest stretches of the erector spinae muscles are likely to reproduce painful lumbar flexion and should be avoided. As a general rule, observe clients and watch them move before making any physical contact.

SEE	MOVE	TOUCH[21]
Observation	*AROM*	*PROM*

Validity
> Degree to which a test measures what it is intended to measure

Reliability
> Degree of consistency with which an instrument or rater measures a particular attribute (expressed as a percentage or decimal e.g. 80% or 0.8)

Sensitivity
> Ability of a test to detect people who actually have a condition (usually recorded as a percentage: sensitivity ≥ 95% rules in a condition)

Specificity
> Ability of a test to correctly identify people who do not have a condition (usually recorded as a percentage: specificity ≥ 95% rules out a condition)

Likelihood ratios
> LR >1 increased probability that a condition is present (the higher the number the better: LR >10 rules in the condition)
> LR < 1 decreased probability that a condition is present (the lower the number the better: LR ≤ 0.1 rules out the condition)

Fig. 2.17 Measuring the diagnostic accuracy of functional tests

Regularly ask clients for feedback and always be alert to non-verbal cues about discomfort or pain.

Passive and resisted tests: Determining tissue types

Active, passive and resisted tests are used initially to indicate the types of tissues that could be involved. They also guide decisions about the need for more specific testing. The results of all functional testing are general guides only (see Table 2.6) and must be interpreted in the light of other assessment findings and of individual responses.

Active tests indicate the region of the body which is a likely source of symptoms. Next passive range of motion (PROM) and resisted range of motion (RROM) tests are carried out to help identify the likely types of tissue involved.

PASSIVE RANGE OF MOTION TESTS (PROM)

PROM tests are performed by the therapist, who moves the joint or body part through its range of motion. Pain and other symptoms reproduced during PROM testing may be related to inert structures including articulating cartilage, joint capsules or ligaments. Muscles are not actively recruited during PROM testing. However, they are passively stretched and resisted range of motion (RROM) testing and palpation may be required to help differentiate the involvement of contractile or inert tissue. PROM tests help detect ligament laxity, joint hypermobility or hypomobility, crepitus and end-feel (the practitioner's interpretation of the feeling of the available movement in the client's tissues at the end of their range of motion). For example, compare the soft end-feel of elbow flexion when muscles are brought together, the hard (bony) end-feel of elbow extension when the olecranon fossa restricts the movement of the ulna, the muscular end-feel of a fully stretched hamstring muscle, and the boggy end-feel when movement is restricted by oedema. Some remedial massage techniques, such as passive joint articulation, are performed near the end of normal physiological range to stretch joint capsules and other tissues around the joint, to prevent the formation of scar tissue and to improve mobility. Stretching beyond the normal physiological limit may result in tissue damage. Sensitivity to tissue tightening near the limits of normal physiological movement is important for safe practice.

Remedial massage therapists are strongly urged to observe AROM before PROM and other assessment and treatment procedures (See-Move-Touch) to determine broad parameters of clients' comfortable movement ranges. Crepitus is sometimes heard and felt and, when related to joint movement, can indicate cartilage wear in the joint space.

Many texts describe capsular patterns of joint limitations in clients with osteoarthritis or joint inflammation (see Table 2.5). They are included here because they have been reported in clinical practice. However, the concept of capsular pattern remains controversial.

Table 2.5 Proposed capsular patterns of joint limitation

Joint	Limitation of range of motion
Cervical spine	Lateral flexion = rotation > extension
Thoracic spine	Lateral flexion = rotation > extension
Lumbar spine	Lateral flexion = rotation > extension
Shoulder	Lateral rotation > abduction > medial rotation
Elbow	Flexion > extension
Wrist	Flexion = extension
Metacarpophalangeal	Flexion > extension
Distal interphalangeal	Flexion > extension
Proximal interphalangeal	Flexion > extension
Hip	Flexion, abduction, medial rotation > extension
Knee	Flexion > extension
Ankle	Plantarflexion > dorsiflexion
Subtalar	Inversion > eversion
2nd–5th metatarsophalangeal	Flexion > extension
1st metatarsophalangeal	Extension > flexion

Table 2.6 Direction of treatment following active, passive and resisted range of motion tests

Type of test	Indications	Implications for treatment
Active range of motion (AROM)	Helps locate musculoskeletal region that is the likely source of symptom (e.g. helps determine if symptoms in the upper limb emanate from the cervical spine or shoulder joint)	Long-term management usually involves treatment of the source of symptoms. Client education about the likely source of symptoms
Passive range of motion (PROM)	Inert tissue (e.g. the articulation itself, ligaments, joint capsule, bursae) (Note: muscles are also passively stretched during PROM testing)	Treatment focuses on inert structures: Swedish massage, thermotherapy, passive joint articulation, myofascial release, range of motion exercises for joint mobility, joint stabilisation, client education
Resisted range of motion (RROM)	Contractile tissue (e.g. major muscles performing a movement tested as a group) Normally followed by specific muscle testing to isolate involved muscle(s)	Treatment focuses on muscle function: Swedish massage, thermotherapy, deep transverse friction, trigger point therapy, soft tissue releasing techniques, muscle stretching and strengthening, client education

RESISTED RANGE OF MOTION TESTS (RROM)

RROM tests are used to test contractile tissue in specific ranges of motion. Position the client's body region or joint (usually in mid-range) and instruct the client to hold the position against your resistance. Resistance normally lasts for 3–5 seconds. RROM tests help locate muscle groups according to their actions. For example, performing an RROM test of knee extension tests the integrity of the knee extensor muscles as a group but will not differentiate between the rectus femoris, vastus medialis, intermedialis or lateralis muscles. Further testing, such as resisted tests for specific muscles and palpation, are required to help identify individual muscles.

Tests for specific muscles

Resisted tests and length tests for specific muscles are of particular interest to remedial massage therapists who often focus their treatments on assessing and treating muscle function (e.g. relationships between agonists and antagonists, patterns of kinetic dysfunction, muscle tightness or weakness, impacts on posture and compensatory patterns). Muscles have been classified as mobilisers and stabilisers. Mobilisers tend to be superficial, span two joints and contain fast twitch fibres for power rather than endurance. Stabilisers, on the other hand, are usually deep, cross one joint and are made up of slow twitch fibres for endurance; they contribute to habitual postures. Mobilisers tend to become short and tight and can inhibit the action of stabilisers that may have become weak and long. Commonly shortened muscles include upper trapezius, pectoralis major, sternocleidomastoid, erector spinae, quadratus lumborum, iliopsoas, hamstring muscles and hip adductors. Shortened hamstrings, adductors and hip flexors are often associated with weakened and lengthened transversalis abdominis and posterior gluteal muscles.

Specific muscle testing to identify correctable abnormalities of muscle strength and length may be prompted by (1) postural observation (e.g. hyperlordotic posture may prompt testing bilateral iliopsoas muscles for shortness), or (2) resisted muscle testing (RROM) in an initial screening that suggests contractile tissue as a source of symptoms.

RESISTED TESTS FOR SPECIFIC MUSCLES

Resisted tests are used by many healthcare professionals to test muscle strength, and grading systems, such as the one described in the box below, have been developed. However, in remedial massage, resisted tests for specific muscles are more commonly used to locate possible lesions in specific muscles. Grading muscle strength is often restricted to bilateral comparisons or judgments based on clinical experience.

> A typical grading system rates muscle strength on a scale from 5 to 0:
> 5 Normal strength: movement is possible against maximum resistance by the examiner
> 4 Good: movement is possible against gravity and some resistance by the examiner
> 3 Fair: movement is possible against gravity but not against resistance by the examiner
> 2 Poor: movement is possible when gravity is eliminated (i.e. testing joint in its horizontal plane)
> 1 Trace: muscle tightens but no movement
> 0 Zero: no contraction

In the following example, resisted testing is used to isolate the specific muscles that are likely sources of the presenting symptoms in a client with shoulder pain.

> ▼ The client would be tested for shoulder range of motion (AROM, PROM, RROM). AROM tests help identify the region of the body that is the likely source of symptoms. If active shoulder abduction reproduces the pain, the injury is likely to be related to the shoulder joint or associated muscles (and not referred from the cervical spine, for example). PROM and RROM tests are required to help suggest the likely tissues involved. If PROM tests do not reproduce the pain (i.e. inert structures are probably not involved) but RROM testing for shoulder abduction does, then contractile tissue is implicated. The client's injury is probably related to the shoulder abductor muscles. Further resisted testing is required to discriminate between the two abductor muscles (deltoid and supraspinatus muscles) (see Figure 2.18).

Isolating the injured muscle(s) enables practitioners to develop targeted treatment plans which are likely to produce faster and better outcomes for clients. Resisted tests for muscles implicated in commonly occurring conditions are detailed in Chapters 10–20. (For further information see Avens and Brown[22].)

Fig. 2.18 Differentiating (a) supraspinatus and (b) middle deltoid strains

MUSCLE LENGTH TESTS

Muscle length and flexibility both refer to the ability of a muscle to be lengthened to the end of its range of motion.[23] There are many reasons why muscles become shortened, including maintaining postures for excessively long periods (e.g. hip flexors may become shortened after prolonged periods of sitting), adaptive responses to other conditions (e.g. the presence of a trigger point, scoliosis or a leg length discrepancy) and ageing. When a shortened muscle is identified, muscle-stretching techniques are usually applied to restore its normal length. Stretching can be performed as part of the consultation and/or prescribed as home exercises. For example, the length of the hamstring muscles can be assessed by straight leg raising when the client is supine. Shortness is assessed by comparison to population norms (normal hamstring length permits approximately 65–80° straight leg raising) and/or by bilateral comparison. A range of stretching techniques can be applied to the posterior thigh after Swedish massage or heat application has warmed the area (see Chapter 5). Length tests of some of the major muscles of the body are included in Table 2.7.

Positioning the client
- Muscle should be placed in the fully elongated position.
- As far as possible isolate the muscle across one joint.
- Bony landmarks that are used for measuring muscle length should be readily palpable.
- Movement should not be blocked by external supports or pillows.
- Client must be able to assume the position.

Stabilisation of proximal bony segment of the associated joint
- Required to isolate intended motion.
- Avoids the client substituting another muscle to perform the motion.

Note the end-feel
- Bony (e.g elbow extension).
- Capsular (e.g. medial hip rotation).
- Muscular (e.g. knee extension with hip flexion).
- Soft tissue (e.g. knee flexion).

Special (orthopaedic) tests

A range of special (orthopaedic) tests can be used by remedial massage therapists to help identify specific conditions. Remember that findings from special tests should be interpreted cautiously, especially where the specificity or sensitivity of the tests are less than 95%, or where likelihood ratios (LR) are in the range $0.1 \geq LR \geq 10$.

Some commonly used special tests are listed in Table 2.8. Details of relevant tests will be discussed in Chapters 10–20.

PALPATION

Palpation is considered by many to be the most important assessment tool of massage therapists. Palpatory assessment continues throughout the treatment as an inherent function of manual therapy. Beginning students can rapidly learn to detect differences in muscle tone as they massage. With practice, palpation can be used to identify specific tissues (see Table 2.9) and to assess tissues for pathological states and stages of healing using the following indicators:

- Temperature: use the dorsum of the hand just above or lightly touching the skin to identify changes in temperature (e.g. increased temperature in acute inflammation, decreased temperature in impaired circulation).
- Changes in normal tissue (e.g. fibrotic cords in muscles, hard pea-shaped painful trigger points, muscle flaccidity, microtears in musculotendinous junctions and muscle bellies).
- Presence of oedema (e.g. sponginess of tissues in acute inflammation, pitting and non-pitting[i]).

The chiropractic, osteopathic and physiotherapy literature contains a number of studies on the efficacy of palpation. One annotated bibliography found only slight interexaminer reliability and moderate intraexaminer reliability for palpation.[26] Inter- and intraexaminer discrepancies were also found in a small study in which two physiotherapists identified 12 anatomical landmarks that enabled measurement of eight joint angles.[27] Joensen et al,[28] on the other hand, found strong agreements between palpation for tendon hypertrophy. Static palpation was moderately reliable for identifying segmental thoracic spine stiffness and tenderness.[29] and inter-rater reliability was good between two clinicians for the stiffest site in each region of the spine.[30] A review to statistically estimate the agreement of manual palpation for identifying myofascial trigger points found moderate inter-rater agreement.[31] This was confirmed by another small study of 21 patients to evaluate inter- and intra-tester reliability of myofascial trigger points in hip and thigh muscles. The study found moderate to substantial intra-rater reliability of active and latent myofascial trigger point evaluation.[32] As with many other aspects of massage assessment practices, further research is needed to confirm the efficacy of palpation as an assessment strategy for remedial massage practice.

Palpatory findings must also be recorded on clients' files. There have been several attempts at categorising palpatory findings but none has been widely taken up. Recording the tissue type and any abnormal temperature, tissue quality or water content is usually sufficient (e.g. fibrotic left upper trapezius, hot swollen right lateral ankle joint, trigger point right supraspinatus muscle).

LEGAL AND ETHICAL REQUIREMENTS FOR REMEDIAL MASSAGE ASSESSMENT

Issues of privacy, confidentiality, child protection and the safe and efficient use of equipment and resources are of paramount importance in all aspects of remedial massage

---

[i]Pitting oedema results when a swollen area is pressed and an indentation persists after the pressure is released. This is the most common form of oedema. It is caused by any form of pressure (e.g. from tight socks). In non-pitting oedema pressure applied to a swollen area does not create a persistent indentation. Non-pitting oedema occurs in disorders of the lymphatic system (e.g. lymphoedema after lymph-node surgery or congenitally). It is usually observed in the arms or legs. It can also be associated with hyperthyroidism.

Table 2.7 Length tests of major muscles[23, 24]

Muscle – upper extremity	Length test	
Levator scapulae	The client lies supine. The practitioner stabilises the client's shoulder with one hand and flexes, sidebends and rotates the occiput to the opposite side.	
Upper trapezius	The client lies supine. The practitioner stabilises the client's shoulder with one hand. With the other the occiput is laterally flexed to the opposite side and rotated to the side of testing.	
Latissimus dorsi	The client lies supine and fully flexes the extended arm. Observe the distance between the extended arm and the table.	
Pectoralis major	The client lies supine with hand behind head. Observe the distance between the elbow and the table.	
Pectoralis major – sternal (lower) portion	The client lies supine and abducts the extended arm to about 135°. The arm is allowed to fall into maximum horizontal abduction.	
Pectoralis major – clavicular (upper portion)	As above except that the arm is abducted to 90°.	

Table 2.7 Length tests of major muscles—cont'd

Muscle – upper extremity	Length test	
Pectoralis minor muscle	The client lies supine with arms by sides. Observe the distance between the shoulders and the table.	
Triceps brachii	The client is seated and tries to touch the back of their shoulder with their hand keeping their humerus fully flexed.	
Biceps brachii	The client lies supine with their shoulder level with the edge of the table, elbow extended and forearm pronated. The client extends their shoulder to their comfortable limit, keeping their elbow fully extended.	
Flexor digitorum superficialis, flexor digitorum profundus, flexor digiti minimi	The client lies supine with shoulder abducted to 70–90°, elbow extended, forearm supinated and fingers extended. The practitioner fully extends the client's wrist.	
Extensor digitorum, extensor indicis, extensor digiti minimi	The client lies supine with shoulder abducted to 70–90°, elbow extended, forearm pronated and fingers flexed. The practitioner fully flexes the client's wrist.	
Trunk		
Lumbar erector spinae	The client is seated on the table, keeping the pelvis as vertical as possible. The client bends forward as far as possible from the lumbo-pelvic region.	

Continued

Table 2.7 Length tests of major muscles—cont'd

Trunk	Length test	
Quadratus lumborum	The client lies on their side with their back near the edge of the table. The client bends their lower leg slightly and holds on to the table for stability. The client extends the upper leg beyond the edge of the table letting the leg drop towards the floor.	

Muscle – lower extremity		
Iliopsoas – supine	The client lies supine at the end of the table so that the hips can fully extend. The client fully flexes one knee. Observe the distance between the extended thigh and the level of the table.	
Iliopsoas – prone	The client lies prone with knee flexed to 90°. The practitioner stabilises the pelvis with one hand. The practitioner lifts the client's thigh as far as possible without moving the pelvis.	
Rectus femoris – supine	The client's position is the same as for the supine ilio psoas test. Observe the degree of knee flexion on the side of the extended thigh.	
Rectus femoris – prone	The client lies prone, knee flexed and the foot is taken towards their buttock.	
Hamstring	The client lies supine and the extended leg is raised. The test may also be performed with the knee slightly flexed.	

Table 2.7 Length tests of major muscles—cont'd

Muscle – lower extremity	Length test	
Hip external rotators	The client lies prone, knee flexed to 90°. The client's leg drops laterally as far as possible.	
Hip internal rotators	As above, except that the client's leg drops medially as far as possible.	
Iliotibial band and tensor fasciae latae muscle length (Ober's test)	The client lies on their side, lower knee slightly flexed. The upper knee is flexed to 90°. The practitioner abducts and slightly extends the upper thigh. The client then allows the upper leg to drop towards the table. A shortened iliotibial band prevents the leg from reaching the table.	
Hip adductors	The client lies supine with knees bent and feet flat on the table. The practitioner stabilises the pelvis on one side as the opposite knee drops to the side as far as possible.	
Gastrocnemius	The client lies supine, knees extended. The practitioner dorsiflexes the client's ankle.	
Soleus	The client lies prone, knee flexed to 90°. The practitioner dorsiflexes the client's ankle.	

Table 2.8 Special tests commonly used by remedial massage therapists (see Chapters 10–20 for specific regional orthopaedic tests)

Adam's test	Test to discriminate idiopathic and functional scoliosis
Anterior draw (knee)	Test for integrity of anterior cruciate ligament of the knee (SN 18–95, SP 86–100, LR+ 1.8–8.3, LR– 0.1–0.5)
Anterior draw (ankle)	Test for anterior talofibular instability (SN 78–95, SP 74–84, LR+ 3.1, LR– 0.29)
Apley's test	Test for meniscal tear in the knee (R 0.95, SN 13–16, SP 86–100, LR+ 0.8–5.9, LR– 0.63–1.1)
Cervical compression test	Test for pressure on a nerve root (increased peripheral pain), joint damage or ligament strain (increased local pain)
Cervical distraction	Pressure on a nerve root relieved by distraction. Increased local pain suggests muscle, ligament or joint capsule damage (R 0.82, SN 40–50, SP 80–100, LR+ 4.4; LR– 0.62)
Drop arm test	Useful to rule in rotator cuff tear (R 0.28–0.66, SN 8–27, SP 88–100, LR+ 2.6–5 LR– 0.83–0.94)
Elbow extension test	Useful to rule out bony or joint injury (SN 97, SP 69, LR+ 3.1, LR– 0.04)[25]
Elevated arm stress test (Roo's test)	Test for thoracic outlet syndrome (SN 82, SP 100)
Empty can test	Pain or weakness suggests supraspinatus damage (SN 44–89, SP 50–90, LR+ 1.8–4.2, LR– 0.22–0.63)
Finkelstein's test	Test for tenosynovitis of the abductor pollicis longus and extensor pollicis brevis (SN 81, SP 50, LR+ 1.6, LR– 0.38)
Hip impingement/FADIR test	Test for femoroacetabular impingement. (SN 78, SP 10, LR+ .86, LR– 2.3)
Iliac compression test	Test for sacroiliac lesion
Kemp's/quadrant test	Leg pain suggests nerve root compression or radiculopathy; low back pain suggests local sprain/strain or facet syndrome
Lachman test	Test for the integrity of the anterior cruciate ligament (SN 86, SP 91)
Morton's test	Test for Morton's neuroma, metatarsal joint arthritis, fracture of the metatarsal heads or metatarsalgia
Moving patella apprehension test	Test for patella instability (SN 100, SP 88.4)
Painful arc	Test for impingement syndrome, rotator cuff or AC pathology (SN 33–98, SP 10–81, LR+ 1.1–3.9, LR– 0.2–0.82)
Patella apprehension test	Test for dislocation or subluxation of the patella (SN 7–37, SP 86–100, LR+ 0.9–2.3, LR– 0.8–1.0)
Patellofemoral grind test	Test for patellofemoral syndrome, osteoarthritis, osteochondritis of the patella, patella fracture (SN 29–49, SP 67–75, LR+ 0.9–1.9, LR– 0.7–1.1)
Patrick's/FABERE test	Test for hip joint pathology, osteoarthritis, sprain/strain, fracture, tight hip adductors (SN 88)
Phalen's test	Test for carpal tunnel syndrome (compression of median nerve) (R 0.79, SN 10–88, SP 33–100, LR+ 0.7–41.5, LR– 0.1–1)
Posterior draw (knee)	Test for the integrity of the posterior cruciate ligament (SN 22–100, SP 99, LR+ 90, LR– 0.1)

Table 2.8 Special tests commonly used by remedial massage therapists—cont'd

Posterior draw (ankle)	Test for the integrity of the posterior ankle ligaments
PSIS asymmetry	Test for sacroiliac lesion, anatomical variation (R 0.7, SN 69)
Shoulder (anterior) apprehension test	Test for anterior glenohumeral instability (SN 53, SP 99, LR+ 53, LR– 0.47)
Shoulder impingement test	Test for shoulder impingement syndrome: shoulder impingement suggested if pain during active flexion; supraspinatus impingement suggested if pain when shoulder internally rotated; biceps long head implicated if pain when shoulder externally rotated.
SI compression test	Test for SI sprain, fracture, joint dysfunction (R 0.64–0.79, SN 25–69, SP 63–100, LR+ 1.6–2.2, LR– 0.4–0.63)
SI distraction test	Test for anterior SI or pubic symphysis sprain, pelvic fracture (R 0.36–0.94, SN 11–60, SP 74–100, LR+ 1.1–3.2, LR– 0.5–0.98)
Sign of the buttock	Test to distinguish whether pain on straight leg raising arises from SI joint dysfunction, bursitis, gluteal muscle strain or from lumbar spine pathology, nerve root pressure or hamstring tension
Slump test	Leg symptoms suggest nerve root tension, radiculopathy, disc herniation. Local lumbosacral pain suggests lumbosacral sprain or strain (SN 83, SP 55, LR+ 1.8, LR– 0.3)
Straight leg raising	Test to distinguish sciatic nerve impingement, disc herniation, piriformis syndrome from SI/lumbar strain or sprain (R 0.92, SN 78–98, SP 11–64, LR+ 1.03–2.2, LR– 0.05–0.86)
Thessaly test	Test for meniscal tears (knee) (SN 90, SP 98)
Thomas test	Test for hip contracture, tight hip flexors (R 0.91, SN 89, SP 92, LR+ 11.123, LR– 0.12)[34]
Thompson test	Test for the integrity of the Achilles tendon (SN 96, SP 93, LR+ 13.47, LR– 0.04)
Tinel's sign	Test for neuropathy Tinel's sign at elbow (SN 70, SP 98, LR+ 35, LR– 0.31) Tinel's sign at wrist (R 0.5–0.8, SN 23–97, SP 53–100, LR+ 0.7–11, LR– 0.03–1.0)
Trendelenburg test	Test for gluteus medius weakness or paralysis, Legg-Calve-Perthes disease, poliomyelitis, hip dislocation, fracture (R 0.68, SN 73, SP 77, LR+ 3.15, LR– 0.36)
Valgus/varus elbow stress test	Test for medial/lateral collateral ligament sprain
Valgus/varus stress test (knee)	Test for medial/lateral collateral ligament sprain (R 0.16, SN 86–100, SP 100)
Valsalva	Test for space occupying lesion, disc herniation, IVF encroachment (R 0.69, SN 22, SP 94, LR+ 3.67, LR– 0.82)
Windlass test	Test for plantar fasciitis (SN 100, SP 32)
Yergason's test	Test for biceps brachii tendonitis or strain, glenoid labrum pathology, torn transverse humeral ligament (SN 9–50, SP 79–93, LR+ 1.3–3.0, LR– 0.72–0.94)

(R) = reliability, (SN) = sensitivity, (SP) = specificity, (LR) = likelihood ratios
Adapted from Visniak[35]

Table 2.9   Palpating tissue layers

Epidermis	Place dorsum of hands lightly on the skin and compare the temperature of different parts of the body. Slide hand over the skin and note the dryness/moistness and texture of the skin. Slide fingers over the skin so that it wrinkles and note any resistance between the epidermis and the underlying tissue.
Muscle	Muscle tissue feels firmer than subcutaneous tissue. Postural muscles often palpate as tight bundles of fibres. Fibrotic tissue feels ropey.
Tendons	Tendons feel like thin firm movable cords.
Ligaments	Ligaments feel like flat bands of tissue, less mobile and elastic than tendons.
Joint capsules	Not palpable unless thickened. Articular disorders are often associated with joint line tenderness.
Peripheral nerves	Peripheral nerves feel like small threads, thinner and less elastic than tendons, often fairly mobile.
Lymph glands	Small soft rubbery nodes, rarely bigger than 0.5 cm.
Blood vessels	Superficial blood vessels feel like soft tubes, pulses are often detected.

Adapted from Chaitow[36]

practice, including assessment. Remedial massage assessments must be recorded accurately and in a well-organised manner so as to be easily interpreted by others. Lack of standard abbreviations of key terms and recordings of remedial massage assessments confounds the transparency of record keeping. SOAP[j] and other similar charting methods are useful guides for massage therapists, however they often lack the capacity for recording the range of assessments commonly used in remedial massage practice. Practice management software can also be used to record assessments, diagnostic imaging and other medical reports and correspondence.

Figure 2.19 is an extract from a sample client assessment form which accommodates commonly used remedial massage assessments.

Another simple method for recording trunk ranges of motion involves drawing a star diagram to represent cervical, thoracic or lumbar motion as if observed from above (see Figure 2.20). Each line represents normal ROM for the movement. Restrictions in ranges of motion are indicated by drawing dashes, and pain is indicated by recording P on the lines of the star diagram. The closer to the centre of the star, the more marked the restriction or the earlier the onset of pain.

KEY MESSAGES

Remedial massage assessments determine the suitability of clients for remedial massage through screening for red flags.

Those deemed suitable for remedial massage undergo further assessments to identify potential sources of symptoms, to understand clients' perceptions of their own functional impairments and to develop effective therapy plans.

For safe practice, all assessments should adhere to the following principles:

1. See-Move-Touch; that is, observe clients and perform active range of motion tests before any physical contact is made with clients.
2. Assessments should be performed slowly and carefully especially when using tests that can reproduce symptoms.

Remedial massage assessments include:

- Case history
  - Identify red and yellow flags
  - Is the client's condition mild, moderate or severe?
- Outcome measures
  - Monitor progress towards treatment goals
- Postural observation
  - Look for underlying predisposing factors to presenting symptoms
- Gait assessment
  - Observe changes in symmetry, rate and rhythm of normal gait
- Functional tests
  - Active range of motion (AROM)
    - indicates source of lesion
  - Passive range of motion (PROM)
  - Resisted tests (RROM)
  - Specific muscle tests (where appropriate)
    - Resisted tests and length tests for specific muscles
  - Special (orthopaedic) tests
- Palpation
  - Identify tissues involved, stage of healing

[j]SOAP charting encourages therapists to record subjective (S) and objective (O) assessments, assessment or analysis (A) and their therapy plan (P).[33]

Postural observation

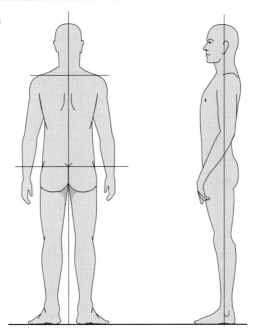

Gait assessment

Rate   Rhythm   Symmetry

Phase

	Heel strike	Foot flat	Midstance	Push off	Acceleration	Mid Swing	Deceleration
Joint							
Muscle							

Palpatory findings

_____

_____

_____

_____

Cervical

AROM	Flexion	Extension	R lat flexion	L lat flexion	R rotation	L rotation

PROM	Flexion	Extension	R lat flexion	L lat flexion	R rotation	L rotation

RROM	Flexion	Extension	R lat flexion	L lat flexion	R rotation	L rotation

Specific muscle tests						
Special tests	Compression		Distraction		Valsalva	

Fig. 2.19 Sample client assessment form

Continued

Thoracic

AROM	Flexion	Extension	R lat flexion	L lat flexion	R rotation	L rotation
PROM	Flexion	Extension	R lat flexion	L lat flexion	R rotation	L rotation
RROM	Flexion	Extension	R lat flexion	L lat flexion	R rotation	L rotation
Specific muscle tests						
Special tests	Adam's test		Deep breathing		Elevated arm stress test	

Shoulder

AROM	Flexion		Extension		Abduction		Horiz adduc		Med rot		Lat rot	
	L	R	L	R	L	R	L	R	L	R	L	R
PROM	L	R	L	R	L	R	L	R	L	R	L	R
RROM	L	R	L	R	L	R	L	R	L	R	L	R
Specific muscle tests												
Special tests	Apley's scratch L R			Impingement L R			Apprehension L R					
	Drop arm L R			Yergason's L R			Empty can test L R					

Elbow

AROM	Flexion		Extension		Supination		Pronation	
	L	R	L	R	L	R	L	R
PROM	L	R	L	R	L	R	L	R
RROM	L	R	L	R	L	R	L	R
Specific muscle tests								
Special tests	Valgus stress L R		Varus stress L R			Extension test L R		
	Resisted wrist flexion L R			Resisted wrist extension L R				

Wrist

AROM	Flexion		Extension		Abduction		Adduction		Supination		Pronation	
	L	R	L	R	L	R	L	R	L	R	L	R
PROM	L	R	L	R	L	R	L	R	L	R	L	R
RROM	L	R	L	R	L	R	L	R	L	R	L	R
Specific muscle tests												
Special tests	Phalen's test L R			Tinel's test L R			Finkelstein's test L R					

Fig. 2.19, cont'd

Lumbar

AROM	Flexion	Extension	R lat flexion	L lat flexion	R rotation	L rotation
PROM	Flexion	Extension	R lat flexion	L lat flexion	R rotation	L rotation
RROM	Flexion	Extension	R lat flexion	L lat flexion	R rotation	L rotation

Specific muscle tests			

Special tests	Kemp's test L R	Valsalva	SLR L R
	Centralisation peripheralisation	Patrick's test L R	SI compression L R
	SI distraction L R	Short leg L R	

Hip

AROM	Flexion		Extension		Abduction		Adduction		Med rot		Lat rot	
	L	R	L	R	L	R	L	R	L	R	L	R
PROM	L	R	L	R	L	R	L	R	L	R	L	R
RROM	L	R	L	R	L	R	L	R	L	R	L	R

Specific muscle tests		

Special tests	Patrick's test L R	Thomas test L R	Trendelenburg L R
	Ober's test L R		

Knee

AROM	Flexion		Extension		Med rot		Lat rot	
	L	R	L	R	L	R	L	R
PROM	L	R	L	R	L	R	L	R
RROM	L	R	L	R	L	R	L	R

Specific muscle tests		

Special tests	Patellofemoral grind L R	Patella apprehension L R	Valgus stress test L R
	Varus stress test L R	Anterior draw L R	Posterior draw L R
	Apley's compression L R		

Fig. 2.19, cont'd

Continued

Ankle and foot

AROM	Flexion		Extension		Inversion		Eversion	
	L	R	L	R	L	R	L	R
PROM	L	R	L	R	L	R	L	R
RROM	L	R	L	R	L	R	L	R
Specific muscle tests								
Special tests	Anterior draw L R			Posterior draw L R			Lat stability L R	
	Morton's test L R							

Fig. 2.19, cont'd

Star diagram

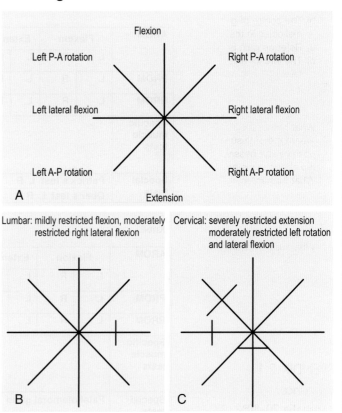

A

Flexion
Left P-A rotation
Right P-A rotation
Left lateral flexion
Right lateral flexion
Left A-P rotation
Right A-P rotation
Extension

B — Lumbar: mildly restricted flexion, moderately restricted right lateral flexion

C — Cervical: severely restricted extension, moderately restricted left rotation and lateral flexion

Fig. 2.20 Recording trunk ranges of motion: (a) the star diagram, (b) and (c) are examples showing how to use the star diagram.

Review questions

1. Complete the following sentences with a word or phrase:
   a) Red flags are _____
   b) A common cause of increased kyphosis of the cervicothoracic spine is _____
   c) Passive range of motion tests are used to test _____
   d) A dermatome is _____
   e) _____ test is used to discriminate between idiopathic and functional scoliosis.

2. What would you do if a client came to your clinic for assessment and treatment of pain in the upper thoracic spine, bilateral shoulders and hands, and with a history of night sweats?

3. Circle the correct answer:
   A client is observed to have a mild scoliosis with the right iliac crest lower than the left. It is likely that:
   a) the right gluteal fold is lower/higher on the right
   b) the gluteal cleft deviates to the left/right
   c) the left PSIS is lower/higher than the right PSIS
   d) the right foot is anterior/posterior to the left foot
   e) the left/right knee is slightly flexed
   f) the waist curve on the right appears to increase/decrease

4. Indicate True or False for each of the following statements.
   a) Using the principle of See-Move-Touch, passive tests are conducted before active tests. True/False
   b) The centre of gravity passes anterior to the lateral malleolus in the erect posture. True/False
   c) Referred pain is sharp and poorly localised. True/False
   d) The inferior angle of the scapula is approximately at the level of T5 spinous process. True/False

5. What type of tissue is implicated if active shoulder flexion is positive and resisted shoulder flexion is positive but passive shoulder flexion is not?
   What further testing, if any, is required?

6. What type of tissue is implicated if active hip abduction is positive and passive hip abduction is positive but resisted hip abduction is not?
   What further testing, if any, is required?

7. How would you interpret the following assessment findings for the lumbar spine: active right lateral flexion positive, resisted right lateral flexion positive, and passive right lateral flexion positive?
   What further testing, if any, is required?

8. Describe a test for the length of the hamstring muscle.

9. What type of tissue is suggested by the following palpatory findings:
   a) Soft, rubbery, pea-shaped, less than 0.5 cm diameter
   b) Tight cord
   c) Small threads
   d) Small pulsing tubes

10. Name a possible cause for the following observations of gait:
    a) steppage gait
    b) heavy heel strike
    c) back knee gait
    d) excessive hip rotation in acceleration phase

11. What are the implications for practice of using a functional test with a sensitivity of 95%?

12. How would you interpret the lumbar ranges of motion indicated by the following star diagram?

APPENDIX 2.1

Skin cancer

In Australia 70–80% of all skin cancers are basal cell carcinomas, 15–20% are squamous cell carcinomas and less than 5% are melanomas.

Basal cell carcinomas usually occur in people over 40 years of age, although they may occur in younger people. They are slow growing and present as either small, raised pearly tumours with small blood vessels on the surface or a red plaque. The latter is more common on the trunk.

Squamous cell carcinomas may develop as a slowly enlarging, scaly nodule or an ulcerated sore with raised, rolled edges or a red, scaly plaque.

Malignant melanoma is a malignant change in the pigment cells of the skin. It can develop in normal skin as a flat, coloured spot or appear as a change in an existing pigmented lesion such as a mole. They can appear anywhere on the body. In the early stages, a melanoma is a flat, coloured spot.

Encourage clients to seek medical attention for pigmented lesions which are either new or changing, especially if their size, colour or shape is changing.

The following checklist may be useful:[37]

a. Asymmetry – one half of the lesion is dissimilar to the other

b. Border irregularity – a spot with a spreading or irregular edge (notched)

c. Colour change – blotchy spots with a number of colours such as black, blue, red, white and/or grey

d. Evolving - spots that are changing and growing

Seborrhoeic keratoses are raised, pigmented lesions which are common benign tumours occurring in people over 40 years old. **Solar keratoses** are scaly lesions which may come and go. They occur on the sun-exposed areas of the body and are seen in 40–50% of people over 40 years old. These lesions are often confused with melanomas. However, their presence indicates that a person has had sufficient sun exposure to be at high risk of having either a basal cell or squamous cell carcinoma somewhere on the sun-exposed areas of their body.

What to look for

Any mole or freckle that has:

1. changed colour. Melanomas often develop a blue or black colour. Sometimes areas may become lighter and many different colours such as reds, greys, blues may be found.
2. changed shape or increased in size. The change in shape is usually from an oval or round mole to an irregular 'coastline' appearance. The increase in size can be overall or simply an elevation above surrounding skin. React quickly to a flat mole that becomes elevated, especially if the elevation is dark or a different colour from the original mole.
3. an irregular border. Most harmless moles have smooth, regular borders. Melanomas often have irregular borders.
4. become itchy or bleeds. A mole that bleeds without any significant injury should be examined by a doctor. Itch may be an important symptom but only if there are other changes.
5. appeared recently from normal-looking skin, especially if it is dark or is rapidly growing.

Any pigmented lesion that looks different from the others on an individual's skin should be examined closely and biopsied if diagnosis is uncertain. (Most moles or pigmented spots on an individual resemble each other – show a family resemblance.)

Clinical features suggestive of malignancy

- size greater than 6 mm
- irregular shape
- variation in colour within the mole
- noticeable increase in size over 3–18 months
- unexplained inflammation in and around the mole (redness and/or tenderness around a mole for longer than two months is suspicious)
- bleeding and itching (repeated bleeding with minor injury is unusual)

REFERENCES

1. Chow R. Complementary medicine: impact on medical practice. Curr Ther 2000;41(7):76–9.
2. Grace S, Vemulpad S, Beirman R. Training in and use of diagnostic techniques among CAM practitioners: an Australian study. J Altern Complement Med 2006;12(7):695–700.
3. Posadzki P, Ernst E. The safety of massage therapy: an update of a systematic review. Focu Altern Complement Ther 2013;18. Doi 10.1111/fct.12007.
4. Yin P, Gao N, Wu J, et al. Adverse events of massage therapy in pain-related conditions: a systematic review. Evid-Based Compl Alt Med 2014. Article ID 480956. http://dx.doi.org/10.1155/2014/480956.
5. Hartvigsen J, Hancock MJ, Kongsted A, et al. What low back pain is and why we need to pay attention. Lancet 2018;391:2356–67.
6. Ge J, Fishman J, Vapiwala N, et al. Patient-physician communication about complementary and alternative medicine in a radiation oncology setting. J Radiat Oncol Biol Phys 2013;85(1):e1–6.
7. Foster NE, Anema JR, Cherkin D, et al. Prevention and treatment of low back pain: evidence, challenges, and promising directions. Lancet 2018;391:2368–83.
8. WorkCover NSW. Training manual for providers of remedial massage therapy to injured workers. Gosford: WorkCover NSW; 2010.
9. New Zealand Guidelines Group. New Zealand acute low back pain guide. Online. Available: www.nzgg.org.nz/guidelines/0072/acc1038_col.pdf; 2004.
10. Posadzki P, Ernst E. The safety of massage therapy: an update of a systematic review. Focu Altern Complement Ther 2013;18:27–32.
11. Weir M. Law and ethics in complementary medicine: a handbook for practitioners in Australia and New Zealand. 4th edn. Crows Nest, NSW: Allen & Unwin; 2011.
12. Cella D, Riley W, Stone A, et al. The Patient-Reported Outcome Measurement Information System (PROMIS) developed and tested its first wave of adult self-reported health outcome item banks: 2005-2008. J Clin Epidemiol 2010;63:1179–94.
13. Fritz S, Chaitow L, Hymel GM. Clinical massage in the healthcare setting. St Louis, MI: Mosby Elsevier; 2008.
14. Adams JA, Cerny K. Observational gait analysis. A visual guide. Thorofare, NJ: Slack; 2017.
15. Latt M, Menz H, Fung V, et al. Walking speed, cadence and step length are selected to optimize the stability of head and pelvic accelerations. Exp Brain Res 2008;184:201–9.
16. Hoppenfeld S. Physical examination of the spine and extremities. 2nd edn. Upper Saddle River, NJ: Prentice Hall; 2010.
17. Magee D. Orthopedic physical assessment. 6th edn. Philadelphia: Saunders; 2013.
18. Chaitow L. Muscle energy techniques. 4th edn. Edinburgh: Churchill Livingstone; 2013.
19. Vizniak N. Physical assessment. Burnaby, B.C.: Professional Health Systems; 2008.
20. Bussieres A, Stewart G, Al-Zoubi F, et al. Spinal manipulative therapy and other conservative treatments for low back pain: a guideline from the Canadian Chiropractic Guideline Initiative. J Manipulative Physiol Ther 2018;41(4):265–93.
21. Esposito S, Phillipson S. Spinal adjusting technique: the chiropractic art. Sydney: Well-Adjusted Publishing; 2005.
22. Avers D, Brown M. Daniels and Worthingham's muscle testing: techniques of manual examination and performance. 10th edn. Oxford: Saunders Elsevier; 2018.
23. Reese N, Bandy W. Joint range of motion and muscle length testing. 2nd edn. Philadelphia: W.B. Saunders; 2009.
24. Reiman M, Manske R. Functional testing in human performance. Champaign, IL: Human Kinetics; 2009.
25. Cleland J, Koppenhaver S. Netter's orthopaedic clinical examination: an evidence-based approach. 2nd edn. Philadelphia: Saunders; 2011.
26. Haneline M, Cooperstein R, Young M, et al. An annotated bibliography of spinal motion palpation reliability studies. J Can Chiropr Assoc 2009;53(1):40–58.
27. Moriguchi C, Carnaz L, Silva L, et al. Reliability of intra- and inter-rater palpation discrepancy and estimation of its effects on joint angle measurements. J Can Chiropr Assoc 2009;53(1):40–58.
28. Joensen J, Couppe C, Bjordal J. Increased palpation tenderness and muscle strength deficit in the prediction of tendon hypertrophy in symptomatic unilateral shoulder tendinopathy: an ultrasonographic study. Physiotherapy 2009;95:83–93.

29. Beynon AM, Hebert JJ, Walker BF. The interrater reliability of static palpation of the thoracic spine for eliciting tenderness and stiffness to test for a manipulable lesion. Chiropr Man Therap 2018;26:49.

30. Holt K, Russell D, Cooperstein R, et al. Interexaminer reliability of seated motion palpation for the stiffest spinal site. J Manipulative Physiol Ther 2018;41(7):571–9.

31. Rathbone ATL, Grosman-Rimon L, Kumbhare DA. Interrater agreement of manual palpation for identification of myofascial trigger points: a systematic review and meta-analysis. Clin J Pain 2017;33(8):715–29.

32. Rozenfeld E, Finestone AS, Moran U, et al. Test-retest reliability of myofascial trigger point detection in hip and thigh areas. J Bodyw Mov Ther 2017;21(4):914–9.

33. Fritz S. Mosby's essential sciences for therapeutic massage. Anatomy, physiology, biomechanics, and pathology. 5th edn. St Louis, MO: Mosby Elsevier; 2017.

34. Reiman M, Manske R. Functional testing in human performance. Champaign, IL: Human Kinetics; 2009.

35. Fritz S. Mosby's essential sciences for therapeutic massage. Anatomy, physiology, biomechanics, and pathology. 5th edn. St Louis, MO: Mosby Elsevier; 2017.

36. Chaitow L. Palpatory literacy: the complete instruction manual for the hands on therapist. London: Thorsons Element; 1991.

37. Australian Cancer Council. Check for signs of skin cancer. Online. Available: https://www.cancer.org.au/preventing-cancer/sun-protection/check-for-signs-of-skin-cancer.html; 2019.

Useful Websites

http://www.pennchiro.org/files/clinical/doctor/Oswestry.pdf

3

Planning remedial massage therapy

PRINCIPLES OF TREATMENT

Treatment plans are co-produced by practitioners and clients from negotiations between them: the practitioner informing the client of the assessment findings, the range of available approaches and their rationale and the client negotiating options that fit their preferences and values. A broad range of techniques is available within the scope of remedial massage therapy, and practitioners individualise treatments based on their preferred techniques and personal treatment style. Client safety and treatment effectiveness are always prioritised. Strategies to ensure safe treatment include warming the area to be treated with Swedish massage before applying deeper techniques, and working within the client's pain tolerance. Treatment effectiveness derives from treatment protocols based on the best available evidence, the type of tissue(s) to be treated, the severity of the condition, the stage of inflammation and individual client needs.

PRIORITISING CLIENT SAFETY

Practitioners have a duty of care to promote their clients' wellbeing and to keep them from harm. The following strategies are used by remedial massage therapists to ensure their clients' safety.

SWEDISH MASSAGE BEFORE REMEDIAL MASSAGE

Most remedial massage begins with Swedish or basic massage to the area to be treated. This practice enables the targeted area to be warmed in preparation for deeper techniques. It also relaxes the client and alerts the practitioner to the client's responses to pressure. In some cases Swedish massage constitutes the whole treatment. This may be because the practitioner and client decide to focus on relaxation therapy or because the practitioner is unsure of the underlying condition and chooses to take a conservative approach.

ACTIVE MOVEMENTS BEFORE PASSIVE

As discussed in Chapter 2, the guiding principle, See-Move-Touch, underpins safe practice; that is, observation and active movements precede any physical contact in assessment or treatment. In treatment this principle dictates that active muscle stretches precede passive muscle stretches, that active soft tissue releasing techniques precede passive soft tissue releasing techniques and so on.

TREATING WITHIN PAIN TOLERANCE

Assessments often aim to locate the source of symptoms and to achieve this clients are asked to perform movements that could reproduce symptoms. The See-Move-Touch principle helps practitioners assess and treat clients within a pain-free or tolerable pain range and minimises the risk of aggravating symptoms. Client history and active range of motion assessments, in particular, guide the application of techniques. For example, if a client reports pain when they turn their head 30° to the right, techniques that involve passive rotation of the cervical spine to the right to 30° or beyond may reproduce or aggravate symptoms. There are many remedial massage techniques, including muscle energy and assisted stretching techniques, that could be used to treat limited cervical rotation within the client's pain-free range.

Techniques like trigger points rely on reproducing symptoms to locate their source and to treat the condition. Pain elicited during trigger point and other deep techniques is monitored by using a pain scale to ensure that the practitioner works within the client's tolerable pain range (usually not beyond 7 or 8 on a pain scale of 0 to 10).

OVERVIEW OF A REMEDIAL MASSAGE TREATMENT APPROACH

Remedial massage clients may require a course of treatment designed to address presenting conditions and that prioritises self-help and health-promotion strategies. Key features of this approach are planning for optimal outcomes for clients in the long term, the central role of educating clients to be active participants in their treatment, and respect for clients' health-care preferences.

SHORT- AND LONG-TERM TREATMENT PLANS

It is helpful to develop short-term and long-term plans for each client. The short-term plan directs treatment to the highest priority (usually determined by symptoms). The long-term plan focuses on contributing or predisposing factors such as underlying structural features and lifestyle factors and client education. There may be a number of healthcare providers involved in clients' care. Good communication with all key stakeholders, including other healthcare providers, is likely to promote better outcomes for clients.[1]

CLIENT EDUCATION AND SELF-HELP

An important part of remedial massage treatment involves educating clients about likely causal or aggravating factors and guiding their management of these factors. Encourage clients to become directly engaged in their recovery from the outset by taking an active role in rehabilitation and health promotion activities (e.g. regular walks to reduce stress and strengthening and stretching exercises to improve range of motion). Most soft tissue injuries resolve within four weeks, although a small number go on to cause permanent disability. Psychosocial factors (yellow flags) can influence return to normal activities. Clients are encouraged to stay active and resume normal activities as soon as possible. It is good practice to include a self-help program, such as home exercises, posture correction and lifting advice in all treatments. Transition from more passive care to increased client activity in exercise rehabilitation, postural and ergonomic correction, weight-loss programs and lifestyle modification within 4 to 6 weeks after injury helps prevent long-term disability and time off work.[2] Strategies such as realistic goal setting and enlisting family support may help motivate clients to participate in self-help programs.

CLIENTS' PREFERENCES

Clients are actively involved in discussions about their treatment. Effective communication skills are required to build rapport with clients and to guide the consultation. Attention to the way clients approach the assessment process provides other important information including their psychological states and value systems which must also be taken into account when formulating treatment plans. Clients must be fully informed of proposals for therapy, the reasons for such proposals and their likely prognoses, and they must give their consent to a negotiated plan before treatment begins.

Figure 3.1 is designed as a guide for developing therapy plans. Provisional assessments are based on a synthesis of findings (e.g. from case history, postural observation, functional testing and palpation). Provisional assessments could

---

Planning Remedial Massage Therapy

1. Provisional assessment
_____
_____

Red or yellow flags? If yes, give details
_____
_____
_____

2. Short-term treatment plan
Massage therapy plan:

Aim:_____

Techniques:_____
_____
_____
_____

Recommendations
Home exercise program
_____

Other (e.g. heat/cold, posture correction, lifestyle modification)
_____
_____

Referral (if required)
_____

Proposed treatment schedule
_____

3. Long-term treatment plan
Massage therapy plan:

Aim:_____
_____

Techniques:_____
_____
_____
_____

Recommendations
Home exercise program
_____

Other (e.g. heat/cold, posture correction, lifestyle modification)
_____
_____

Referral (if required)
_____

Proposed treatment schedule
_____
_____

Fig. 3.1 Developing short- and long-term therapy plans

include stage of injury, severity, affected tissues, condition and likely cause (e.g. acute mild right supraspinatus tendinitis or chronic cervicogenic headache secondary to right C-shaped thoracic scoliosis). Clear aims for both short-term and long-term management help focus the treatment. Short-term aims are usually directed to decreasing or to eliminating symptoms (e.g. decrease pain from 7/10 to 4/10 in two weeks). Long-term aims usually address underlying or predisposing conditions (e.g. improve muscle function associated with hyperlordosis). All plans prioritise staying active and timely return to normal activities where possible.

TREATMENT PROTOCOLS

The evidence base for remedial massage is discussed in Chapter 1. The efficacy of many assessment and treatment techniques used in clinical practice remains unconfirmed by scientific study, despite an increasing number of high-quality studies in massage therapy. Clinical Guidelines have been developed for some musculoskeletal conditions based on the best available evidence. Massage therapists should use Clinical Guidelines where they exist to inform their treatment practice. (See, for example, clinical guidelines for low back pain.[3, 4]) To keep abreast of recent developments, practitioners should regularly consult professional associations' websites, relevant journals, research websites and attend conferences where current research is presented.

In the absence of evidence-based clinical guidelines specifically for remedial massage, therapists rely on treatment protocols derived from clinical practice and based on the best available evidence. Treatment protocols can be modified to suit the needs of individual clients. Treatment protocols for a range of clinical presentations including acute and chronic inflammatory conditions, grade 1, 2 or 3 injuries, and for a variety of tissue types are presented in this chapter. For example, a typical remedial massage protocol for a chronic mild or moderate soft tissue injury would be:

- Begin with Swedish or basic massage to the injured site, surrounding or compensatory areas and areas of the spine from which the nerve supply to the injured area emanates.
- Apply specific remedial massage therapy techniques appropriate to the tissue type (e.g. muscle stretching and deep transverse friction for muscle injuries, passive joint mobilisation for joint conditions) and phase of inflammation.
- Educate clients about self-help activities (e.g. home exercise program and advice about posture) and negotiate a schedule for ongoing remedial massage therapy.

ALIGNING TREATMENT TO ASSESSMENT FINDINGS

Remedial massage therapy plans take into account tissue type, stage of inflammation and severity of the condition when treatment techniques are being considered. It is essential that red and yellow flags[a] are identified (see Chapter 2). A definitive diagnosis is not always possible or necessary for many musculoskeletal conditions. However, a provisional diagnosis that directs treatment according to assessment findings (e.g. tissue type, stage of inflammation, severity of injury) is often used to direct treatment.

Tissue type

As discussed in Chapter 2, active range of motion (AROM) tests are designed to locate a possible source of symptoms and identify the quality and range of movement. For example, clients with shoulder pain could be experiencing referred pain from the lower cervical spine (C5 dermatome) or from a local shoulder injury (among other things). If AROM of the cervical spine reproduces the symptoms, but AROM of the shoulder does not, then the source of the problem is likely to be the lower cervical spine and clients are likely to respond to treatments directed to that area. However, active movements do not discriminate between inert and contractile components of the joint complex. Passive range of motion (PROM) and resisted range of motion (RROM) tests usually follow active tests to help identify the type of tissue that could be involved.

PROM tests are designed to test the integrity of joints and non-contractile structures like joint capsules, ligaments and cartilage.[b] If symptoms are reproduced by PROM consider the following treatments for chronic conditions:

- Swedish massage and/or heat therapy to increase blood flow to the area, to relieve pain and to prepare tissues for more specific techniques.
- Passive joint mobilisation for joint conditions like osteoarthritis (see Chapter 7).
- Deep transverse friction for ligament sprains (see Chapter 4).
- Myofascial releasing techniques for associated fascial restrictions (see Chapter 8).

RROM tests are designed to test the integrity of contractile tissue. If symptoms are reproduced on resisted muscle tests, consider the following treatments for chronic conditions:

- Swedish massage and/or heat therapy to increase blood flow to the area, relieve pain prepare tissues for more specific techniques.
- Muscle-specific techniques including deep gliding, cross-fibre frictions, deep transfers frictions and soft tissue releasing techniques (see Chapter 4), muscle stretching (see Chapter 5) and trigger point therapy (see Chapter 6).
- Myofascial releasing techniques for associated fascial restrictions (see Chapter 8).

Stage of inflammation

Our understanding of inflammation has continued to evolve with advances in molecular biology. We now know that inflammation involves a broad range of inflammatory conditions that are initiated by different stimuli.[5] Inflammation activates a wide range of complex biological processes but these processes are not yet fully understood.

Acute inflammation is a protective response to harmful bacterial or viral infection or injury. It is designed to remove the initial cause of cell injury, dilute or destroy the harmful agents, remove damaged tissue and generate new tissue. The

---

[a]Red flags are indicators of a serious underlying physical condition. Such conditions include cancer, and infection, fractures and neurological damage. Yellow flags are indicators of underlying psychosocial and occupational factors that may impede recovery. They include attitudes and beliefs about pain, compensation issues, emotions, family and work.

[b]During passive range of motion tests, muscles are also passively stretched. Resisted tests will usually confirm any specific muscle involvement.

process is characterised by immediate vascular changes followed by an influx of inflammatory cells (neutrophils) and the widespread effects of inflammatory mediators.

The acute inflammatory response is initiated and propagated by several inflammatory chemicals including histamine and kinins that are released from damaged cells. These inflammatory mediators dilate blood vessels and attract neutrophils, monocytes and macrophages to the injury site. Clearing the area of infectious and toxic substances and tissue debris is an important function of the inflammatory response. Within about an hour of the injury, neutrophils migrate from capillaries into interstitial spaces to ingest damaged cells, bacteria and other inflammatory agents. Monocytes which mature into macrophages follow in the next 8 to 12 hours. Released histamine also increases capillary permeability and blood plasma leaks into the interstitial spaces. Plasma proteins such as clotting and anti-clotting factors and proteins in the complement system that are vital for the immune response also escape to the injury site. The area becomes red, warm and swollen. Pain receptors are activated by inflammatory mediators and by local oedema. Clotting proteins lay down fibrin to wall off the injured area and prevent the spread of pathogens.

Within 2–4 days of the injury, the repair and healing phase begins. As tissues heal, capillary beds grow into the area bringing nutrients and oxygen to the area and removing waste products. New cells rapidly develop to restore normal function. In non-regenerative tissue such as nerve and muscle, injured cells are replaced by scar tissue which is less elastic and less strong than the tissue it replaces. Collagen, the main component of scar tissue, is secreted by rapidly dividing fibroblasts. It is laid down in a random and disorganised way and in this immature form is less dense and more easily injured than the mature collagen that develops over the ensuing 2 months. Collagen also develops abnormal cross-links, decreasing the flexibility of the tissue. The inflammatory exudate that accumulates at the injury site is slowly removed through the lymph vessels. Any remaining bacteria or tissue debris are destroyed by white blood cells in lymph nodes (see Figure 3.2 on p 46).

Chronic inflammation begins 2 to 3 weeks after an injury and can last from 6 weeks to months or years where repeated microtrauma or chronic irritation persists. It is characterised by the presence of mononuclear cells rather than neutrophils at the injury site and by simultaneous destruction and healing of tissue from the inflammatory process. Continued fibroblast activity can lead to tissue fibrosis, accompanied by loss of flexibility and strength (scar tissue never achieves more than about 70–80% of the strength of the original tissue).[6]

Conditions like asthma, allergies, arthritis, and autoimmune disorders have an inflammatory component. Chronic inflammation is also associated with cardiovascular disease, diabetes, cancer, depression and Alzheimer's disease and may accelerate the ageing process.[7] The link between lifestyle choices and inflammation has led to such recommendations as a diet rich in Omega-3 fatty acids, fruit and vegetables, regular exercise and relaxation.

ACUTE INJURY MANAGEMENT

For many years the recommended treatment for acute injuries has been 'RICE': Rest or restrict movement of the injured area; Ice the injured area; Compress the injured area; and Elevate the injured area. However, there is insufficient evidence to support its use. One study found insufficient evidence to determine the relative effectiveness of RICE therapy for acute ankle sprains in adults.[8] The authors found moderate evidence that some type of immediate post-traumatic mobilisation was beneficial for acute ankle sprains. There was limited evidence supporting the use of ice or compression and no evidence could be found to support or reject the use of elevation in the treatment of acute ankle sprains.

A Cochrane review on the use of superficial heat and cold could only locate three poor-quality trials and could not draw any conclusions about the effects of cold applications for low back pain.[9]

A range of massage techniques including reflexology[c], acupressure, aromatherapy and other complementary therapies (e.g. Reiki, acupuncture, homoeopathy, herbal and nutritional supplementations including vitamin C, bromelain and calcium) may be indicated for acute inflammation. Light lymphatic drainage proximal to the injury site and midrange passive movements may be suitable.[10] The rate of recovery of an injury to soft tissue can be increased by early mobilisation with careful supervision. The nature of the injury determines when mobilisation may begin.[11] Introduce pain-free AROM and/or isometric exercises as soon as possible to assist fibrous repair.

In current clinical practice treatment decisions are based on needs of individual clients. A review of the mechanisms of heat and cold therapies for musculoskeletal injuries[12] found some limited evidence supporting the use of cryotherapy (cold therapy) following acute musculoskeletal injury and delayed-onset muscle soreness and limited overall evidence to support the use of topical heat in general. Remedial massage therapists who use heat and/or ice in their clinical practices are advised to keep abreast of evolving research in the field.

Cryotherapy

Cryotherapy is the local, regional or whole-body application of cold for therapeutic purposes. In remedial massage cryotherapy commonly refers to local applications of ice. For acute soft tissue injuries ice applied to the affected area can provide pain relief.[5] It can be applied immediately after injury for 10–15 minutes and every 60 minutes thereafter until pain subsides. Its physiological effects also include reductions in blood flow, oedema, muscle spasm, and metabolic demand.[12]

Contraindications and precautions
Never apply cold:

- if the client has cold hypersensitivity
- to an open wound
- directly to the skin (unless applying ice massage)
- if the client is taking analgesics
- if the client has circulatory insufficiency (e.g. Raynaud's disease[d], diabetes mellitus)

Methods of application
Cryotherapy can be applied using immersions in buckets of ice or ice-cold water. Ice packs are commonly used in remedial massage practice.

---

[c]Note that reflexology is contraindicated in acute injuries of the foot and ankle where pressure applied to the injured area is likely to cause further inflammation.
[d]Raynaud's phenomenon (or disease) refers to digital ischaemia brought on by cold or emotional stress. Affected digits turn white (digital artery spasm or obstruction), blue (deoxygenation of static venous blood) and red (reactive hyperaemia).[13]

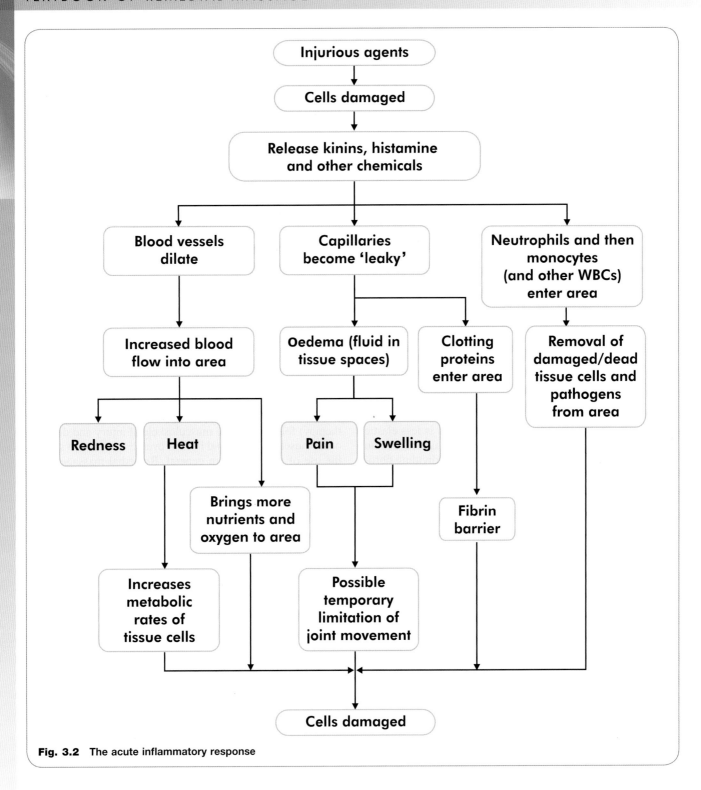

Fig. 3.2 The acute inflammatory response

Ice packs should be kept refrigerated in the clinic and ready to use. Wrap the ice pack in a towel and apply it to the injured area as soon as possible. If required, use an elastic wrap or tape to keep the ice pack in place. If no ice is available, use a packet of frozen peas, wet cold sponges, cold running water or ice blocks. Apply ice for 10–15 minutes at a time.

CHRONIC INJURY MANAGEMENT

Most clients of remedial massage have chronic conditions. Treatment for chronic conditions includes such remedial massage techniques as heat application, deep transverse friction (see Chapter 4), myofascial release (see Chapter 8) and exercise therapy, which are designed to produce strong mobile scar tissue. Rehabilitation exercises help realign collagen fibres to make the scar tissue as strong as possible. Remedial massage therapy is also directed to musculoskeletal compensations that are often associated with chronic inflammation (e.g. hypertonic flexor muscles and weakened extensor muscles associated with chronic arthritis of the knee[14]).

Thermotherapy

Thermotherapy is the local or systemic application of heat to the body. It is mainly used for pain relief and psychological relaxation. It accelerates tissue metabolism, increases vasodilation, elasticity of connective tissues and reduces viscosity of synovial fluid.[12] In remedial massage, thermotherapy commonly refers to local applications of heat. There is scant evidence for the use of superficial heat. One systematic review concluded that heat wrap therapy appears to reduce pain and disability for clients with back pain of less than three months' duration, although the effect is small and only lasts for a short time after the application has been removed.[9]

Contraindications and precautions
Never apply heat:

- immediately after an injury (acute phase)
- where there is loss of sensation (skin test first) or sensitivity to heat (consider skin type: fair-skinned people may be sensitive to heat)
- where there is decreased circulation
- directly to eyes or genitals
- directly to the abdomen during pregnancy or menstruation
- if the client has a fever
- on skin infections, open wounds or if a client has frail skin
- if a client is using analgesics
- if a client has cardiac disease, cancer or hypertension.

Use cautiously where bone is close to the surface (e.g. anterior leg).

Methods of application
A wide range of thermotherapy products are available including:

- hydrocollator or microwave for sandbags, volcanic sand, chemical gel packs, wheat packs and therabead packs
- chemically activated packs
- paraffin wax baths
- oriental methods such as moxa sticks and cupping
- creams, rubs and ointments (e.g. Dencorub, Deep Heat, Capsolin, Tiger Balm, Zheng Gu Shui). Many of these products contain methyl salicylate and camphor.

Do not apply heat packs directly to the skin. Wrap the pack in a pillow case or towel to avoid burning the skin. Heat applications are usually applied for 20–30 minutes. If required, secure the application with an elastic bandage, towel or Velcro belt to ensure that it cannot slip during treatment.

Precautions associated with the use of heat creams
Check the composition of all topical products. Be aware of interactions between creams, rubs and ointments with massage oil and remember that vigorous massage increases surface heat which potentiates some heat creams. Clients with chronic conditions often suffer long-term pain and may look for relief at any cost. Be especially careful with the home use of practitioner-only products and essential oils (see Table 3.1).

Considerations for applications of heat creams

- Test the area to be warmed with a skin sensation test.
- Warn clients of possible side effects (e.g. burning).
- Some heat creams/gels can be reactivated hours after use (e.g. when showering).
- Warn clients not to touch areas treated with creams to avoid transferring products to eyes, mouth or genitals.
- Check the client's response often.
- Use a wooden stick for individual applications of creams/gels to avoid contaminating stock.
- Transfer ointments and creams to small jars and store the main stock in a dark and cool environment.

Severity of injury

Injuries are often graded according to severity which determines the most appropriate treatment. Characteristics of injuries to muscles, tendons and ligaments according to severity are described in Table 3.2 and illustrated in Figure 3.3.

Grade 1 and 2 injuries (mild and moderate) are generally suitable for remedial massage therapy. Severe injuries (Grade 3) require referral to a medical practitioner for surgical repair. However, remedial massage can contribute to the treatment of Grade 3 injuries in the rehabilitation phase when techniques like deep transverse friction, resisted muscle stretches and passive joint mobilisation can be applied. Treatment is directed to the injury itself and to compensatory movement patterns. Therapists can educate clients about causative and predisposing factors from a remedial massage perspective and develop and/or monitor exercise rehabilitation programs (see Table 3.3).

MONITORING AND REVIEWING TREATMENT PLANS

Initial assessments are important for establishing baseline data against which repeated assessments can be measured. Clients are continually assessed, both during treatments and at the end of a single treatment or a course of treatments. Changes in assessment findings are crucial for monitoring treatment progress and form the basis of regular reviews of treatment plans. An essential part of monitoring and reviewing treatment is explaining to clients the rationale for, and outcomes of, treatment and encouraging clients to ask questions about their treatment. Practitioners also negotiate treatment schedules, from frequent to less frequent consultations as recovery progresses, and the transition from rehabilitation to a health maintenance or promotion plan. As a general guideline, massage for mild or moderate conditions is usually performed weekly; acute conditions could require two or three treatments a week. Most soft tissue injuries recover within 6 weeks. Maintenance treatments become progressively less frequent until a schedule that prevents deterioration and promotes health is determined.

The frequency and duration of treatment ultimately depends on a number of factors including:

- how quickly the condition responds to treatment (influenced by age, nature and severity of injury and previous history)

Table 3.1 Massaging with essential oils: Contraindications and precautions

Major hazardous oils – do not use (potential for dermal toxicity, skin sensitisation and skin irritation)	ajowan, bitter almond, bitter fennel, boldo leaf, buchu, calamus, camphor, cassia, cinnamon bark, costus, elecampane, horseradish, mugwort, mustard, origanum, pennyroyal, rue, thuja, dwarf pine, sassafras, savin, winter savory, summer savory, southernwood, tansy, wormseed, wormwood, clove (leaf, stem and bud), parsley seed, wintergreen
Essential oils that can cause skin reactions (may irritate the skin when used in baths or massage; do not use if client is known to have sensitive skin or is susceptible to reactions)	sweet basil, peppermint, lemon, lemongrass, tea tree, Virginian cedarwood, juniper berry, sweet orange, clary sage
Essential oils that can cause sensitisation (avoid if positive patch test for sensitive skin or history of allergies)	basil, geranium, sweet orange, tea tree, bergamot, lemon expressed, peppermint, ylang ylang, Virginian cedarwood, lemongrass, rose absolute
Essential oils that may cause dermatitis	basil, geranium, damask rose, Virginia cedarwood, bergamot, lemon, rosemary CT2, sweet orange, ylang ylang
Phototoxic essential oils (avoid UV light and sunbeds for 12 hours after application)	bergamot expressed, lemon expressed, bitter orange expressed, Virginia cedarwood, sweet orange expressed
Essential oils which should not be used during pregnancy	aniseed, basil, birch, cajeput, atlas cedarwood, Virginia cedarwood, clary sage, cypress, sweet fennel, frankincense, geranium, jasmine absolute, juniper berry, lemongrass, sweet marjoram, may chang, melissa, myrrh, peppermint, damask rose, rosemary, sage, spearmint, thyme, valerian
Essential oils which should not be used by people with epilepsy	fennel (sweet), hyssop, sage, rosemary, spike lavender, eucalyptus
Essential oils which should not be used by people with high blood pressure	hyssop, rosemary, sage, thyme, spike lavender, sweet basil, eucalyptus

Adapted from Battaglia[15]

- the client's level of compliance with a self-help program
- the occurrence of setbacks such as falls, injuries or emotional stress during the course of treatment
- the presence of pre-existing or complicating factors (e.g. underlying disease, yellow flags).

Approximate healing times for soft tissue injuries are illustrated in Table 3.4.

RECORDING REMEDIAL MASSAGE TREATMENTS

Treatment records should include the major techniques used in treatment, the specific locations of their application and recommendations made to clients. Records should also reflect relevant responses to treatment. There are currently no standardised recording procedures. The example in Table 3.5 is a possible model.

KEY MESSAGES

- Client safety is a priority. Strategies to ensure client safety include:
  - beginning treatment with Swedish massage before applying deeper more specific remedial techniques
  - using active movements to gauge client's range of motion before applying passive techniques

- using a pain scale and working within the client's pain tolerance.
- A remedial massage treatment approach involves:
  - planning for both short- and long-term management of clients
    - short-term therapy plans often focus on presenting symptoms
    - long-term therapy plans often focus on potential contributing factors (e.g. lifestyle factors, underlying structural features, or underlying disease processes)
  - educating clients about likely causal and predisposing factors
  - promoting the self-help component of treatment wherever possible (to reduce likelihood of recurrence and/or to promote health maintenance and illness prevention)
  - taking the client's preferences and value system into account.
- Consider the best, available evidence (e.g. refer to Clinical Guidelines) when planning therapy. Treatment protocols can be used to guide remedial massage treatment and modified to suit the needs of individual clients. Treatment protocols take into consideration:
  - tissue type: assessment findings suggest appropriate techniques for particular tissue types (e.g. passive joint mobilisation for joint conditions, deep transverse friction and other muscle-specific techniques for muscle lesions)

Table 3.2 Grading injuries: Characteristics of injuries

a) Grading muscle strains

Muscle strains	Definition	Characteristics
Grade 1	A small number of fibres are torn.	Localised pain. No loss of strength.
Grade 2	A significant number of fibres are torn.	Pain and swelling. Pain is reproduced on muscle contraction. Strength is reduced and movement is limited by pain.
Grade 3	A complete tear of the muscle.	Significant pain and swelling. Significant loss of strength. Most often occurs at the musculotendinous junction.

Grade 1   Grade 2   Grade 3

Fig. 3.3 Grades of muscle strain

b) Grading ligament sprains

Ligament sprain	Definition	Characteristics
Grade 1	A small number of fibres are torn.	Pain is felt on stressing the ligament with no increase in joint laxity.
Grade 2	A significant number of fibres are torn.	Pain is felt on stressing the ligament and joint laxity increases.
Grade 3	A complete tear of the ligament.	Pain may be present with gross joint laxity.

c) Grading tendon injuries

Tendon injury	Definition	Characteristics
Grade 1	A small number of fibres are torn.	Pain after activity only.
Grade 2	A few fibres are torn.	Pain at start of activity. Pain disappears during activity and returns after activity.
Grade 3	A considerable number of fibres are torn.	Pain at the start of the activity that persists during and after activity. Restriction of activity.
Grade 4	A significant number of fibres are torn.	Pain during everyday activities. Pain progressing and worsening.

Adapted from Douglas et al[11]

■ stage of inflammation:
   – acute soft tissue injuries are treated with cold therapy, gentle lymphatic drainage, gentle active followed by passive range of motion exercises and gentle mobilisation of scar tissue
   – chronic soft tissue injuries are treated with heat application and other remedial massage techniques (e.g. deep transverse friction, cross-fibre frictions, trigger point therapy), myofascial releasing techniques and exercise therapy

■ severity of the injury: no referral is required to treat grade 1 and mild to moderate grade 2 injuries; severe grade 2 and grade 3 injuries may be treated after surgical repair.
■ Continuously monitor and review treatment plans.

Table 3.4 Approximate healing times[16]

Muscle soreness	Several days
Grade 1 muscle tears	2-3 weeks
Grade 2 muscle tears	3-4 weeks
Grace 3 muscle tears	2 months
Fracture	6-12 weeks
Nerve root lesion	Weeks or months depending on severity

Table 3.3 Treatment approach according to injury grade

Grade 1 and 2 injuries	Acute injury management	First aid management (e.g. cryotherapy, acupuncture, homoeopathy) Exercise advice
	Chronic injury management	Remedial massage therapy Heat therapy Joint mobilisation Exercise rehabilitation and training
Grade 3 injuries	Acute injury management	First aid management (e.g. cryotherapy, acupuncture, homoeopathy) Referral for surgical repair
	Chronic injury management	Remedial massage therapy Heat therapy Joint mobilisation Exercise rehabilitation and training

Table 3.5 A three-stage method of recording remedial massage treatment

	Record	Treatment technique
1	Swed mass lower back, BL lower limbs	Remedial massage usually begins with a Swedish or basic massage to a region
2	L up traps TP L lev scap XFF distal attach L up traps act rel	List two or three of the major techniques used: ■ Left upper trapezius; trigger point ■ Left levator scapulae: cross fibre frictions at the distal attachment ■ Left upper trapezius active releasing technique
3	Home ex: L up traps, lev scap stretches 3 × 3/24	Self-help program: ■ Left upper traps and left levator scapulae stretches 3 repetitions, 3 times per day

Review questions

1. Match the following descriptions with their injury grade:

Pain may be present with gross joint laxity.	Grade 1 muscle strain
Significant pain and swelling. Significant loss of strength. Most often occurs at the musculotendinous junction.	Grade 2 tendon strain
Pain is felt on stressing the ligament with no increase in joint laxity.	Grade 1 ligament sprain
Pain at start of activity. Pain disappears during activity and returns after activity.	Grade 3 ligament sprain
Pain during everyday activities. Pain progressing and worsening.	Grade 3 muscle strain
Localised pain. No loss of strength	Grade 4 tendon strain

2. List five precautions for the use of ice.
3. A client presents with neck pain. On active cervical flexion and right rotation the client reports pain. The practitioner performs resisted tests for cervical flexion and right rotation. The client reports pain on resisted right rotation of the cervical spine. It is likely that the pain is related to *inert/contractile* tissue.
4. a) How would you identify an acute soft tissue injury?
   b) What is the usual treatment for acute soft tissue injuries?

5. How soon after an injury can exercise rehabilitation start?
6. For client safety, it is recommended that active movements be performed before passive movements. Explain the rationale for this treatment approach.
7. Name three essential oils that could cause skin reactions.
8. Describe a typical treatment schedule for a client who has recently sprained his ankle (grade 1).
9. Complete the following:
When tissue is injured two immediate responses occur in blood vessels near the injury: i) vasodilation and ii) increased _____ of capillaries so that antibodies and clotting factors can enter the injured area. This response is initiated and propagated by several inflammatory chemicals including _____ and _____. Within an hour neutrophils squeeze through the blood vessel walls to reach the injury site. Neutrophils dominate initially, followed by _____ and _____ which contribute to phagocytic activity. The main function of the inflammatory response is to _____ _____. Plasma proteins including _____ also arrive at the injury site. The area is walled off by _____ laid down by clotting proteins. During the repair phase new blood vessels supply nutrients and oxygen to the area and remove waste products. In muscle tissue new cells form _____ which is less dense and more easily injured than the tissue it replaces.

REFERENCES

1. Grace S, Bradbury J, Avila C. 'The healthcare system is not designed around my needs': How healthcare consumers self-integrate conventional and complementary healthcare services. Complement Ther Clin 2018;32:151–6.
2. WorkCover NSW. Overview. Improving outcomes: Integrated, active management of workers with soft tissue injury. Online. Available: https://docplayer.net/19310953-Overview-improving-outcomes-integrated-active-management-of-workers-with-soft-tissue-injury.html; 2019.
3. Almeida M, Saragiotto B, Richards B, et al. Primary care management of non-specific low back pain: key messages from recent clinical guidelines. Med J Australia 2018;208(6):272–5.
4. Stochkendahl MJ, Kjaer P, Hartvigsen J, et al. National clinical guidelines for non-surgical treatment of patients with recent onset low back pain or lumbar radiculopathy. Eur Spine J 2018;27:60–75.
5. Duchesne E, Dufresne S, Dumont N. Impact of inflammation and anti-inflammatory modalities on skeletal muscle healing: from fundamental research to the clinic. Phys Ther 2017;97(8):807–17.
6. Joiner MC, van der Kogel A. Basic clinical radiobiology. 5th edn. Boca Radon, FL: CRC Press; 2019.
7. You T, Nicklas BJ. Chronic inflammation: role of adipose tissue and modulation by weight loss. Curr Diabetes Rev 2006;2(1):29–37.
8. van den Bekerom MP, Struijs PA, Blankevoort L, et al. What is the evidence for Rest, Ice, Compression and Elevation therapy in the treatment of ankle sprains in adults? J Athlet Train 2012;47(4):435–43.
9. French SD, Cameron M, Walker BF, et al. Superficial heat or cold for low back pain. Cochrane Database Syst Rev 2006;(1):CD004750.
10. Fritz S. Mosby's essential sciences for therapeutic massage. Anatomy, physiology, biomechanics, and pathology. 5th edn. St Louis, MO: Mosby Elsevier; 2017.
11. Brukner P, Clarsen B, Cook J, et al. Brukner and Khan's clinical sports medicine: injuries. 5th edn. North Ryde, NSW: McGraw Hill; 2017.
12. Malanga GA, Yan N, Stark J. Mechanisms and efficacy of heat and cold therapies for musculoskeletal injury. Postgrad Med 2015;127:1, 57–65, Doi: 10.1080/00325481.2015.992719.
13. Douglas G, Nichol F, Robertson C. McLeod's clinical examination. 13th edn. Edinburgh: Churchill Livingstone; 2013.
14. Fritz S, Chaitow L, Hymel GM. Clinical massage in the healthcare setting. St Louis, MI: Mosby Elsevier; 2008.
15. Battaglia S. The complete guide to aromatherapy. 2nd edn. Virginia, Qld: Perfect Potion; 2004.
16. WorkCoverSA. Recovery timeframes for common injury types. Online. Available: http://www.workcover.com/site/treat_home/guidelines_by_injury_type/recovery_timeframes_for_common_injury_types.aspx?str=Recovery%20timeframes; 2009.

4

Remedial massage techniques for muscles

INTRODUCTION

Just about everyone will experience a muscle strain at some time in their life. Any sport that involves high-intensity sprinting efforts (e.g. football, tennis, cricket) will have a high incidence of muscle strains. Muscle strains also have high recurrence rates: for example, having a previous identical injury in the preceding season increased injury rates significantly for professional athletes.[1, 2] Such conditions as a quadriceps contusion incurred on a football field, a fibrotic tangle of muscle left years after a bone fracture, muscles and joints aching from postural overload or a triceps head strained during a motorcycle accident are typical presentations to remedial massage therapists. Much can be done to assist restoration of normal muscle function. One of the key roles of remedial massage therapists is to assess and treat muscle strains and compensatory movement patterns and to work with other health professionals to restore optimal function.

The aim of this chapter is to explore some approaches to the assessment of muscle lesions and dysfunctions and to examine techniques which are often incorporated into remedial massage treatment regimens. Techniques presented in this chapter are based on the best available research.

ASSESSING MUSCLE FUNCTION

Several approaches to the assessment of muscles are presented in this chapter:[3–8]

- functional deficit demonstration (active functional range of motion)
- postural assessment

- muscle length testing
- muscle strength testing
- palpation.

FUNCTIONAL DEFICIT DEMONSTRATION

During the history-taking interview, ask the client if their pain or restriction stops them from doing anything that they want or need to do.[5] The inability to bend far enough to tie shoes or to reach high enough to wash and dry one's hair can be significant problems for clients. The therapist can interpret the functional deficit more accurately by observing the movements it affects. Range of motion examination should be familiar to the reader. The joints of the body can move through various planes of motion and through certain ranges within those planes. Normative data has been collected for joint range of motion and can be used when assessing clients. In active range of motion (AROM) tests, the client performs the movements to their comfortable limit, which necessarily involves the use of muscles. AROM tests are usually performed in single planes. However, some tests like Apley's scratch test (see Figure 15.21 on p 274) and the standing ankle AROM tests assess multiplanar movements that mimic everyday functions which are rarely performed in only one plane (see Figure 4.1). It should also be noted that AROM or active functional deficit tests may need to be repeated a number of times to reproduce symptoms.

POSTURAL ASSESSMENT

A common cause of soft tissue dysfunction and pain is postural distortion.[9] Our bodies are often required to maintain positions for extended periods, sometimes due to occupational demands. Our responses to these demands are reflected in our musculoskeletal framework and an assessment of posture is a common part of clinical examination.

A common postural distortion is forward carriage of the head, rounded shoulders, increased thoracic kyphosis, elevated and protracted scapulae, internally rotated glenohumeral joints, and hyperextended cervical spine. Such postures are maintained by muscular effort (e.g. cervical extensor muscles, sternocleidomastoid, levator scapulae, pectoralis major, possibly pectoralis minor and others), and permitted by muscular weakness (e.g. rhomboids, middle and lower trapezius, infraspinatus, deep flexors of the cervical spine and others). This postural distortion is referred to as upper-crossed syndrome (see Figure 12.21 on p 220).[10, 11] Other occupational distortions include the externally rotated femurs of a long-distance driver or dancer, and the spinal rotation and lateral flexion of a sedentary worker whose work station is positioned to the side (see Figure 4.2). It has been estimated that the average Australian adult takes about 7400 steps a day.[12] With such demands on the body, even a small distortion of normal gait or posture amplifies over time.

A muscle or functional group of muscles may become structurally shortened either as a result of spasm or contracture (*locked short*); a muscle or functional group of muscles, often antagonistic, may are overstretched (*locked long*) and are usually functionally weak.[9, 13, 14] There has been some discussion between researchers regarding the tendency of certain muscles to become hypertonic when overstressed (e.g. upper trapezius, levator scapulae, quadratus lumborum, rectus femoris, iliopsoas, hamstrings), while others typically tend towards hypotonicity under the same conditions (e.g. middle and lower trapezius, serratus anterior, rhomboids, rectus abdominis, gluteals).[14, 15] These muscles have been categorised as *postural* (or *antigravity*) and *phasic* respectively[4, 14] although there is disagreement about classifications of some muscles, including the scalenes.[14] Each muscle or muscle group should be assessed to determine its functional state which may differ in different individuals. Figure 4.3 shows major postural and phasic muscles.

Case study: The forklift driver (part 1)

Consider John, 34 years of age, with no significant injury history. He played soccer and cricket (mainly as a batter) until his early twenties when he married and had children. Since then he has worked in various jobs, mostly assisting in warehouses and workshops, with no major physical complaints.

Over the past 2–3 months, John has been experiencing headaches, neck stiffness, some upper back discomfort and sometimes a feeling of tightness across the chest. He also reports that taking deep breaths is not as easy as it used to be. He has seen his doctor and had stress tests for his heart, which showed nothing unusual. He has had his eyes tested by an optometrist and his vision is fine. The doctor prescribed some NSAIDs for his neck and back pain and referred him to you for treatment.

On questioning you learn that John obtained his forklift ticket about four months ago and secured a full-time position in a warehouse about a month later. This was about the time when his symptoms began.

Do some research on forklift driving. Are there occupational or ergonomic conditions that could contribute to John's symptoms?

Fig. 4.1 Functional multiplanar tests for ankle range of motion

---

Fig. 4.2 Sedentary worker whose work station is positioned to the side

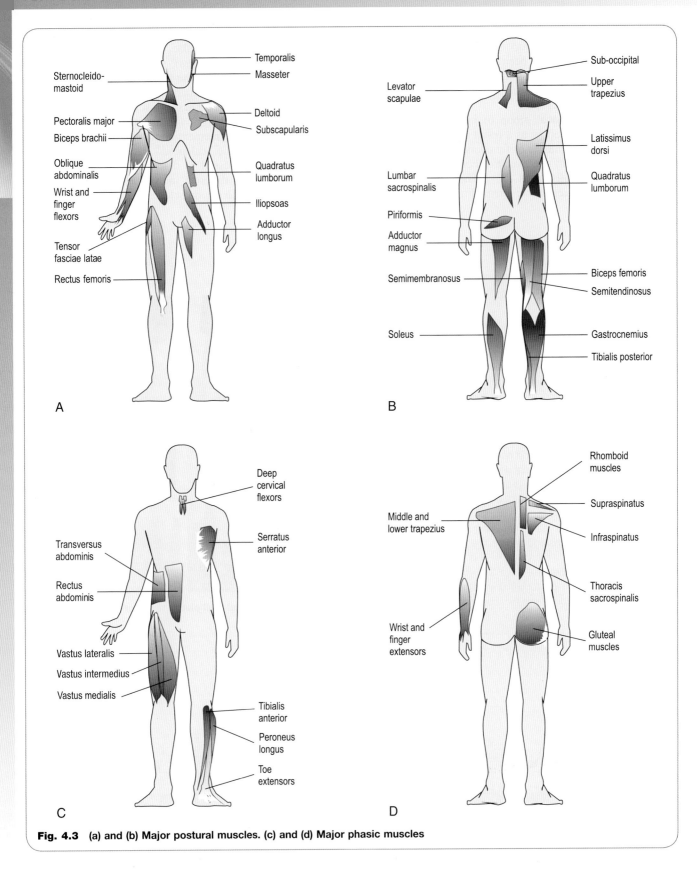

Fig. 4.3   (a) and (b) Major postural muscles. (c) and (d) Major phasic muscles

Case study: The forklift driver (part 2)

If you have looked at the way in which forklifts are operated, you may have noticed that there are some common hazards that need to be avoided. These include continuously or repeatedly looking up to stack high shelves, continuously or repeatedly looking behind to reverse and driving on uneven surfaces.[16]

Now, consider the signs and symptoms. Think about individual muscles or functional groups of muscles which could be involved. See if you can predict which muscles are likely to be locked short and which are likely to be locked long from extended periods of forklift driving. How would you confirm or disprove your predictions? What would you recommend to the driver to minimise the risk of muscle strains at work?

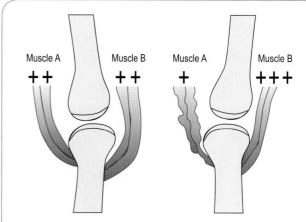

Fig. 4.4 Relationship between muscle function and joint range of motion

---

Postural flexibility is our capacity to adapt to postural stresses. Muscles in the immediate vicinity of injuries and/or painful sites, for example, will often spasm in an effort to immobilise or protect the damaged structure.[14] An injured person will often adjust their posture to allow continued use of the rest of the body, as in the case of a limp due to an ankle sprain. Posture can also reflect the overall attitude and mood of a person. For example, a depressed person may cast their eyes to the floor, dropping their head and rounding their shoulders. Postural observations should always be interpreted in the light of the client's presenting condition, history and other assessment findings.[9, 14, 17]

TESTING MUSCLES FOR LENGTH

History and questioning provide clues about causes and perpetuating factors[6] and help guide advice and recommendations given to clients. Postural assessment reveals the more visible problem areas and suggests muscles to target. Specific muscle tests help confirm or rule out the involvement of individual muscles.

As mentioned previously, in many cases the muscles which have become hypertonic (locked short) or hypotonic (locked long) are fairly predictable.[4, 14, 15] Next we use assessments which can give valuable information as to the form the treatment might take.

For passive range of motion (PROM) tests, the therapist moves the client's body with no assistance from contracting muscles.[4, 18] In general, AROM is smaller than PROM because contracting muscles tend to limit bony approximation.[4] There are several things which can limit PROM at any given joint. These include inflammation, instability and changes in any of the structures surrounding or inside the joint itself.[7] Because of this and also because of limitations in reproducibility, PROM measurements are sometimes seen as unreliable and of limited clinical use.[19, 20]

Muscle tissue which is locked short from either spasm or contracture will often restrict the joint by not allowing it to reach its normal range (see Figure 4.4).[4, 6] Spasms in these shortened muscles can be responsible for weakness in their antagonistic groups. When an agonist is contracting, its antagonist will be neurally inhibited in order to allow unopposed joint motion.[4, 21] It is thought that relieving the spasm in the shortened muscle may lead to the withdrawal of the neural inhibition of the locked long muscle with an immediate improvement in function testing results.

Full range of motion depends on both joint range of motion and muscle length. For example, to measure knee flexion range of motion, the client lies supine and the hip is flexed to put rectus femoris in a shortened position so that full joint range of motion can be achieved. To measure the length of rectus femoris, on the other hand, the client lies prone to extend the hip and lengthen the rectus femoris (see Figure 4.5). (See Table 2.7 on p 16, which illustrates length tests of major muscles of the body.)

TESTING MUSCLES FOR STRENGTH

Therapists use strength testing to gauge the ability of a hypotonic muscle to contract. Moreover, a muscle which is locked short, but is actually in contracture (electrically silent) rather than in spasm (electrically active), will usually also test weak during function testing. Hammer[4] suggested that a muscle shortened due to spasm often tests weak due to the number of myosin crossbridges already engaged and because pain associated with muscle spasm may inhibit contractile power.

Acute injuries may involve damage to the fabric of the muscle and/or tendon.[22] Whereas injury or pain in inert structures around a joint can often be identified through PROM testing, resisted muscle testing usually elicits pain from dynamic/contractile tissue injuries, often within the musculotendinous units, and can be used to grade these injuries.[4]

To perform resisted tests for specific muscles the therapist applies resistance as the client contracts the muscle.[4, 9, 11, 18] The amount of resistance matches the client's force so that no movement occurs; that is, an isometric contraction is performed. Contracting a muscle moves its attachment points into closer approximation. To perform a resisted test, the

Fig. 4.5 Length test for rectus femoris

Fig. 4.6 Resisted test for rhomboids

relevant joints and muscles are positioned carefully, proximal regions are stabilised and the client is instructed to perform a movement[11] or to hold the position[9] against resistance. This procedure is carried out initially on the uninjured limb or side wherever possible, to provide a reference for test results on the target muscle. Figure 4.6 shows a resisted muscle test for the rhomboids. Resisted tests for major muscles are described in Chapters 10–20.

Two of the more widely used grading systems for muscle strength are those of Kendall et al[9] and Janda.[11] Differences between the two systems are illustrated in Table 4.1. Note that break testing[a] should be avoided, partly because heavy contraction may damage a compromised muscle, and also because it can be very difficult for the therapist to control accessory movements by the client and accuracy will therefore suffer.[9]

PALPATION

Although palpation is one of the key assessment procedures used by remedial massage therapists, its findings need to be integrated with others in order to reveal the whole clinical picture.[18, 23] Palpation can be used to locate and identify soft tissues lesions, to detect activity (or lack of it) in

Table 4.1 Comparison of muscle strength testing systems of Kendall et al[9] and Janda[11]

Feature	Kendall[9]	Janda[11]
Grading system	12 grades	6 grades
Client positioning	For best fixation and access	For best fixation and access
Stabilisation	Yes	Yes
Therapist resistance	Against line of action, equal and opposite to contraction	Against movement direction, but not overcoming movement
Contraction type	Isometric, against equal resistance	Isotonic, through range
Tests	Muscle, rather than movement	Movement, rather than individual muscle
Tests very weak muscles	Yes	Yes

---

[a]Break testing refers to resistance applied at the end of a range of motion in the opposite direction to the concentrically contracting muscle.

Table 4.2 Palpatory findings

Condition	Temperature	Pain/tenderness	Hard/soft	Smooth/gritty/crepitation
Acute injury (sprain or strain)	Warm–hot	Yes, on lesion and usually associated with spasm	Palpable defect in Grade 3 injuries, otherwise usually hard (protective spasm)	Normally smooth
Spasm	Varies	Yes, often tender	Hard	Normally smooth
Tendinosis (chronic)	Cool–cold	Not always	Often a thickened area is palpable	May be crepitus on movement Often feels gritty
Fibrosis (muscle)	Cool–cold	Not always	Hard, sometimes stringy/ropey	Often feels gritty
Weakness/ inhibition	Cool–warm	Sometimes (often develop trigger point activity)	If overstretched, may palpate firm; otherwise soft, spongy	Often ropey but may be smooth
Oedema	Hot if acute; variable if chronic	Not always	Spongy, often with some resistance; may retain indent after removal of finger	Usually smooth, but may become gritty over time

muscle tissue, and to elicit symptoms, including pain.[4, 9, 17, 18, 24] Massage therapists should be experts in palpation and need to continually refine their skills by practice.[24] Many palpation exercises have been devised to develop fine discrimination and other aspects of palpation skill. The exercise made famous by Gray's *Anatomy*, for example, requires the therapist to develop their skills by palpating a hair through an increasing number of sheets of paper.[24] Researchers are also working on devices, such as a palpation trainer,[25] to enable greater validity and reliability in assessment findings based on palpation.

A good way to begin the development of palpation skills is to palpate normal undamaged muscle which is usually painless to palpation and should feel smooth, soft and resilient when the muscle is relaxed. When the muscle is contracted the therapist can palpate its tension. The muscle will become firmer to the touch. Tendons tend to feel less leathery or resilient than muscles and feel strong and hard when under tension. Bony landmarks may feel the hardest of all, depending upon the tissues which separate them from the skin. The intervening bursae, fat pads, fascia and other tissues will all have their signature quality. After much practice at palpating normal tissues, you will be well equipped to identify damaged or otherwise abnormal tissue.

It is useful to have a wide vocabulary of descriptive terms for palpation findings. These may include terms like *firm, tense, resistant, hard, spongy, springy, warm, cold, dense, ropey, cordlike, stringy* and *puffy*.[4, 18, 24] Table 4.2 lists some palpatory findings. This table is not exhaustive. Palpatory findings should always be interpreted with caution and correlated with case history and other assessment findings.

REMEDIAL MASSAGE TECHNIQUES

The following section presents some of the most useful and widely used remedial massage techniques for treating muscle injuries and facilitating postural flexibility. These techniques are known by several names. The following terms and abbreviations are used in this book:

Fig. 4.7 Deep gliding friction to the hamstring muscle

- Deep gliding friction (DG)
- Cross-fibre friction (XFF)
- Deep transverse friction (DTF)
- Soft tissue release (STR)

DEEP GLIDING (WITH-FIBRE) FRICTIONS AND CROSS-FIBRE FRICTIONS

The technique referred to here as deep gliding frictions (DG) is also known as *with-fibre frictions*. Cyriax and Russell[26] called it *deep effleurage*, as did Goats.[27] Lowe[28] discussed *deep longitudinal stripping* and *deep tissue massage*. The basic stroke is performed parallel to the muscle fibres in the direction of venous flow. The therapist uses fingers, thumbs, palms, loose fists, forearms or elbows, depending upon the location and the depth required[22, 26, 28] as illustrated in Figure 4.7. Some lubrication is normally used and some measure of discomfort or even pain (always within tolerance, say below 7 out of 10 on a pain scale) is to be expected, but if the client's muscles begin to contract in an attempt to protect the muscle then too much pressure is being applied.[28]

Fig. 4.8 Cross-fibre friction to the gastrocnemius muscle

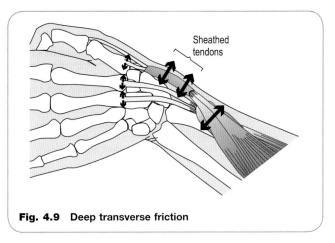

Fig. 4.9 Deep transverse friction

Claims about the effect of deep gliding frictions have included:

- relief of congestion and swelling[22, 26, 28]
- relief of muscle spasm[27, 28]
- acceleration of lymph and blood flow[22, 27]
- localised stretching[27, 28]
- inactivation of trigger points.[28]

Cross fibre friction (XFF), like DG, is a technique that may be performed as part of a Swedish massage routine. As with DG, a lubricant allows the fingers or palms to glide across the skin surface. The difference between the techniques lies in the direction of application: XFF is angled across the muscle fibres, rather than along them (see Figure 4.8). Pressure varies according to the needs of individual clients. The stroke is usually delivered with the fingers together as a unit or the thumb (although therapists should be cautious about overuse of the thumb which can lead to injury and the premature end of a massage career).

The massage literature has claimed that XFF can:

- separate and broaden muscle fibres[28]
- reduce tension in the muscle[28]
- improve or preserve relative mobility of muscle and connective tissue.[29]

Evidence for the effectiveness of DG and XFF

The scientific literature has few studies specifically addressing the effectiveness of either DG or XFF. There are very few randomised controlled trials which use only these massage techniques as interventions.[30, 31] It seems that many of the claimed effects are extrapolated from physiological phenomena which may or may not be directly related to the application of these specific techniques.

Relevant studies on the effectiveness of DG or XFF include:

- Field et al[32] found that objective measures for stress in adults were reduced by massage strokes of moderate pressure, possibly due to increased vagal activity.
- Lewis and Johnson[33] reviewed 20 studies of massage therapy and muscle pain and found that evidence is inconclusive for any effect. The authors suggested that low-quality studies and small sample sizes may have been partly responsible for the inconclusive findings.

- Best, Hunter, Wilcox et al[34] looked at studies of sports massage (some including friction techniques) and found inconsistent results from case study reports, but moderate evidence from 10 randomised controlled trials.

While it would appear that the evidence does not consistently support claims made for the effects of DG or XFF, we must remember that the paucity of studies and the quality of those studies that do exist may be partly responsible for this. Clearly there is a need for further high-quality research to support or refute claims about the effectiveness of DG and XFF.

CONTRAINDICATIONS

The contraindications for DG and XFF techniques are similar to those for Swedish massage. They include:

- acute injury to tissue, including recent surgery
- active inflammation (redness, pain, swelling, heat, loss of function)
- systemic infection or uncontrolled medical condition
- undiagnosed cancer or swelling
- possibility of thrombosis
- skin infections which may spread (e.g. impetigo)
- osteoporosis.

This list is not exhaustive. Therapists should avoid massage in cases where the pathology involved is either unknown or poorly understood.[35]

DEEP TRANSVERSE FRICTION (DTF)

Deep transverse friction (DTF) has long been held to be one of massage therapy's most powerful tools. Pioneered by James Cyriax, DTF became the technique of choice for the treatment of tendinosis and various other scarring and adhesive conditions in muscles, tendons and ligaments.[4, 26, 28, 29] The term *deep transverse friction* is used because of its currency and wide acceptance by the massage profession. A more appropriate term is yet to emerge.

DTF differs from XFF in several ways. First, no lubricant is used. The finger and the skin move together, generating a friction force over the tissues beneath. The stroke is typically applied at 90° to the predominant fibre direction (see Figure 4.9). Care should be taken to ensure sufficient sweep;

that is, the stroke should cover the entire lesion although this would normally be less than a centimetre. Pressure usually varies from light to very deep during the specific application.[4, 22, 26, 28, 35, 36]

A number of claims have been made about the effectiveness of the technique. Cyriax and Russell list 22 separate disorders which are intractable except by DTF.[26] Some of the apparent effects of DTF are thought to be due to:

- separation of adhesions and broadening of muscle tissue[26, 29]
- analgesia, possibly by activation of the pain gate mechanism[4, 28, 29] or by enhancement of circulation to the area (traumatic hyperaemia)[26]
- stimulation of fibroblastic activity in cases of tendinosis.[4, 28]

Evidence for the effectiveness of DTF

The following research into the effectiveness of DTF found inconclusive support for the technique.

- Joseph et al[37] conducted a systematic review to assess the efficacy of deep friction massage in the treatment of tendinopathy. Nine studies met the inclusion criteria. However, no firm conclusions could be drawn for the benefits of DTF used alone or compared to other techniques and control. However, the authors noted that 'excellent anecdotal evidence remains along with a rationale for its use that fits the current understanding of tendinopathy'.

- Loew[38] examined the effectiveness of deep transverse friction in the treatment of lateral elbow or lateral knee tendinitis and found insufficient evidence to draw conclusions on its effect on pain, grip strength, and functional status for patients.
- A Cochrane review of DTF and tendinitis[39] found inconsistent results across a number of studies and stated that no conclusions could be drawn about the effectiveness of DTF.

Further research is needed to inform the use of DTF in clinical practice. Some applications of DTF are illustrated in Figure 4.10.

CONTRAINDICATIONS

The literature lists a number of contraindications to DTF application, including:

- active inflammation or infection
- calcification or ossification within tendons, muscles or ligaments
- haematomas
- directly to a peripheral nerve
- rheumatoid arthritis
- bursitis (note that Cyriax and Russell[26] do not recommend DTF for any bursitis. Hammer,[4] on the other hand, states that DTF can be very helpful in chronic cases of hip and subacromial bursitis).

Fig. 4.10   **Examples of deep transverse friction in practice**

This list is not exhaustive. Avoid DTF in cases where the pathology involved is either unknown or poorly understood.[4, 26]

SOFT TISSUE RELEASE (STR)

Soft tissue release is a group of techniques known by several names and there are small variations in their application. This section describes a myofascial lengthening technique known variously as soft tissue release, directional release, pin and stretch technique[28] or lock and load technique. A patented treatment regimen known as active release technique claims very high success rates with a multitude of soft tissue problems.[40]

Soft tissue release (STR) is applied by fixing specific areas of palpable fibrosis or tension within a muscle and then lengthening the muscle while holding the fixed area still. Two variations within the technique are the passive and active forms. In both of these, the muscle is initially placed in a shortened position and the target area is palpated and pinned or locked by the therapist. This can be done with different parts of the hand, forearm or elbow. The smaller the contact point, the more precise the technique, but the more difficult to maintain control over the tissue.[28, 41]

In the passive variant, move the limb/joint to stretch the target muscle while applying pressure with the other hand (see Figure 4.11). The client can also generate some tension within the target muscle by performing an isometric contraction while the therapist pulls the muscle into an eccentric contraction and maintains the locked tissue.[28] In active STR the client moves the limb/joint through its range of motion while the therapist maintains pressure on the targeted tissue (see Figures 4.12 and 4.13). A good way to think about this technique is to consider that the fixation of the muscle at the selected point creates a false attachment point and the limb/joint movement sets up a new line of stretch, which selectively elongates the desired tissue.[41]

Another variant of this technique involves performing DG frictions or XFF instead of fixing the tissue. This technique is sometimes referred to as *stripping*, especially in sports massage literature.[28, 42] This is a favoured technique when working with athletes as it is considered useful for reaching hard-to-stretch muscles like infraspinatus and the peroneals.[41]

Fig. 4.11   Soft tissue release: passive

Fig. 4.12   Soft tissue release: active

Fig. 4.13 Soft tissue release: active

Claims made for the effectiveness of STR include:

- decreasing muscle tension
- stretching contractile and connective aspects of the tissue
- reducing irritation in trigger points.[28, 41]

Evidence for the effectiveness of STR

There is a paucity of research on STR techniques despite its widespread use and acceptance, and much of the evidence underpinning STR appears to be anecdotal. Kim et al[43] compared the effect of active release technique and joint mobilisation in 24 patients with chronic neck pain. The active release and joint mobilisation groups demonstrated significant improvements in both pain and range of motion compared to the control group. Another study looked at the effects of STR on delayed onset muscle soreness (DOMS). The findings suggested that in 20 subjects, the application of STR technique post-exercise actually increased the pain reported due to DOMS and that recovery was not accelerated within the first 48 hours.[44] Clearly, there is a need for more research to support or refute the effectiveness of this technique.

CONTRAINDICATIONS

Contraindications to the technique include those for Swedish massage. In addition,

- easy bruising (stripping, especially, may bruise clients)
- hypermobility in relevant joints.[41]

This list is not exhaustive. Avoid massage in cases where the pathology involved is either unknown or poorly understood.[4, 26]

Table 4.3 summarises the remedial massage techniques for muscles discussed in this chapter. These techniques are perhaps the most widely used by remedial massage therapists. Students and remedial therapists are encouraged to explore further muscle function assessments, like muscle-firing patterns,[44] that are beyond the scope of this book.

KEY MESSAGES

- Remedial massage therapists apply specific techniques to treat muscle injuries and to promote postural flexibility.
- Assessment of muscle function includes case history, postural assessment and functional testing (including functional deficit demonstration and tests for the strength and length of specific muscles).
- Commonly used remedial massage techniques for muscle tissue include deep gliding (DG), cross-fibre frictions (XFF), deep transverse frictions (DTF) and soft tissue release (STR).
- There is insufficient evidence to support or refute the effectiveness of these muscle-specific techniques.

Table 4.3 Major remedial massage techniques for muscles

Technique		Indications	Contraindications
Deep gliding	Deep slow stripping movement along the line of muscle fibres with fingers, knuckles, thumbs, elbows, forearms	Muscle strains, overload	As for Swedish massage, including ■ acute injury ■ recent surgery ■ acute inflammation ■ systemic infection or uncontrolled medical condition ■ undiagnosed cancer ■ possible thrombosis ■ skin infections ■ osteoporosis
Cross-fibre friction	Deep slow gliding movements perpendicular to the muscle fibres with thumbs, fingers, knuckles, palms, forearms		
Deep transverse friction*	No lubricant Deep friction applied perpendicularly to the line of fibres over the entire lesion (usually <1 cm) with thumbs, fingers, single knuckle, massage tool (e.g. T-bar)	Muscle strains, especially to break down scar tissue/ adhesions	As for Swedish massage including ■ acute inflammation ■ acute infection ■ calcification or ossification within tendons, muscles or ligaments ■ haematomas ■ peripheral nerves ■ rheumatoid arthritis ■ bursitis
Soft tissue release	Practitioner's contacts either static (apply static pressure to lesion with fingers, thumbs, knuckles, elbow) or dynamic (apply deep gliding** with thumbs, fingers, knuckles, forearm) Movement of affected limb either passive (i.e. practitioner moves limb/part) or active (client moves limb/part) Four variations: i) passive, static ii) passive, dynamic iii) active, static iv) active, dynamic	Muscle strains, overload	As for Swedish massage including ■ easy bruising ■ joint hypermobility

*DTF need not be restricted to transverse strokes.
**In the dynamic version of STR, deep gliding could be replaced with cross-fibre friction or diagonal gliding.

Review questions

1. Name five procedures that can be used to assess the function of muscles.
2. Give an example of an active functional deficit assessment procedure. Why do some authors prefer active functional deficit assessments to active range of motion assessments in single planes of motion?
3. Why are AROM ranges generally smaller than PROM ranges?
4. What happens to the antagonist when the agonist is contracting? Give an example of how this could be used in remedial massage practice.
5. How would you test the length of:
   i) latissimus dorsi?
   ii) pectoralis major?
   iii) pectoralis minor?
   iv) quadriceps?
6. What is the difference between the response of postural and phasic muscles to fatigue? How would this fact influence your treatment plan?
7. What do the terms *locked short* and *locked long* mean?
8. What is the difference between a muscle spasm and a contracture? What does this difference mean for treatment of shortened muscle tissue?
9. Joint ranges of motion differ, often markedly, from normative data. This may result from previous conditions or injuries, for instance poorly treated dislocations, or even from training. Name two sports which are associated with either an increased or reduced ROM in specific joints.
10. When assessing a client's right elbow both active and passive ranges of motion appear to be restricted in extension. What can you do to ascertain whether this range is normal for the client?
11. Match Column A (condition) with their palpatory characteristics in Column B.

Column A	Column B
Fibrotic tissue	Tender
Oedema	May be crepitus
Acute strain	Hard, sometimes stringy
Chronic tendinosis	Spongy

12. Answer the following questions about deep transverse friction:
   i) What was the technique originally thought to achieve?
   ii) What have we learned from recent research?

REFERENCES

1. Eckhard T, Padua D, Dompier T, et al. Epidemiology of hip flexor and hip adductor strains in national collegiate athletic association athletes, 2009/2010-2014/2015. Am J Sports Med 2017;45(12):2713–22.

2. Hägglund M, Waldén M, Ekstrand J. Risk factors for lower extremity muscle injury in professional soccer: the UEFA Injury Study. Am J Sports Med 2013;41:327–35.

3. Konin JG, Lebsack D, Snyder Valier A, et al. Special tests for orthopedic examination. 4th edn. New Jersey: Slack; 2015.

4. Hammer WI. Editor. Functional soft-tissue examination and treatment by manual methods. 3rd edn. Sudbury, MA: Jones and Bartlett; 2007.

5. Chaitow L, Delaney J. Clinical application of neuromuscular techniques – practical case study exercises. Edinburgh: Elsevier; 2005.

6. Travell J, Simons D. Myofascial pain and dysfunction: the trigger point manual. Vol. 1: the upper extremities. Baltimore: Williams and Wilkins; 1983.

7. Cook CE, Hegedus EJ. Orthopedic physical examination tests – an evidence-based approach. 2nd edn. Essex: Pearson; 2014.

8. Cook CE, Hegedus EJ. Orthopedic physical examination tests – an evidence-based approach. New Jersey: Pearson Prentice Hall; 2008.

9. Kendall FP, McCreary EK, Provance PG, et al. Muscles – testing and function. 5th edn. Maryland: Williams and Wilkins; 2005.

10. Chaitow L. Muscle energy techniques. Edinburgh: Churchill Livingstone; 2006.

11. Janda V. Muscle function testing. London: Butterworths; 1983.

12. Australian Bureau of Statistics. 4364.0.55.004 – Australian Health Survey: Physical Activity, 2011-12. Online. Available: http://www.abs.gov.au/ausstats/abs@.nsf/Lookup/4364.0.55.004Chapter 5002011-12; 2013.

13. Myers T. Anatomy trains – myofascial meridians for manual and movement therapists. Edinburgh: Churchill Livingstone; 2014.

14. Chaitow L, Delany JW. Clinical application of neuromuscular techniques. Vol 2: the lower body. 2nd edn. Edinburgh: Churchill Livingstone; 2011.

15. Mohamed SHP, Alagesan S, Subbarayalu AV. Management of postural low back pain among the information technology professionals: a multiple therapeutic intervention approach. Int J Physiother Res 2015;3(6):1271–83. Doi: 10.16965/ijpr.2015.191.

16. Workplace Standards Tasmania. Forklift safety: Reducing the risks Rosny Park, Tasn.d. Available from: https://www.worksafe.tas.gov.au/__data/assets/pdf_file/0003/168141/nhp001.pdf.

17. Chaitow L, Delany JW. Clinical application of neuromuscular techniques. Vol. 1: the upper body. Edinburgh: Churchill Livingstone; 2000.

18. Cyriax J. Textbook of orthopedic medicine. Vol. 1: diagnosis of soft tissue lesions. London: Baillière Tindall; 1982.

19. Gracovetsky SA. Range of normality vs range of motion: a functional measure for the prevention and management of low back injury. J Bodyw Mov Ther 2010;14:40–9.

20. Muir S, Corea C, Bearpre L. Evaluating change in clinical status: reliability and measures of agreement for the assessment of glenohumeral range of motion. North Am J Sports Phys Ther 2010;5:98–110.

21. Chaitow L. Muscle energy techniques. 4th edn. Edinburgh: Churchill Livingstone; 2013.

22. Hutchinson M. Brukner & Khan's clinical sports medicine. 5th edn. Vol 1. Injuries. Sydney: McGraw Hill; 2017.

23. Muscolino J. The muscle and bone palpation manual: with trigger points, referral patterns and stretching. St Louis, MO.: Mosby/Elsevier; 2009.

24. Chaitow L, Chambers G, Frymann V. Palpation and assessment skills. Edinburgh: Churchill Livingstone; 2003.

25. Holsgaard-Larsen A, Myburgh C, Hartvigsen J, et al. Standardized simulated palpation training – development of a palpation trainer and assessment of palpatory skills in experienced and inexperienced clinicians. Man Ther 2010;15:254–60.

26. Cyriax J, Russell G. Textbook of orthopaedic medicine. Vol 2: treatment by manipulation, massage and injection. London: Baillière Tindall; 1980.

27. Goats GC. Massage – the scientific basis of an ancient art. Part 1: the techniques. Br J Sp Med 1994;28(3):149–52.

28. Lowe W. Orthopedic massage: theory and technique. 2nd edn. Edinburgh: Mosby Elsevier; 2009.

29. Goats GC. Massage – the scientific basis of an ancient art. Part 2: physiological and therapeutic effects. Br J Sp Med 1994;28(3):153–6.

30. de las Penas CF, Sohrbeck Campo M, et al. Manual therapies in myofascial trigger point treatment: a systematic review. J Bodyw Mov Ther 2005;9:27–34.

31. Miake-Lye I, Lee J, Lugar T, et al. VA Evidence-based synthesis program reports. Massage for pain: an evidence map. Washington (DC): Department of Veterans Affairs (US); 2016.

32. Field T, Diego M, Hernandez M. Moderate pressure is essential for massage therapy effects. Int J Neurosci 2010;120(5):381–5.

33. Lewis M, Johnson MI. The clinical effectiveness of therapeutic massage for musculoskeletal pain – a systematic review. Physiotherapy 2006;92(3):146–58.

34. Best TM, Hunter R, Wilcox A, et al. Effectiveness of sports massage for recovery of skeletal muscle from strenuous exercise. Clin J Sport Med 2008;18(5):446–60.

35. Benjamin P. Tappan's handbook of massage therapy. Blending art with science. 6th edn. Upper Saddle River, N.J.: Pearson/Prentice Hall; 2015.

36. Mellion MB, Putukian M, Madden CC. Sports medicine secrets. 3rd edn. Philadelphia: Hanley and Belfus; 2003.

37. Joseph MF, Taft K, Moskwa M, et al. Deep friction massage to treat tendinopathy: a systematic review of a classic treatment in the face of a new paradigm of understanding. J Sport Rehabil 2012;21(4):343–53.

38. Loew LM, Brosseau L, Tugwell P, et al. Deep transverse friction massage for treating lateral elbow or lateral knee tendinitis. Cochrane Database Syst Rev 2014;11:CD003528.

39. Brosseau L, Casimiro L, Milne S, et al. Deep transverse friction massage for treating tendinitis. Cochrane Database Syst Rev 2002;(4)CD003528.

40. Leahy M. Active release techniques: logical soft tissue treatment. In: Hammer WI, editor. Functional soft-tissue examination and treatment by manual methods. 3rd edn. Jones Sudbury, MA: Jones and Bartlett; 2011.

41. Johnson J. Soft tissue and trigger point release: hands-on guides for therapists. 2nd edn. Champaign: Human Kinetics; 2019.

42. Walden M, editor. Sports massage tutorials. Accessed: 31 July 2010. Online. Available: http://www.sportsinjuryclinic.net/sports-massage/legs-and-back-sports-massage.php.

43. Kim J, Lee H, Park S. Effects of active release technique on pain and range of motion of patients with chronic neck pain. J Phys Ther Sci 2015;27(8):2461–664.

44. Micklewright D. The effect of soft tissue release on delayed onset muscle soreness: a pilot study. Phys Ther Sport 2009;10:19–24.

5

Muscle stretching

Learning Outcomes

- Assess clients' suitability for muscle stretching.
- Describe the current evidence for the effectiveness of muscle stretching.
- Briefly describe the neurophysiology of muscle reflexes involved in stretching.
- Apply muscle-stretching techniques effectively and safely to a range of clients.
- Advise clients who have been treated with muscle stretching about home exercise.

INTRODUCTION

Therapeutic stretching involves elongating contractile tissue (muscle and associated tendon and connective tissue) within its elastic range of motion. It requires the skilful application of knowledge of anatomy, neuromuscular physiology and biomechanics blended with sound clinical judgment to achieve an optimum predictable outcome. Stretching techniques range from simple stretches of a body part through to re-educating the neuromuscular system of the central nervous system. Although stretching is relatively safe, inappropriate or ill-judged use of stretching techniques can result in injury.[1] When considering the potential benefits of stretching, practitioners should take the many functions performed by muscle into account. How may stretching assist in the execution of these functions? What criteria do we use to determine a client's suitability for stretching? Should a stretching regimen be part of this client's overall management plan? How can stretching be performed effectively and safely?

FUNCTIONAL ANATOMY

Skeletal muscle is made up of bundles of muscle fibres called fasciculi. Each muscle fibre contains hundreds of myofibrils that are surrounded by sarcoplasm. The sarcoplasm contains mitochondria and is the storage site for glycogen, fat particles and enzymes. Each myofibril is arranged lengthwise in sarcomeres. Sarcomeres are the basic functional unit of skeletal muscle. They contain protein filaments actin (thin filaments), myosin (thick filaments), and titin that enable muscular contraction and elongation. Titin is a giant protein in sarcomeres that keeps actin and myosin in place as muscles contract and relax.[2]

Stretching takes advantage of four properties of muscle:

- Excitability (also called irritability) – the ability to receive and respond to stimuli. The response is contraction of muscle fibres.
- Contractility – muscle can actively shorten its length. This is a unique property of muscle tissue.
- Extensibility – muscle can be stretched beyond its resting length.
- Elasticity – muscle fibre can recoil and resume its resting length after being stretched.

A contractile unit consists of a muscle fibre, tendon and the connective tissue that binds these tissues together (see Figure 5.1 on p 65).

TISSUE RANGE OF MOTION

All soft tissue of the body has an inherent range of motion. Joints, contractile units and structures that are involved with gross movement are the focus of interest in stretching regimens. However, it is important to consider the influence of a stretching routine on all tissue and the mechanical properties of the affected tissues when developing a routine. For example, a neck-stretching routine must take into account the impact of stretching delicate nerve and vascular tissue within the neck. The type of stretching procedure delivered to the neck must be appropriate for these structures and at the same time must be effective in its primary purpose. Healthy tissue can generally tolerate stretching through a normal range of motion. However, a person suffering vascular disease may be considerably less tolerant of the 'normal' expected range of motion. Give priority to the most at-risk tissue that could be affected by the stretch when planning a stretching routine.

Tissues like bone undergo almost no deformity under tensile loading (stretching) before they fracture. Other tissues are ductile; that is, they undergo plastic (permanent) deformity of shape before they rupture when under load. If stretching allows a ductile tissue (e.g. a ligament) to undergo repeated or prolonged stretch beyond its elastic limit then permanent deformity will ensue. This results in joint hypermobility due to elongation of the ligaments that support the joint and maintain the normal proximity of the congruous articular surfaces. A joint will develop hypermobility only in the directions of excessive stretch. In determining the impact of excessive stretching consider also the mechanical properties of joints including the concept of 'coupled motion' of joints; that is,

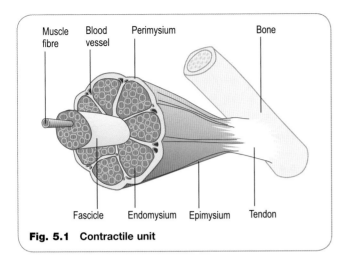

Fig. 5.1   Contractile unit

Labels: Muscle fibre · Blood vessel · Perimysium · Bone · Fascicle · Endomysium · Epimysium · Tendon

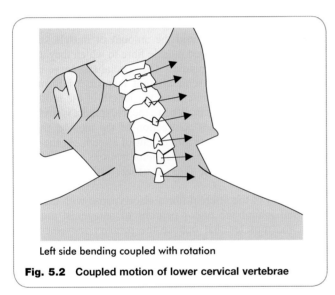

Left side bending coupled with rotation

Fig. 5.2   Coupled motion of lower cervical vertebrae

motion in which translation or rotation about an axis is associated with simultaneous translation or rotation about another axis.[3] Normal cervical movement, for example, involves coupled movement: lateral flexion of the lower cervical spine invokes simultaneous ipsilateral rotation of the vertebrae (see Figure 5.2).[4]

MUSCLE FUNCTIONS

Muscles produce movement, maintain posture, stabilise joints, generate and maintain body heat, guard orifices and support and protect tissue.

Produce movement

Muscles are responsible for:

- all locomotion of the skeleton and manipulation of the external environment
- movement of fluids via muscle pumping actions. The movement of blood through the body reflects the work of the rhythmically beating cardiac muscle and smooth muscle in the walls of blood vessels. Movement of lymph fluid, urine, bile and faeces results from muscle contractions.

Maintaining posture and position

Adjusting muscles enable us to maintain posture despite external forces acting on the body and the never-ending downward pull of gravity. Righting reflexes are involuntary muscle contractions of the voluntary muscle system that automatically adjust posture and position.

Stabilising joints

Muscles not only pull on bones to create movement, but they also stabilise joints. Muscle tone is a major factor in joint stability.

Generating and maintaining body heat

Muscles generate heat as they contract which is vitally important in maintaining normal body temperature. Involuntary muscles cause the redistribution of heat via the systematic contraction of smooth muscle in blood vessels.

Guard orifices

Sphincter muscles form valves to control passage of substances.

Support and protect soft tissues

Muscle often protects adjacent delicate soft tissue like blood and lymph vessels and peripheral nerves. Strengthening programs are often prescribed to protect hypermobile joints, disc lesions and other tissue injury sites.

TYPES OF MUSCLE CONTRACTIONS

Most body movements are a mixture of both isotonic and isometric contractions.

Isotonic contractions

The tension or tone in a muscle remains the same while the muscle length changes; that is, the muscle shortens or lengthens while it contracts (e.g. lifting an object overhead, throwing a ball).

- A concentric contraction occurs when the muscle shortens as tension is applied, as in lifting an object or performing a biceps curl.
- In an eccentric contraction the muscle lengthens as it contracts, as when a load is lowered to the ground or running downhill.

Isometric contractions

The muscle length remains the same while the muscle tension increases; that is, a static contraction occurs (e.g. pushing arms against a wall, trying to lift an immovable object).

PHYSICAL CHARACTERISTICS AND NEUROLOGICAL REFLEXES ASSOCIATED WITH STRETCHING

The physical properties of muscle, particularly its limits of shortening and lengthening, are important factors in stretching. The ideal length–stretch relationship within a muscle

Fig. 5.3   Muscle stretching

Fig. 5.4   Stretch reflex

occurs when a muscle is slightly stretched beyond its normal resting length. At this length, the actin and myosin filaments within the muscle barely overlap. This permits sliding along the entire length of the filaments. If a muscle is stretched to the extent that the myofilaments do not overlap at all, the muscle cannot generate tension and therefore cannot contract. Conversely, if the muscle is so compressed that the myofilaments are completely overlapping then further shortening is impossible (see Figure 5.3). Muscles have an optimum operational range of length of 80% to 120% of their normal resting length.[4]

ACTIVE AND PASSIVE INSUFFICIENCY

When multiarticular muscles (i.e. muscles that span more than one joint) contract, they exert force on all the joints they span so that movement can occur at more than one joint simultaneously. Because of limitations in the length of the muscle, these muscles cannot exert enough tension to shorten sufficiently for both joints to achieve full end range movement at the same time. This is called *active insufficiency*. Conversely, it is very difficult for a multiarticular muscle to be stretched enough to allow full end range movement in both joints simultaneously. This is called *passive insufficiency*. These physical properties of muscle should be considered when devising stretching and rehabilitation programs for clients. An example of this principle can be observed in practice when stretching the hamstring muscle. Clients with shortened hamstrings can stretch the muscle by extending the knee with the hip flexed to 90° (i.e. the muscle is stretched across one joint – the knee). For clients with greater hamstring flexibility, flexing at the hip with the knee extended (i.e. stretching the muscle over two joints) may be required to achieve further muscle stretch.

NEUROLOGICAL EVENTS THAT MEDIATE STRETCHING

The neurological events that mediate stretching are briefly reviewed below.

Myotatic reflex (stretch reflex)

This is a protective reflex guarding against overstretching muscles. It is mediated within the spinal cord and occurs quickly (1–2 milliseconds). All muscles contain nerve endings that respond to the rate and the amount of muscle stretch. Together with the modified muscle fibre to which they attach, they form the muscle spindles. The specialised nerve receptors of these spindles send afferent (sensory) information regarding the rate of stretch and the length of the muscle to the central nervous system. When a muscle spindle is stretched, the stretch reflex causes contraction of the muscle, thereby limiting the muscle's rate and extent of stretch. At the spine the afferent stimuli excite alpha motor neurons which activate the muscle to contract, thus resisting further stretch (see Figure 5.4).

Branches of the afferent fibres also synapse with interneurons that inhibit the motor neurons of antagonist muscles. Thus, the muscles that oppose the primary movement are stopped from resisting that movement. This is called *reciprocal inhibition*.[5]

Deep tendon reflex

When muscle tension increases during contraction or passive stretching, golgi tendon organ (GTO) receptors within the muscle's tendon are activated. The GTO send afferent impulses to the spinal cord and cerebellum. Motor neurons in the spinal cord that supply the contracting muscle are inhibited and neurons to the antagonist muscles are activated. This process is called *reciprocal activation*.[5] Fine control of muscle coordination is achieved with the help of this system (see Figure 5.5 on p 67).

TYPES OF MUSCLE STRETCHING

Numerous stretching techniques have been developed, including practitioner-assisted stretching and active stretching where the client performs the stretch independently. Some of the major muscle-stretching techniques include:

1. PASSIVE STRETCH

An assistant/practitioner performs a stretch on a client to increase tissue range of motion.

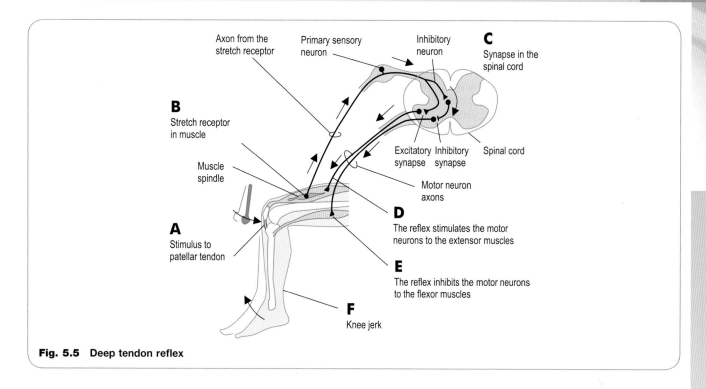

Fig. 5.5 Deep tendon reflex

*(Figure labels:)*

A — Stimulus to patellar tendon

B — Stretch receptor in muscle

Muscle spindle

C — Synapse in the spinal cord

Axon from the stretch receptor

Primary sensory neuron

Inhibitory neuron

Excitatory synapse   Inhibitory synapse   Spinal cord

Motor neuron axons

D — The reflex stimulates the motor neurons to the extensor muscles

E — The reflex inhibits the motor neurons to the flexor muscles

F — Knee jerk

2. ACTIVE, ACTIVE-ASSISTED STRETCH

Active stretches or self-stretches are inherently safer than passive stretching as the client can judge when the muscle being stretched has reached its comfortable limit.

3. MUSCLE ENERGY TECHNIQUE[5]

Muscle energy technique (MET) involves isometric contraction before stretching. The client uses minimal force during the isometric contraction and this is followed by passive stretching. The main goal of MET is joint mobilisation. The technique uses both reciprocal inhibition and post-isometric relaxation.[6] In post-isometric relaxation the muscle is passively stretched and minimal resistance applied against isometric contraction. When the contraction is released the muscle is taken gently into a further stretch.

4. ACTIVE ISOLATED STRETCH[2]

In this technique, the client actively lengthens the muscle to the point of light irritation and holds for 2 seconds before returning to the starting position. This sequence is repeated 8 to 10 times. The technique is designed to prevent activation of the stretch reflex while activating reciprocal inhibition.

5. BALLISTIC STRETCH

Ballistic stretching involves rapid bouncing performed at the end range of joint motion. It can be an active or passive stretch. Popularised by Beaulieu in 1981[7] ballistic stretching has now fallen out of favour because of the risk of tearing muscle. It produces a strong myotonal reflex, leaving the muscle shorter than before the stretch.[8]

6. DYNAMIC STRETCH

This type of stretching usually occurs in dynamic range of motion warm-up routines. The limbs are moved through their full range of motion slowly in a controlled and comfortable manner. Speed is increased with repetitions.[9]

7. STATIC STRETCH

In static stretching the client stretches the muscle to a point of mild discomfort. Bob Anderson, in his book *Stretching*, gives a comprehensive description of static stretching methods for sports, activities of daily living and occupational activities.[10] His method employs slow lengthening of a muscle which is held for 15 to 30 seconds and then repeated, increasing range of motion as the muscle relaxes. Various authors suggest different time intervals for maintaining a static stretch, usually between 15 and 60 seconds that may be repeated 2–4 times.[2] In one variation, the client holds the position for 30 seconds to two minutes which gradually lengthens a muscle. A study by Ford et al[11] investigated the effect of four different durations (30, 60, 90 and 120 seconds) of static hamstring stretch on passive knee extension range of motion in healthy subjects and found that similar benefits were achieved regardless of the stretch duration. Another study investigating the effect of static stretching (10, 20 and 30 seconds) combined with a 90-second dynamic stretching routine found that the longer durations (20- and 30-second static stretching) had a significant positive effect on sit and reach scores but not on repeated sprint times or change of direction results.[12] It is thought that static stretching slightly lessens the sensitivity of muscle spindle receptors which allows the muscle to relax and to be stretched to greater length.

8. PROPRIOCEPTIVE NEUROMUSCULAR FACILITATION

Developed in the 1940s, proprioceptive neuromuscular facilitation (PNF) techniques are the result of the work of Kabat, Knott and Voss.[13–14] They combined their analysis of functional movement with theories from motor development, motor control, motor learning and neurophysiology.[14] PNF can be a valuable part of rehabilitation programs. Most clinicians use PNF to promote muscle elasticity, functional movement and performance,[15] although it was originally used to develop muscular strength and endurance, improve joint stability or increase neuromuscular control and coordination.[16]

PNF stretching techniques

PNF stretching has been found to be an effective stretching technique, particularly for immediate improvements in range of motion.[9, 17] In PNF stretching neuromuscular inhibition procedures reflexively relax the contractile components of shortened muscles so clients can increase their range of movement.[15, 16] Various techniques are used, among them:

Hold-Relax

This technique is also known as *Contract-Relax*. First, the practitioner passively lengthens a tight muscle to its comfortable limit, then the client isometrically contracts it for several seconds. When the contraction is released, the practitioner further lengthens the muscle and holds the stretch at the new end range of motion. Reflexive muscle relaxation occurs as a result of the firing of the golgi-tendon organ (GTO). Hold-relax technique is easy to perform in clinic and is suitable for home exercises and muscle injury prevention programs.

It is important to be aware that although activating the GTO can increase flexibility, it may also predispose to injury. PNF stretching applied directly before activity can predispose clients to musculotendinous injury if a sudden stretch occurs during functional activity. Research into the effects of PNF stretching does not generally report significant gains in muscle strength or power. In fact, some studies found that peak power was reduced after PNF. However, PNF is a reliable option for increased flexibility.[2]

Hold (or Contract)-Relax with Agonist Contraction (CRAC)

This technique follows the same procedure as the Hold-Relax technique except that, after the tight muscle is contracted isometrically against the practitioner's resistance, the client concentrically contracts the muscle opposite the tight muscle to actively move the joint through the increased range.[14] A static stretch is then applied at the end of this new range of motion. The process can be repeated several times. Figure 5.6 shows a CRAC stretch for latissiumus dorsi.

Agonist contraction First, the practitioner passively lengthens the tight muscle (antagonist) to its end range; then the client concentrically contracts the muscle opposite the tight muscle (agonist) to move the joint to a new position in the range of motion.[14] Next, the practitioner applies mild resistance during this contraction, taking care to allow for movement through the available functional range of motion. This technique uses reciprocal inhibition to encourage the tight muscle to lengthen during agonist muscle contraction.

There is much inconsistency in the use of PNF-related terminology and implementation among practitioners. For example, some practitioners also incorporate a concentric contraction of the tight muscle against minimal resistance before applying a second stretch. This procedure, however, does not allow for maximum gains in flexibility; any firing of GTO is negated by the

Fig. 5.6 CRAC stretching
[1] Throughout this book, → represents the direction of the practitioner's pressure; ⇒ represents the direction of the clients' pressure.

time the client moves the extremity back to the starting point of the concentric contraction. There are also varying opinions on the duration and number of repetitions. For example, Walker[18] recommended contracting the muscle for 5–6 seconds at a comfortable starting stretch, relaxing the contraction and then further passive stretching for 30 seconds. This was followed by a 30-second recovery period out of the stretch. The sequence was repeated 2–4 times. Most PNF techniques use 75–100% of a maximal contraction.[9] However, one study found that sub-maximal contractions of 20% or 60% were equally effective.[19]

Laughlin[20] developed a method of stretching that focuses on injury prevention and rehabilitation. This method uses a contract-relax (C-R) approach. The contract phase involves contracting the muscle for an interval of 2 to 30 seconds depending on its size and location. The intensity of this contraction also depends on the same two variables. The relax phase is composed of two intervals: relaxation of the whole body followed by re-stretch of the muscle in order to exaggerate the stretch. The new stretch is commonly held for a period of 15 to 45 seconds depending on the size and location of the muscle. The C-R stretch can then be repeated. According to the author, no improvement in range of motion is usually found beyond three repetitions.

PNF strengthening techniques

Spiral-diagonal patterns are observed in normal movements such as swinging the arms across the body during walking. PNF techniques that use spiral-diagonal patterns are designed to restore and enhance coordinated movements through multiple planes and axes of motion.[8] PNF strengthening techniques use spiral-diagonal patterns, often referred to as D1 and D2 patterns. They also apply sensory cues, specifically proprioceptive, cutaneous, visual and auditory feedback, to improve muscular responses.[14] The diagonal movements associated with PNF involve multiple joints moving through various planes of motion. These patterns incorporate rotational movements of the extremities, but also require core stability if patients are to successfully complete the motions.

D1 and D2 patterns can be performed in either flexion or extension.[21, 22] They are referred to as D1 flexion, D1 extension, D2 flexion or D2 extension techniques for the upper or lower extremity.[14] In practitioner-assisted PNF strengthening the practitioner applies manual resistance throughout a range of motion using precise hand positioning while guiding the client through the appropriate range of movement.[14] The practitioner can make minor adjustments as the client's coordination improves or fatigue occurs during the rehabilitation session. In general, the practitioner applies the maximum amount of resistance that allows for smooth, controlled, pain-free movement throughout the range of motion.[21] In addition to manual resistance strengthening, PNF diagonal patterns are thought to enhance proper sequencing of muscular contraction, from distal to proximal. This promotes neuromuscular control and coordination.[14]

Variations of PNF technique

To enhance coordination, movement and stability, practitioners use numerous techniques during PNF exercises, among them:

Rhythmic stabilisation

This technique, which incorporates passive movement of the joint through the desired range of motion, is used to re-educate the neuromuscular system to initiate the desired movement. The practitioner passively moves the extremity several times through the movement pattern at appropriate speed. Active assistive and then active movement with resistance are progressively introduced through the same pattern to improve the client's coordination and control.

Slow reversal

This technique involves a dynamic concentric contraction of a strong agonist muscle group, which is immediately followed by a second dynamic concentric contraction of a weak antagonist muscle group.[14] Because rest periods do not occur between contractions this technique promotes the rapid, reciprocal motion that these muscle groups need for coordinated activities.

Slow reversal hold

This technique supplements the technique above with an isometric contraction (hold) at the end range of each muscle group. It is used to enhance dynamic stability of the larger proximal muscle groups (e.g. hip flexors, quadratus lumborum, lower trapezius). This adds a sustained contraction to enhance the tone of proximal stabilising muscles.

Alternating isometrics

This technique encourages stability in postural trunk muscles and stabilisers of the hip and shoulder girdle. The practitioner applies manual resistance to the involved limb in a single plane from one side of the body to the other while the client holds the starting position using alternating isometric contractions. This technique can be used to strengthen muscles of the trunk, upper limbs or lower limbs. It can be applied with the limbs in an open kinetic chain (i.e. the hand or foot free to move) or closed kinetic chain position (i.e. the hand or foot fixed).

Alternating rhythmic stabilisation

This technique is an extension of alternating isometrics in which the involved muscle groups co-contract. Rhythmic stabilisation is most commonly performed in a closed kinetic chain position to further enhance muscular co-contraction and joint stability. The practitioner may apply simultaneous manual resistance in a multidirectional pattern, forcing different muscle groups to contract simultaneously to support and stabilise the extremity. This technique is particularly beneficial for isometrically contracting the proximal joint rotators.[14]

STRETCHING TREATMENT GOALS

Using the acronym SMART (Specific, Measurable, Acceptable, Realistic, Time Related), we can develop therapeutic goals that the practitioner and client mutually understand and agree to at the commencement of therapy. This approach facilitates communication and motivates the client to self-assess their needs and re-evaluate any preconceived ideas.

Some defined goals will be almost universal, such as decreasing pain, increasing range of motion, increasing strength and endurance and developing balance between motion and stability. Other goals will be client-specific. Examples are specific performance goals such as walking or running a certain distance in a certain time. Incremental goals established to act as landmarks throughout the course of recovery are particularly helpful.

ASSESSING CLIENTS' SUITABILITY

HISTORY

Clients may complain of muscle aches, pain or stiffness. In some cases clients are not aware of the muscle contractures that have preceded the development of many musculoskeletal complaints, such as headaches from tight upper trapezius and sub-occipital muscles, or knee pain from an overly tight vastus lateralis muscle. Correlating the client's history with other assessment findings helps identify functional limitations that may underlie presenting conditions.

POSTURAL ANALYSIS

Postural analysis gives a great deal of information about the way an individual uses their body (see Chapter 2). Common posture distortions like scoliosis, upper crossed and lower crossed syndrome and hyperlordosis are associated with muscle contractures and weaknesses.

GAIT ANALYSIS

Gait analysis contributes to the functional assessment of the client, enabling identification of muscles requiring stretching and strengthening. For example, walking on the balls of the feet may indicate shortened gastrocnemius and soleus muscles; abnormal hip rotation in the acceleration phase of gait may indicate weak quadriceps. Assess gait for focal dysfunction and for a global view of the whole kinematic chain affecting the client's gait (see Chapter 2). Reassessing gait at a later date will inform modification to the initial routine as the client's kinematics alter over time.

FUNCTIONAL TESTS

Muscle strains are identified by pain and impaired function which may include decreased strength and impaired ability to lengthen. Muscle length tests help identify muscles requiring stretching. Compare findings to the unaffected side or to population norms (see Chapter 2, Table 2.7).

PALPATION

Palpation is a useful tool for assessing muscle tone. Use palpation to confirm findings from postural observation and gait analysis. Assess the perceived level of tension in muscle and tendon. Taut muscle that feels like a stretched fibrous rope suggests chronic hypertonicity. Muscle with a soft, unresponsive, flaccid feel suggests a mechanical dysfunction of the kinematic chain associated with that muscle or neurological deficit.

The WHO's International Classification of Function, Disability and Health (ICF) provides a systematic process which is designed to provide and/or maintain the greatest level of functionality available for that individual.[23] It is a useful guide which integrates findings from a range of assessments. At the end of remedial massage assessment the practitioner should be able to describe:

- Functioning and Disability:
  - Body functions, including mental functions, sensory functions and pain, neuromusculoskeletal and movement-related functions
  - Body structures
  - Activities and Participation, including general tasks and demands, communication, mobility, domestic life, interpersonal interactions and relationships
- Contextual Factors:
  - Environmental Factors, including products and technology, natural environment and human-made changes to environment, support and relationships, services
  - Personal Factors

EVIDENCE FOR EFFECTIVENESS

Many people, both lay and professional, believe that static stretching may benefit the user to better prepare the body for activity, reduce the likelihood of injury and post-event muscle soreness, and enhance performance. To date, none of these beliefs can be substantiated by scientific research. Indeed, the clinical effectiveness of many different types of stretching remains unclear. It may be that we have individualised responses to stretching that are influenced by our genetics, level of training and so on.[2, 24, 25] There is a need for rigorous scientific investigation to underpin many stretching techniques commonly used in sports medicine practices.

Research generally recommends all types of stretching for increasing ROM, although PNF stretching appears to produce the most immediate results.[2] The effectiveness of stretching appears to vary with age and gender. For example, older adults may receive greater improvements in flexibility with long duration stretches (60 seconds) compared to short duration ones.[26] Elderly women showed improved gait adaptations associated with reduced falls risk after a daily stretching routine.[27] Men appear to respond better to contract-relax stretching compared to women.[9]

A number of studies have found that static stretching impaired strength and performance[28, 29] and may therefore only be suitable for athletes requiring flexibility for their sport (e.g. gymnastics, dance). Dynamic stretching is recommended as a warm-up for athletes requiring running or jumping performance.[30] Stretching has not been shown to be effective at reducing the incidence of overall injuries, although it may reduce musculotendinous injuries.[31]

Stretching is often used in rehabilitation to increase muscle length and joint ROM.[32, 33] For example, static and PNF stretching increased knee ROM in patients with knee osteoarthritis.[17, 34] Another study found that 2 weeks of static, dynamic or PNF stretching increased knee ROM in knee replacement patients.[35] Active isolated stretch does not appear to elicit exercise performance gains, but has shown success in rehabilitation settings.[2] Stretching is often included in pain management programs, including for the low back, knee and shoulder.[36, 37] A year of stretching was found to be as effective as strengthening exercises or manual therapy in patients with chronic neck pain.[38, 39] Trigger point pain was immediately reduced after stretching, according to Lewit and Simons.[40] Patients with joint contractures do not appear to benefit from stretching. Stretching that sustained the soft tissues in a lengthened position for at least 20 seconds on more than one occasion appears to have no benefit for neurological patients who have had a stroke or spinal cord injury.[41]

CONTRAINDICATIONS AND PRECAUTIONS

Contraindications and precautions for muscle stretching include:

- joint instability
- pain in the region of treatment
- pre-existing injury in muscle or tendon being treated
- active local inflammation of tissues
- geriatric clients – connective tissue begins losing elasticity from around the age of 30 years so that organs, blood vessels, and airways become more rigid with age.
- children – PNF stretching is not recommended when bones are still growing
- post surgery
- pre-event and post-event athletics
- recent or unresolved haematoma
- advanced osteoporosis and conditions that weaken bone such as osseous cancer and osteomalacia
- muscle fatigue or weakness.

APPLYING MUSCLE STRETCHING IN REMEDIAL MASSAGE

Muscle stretching is a common component of remedial massage, not only for treating specific muscle strains but also for releasing muscle contractures associated with chronic conditions like osteoarthritis and postural deviations like upper and lower crossed syndrome. Swedish massage or heat application to the area usually precedes muscle stretching and other remedial techniques. Stretches performed during the consultation are often supplemented by a stretching program performed by the client at home.

ADAPTING STRETCHES FOR INDIVIDUAL CLIENTS

Stretches can be performed in a number of ways. Consider, for example, hamstring stretches which can be performed in various positions including sitting with legs straight and touching toes, lying and raising a straight leg or standing and bending forward towards the toes. Characteristics of individual clients, including age, fitness and history of previous injury need to be taken into account when performing or recommending stretches. Use the See-Move-Touch principle described in Chapter 2: passive techniques are performed after observing the client move the muscle/joint through its active range of motion. This principle alerts you to the client's functional range of motion and helps ensure that further assessments and treatments are performed safely.

THERAPIST'S POSITION

When applying stretching in remedial massage, consider your position as the therapist relative to the client, to the equipment and to gravity. You must ensure at all times that your own position is stable, supported and able to transmit force from your body to the client's body in the most efficient manner possible. This will minimise the load on your body and the energy expenditure required to perform the technique while maintaining the client's confidence and comfort.

A stretching routine should form part of a health promotion program for massage therapists, who may be prone to repetition strain injury, particularly of the lower back, upper back, wrist and hand.[42] Using a variety of techniques and a variety of contacts (in particular substituting forearms and elbows for thumbs) and maintaining correct posture and table height are imperative. Stretches for the pectoral muscles, shoulder internal rotators, elbow flexors and wrist extensors are advisable and may be accompanied by strengthening exercises for the middle trapezius, rhomboids, serratus anterior as well as lumbar exercises tailored to the needs of individual practitioners.

RECOMMENDATIONS

Recent research suggests that passive treatments like remedial massage (including passive stretching) are most beneficial in the first few weeks after injury.[43] From about 6 weeks post injury, clients have been shown to have better outcomes if they take an increasingly active part in their rehabilitation. Home exercise programs to support remedial massage treatment are recommended. Some forms of yoga are considered to be stretching routines for the whole body and are recommended by some practitioners.

Guidelines for active stretching:[9]

For a general fitness program:

- an active warm-up precedes static stretching
- at least 2–3 days per week
- hold each stretch 15–30 seconds and repeat 2–4 times

Warm up for sports and exercise

- static stretching for flexibility
- dynamic stretching for running or jumping performance

MUSCLE STRETCHING IN PRACTICE

The choice of specific technique depends on the functional requirements and personal characteristics of individual clients (e.g. age and agility). The range of stretching techniques includes simple active stretches performed by clients, passive stretches which are designed to elongate the contractile unit and soft tissue around the joint to increase joint mobility and connective tissue flexibility, and facilitated neuromuscular coordination techniques such as CRAC variations to induce proximal muscle stability. When recommending home exercises you should demonstrate or carefully explain them and observe clients performing them correctly before they leave

Fig. 5.7 Scalene stretch

Fig. 5.8 Upper trapezius stretch

the clinic. The following examples have been selected to demonstrate the wide range of stretching techniques in the clinical setting.

Scalene group

Hypertonicity is common in the scalene muscles. This can result in functional impairment of the ability to spontaneously respond to mechanical vectors and loading; for example, for maintaining efficient head carriage. An appropriate stretching technique in this case could be CRAC which involves neurological co-ordination.

For the posterior and medial fibres, gently move the client's head to approximately a third of their available range of lateral flexion (i.e. close to neutral). Your hand is placed on the side of the head to isolate the involved muscle. The client tries to further laterally flex their neck against your resistance (i.e. the muscle is isometrically contracted) for 5 seconds. Passively move the client's head to stretch the involved muscle as far as possible within its comfortable range and hold the stretch for 10 seconds. The procedure is repeated but this time starting at two-thirds of the client's available range of lateral flexion. A final repetition starts at the fully stretched position (see Figure 5.7).

Upper trapezius

A number of practitioner-assisted stretches of the upper trapezius can be performed. In one example, a practitioner-assisted stretch may be performed with the client supine. Stand at the head of the table. Place your ipsilateral hand medial to

the acromioclavicular joint over the top of the shoulder; the contralateral hand supports the occiput. Slowly move the client's neck into contralateral lateral flexion and slight ipsilateral rotation. Your ipsilateral forearm can be used as a pivot against the head to assist lateral flex.

For an active stretch for the upper trapezius the client sits on a chair and holds the seat of the chair with the ipsilateral hand. The client's contralateral hand reaches over their head and contacts the side of the head around the temple. The client uses their contralateral hand to laterally flex their neck and simultaneously lift their head (see Figure 5.8). Further lateral flexion can be obtained by leaning the body contralaterally against the resistance of the hand holding the chair.

Pectoral muscles

Chronic shortening of the pectoral muscles is associated with protraction of scapulae in upper crossed syndrome (see Chapter 12). An active stretch for the pectoral muscle group is the doorway stretch. The client stands side-on in a doorway and places the arm in the stop sign position with the forearm against the doorframe. The body is turned away from the doorframe until a comfortable stretch is felt across the front of the shoulder. The position is held for 20 seconds (see Figure 5.9 on p 73).

This stretch can be enhanced by introducing PNF. The starting position is similar to the position described above except that the client's arm position is more anterior. The client pushes the forearm against the doorframe to isometrically contract the pectoral muscles. This is held for 5 seconds before relaxing. The muscle is stretched to its new comfortable limit by progressively turning the body away from the doorframe after each contraction is released. The procedure can be repeated three times.

Levator scapulae

This stretch is similar to the active upper trapezius stretch. With the ipsilateral hand holding under the seat of the chair,

Fig. 5.9   Pectoralis major stretch: Doorway stretch

Fig. 5.10   Levator scapulae stretch

the client leans their body diagonally forward. The contra-lateral hand reaches over the top of the head and holds the lateral aspect of the occiput behind the ear. The client simultaneously flexes and laterally flexes the neck so that the stretch can be localised to the scapula insertion of the muscle. Hold for 10 seconds (see Figure 5.10).

Wrist flexors/extensors

Actively stretching the wrist flexor and extensor muscles stretches fibrous repair tissue along lines of pull which contributes to normal fibre orientation.

To perform a PNF stretch to the wrist extensors, the client's elbow is extended. The wrist is flexed by the client's other hand holding the dorsum of the hand on the side to be stretched. The client pulls the wrist to exaggerate wrist flexion. The stretch is held for 15 seconds before releasing. The stretch can be repeated in several positions by rotating the forearm around an arc to find the position that maximally stretches the lesion. Each stretch is held for 15 seconds, released for a minimum of 5 seconds and repeated. Note: stretching is always performed within the client's pain tolerance.

A similar procedure is used to stretch the wrist flexors except that the wrist is extended to stretch the flexor muscles. Active stretches for the wrist extensor and floxor muscles are demonstrated in Figures 5.11 and 5.12 respectively.

Piriformis

When trigger points are present in the muscle or if the client has piriformis syndrome (see Chapter 10) stretching is an

Fig. 5.11   Wrist extensor stretch

appropriate treatment. Passive stretching is commonly used in clinical practice and active stretches are prescribed for home.

For a practitioner-assisted stretch, the client is supine with their knee flexed and foot placed over the opposite leg just below the knee. Guide the client's flexed knee to the opposite side (laterally) with one hand stabilising the pelvis on the involved side by holding the ipsilateral anterior superior iliac spine. Hold the stretch for 20 to 40 seconds. Repeat the stretch three or four times (see Figure 5.13).

Do not use PNF if the client has piriformis syndrome to avoid irritation of the sciatic nerve. However, in chronic cases, PNF can be used to enhance the muscle's range of motion.

Fig. 5.12 Wrist flexor stretch

Fig. 5.13 Piriformis stretch

Fig. 5.14 Psoas stretch

Stretch the muscle to mid range and perform a resisted submaximal contraction against your resistance for 15 seconds. When the client relaxes the muscle is passively stretched to its full range. Release the stretch slightly and repeat resistance and stretch.

Psoas

Psoas is commonly treated to maintain optimal lumbar and pelvic biomechanical function. An active stretch is performed by the client in a lunge position. The client adopts a fencer's stance with one foot in front of the other, feet pointing forward. The feet should be shoulder width apart. The pelvis should face the front; the low back straight. Body weight is transferred to the front foot and the psoas stretch should be felt in the groin region on the back leg. The stretch can be held for 10 seconds, then repeated four times on each leg (see Figure 5.14).

Quadriceps

HIP FLEXOR STRETCH (RECTUS FEMORIS AND ILIOPSOAS)

For a practitioner-assisted stretch, the client lies prone, knee flexed to 90°. Hold the distal thigh with the caudal hand. With the other hand, contact the posterior aspect of the hip to stabilise the pelvis. The client's knee should be maintained at 90° flexion. Raise the thigh until the client feels a comfortable stretch of rectus femoris. Hold the stretch for 20 seconds (see Figure 5.15a on p 75).

HIP FLEXORS, VASTUS LATERALIS, VASTUS INTERMEDIALIS AND VASTUS MEDIALIS

Alternatively, with the client prone, a pillow can be placed under the distal thigh to extend the hip. Move the client's heel towards their buttock until they feel a comfortable stretch (see Figure 5.15b on p 75).

Hamstrings

For a PNF stretch, the client lies supine and flexes their hip and knee to 90°. Support the anterior aspect of the knee with the cephalad hand; the other hand holds the Achilles region. Extend the knee to stretch the hamstrings to a comfortable limit. Hold the stretch for 20 seconds. Maintaining this position, the client contracts the hamstrings against your resistance for 5 seconds and then releases. Passively extend the knee to the new point of comfortable stretch. Repeat this procedure three times (see Figure 5.16 on p 75).

Adductors

For a PNF stretch, the client lies supine. Abduct the client's leg and stand between it and the table distal to client's knee. Hold the ankle of the uninvolved leg to prevent any

Fig. 5.15 (a) Hip flexor stretch, (b) hip flexor and quadriceps stretch

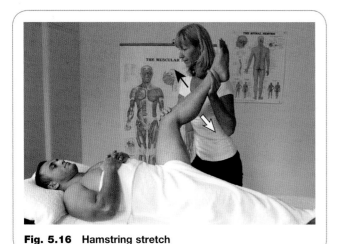

Fig. 5.16 Hamstring stretch

movement. The client tries to bring the abducted leg back to the midline against resistance by your thigh or other hand. The client releases the contraction after 5 seconds and then you abduct the client's leg further. When a comfortable maximum stretch is achieved the client adducts their leg again. Release after 5 seconds and abduct the leg further to the new comfortable maximum stretch (see Figure 5.17).

Fig. 5.17 Hip adductor stretch – draping

Fig. 5.18 Gastrocnemius stretch

Gastrocnemius

For an active home stretch the client rolls a towel to make a rope and loops it around the ball of the foot. Holding the ends of the towel in each hand the client pulls the towel towards their head to stretch the gastrocnemius. The stretch is held for 20 seconds, released for 5 seconds and repeated six times (see Figure 5.18).

Quadratus lumborum

This technique involves contractions of the quadratus lumborum on one side and stretching of the quadratus lumborum on the other.

The client stands upright with knees extended throughout the procedure. The client raises one heel while simultaneously lowering the shoulder on the same side. Instruct the client to maintain their spine in a vertical line. Imagine the shoulder and hip getting closer together while the back remains straight. Lower the heel and level the shoulders and repeat on the other side. This is a repetitive action (do not hold position). Repeat for up to 2 minutes. Stop the exercise if the client experiences any discomfort (see Figure 5.19).

Fig. 5.19 Quadratus lumborum stretch

Fig. 5.20 Latissimus dorsi stretch

Latissimus dorsi

Latissimus dorsi is an important muscle to consider when treating shoulder problems. Latissimus dorsi is commonly involved in rounded shoulder posture involving scapula protraction and internal rotation of the upper limb. When chronically contracted, it inhibits shoulder abduction and external rotation. Latissimus dorsi is also often involved in lumbar and pelvic problems because of its attachments to the lumbosacral fascia and innominate bones. To passively stretch latissimus dorsi, the client lies supine. Abduct and externally rotate the involved arm and laterally flex the trunk contralaterally. The stretch is held for 5 to 40 seconds (see Figure 5.20).

Review questions

1. What are the four properties of muscle?
2. What is the difference between post-isometric relaxation stretching and CRAC stretching?
3. Name four contraindications to stretching.
4. What palpatory findings suggest tissue that will benefit from stretching?
5. Match items in Column A with their function in Column B.

A	B
Hold-relax	muscle stretching
Rhythmic stabilisation	stability in postural trunk muscles and hip and shoulder stabilisers
Muscle energy technique	muscle stretching
CRAC	joint mobilisation
Alternating isometrics	motor coordination and control

6. How would you integrate stretching into your remedial massage plan?
7. How would you modify your recommended home stretch for the hamstring muscles for:
   a) an athlete?
   b) a 35 year old who plays football once a week, does no other exercise and has a sedentary job?
   c) a 70 year old?

8. When running downhill the quadriceps muscles contract:
   a) Concentrically
   b) Eccentrically
   c) Isometrically
9. When a muscle spindle is stretched an impulse is immediately sent to the spinal cord and a response to contract the muscle is received. This is known as:
   a) Post-isometric relaxation
   b) Reciprocal inhibition
   c) Stretch reflex
10. Afferent fibres from muscle spindles send information about the length of a muscle and rate of stretch to the spinal cord. Branches of the afferent fibres synapse with interneurons that inhibit the motor neurons of the antagonist muscle. This is known as:
    a) Post-isometric relaxation
    b) Reciprocal inhibition
    c) Stretch reflex
11. Which form of stretching is generally regarded as the most dangerous?
    a) Static
    b) PNF
    c) Ballistic
    d) Passive
12. Which form of stretching is generally regarded as the most beneficial?
    a) Dynamic
    b) Passive
    c) PNF
    d) Ballistic

REFERENCES

1. Adler S, Beckers D, Buck M. PNF in practice: an illustrated guide. 4th edn. Heidelberg: Springer Medizin; 2014.
2. Bernhart C. A review of stretching techniques and their effects on exercise. Senior Honors Thesis. 383: Liberty University; 2013.
3. Barnes D, Stemper BD, Yogananan N, et al. Normal coupling behavior between axial rotation and lateral bending in the lumbar spine. Biomed Sci Instrum 2009;45:131–6.
4. Kapandji I. The physiology of the joints. 6th edn. Oxford: Churchill Livingstone; 2008.
5. Marieb E, Keller SM. Essentials of human anatomy and physiology. 12th edn. London: Pearsons; 2017.
6. Chaitow L. Muscle energy techniques. 4th edn. Edinburgh: Churchill Livingstone; 2013.
7. Beaulieu J. Developing a stretching program. Phys Sports Med 1981;9(11):59–69.
8. McAtee R, Charland J. Facilitated stretching. 3rd edn. Champaign, IL: Human Kinetics; 2007.
9. Page P. Current concepts in muscle stretching for exercise and rehabilitation. Int J Sports Phys Ther 2012;7(109–19).
10. Anderson B. Stretching: 30th Anniversary edn. Bolinas, CA: Shelter; 2010.
11. Ford G, Mazzone M, Taylor K. The effect of 4 different durations of static hamstring stretching on passive knee-extension range of motion in healthy subjects. J Sport Rehabil 2005;14(2):95–107.
12. Behm DG, Chaouachi A, Lau PWC, et al. Short durations of static stretching when combined with dynamic stretching do not impair repeated sprints and agility. J Sports Sci Med 2011;10(2):408–16.
13. Knott M, Voss D. Proprioceptive neuromuscular facilitation. Philadelphia PA: Harper and Row; 1968.
14. Kisner C, Colby L. Therapeutic exercise: foundations and techniques. 7th edn. Philadelphia PA: FA Davis; 2018.
15. Hindle KB, Whitcomb TJ, Briggs WO, et al. Proprioceptive neuromuscular facilitation (PNF): its mechanisms and effects on range of motion and muscular function. J Hum Kinet 2012;31:105–13.
16. Gidu DV, Ene-Voiculescu C, Straton A, et al. The PNF (Prioprioceptive Neuromuscular Facilitation) stretching technique. A brief overview. Ovidius University Annals 2013;13:623–8.
17. Weng MC, Lee CL, Chen CH, et al. Effects of different stretching techniques on the outcomes of isokinetic exercise in patients with knee osteoarthritis. Kaohsiung J Med Sci 2009;25(6):306–15.
18. Walker B. The stretching handbook. Robina, Qld: Walkerbout Health; 2011.
19. Feland JB, Marin HN. Effect of submaximal contraction intensity in contract-relax proprioceptive neuromuscular facilitation stretching. Br J Sports Med 2004;38(4):E18.
20. Laughlin K. Stretching and flexibility. 2nd edn. Sydney: BodyPress; 2014.
21. Prentice W. Rehabilitation techniques in sports medicine and athletic training. 6th edn. Boston: McGraw-Hill; 2015.
22. Houglum PA. Therapeutic exercise for musculoskeletal injuries. 4th edn. Champaign, IL: Human Kinetics; 2016.
23. World Health Organization. International Classification of Functioning, Disability and Health. Online. Available: https://www.cdc.gov/nchs/data/icd/icfoverview_finalforwho10sept.pdf; 2017.
24. Curry BS, Chengkalath D, Crouch GJ, et al. Acute effects of dynamic stretching, static stretching, and light aerobic activity on muscular performance in women. J Strength Cond Res 2009;23(6):1811–19.
25. Dalrymple KJ, Davis SE, Dwyer GB, et al. Effect of static and dynamic stretching on vertical jump performance in collegiate women volleyball players. J Strength Cond Res 2010;24(1):149–55.
26. Feland JB, Myrer JW, Schulthies SS, et al. The effect of duration of stretching of the hamstring muscle group for increasing range of motion in people aged 65 years or older. Phys Ther 2001;81(5):1110–17.
27. Rodacki AL, Souza RM, Ugrinowitsch C, et al. Transient effects of stretching exercises on gait parameters of elderly women. Manual Ther 2009;14(2):167–72.
28. Nelson A, Driscoll N, Landin D, et al. Acute effects of passive muscle stretching on sprint performance. J Sports Sci 2005;23(5):449–54.
29. Marek S, Cranmer J, Fincher A, et al. Acute effects of static and PNF stretching on muscle strength and power output. J Athlet Train 2005;40(2):94–103.
30. Behm DG, Kibele A. Effects of differing intensities of static stretching on jump performance. Eur J Appl Physiol 2007;101(5):587–94.
31. Small K, Mc Naughton L, Matthews M. A systematic review into the efficacy of static stretching as part of a warm-up for the prevention of exercise-related injury. Res Sports Med 2008;16(3):213–31.
32. de Weijer VC, Gorniak GC, Shamus E. The effect of static stretch and warm-up exercise on hamstring length over the course of 24 hours. J Orthop Sports Phys Ther 2003;33(12):727–33.
33. Davis DS, Ashby PE, McCale KL, et al. The effectiveness of 3 stretching techniques on hamstring flexibility using consistent stretching parameters. J Strength Cond Res 2005;19(1):27–32.
34. Reid DA, McNair PJ. Passive force, angle, and stiffness changes after stretching of hamstring muscles. Med Sci Sports Exerc 2004;36(11):1944–8.
35. Chow TP, Ng GY. Active, passive and proprioceptive neuromuscular facilitation stretching are comparable in improving the knee flexion range in people with total knee replacement: a randomized controlled trial. Clin Rehabil 2010;24(10):911–18.
36. Davis DS, Ashby PE, McCale KL, et al. The effectiveness of 3 stretching techniques on hamstring flexibility using consistent stretching parameters. J Strength Cond Res 2005;19(1):27–32.
37. Depino GM, Webright WG, Arnold BL. Duration of maintained hamstring flexibility after cessation of an acute static stretching protocol. J Athlet Train 2000;35(1):56–9.
38. Hakkinen A, Kautiainen H, Hannonen P, et al. Strength training and stretching versus stretching only in the treatment of patients with chronic neck pain: a randomized one-year follow-up study. Clin Rehabil 2008;22(7):592–600.
39. Ylinen J, Kautiainen H, Wiren K, et al. Stretching exercises vs manual therapy in treatment of chronic neck pain: a randomized, controlled cross-over trial. J Rehabil Med 2007;39(2):126–32.
40. Lewit K, Simons DG. Myofascial pain: relief by postisometric relaxation. Arch Phys Med Rehabil 1984;65(8):452–6.
41. Katalinic OM, Harvey LA, Herbert RD, et al. Stretch for the treatment and prevention of contractures. Cochrane Database Syst Rev 2010;9:CD007455.
42. Albert W, Currie-Jackson N, Duncan C. A survey of musculoskeletal injuries amongst Canadian massage therapists. J Bodyw Mov Ther 2008;12(1):86–93.
43. Cosio D, Lin E. Role of active versus passive complementary and integrative health approaches in pain management. Glob Adv Health and Med 2018;7:1–7.

Myofascial trigger points

Learning Outcomes

- Assess clients for the presence of myofascial trigger points.
- Describe current theories posited to explain the pathogenesis of trigger points.
- Apply myofascial trigger point therapy effectively and safely to a range of clients, adapting the therapy to suit individual client needs.
- Advise and resource clients who have been assessed and treated for myofascial trigger points.

INTRODUCTION

Myofascial trigger points were first described in 1952 by Janet Travell and Seymour Rinzler in an article entitled *The Myofascial Genesis of Pain.*[1] During her long and productive career Travell helped develop new techniques for treating muscle pain using procaine injections and vapocoolant sprays. Today myofascial trigger point therapy is widely used by many physical therapists, including chiropractors, physiotherapists, osteopaths and remedial massage therapists. This chapter presents a brief overview of the identification and treatment of common myofascial trigger points. Remedial massage therapists who plan to use trigger point therapy in their practices should consult the original texts, *Myofascial Pain and Dysfunction: The Trigger Point Manual (Volume 1: The upper half of body* (Simons, Travell and Simons)*; Volume 2: The lower extremities* (Travell and Simons)).[2, 3] Travell's books contain very practical information on postural corrections and rehabilitation exercises to accompany manual trigger point therapy.

WHAT IS A TRIGGER POINT?

A trigger point is a focus of hyperirritability in a tissue that is locally tender when compressed and if sufficiently tender refers pain in a particular pattern that is similar in all clients. It is thought that pain is initiated when the trigger point area is stimulated by stressors like cold, postural distortions and emotional stress which set up a self-perpetuating pain cycle that long outlasts the initiating stimulus. Trigger points are commonly misdiagnosed as muscular rheumatism, myalgic

spots and fibrositis.[2, 4] There is also much interest in the relationship between acupuncture points and trigger points, a number of studies reporting considerable overlap.[5, 6] One study, for example, reported that 95% of trigger points (225 out of 255) corresponded to acupuncture points in anatomical location and indications. On the other hand, Chen et al,[7] noted a number of differences between traditional Chinese medicine's ashi points (the most tender points in the muscles) and myofascial trigger points, including: ashi points are generally located in the muscle region of acupuncture meridians on the boundaries between muscles and reflect disorders of internal organs and soft tissue; trigger points develop in a range of soft tissues (e.g. muscles, ligaments, fascia) and rarely reflect disorders of internal organs.

LOCATING TRIGGER POINTS

Trigger points can be found in skeletal muscles and tendons, joint capsules, ligaments, fascia, periosteum and skin (usually in scar tissue). They tend to develop more readily in postural muscles (e.g. upper trapezius, levator scapulae, quadratus lumborum, iliopsoas, piriformis and tensor fasciae latae) than in phasic muscles,[8, 9] and in high-demand muscles more than in low-demand muscles. Trigger points in skeletal muscles usually develop at the origins and insertions (attachment trigger points), and bellies of muscles, particularly at the neuromuscular junction (central trigger points). Trigger points tend to be found near origins and insertions in long eccentrically contracted muscles, and in muscle bellies in short concentrically contracted muscles.[10] Areas of muscles that are prone to mechanical strain, impaired circulation and muscular or fascial adhesions are also common sites.

CLASSIFYING TRIGGER POINTS

ACTIVE AND LATENT TRIGGER POINTS

The main difference between active and latent trigger points is the presence of pain. Active trigger points are always painful and refer pain at rest and/or when the specific muscle containing the trigger point is moved.[11] Active trigger points prevent full lengthening of muscles and weaken the muscle. They can mediate a local twitch response (i.e. a brisk contraction of a taut band of skeletal muscle fibres elicited by snapping palpation of a trigger point[12]) and often produce autonomic phenomena such as local sweating and vasomotor activity,

Table 6.1 Key trigger points

Key trigger point	Associated satellite trigger point
sternocleidomastoid	temporalis, masseter
upper trapezius	temporalis, masseter
scalene	deltoid, extensor carpi radialis, extensor digitorum communis
splenius capitis	temporalis
supraspinatus	deltoid, extensor carpi radialis
infraspinatus	biceps brachii
pectoralis minor	flexor carpi radialis, flexor carpi ulnaris
latissimus dorsi	triceps brachii, flexor carpi ulnaris
serratus posterior superior	triceps brachii, extensor digitorum communis, extensor carpi ulnaris
quadratus lumborum	gluteus maximus, piriformis
piriformis	hamstrings
hamstrings	gastrocnemius, soleus

generally in the pain reference zone. Active trigger points are likely to be found in postural muscles of the neck, shoulder and pelvic girdle and the muscles of mastication.

Latent trigger points do not refer pain until pressed but are tender on palpation. They may become active through physical events such as sleeping position, chilling or viral disease or through emotional events. Latent trigger points are often found incidentally during routine massage.

Satellite and secondary trigger points

Simons et al[2] also described associated trigger points, which can be either:
i. Satellite trigger points which are activated because the muscle in which they are located is in the referral zone of another muscle; or
ii. Secondary trigger points which are activated because the muscle is a synergist or an antagonist of the muscle with the primary trigger point and becomes overloaded.

Key trigger points

Key trigger points have also been identified. It appears that by treating key trigger points, satellite trigger points may also be reduced or eliminated.[13, 14] Key trigger points are listed in Table 6.1.

WHAT CAUSES TRIGGER POINTS?

A number of theories have been proposed to explain possible causes of myofascial trigger points. However the pathogenesis of myofascial pain syndrome remains unclear. Simons et al[2] posited a perpetuating cylce of damage to small blood vessels and release of proinflammatory substances like serotonin and histamines which in turn further sensitised pain receptors in the region. The pain cycle could be initiated by any stimulus that acts directly or indirectly on the area containing the trigger point (e.g. direct trauma, strain, fatigue, heat, cold, nerve root irritation, visceral dysfunction, emotional factors, chronic conditions or overuse). The *injury pool theory*[2] suggested that trigger points are activated when these trigger events combine with other predisposing factors (see below). Today, it is generally thought that trigger points develop from muscle overload (e.g. from sustained or low-level repeated muscle contractions, eccentric contractions, or maximal/submaximal concentric contractions) or from direct trauma.[11]

Perpetuating factors of trigger points

- Mechanical stresses (e.g. skeletal asymmetry, poor lifting techniques, poor posture, prolonged immobility)
- Nutritional inadequacies (low level of vitamins B_1, B_6, B_{12}, and C, folic acid, calcium, potassium, iron)
- Metabolic and endocrine inadequacies (thyroid underactivity, hyperuricaemia, hypoglycaemia) or any impairment to muscle metabolism (anaemia, hypoxia)
- Psychological factors
- Chronic infection
- Allergy, impaired sleep, radiculopathy, chronic visceral disease

(adapted from Fritz et al[10])

The *integrated hypothesis* is a currently accepted explanation of the pathogenesis of trigger points. It is summarised by Eloqayli[15] as follows:

> *Trigger points are triggered by dysfunction in the neuromuscular unit with aberrant post-synaptic sodium channel mediated action potential generation and abnormal calcium and ATP homeostasis with persistent sarcomere shortening. The sustained localized contractile activity causes local ischemia and hypoxia with cell injury and metabolic alterations that lead to the release of sensitizing inflammatory and pain mediators. These mediators lead to pain by activation of nociceptors (pain receptors) and also lead to autonomic modulation that potentiate abnormal acetylcholine release. Sustaining triggers point need sustained acetylcholine activity.*

There have been a number of studies demonstrating physiological changes at trigger point sites. For example, abnormal spontaneous electrical activity, spike activity and local twitch responses at trigger point sites have been reported.[16, 17] Moraska et al[18] found that trigger point release massage of an active myofascial trigger point affected anaerobic metabolism: there was an increase in dialysate lactate without change in nutritive blood flow or dialysate glucose. Several studies suggest that referred pain and local twitch responses are related to nerve degeneration and disintegration of motor and sensory nerves in the spinal cord. A study by Chang et al[19] found evidence of neuroaxonal degeneration and neuromuscular transmission disorders in trigger point muscles of 23 myofascial pain syndrome patients.

IDENTIFYING TRIGGER POINTS

Likely trigger points are often identified during history (e.g. by descriptions of the nature of pain, location of pain in referral pattern, onset) and confirmed by physical examination. Reliability of physical examination for the presence of trigger points is as yet unconfirmed because of the lack of high-quality studies.[20] A systematic review investigating interrater agreement of manual palpation for identification of myofascial trigger points found moderate agreement and that agreement was higher for experienced examiners.[21]

CHARACTERISTICS OF TRIGGER POINTS

Symptoms

- Deep, dull aching pain
- Pain referred in a specific pattern that is characteristic of each trigger point
- Activated directly by acute overload, overwork, fatigue, trauma, chilling
- Activated indirectly by disease, arthritic joints, emotional stress
- Vary in irritability from hour to hour and day to day
- Symptoms long outlast the precipitating event
- Occasionally autonomic reactions (e.g. sweating, local vasoconstriction, lacrimation, coryza, salivation, pilomotor activity) and proprioceptive disturbances (e.g. dizziness and tinnitus)
- Affected muscles are shortened and weakened

Signs

- Flat or pincer palpation identifies trigger points (circumscribed spots of exquisite tenderness in taut bands of muscle)
- Pressure on an active trigger point usually elicits a jump sign (i.e. the client quickly pulls away when the trigger point is palpated)
- Snapping palpation (rapid movement across the muscle so that fibres snap back) frequently evokes a local twitch response
- Skin sometimes evinces dermographia (elevations or wheals caused by scratching the skin) or panniculosis (sensitive thickenings or nodules in the subcutaneous tissue) in the area overlying trigger points

Strategies to identify trigger points are summarised in Table 6.2.

TREATING TRIGGER POINTS

The most important consideration in the treatment of trigger points is eliminating or reducing causative or aggravating factors. If the aetiology is not addressed, the trigger point may be temporarily deactivated but is likely to recur. When trigger points were first described, Travell and Simons recommended two options for reducing trigger points: (1) injecting trigger points with local anaesthetics, followed by muscle stretching, or (2) spraying the skin overlying the trigger point referral pattern with a vapocoolant spray (see Simons et al[2] and Travell and Simons[3] for directions for spraying specific muscles). Most treatment options that have been developed for trigger points since the 1950s still maintain the original two-phase procedure: (1) hyperstimulation analgesia and counter-irritation to break the pain cycle and (2) stretching the affected muscle to realign the muscle fibres. The following treatment methods are used in a range of practices including physiotherapy, chiropractic, osteopathy, acupuncture, general practice and remedial massage:

1. Injection and stretch. Injection with local anaesthetic, corticosteroids, botulinum A toxin, sterile water and sterile saline followed by stretching of the affected muscle.
2. Vapocoolant spray (e.g. ethyl chloride) and stretch. Spray from the trigger point towards the pain referral zone in a slow sweep (up to 6 seconds) covering the full length of the zone, then stretch the affected muscle. Spray in slow sweeps over the entire width of the muscle, maintaining the passive stretch. Repeat this until the full range of motion of the muscle group is reached, re-warming the area with moist heat at least every three repetitions. Avoid prolonged exposure to the spray and overstretching. This technique was considered by Simons et al[2] to be the most effective non-invasive method to deactivate trigger points.
3. Ice/ice massage (see Chapter 3).
4. Acupuncture. Chou et al[23] studied the effect of acupuncture on pain referred from trigger points and recorded reductions in both subjective reports of pain intensity and changes in endplate noise amplitude in the trigger point region of the upper trapezius during and after acupuncture treatment.
5. Electrical stimulation (e.g. transcutaneous electrical were stimulation (TENS) electrodes are placed at the trigger point site or along the referred pain zone).
6. Muscle energy and other remedial massage techniques. Remedial massage therapists sometimes use muscle energy techniques, positional release and direct muscle manipulation methods such as cross-fibre frictions (see Chapter 4) and a variety of muscle-stretching techniques. Such techniques are particularly useful for trigger points which are not easily accessible (e.g. trigger points in iliopsoas and subscapularis).
7. Dry needling. In this technique an acupuncture needle is inserted into a trigger point. The trigger point is needled many times to elicit a local twitch response and reproduce the patient's symptoms. The needle can remain inserted for 2 minutes.[24] Dr Ma's[25] technique involves inserting a one-inch 32-gauge acupuncture needle perpendicularly through subcutaneous tissue until a density change is encountered. The needle is 'bounced on the muscle' at a rate of 1–3 times per second until the tissues soften. Recent studies suggest that dry needling a primary trigger point may inhibit activity in satellite trigger points situated in the zones of pain referral.[13, 14]

Table 6.2 Identifying trigger points

History	History of onset usually related to trauma or overload of affected muscle.	Patients are rarely aware of the existence of trigger points. They experience pain and/or other symptoms.
	Nature of pain ■ deep, steady, aching ■ varies from hour to hour and day to day ■ outlasts initial event.	Active trigger points produce steady, deep, aching pain. The pain is rarely felt as a burning pain. Occasionally it is described as sharp, lancing pain. (Compare prickling pain, numbness or paraesthesia of peripheral nerve entrapment/nerve root irritation; throbbing pain of vascular origin.)
	Location of pain Characteristic pain referral pattern.	Referred pain differentiates trigger point pain from fibromyalgia and other tender points. Referred pain does not coincide with dermatological or neuronal distributions. Pain usually accompanies muscle function change.
	Muscle function Restricted range of motion. Affected muscle feels tight or weak.	
Physical examination	Palpation Focus of exquisite tenderness in taut band identified by flat or pincer palpation (Figure 6.1). Trigger points tend to be located centrally in the bellies of muscles or at the attachments of muscles.	Trigger points are located in hypertonic muscle fibres. They are common in the neck, shoulder and lower back muscles. Palpation of taut bands requires practice. Less experienced practitioners may need to rely on clients' identification of exquisite pain sites and pain referral patterns until they develop their palpation skills.
	Digital pressure on the trigger point reproduces the client's symptoms.	
	Jump sign.	The client flinches and pulls away from pain; the reaction is out of proportion to the pressure applied.
	Local twitch response when the taut band is snapped near the site of the trigger point.	Brisk contraction of muscle fibres in and around the taut band.
	There can be autonomic signs.	For example, increased vasomotor activity, changes in skin temperature, erythema of overlying skin, lacrimation, coryza, sweating, goose bumps.[22]
	Resisted and length tests for affected muscles.	Affected muscles may have altered length and strength.

8. Direct manual ischaemic compression. Pressure is applied to the trigger point with increasing intensity and maintained until the patient reports a significant reduction in pain or the practitioner palpates a release of the taut band of muscle. After the digital pressure is released, the muscle is stretched.

MANUAL TECHNIQUES

Since the identification of central and attachment trigger points[2] it has become apparent that each requires a different treatment approach. The traditional manual techniques that were previously used to treat all trigger points are now recommended for central trigger points only. Such deep techniques may inflame or irritate tissues near attachment trigger points and cold applications are now recommended for attachment trigger points. A treatment protocol including currently recommended trigger point treatments is presented in Table 6.3. Trigger point therapy should be integrated into a short-term treatment plan that may focus on relieving symptoms and a long-term treatment plan that tries to address the underlying causes.

Typically, Swedish massage is applied to the area before specific trigger points are treated. Remedial massage thera-

pists have commonly used direct ischaemic pressure on the trigger point followed by specific muscle stretching. Steady pressure is applied using the thumb, fingers, elbow or knuckle to the trigger point to within the client's pain tolerance (between 4 and 7 on a pain scale of 0 to 10) for up to 60 seconds. The pressure can be gradually increased until the client reports a 7 or 8 out of 10 on the pain scale, maintaining pressure until the client reports a reduction to 3 or 4 and then increasing the pressure again up to 7 or 8. This process is repeated up to three times or until the therapist feels a tissue change in the trigger point area. Using variable pressure prevents further irritation to the trigger point. The trigger point is pressed onto the underlying bone, or if there is no underlying bone (e.g. sternocleidomastoid muscle), the trigger point can be squeezed using a pincer grip[a]. The aim is to cause mechanical disruption of sensory nerve endings that contribute to trigger point activity. Other authors suggest that pressure need only be sufficient to release contracted sarcomeres and that heavy ischaemic pressure is not required.[2]

---

[a]Special caution is required when treating trigger points in the sternocleidomastoid muscle because of the proximity of the carotid artery, jugular vein, cervical and brachial plexuses, and cervical lymph nodes.

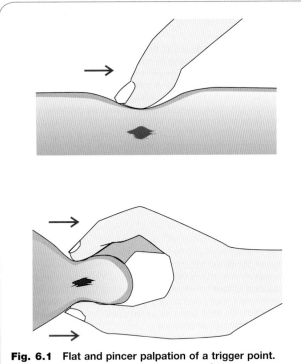

Fig. 6.1 Flat and pincer palpation of a trigger point.
Adapted from Simons, Travell and Simons.[2]

After pressure has been applied to the trigger points in a muscle group, the muscles are gradually stretched to their full range of motion.[8] Most sources describe passive stretching following the hyperstimulation phase of treatment. As discussed in Chapter 2, use active stretching wherever possible before passive stretching. An overview of a remedial massage treatment that incorporates myofascial trigger point therapy is presented in Table 6.3.

Save your body

A lot of strain can be placed on therapists' joints and muscles during sustained ischaemic compression. McMahon et al[26] found that 65% of physiotherapists who responded to a survey had experienced thumb problems at some stage during their working lives. Trigger point therapy was reported as one of the factors that were significantly associated with thumb problems. Vary the contact (use your thumbs sometimes, knuckles and elbows at other times) and avoid flexion and extension, especially of metacarpophalangeal joints or interphalangeal joints when applying pressure (see Figure 6.2). Some therapists use a rubber-capped T-bar made of wood, plastic or metal to save their hands. Another study compared muscle load to the shoulder using three different trigger point therapy techniques: digital ischaemic pressure using a single hand contact, a double hand contact and a treatment tool. The authors found that using the treatment tool decreased the muscle load to the shoulder of the contact arm although they were unable to comment on where the load was redistributed.[27]

Some key trigger points and their associated muscle stretches are illustrated in Appendix 6.1.

Fig. 6.2 (a) incorrect, and (b) and (c) correct ergonomics for intermittent, (c) digital pressure

Table 6.3 Remedial massage treatment of myofascial trigger points

1. Swedish massage	Massage the whole muscle, muscle group or region.	Improves circulation (increased oxygenation, removal of waste products); increases awareness of the body's adaptations to external and internal stressors, locates taut bands in muscles, relaxes the client.
2. Apply a range of remedial massage techniques		
i) *Trigger point techniques* Treat key trigger points first	Usually only two or three and not more than five trigger points are treated at any one time. Treat the most painful, the most medial and the most proximal trigger points first. Key trigger points are closest to the head and to the midline.[8]	Deactivating key trigger points may also deactivate or reduce satellite and attachment trigger points.
Treat central trigger points before attachment trigger points.	A range of massage techniques can be used to treat central trigger points including: *Intermittent digital pressure*	Apply gradually increasing pressure to 7 or 8 out of 10 on the pain scale, maintain the pressure until the client reports 3 or 4 out of 10, then gradually increase the pressure to 7 or 8 again. Repeat the process up to three times. Note: There is no need for heavy ischaemic pressure (only sufficient pressure to release contracted sarcomeres).[2]
	Gliding massage techniques from the muscle belly out towards the muscle attachments.	To lengthen shortened sarcomeres in the belly of the muscle and reduce tension on muscle attachments.
	Mild stretching	Full range of motion stretches could irritate attachment trigger points. Newly activated trigger points can be deactivated by slow passive stretching.[2, 28]
	Thermotherapy	Heat packs to the affected muscles.
	Deep stroking or stripping massage over the trigger point area.[2]	Deep gliding along the line of the fibres and then cross-fibre frictions,[24] 6-12 strokes per trigger point.[29] Thought to be the most effective direct manual treatment.[2]
	Other techniques including joint mobilisation, friction massage, myofascial release, lymphatic drainage massage.	Joint mobilisation has been recommended in the management of trigger points based on indicators that muscle sensitivity reduced after spinal manipulation.[30]
		Avoid deep pressure or friction as it could aggravate surrounding tissues.
Treat attachment trigger points.	Ice massage Short 20-30 second cold applications.[8]	
Return muscle to its normal resting length.	Regardless of the method used to deactivate the trigger point, restoring the normal resting length of the muscle is recommended.[8]	Gradual, gentle, pain-free stretching (especially muscle energy techniques and myofascial release).
ii) *Apply a range of remedial massage techniques to eliminate perpetuating factors where possible.*	Techniques to correct or reduce mechanical factors predisposing to trigger points: (e.g. postural stresses, muscle contractures, joint dysfunction).	Trigger points are a culmination of a number of events. Find and correct the cause if possible. Trigger point treatment techniques can permanently eliminate pain cycles. However, if the cause is remote, such as a visceral or emotional cause, a new stream of noxious stimuli can reactivate the trigger.
3. Client education	Action to eliminate perpetuating factors.	For example, if psychological stress is a perpetuating factor then the client might benefit from referral to a counsellor, yoga teacher or for a course of relaxation massage.
	Advise clients about causes including mechanical stress (e.g. prolonged immobilisation, inadequate training for sport) and systemic factors (e.g. metabolic and endocrine dysfunction, chronic infection, dietary insufficiencies especially vitamin B_{12}, folic acid, vitamin C and iron[2], psychological stress).	
	Home exercise program.	Exercises to stretch and strengthen the affected muscle(s) as required.

EVIDENCE-BASE FOR TRIGGER POINTS

Vernon and Schneider[31] conducted a literature review and summarised the evidence for myofascial trigger point therapy as follows:

- Manipulation and ischaemic pressure for immediate pain relief at trigger points is supported by moderately strong evidence. Long-term pain relief is supported by limited evidence.
- The use of laser therapy for treating myofascial trigger points and myofascial pain syndrome has strong support in the literature.
- Moderate evidence supports the use of electrical nerve stimulation, acupuncture and magnet therapy for treating myofascial trigger points and myofascial pain syndrome.
- The use of electrical muscle stimulation, high-voltage galvanic stimulation, interferential current and frequency-modulated neural stimulation for treating myofascial trigger points and myofascial pain syndrome is supported by limited evidence.
- The use of ultrasound therapy for treating myofascial trigger points and myofascial pain syndrome is supported by weak evidence.

There have been a number of systematic reviews of the effectiveness of myofascial trigger points for a range of conditions. Many were unable to draw definitive conclusions because few high quality trials have been conducted. For example, Denneny et al[32] conducted a systematic review of 19 randomised controlled trials and were unable to recommend trigger point therapy for non-cancer pain because the evidence was weak. Another review found few randomised controlled trials evaluating the effectiveness of manual therapy in the treatment of myofascial pain syndrome and could neither support nor refuted its effectiveness.[33]

Dry needling has been the focus of much research. A systematic review and meta-analysis of seven randomised controlled trials on acupuncture and dry needling in the management of myofascial trigger points found limited evidence: one study found that deep needling directly into trigger points had an overall treatment effect when compared to standardised treatment.[34] Another meta-analysis found that dry needling was better than other interventions and sham therapy for orofacial pain intensity but the quality of evidence was low and the effect size small.[35]

CONTRAINDICATIONS AND PRECAUTIONS

As well as the usual contraindications of massage therapy (e.g. acute inflammation, moles, varicose veins, breast tissue, pregnancy, rheumatoid arthritis), the following special considerations apply when using trigger point therapy:

- The heaviness of digital ischaemic pressure makes it unsuitable for clients with osteoporosis. The technique must be adapted to the size, age and level of fitness of the client.
- Resistance stretching techniques (see Chapter 5) are unsuitable for hypertensive clients.
- Potentially painful massage (including trigger point therapy) has been associated with increased blood pressure and should be avoided in hypertensive clients.[36]
- Muscle stretches, including home exercise programs, must make allowance for age and levels of fitness.
- Where a trigger point is maintaining joint stability in a hypermobile client, a strengthening program may need to be introduced before deactivation of the trigger point.[8]

KEY MESSAGES

- Trigger point therapy is widely used in the treatment of myofascial pain. One current hypothesis about the pathogenesis of trigger points suggests that they are activated by a dysfunctional neuromuscular unit that is associated with an aberrant action potential, calcium and ATP homeostasis and sarcomere shortening. This sustained contractile activity injures the cell, triggering inflammatory and pain mediators. Nociceptor activation and autonomic modulation causes sustained acetylcholine release that sustains the trigger point.[15]
- Trigger points are identified by client history (e.g. deep dull aching pain, pain referral pattern, variability of symptoms) and physical assessment including muscle function tests, palpation (e.g. a hyperirritable and very painful spot in a taut band of muscle) and by eliciting the jump sign and local twitch response.
- Treatment techniques for trigger points include spray and stretch, dry needling, and a range of manual techniques. Treat central trigger points with intermittent digital pressure (or deep gliding, cross-fibre friction, thermotherapy, etc). Attachment trigger points require 20–30-second cold applications. Follow the deactivation of trigger points with gentle pain-free stretching.
- Eliminating key trigger points may also deactivate their associated satellite trigger points. Treat key trigger points first.
- Treat the most painful, the most medial and the most proximal trigger points first.
- Address predisposing or contributing factors to prevent reactivation of trigger points.
- Intermittent digital pressure is suitable for most clients; digital ischaemic pressure is contraindicated in osteoporotic and hypertensive clients.

Review questions

1. What is the difference between an active trigger point and a tender point in a tight band of muscle? List five distinguishing features.
2. What is the difference between an active trigger point and a latent trigger point?

3. List five perpetuating factors of trigger points. Discuss the impact of perpetuating factors on treatment.
4. Draw an X on the following diagrams to indicate the locations of trigger point(s) in each of the following muscles.

i) Levator scapulae

ii) Upper trapezius

iii) Iliopsoas

iv) Piriformis

Continued

Review questions—cont'd

5. On the following diagrams, draw in the pain referral patterns for the trigger points indicated.

i) Quadratus lumborum

ii) Infraspinatus

iii) Rhomboids

iv) Sternocleidomastoid

Review questions—cont'd

6. Draw a stretch of (or otherwise describe a stretch for) the following muscles:
   i) Erector spinae muscles
   ii) Upper trapezius muscle
   iii) Piriformis
7. What is the proposed effect of a trigger point on the function of a muscle?
8. What is the difference between digital ischaemic pressure and intermittent digital pressure?
9. How is a twitch response elicited?
10. Give two examples of autonomic signs associated with the presence of a trigger point.
11. What is a key trigger point? Give an example of a key trigger point and its associated satellite trigger points.
12. A client is found to have trigger points in the right piriformis, gastrocnemius and hamstring muscles. If all three trigger points are described as equally painful, in what order would you treat these trigger points?
13. Briefly describe your treatment for:
    a) a central trigger point in the upper trapezius
    b) an attachment trigger point in the hamstring muscles.

APPENDIX 6.1
Some key trigger points

Muscle	Trigger point	Stretch
Sternocleidomastoid		
Upper trapezius		

Continued

Muscle	Trigger point			Stretch

Scalenes

Splenius capitis

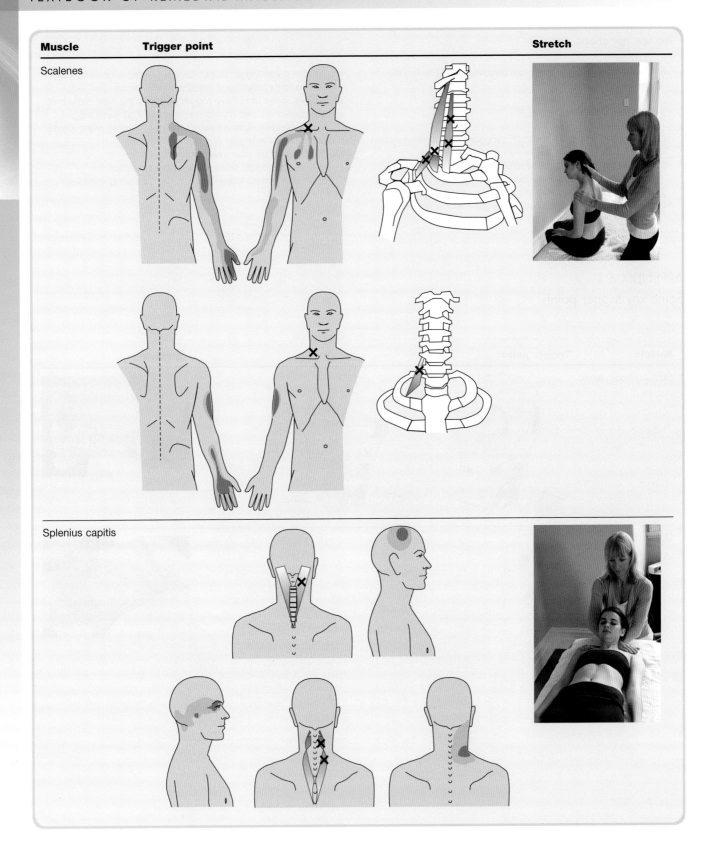

Muscle	Trigger point		Stretch
Supraspinatus			

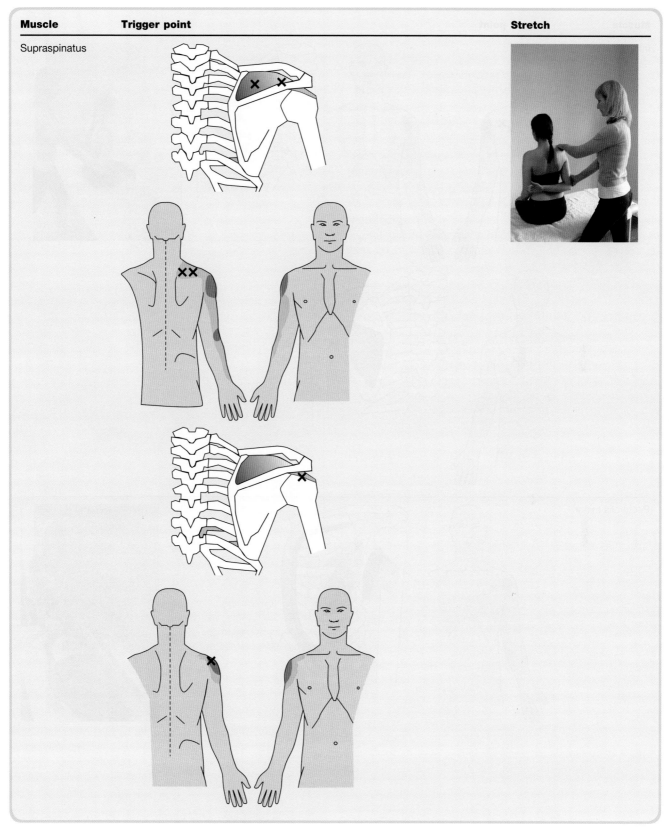

Continued

Muscle	Trigger point			Stretch

Infraspinatus

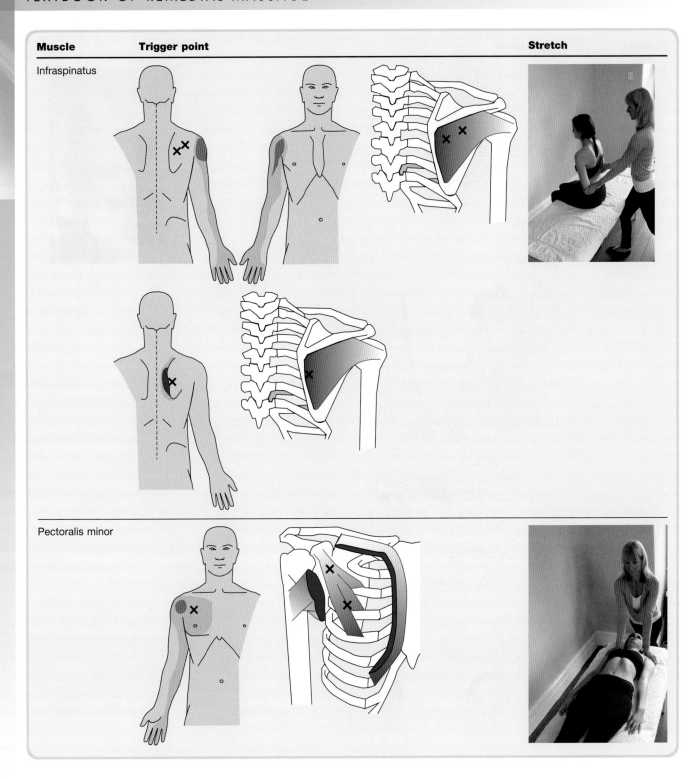

Pectoralis minor

Muscle	Trigger point			Stretch

Latissimus dorsi

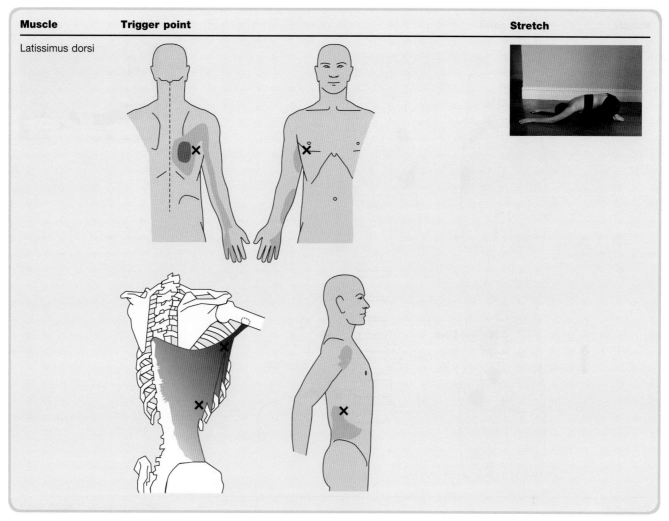

Continued

Muscle	Trigger point	Stretch
Quadratus lumborum		
Piriformis		

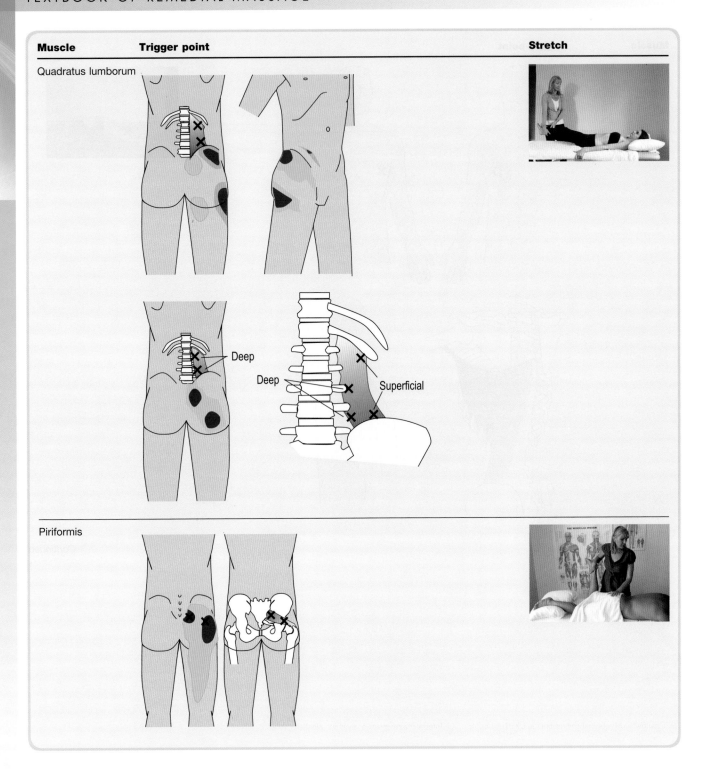

Muscle	Trigger point	Stretch

Hamstrings

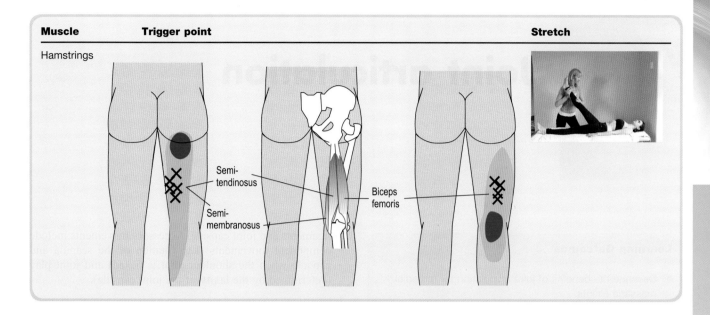

Semi-
tendinosus

Semi-
membranosus

Biceps
femoris

REFERENCES

1. Travell J, Rinzler S. The myofascial genesis of pain. Postgrad Med 1952;11(5):424–34.
2. Simons D, Travell J, Simons L. Myofascial pain and dysfunction: the trigger point manual. Vol 1: Upper half of body. 2nd edn. Philadelphia: Williams and Wilkins; 1999.
3. Travell J, Simons D. Myofascial pain and dysfunction: the trigger point manual. Philadelphia: Lippincott Williams and Wilkins; 1993.
4. Offenbacher M, Stucki G. Physical therapy in the treatment of fibromyalgia. Scand J Rheumatol Suppl [Review] 2000;113:78–85.
5. Dorsher PT, Dorsher PT. Myofascial referred-pain data provide physiologic evidence of acupuncture meridians. J Pain 2009;10(7):723–31.
6. Peng ZF. Comparison between western trigger point of acupuncture and traditional acupoints. Zhongguo zhenjiu. [Comparative Study English Abstract] 2008; 28(5):349–52.
7. Chen D, Yang G, Wang F, et al. Discussing the relationship among the ashi point, tender point and myofascial trigger point. Zhongguo zhenjiu 2017;12; 37(2):212–14. Doi: 10.13703/j.0255-2930.2017. 02.031.
8. Chaitow L, Fritz S. A massage therapist's guide to understanding, locating and treating myofascial trigger points. Edinburgh: Churchill Livingstone, 2006.
9. Chaitow L. Myofascial trigger points. UK: Health Education. Online. Available: http://leonchaitow.com/ trigger_point_videos/; 2014.
10. Fritz S, Chaitow L, Hymel GM. Clinical massage in the healthcare setting. St Louis, MI: Mosby Elsevier; 2008.
11. Bron C, Dommerholt J. Etiology of myofascial trigger points. Curr Pain Headache R 2012;16(439–44).
12. Perreault T, Dunning J, Butts R. The local twitch response during trigger point dry needling: is it necessary for successful outcomes? J Bodyw Mov Ther 2017;21:940–7.
13. Tsai C, Hsieh L, Kuan T, et al. Remote effects of dry needling on the irritability of the myofascial trigger point in the upper trapezius muscle. Am J Phys Med Rehabil 2010;89(2):133–40.
14. Hsieh Y, Kao M, Kuan T, et al. Dry needling to a key myofascial trigger point may reduce the irritability of satellite MTrPs. Am J Phys Med Rehabil 2007;86(5):397–403.
15. Eloqayli H. Subcutaneous accessory pain system (SAPS): a novel pain pathway for myofascial trigger points. Med Hypotheses 2018;111:55–7.
16. Chung J, Ohrbach R, McCall W. Characteristics of electrical activity in trapezius muscles with myofascial pain. Neurophysiol Clinic 2006; 117:2459–66.
17. Kuan T, Hsieh Y, Chen S, et al. The myofascial trigger point region: correlation between the degree of irritability and the prevalence of endplate noise. Am J Phys Med Rehabil 2007;86:183–9.
18. Moraska A, Hickner R, Rzasa-Lynn R, et al. Increase in lactate without change in nutritive blood flow or glucose at active trigger points following massage: a randomized clinical trial. Arch Phys Med Rehabil 2018;99:2151–9.
19. Chang CW, Chen YR, Chang KF, et al. Evidence of neuroaxonal degeneration in myofascial pain syndrome: a study of neuromuscular jitter by axonal microstimulation. Eur J Pain 2008;12(8): 1026–30.
20. Lucas N, Macaskill P, Irwig L, et al. Reliability of physical examination for diagnosis of myofascial trigger points: a systematic review of the literature. Clin J Pain 2009;25(1):80–9.
21. Rathbone ATL, Grosman-Rimon L, Kumbhare DA. Interrater agreement of manual palpation for identification of myofascial trigger points: a systematic review and meta-analysis. Clin J Pain 2017;33(8):715–29.
22. Lavelle ED, Lavelle W, Smith HS, et al. Myofascial trigger points. Anesthesiol Clin [Review] 2007; 25(4):841–51.
23. Chou LW, Hsieh YL, Kao MJ, et al. Remote influences of acupuncture on the pain intensity and the amplitude changes of endplate noise in the myofascial trigger point of the upper trapezius muscle. Arch Phys Med Rehabil [Randomized Controlled Trial] 2009;90(6):905–12.
24. Niel-Asher S. Concise book of trigger points. 3rd edn. Berkeley, CA: North Atlantic; 2014.
25. Ma Y-t. Biomedical acupuncture for sports and trauma rehabilitation: dry needling technique. St Louis, MI: Elsevier; 2011.
26. McMahon M, Stiller K, Trott P, et al. The prevalence of thumb problems in Australian physiotherapists is high: an observational study. Aust J Physiother 2006;52(4):287–92.
27. Smith EK, Magarey M, Argue S, et al. Muscular load to the therapist's shoulder during three alternative techniques for trigger point therapy. J Bodywork Mov Ther [Clinical Trial] 2009; 13(2):171–81.
28. Lewitt K. Manipulation in rehabilitation of the motor system. 3rd edn. London: Butterworths; 1999.
29. Davies C. The trigger point therapy workbook. 2nd edn. Oakland, CA: New Harbinger Publications; 2013.
30. Fernandez-de-Las-Penas C, Alonso-Blanco C, Cuadrado ML, et al. Are manual therapies effective in reducing pain from tension-type headache?: a systematic review. Clin J Pain 2006;22(3): 278–85.
31. Vernon H, Schneider M. Chiropractic management of myofascial trigger points and myofascial pain syndrome: a systematic review of the literature. J Manipulative Physiol Ther 2009; 32(1):14–24.
32. Denneny D, Frawley H, Petersen K, et al. Trigger point manual therapy for the treatment of chronic non-cancer pain in adults: a systematic review and meta-analysis. Arch Phys Med Rehabil 2019;100(3): 562–77.
33. de las Penas CF, Sohrbeck Campo M, Fernandez Carnero J, et al. Manual therapies in myofascial trigger point treatment: a systematic review. J Bodyw Mov Ther 2005; 9(1):27–34.
34. Tough EA, White AR, Cummings TM, et al. Acupuncture and dry needling in the management of myofascial trigger point pain: a systematic review and meta-analysis of randomised controlled trials. Eur J Pain 2009;13(1):3–10.
35. Vier C, de Almeida M, Neves M, et al. The effectiveness of dry needling for patients with orofacial pain associated with temporomandibular dysfunction: a systematic review and meta-analysis. Brazil J Phys Ther 2019;23(1):3–11.
36. Cambron JA, Dexheimer J, Coe P. Changes in blood pressure after various forms of therapeutic massage: a preliminary study. J Altern Complement Med 2006;12(1):65–70.

7

Joint articulation

INTRODUCTION

As part of a remedial massage treatment, articulations of joints are designed to improve range of motion and to reduce pain or other symptoms generated from joint dysfunction. Passive joint articulations move joints beyond their active range of motion until an elastic barrier is reached (see Figure 7.1 on p 95).[1] Such manoeuvres are distinct from manipulative techniques which are thought to overcome the elastic barrier but remain within the limit of anatomical integrity. As with all remedial massage techniques there are some clients for whom joint articulation is not suitable and it is important to assess the particular joint for indications and contraindications before performing the technique. Joint articulation and mobilisation techniques are widely used among manual therapists to treat mobility restrictions and pain.[2]

WHAT IS JOINT ARTICULATION?

Joint articulation involves the practitioner moving a joint through its ranges of motion without active participation on the client's part. Joint movement is described as:

- Physiological; that is, movements that clients can perform themselves. The ranges of motion that are possible for physiological movements are determined by concentric or eccentric muscle contractions.
- Accessory; that is, movements within the joints that are necessary for normal activities but that cannot be performed actively by the client. Accessory movements represent the movement permitted by the articulating surfaces,

ligaments and joint capsule. Accessory movements include component movements (e.g. rotation of the scapula and clavicle when the shoulder joint is flexed) and joint play (determined by the laxity of the joint capsule).

Joint articulation uses accessory movements to improve range of motion and decrease pain. They are specific for each joint. The joint surfaces are slowly moved through an increased range of motion by gentle traction or by slow pressure. The movement can be stopped by the client at any stage. The practitioner attempts to restore normal movement within the joint and normal load to muscles which have been sustained in a shortened or lengthened position.

EVIDENCE FOR THE EFFECTIVENESS OF JOINT ARTICULATION AND MOBILISATION

Joint mobilisation is often included in clinical practice guidelines which are based on the best available evidence.[3, 4] Many studies have investigated multimodal therapeutic approaches that included joint mobilisation. For example, a clinical practice guideline from the Canadian Chiropractic Guideline Initiative on the conservative management of low back pain recommended spinal manipulative therapy and other commonly used treatments including joint mobilisation or both in addition to advice (posture and to stay active) and reassurance.[5] In fact, guidelines for chronic musculoskeletal conditions commonly recommend multimodal therapies, including manual therapies like myofascial therapy, joint mobilisation, spinal manipulative therapy and massage along with usual medical care.[5, 6]

A number of studies have compared the effectiveness of individual components of manual therapy or combinations of them. For example, Ferreira et al[7] compared spinal manipulation (n = 77) including spinal manipulative therapy and joint mobilisation (directed to the lumbopelvic region for up to a maximum of 12 visits) with motor control exercise (n = 73) and general exercise (n = 74) in patients with low back pain of more than 3 months' duration. The authors found that motor control exercise, spinal manipulative therapy and joint mobilisation had slightly better short-term effects than general exercise. Pain relief was most effective within the first 6 months, and functional improvement was most effective at 1 month. A comparison of 'thrust' versus 'non-thrust' mobilisation of the thoracic spine in clients with neck pain by Cleland et al[8] found significantly greater short-term reductions in pain and disability in the thrust group. A systematic review investigating

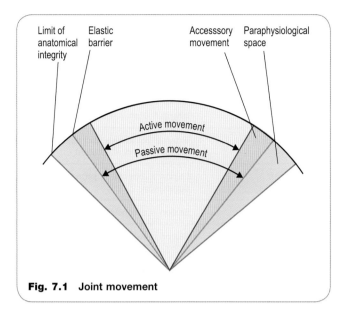

Limit of anatomical integrity

Elastic barrier

Accesssory movement

Paraphysiological space

Active movement

Passive movement

Fig. 7.1 Joint movement

the effectiveness of manual therapy, consisting of deep massage, myofascial release or joint mobilisation, in treating plantar heel pain found that soft tissue mobilisation was an effective modality for treating plantar heel pain.[9] Another trial reported that massage and mobilisation of the feet and ankles made a significant improvement in the balance of 28 elderly adults compared with a placebo.[10] Further studies are needed to evaluate the short- and long-term effect of different soft tissue mobilisation techniques.

The effectiveness of joint mobilisation alone has also been evaluated for specific conditions. For example, Jayaseelan et al[11] conducted a systematic review on the effects of joint mobilisation on people with patellofemoral pain syndrome. The authors found that it was most effective in improving pain and function when used in combination with other therapies, thereby supporting multimodal therapeutic approaches. Another study examining joint mobilisations for the treatment of conditions of the elbow, wrist and hand found moderate evidence for its inclusion in the treatment of lateral epicondylalgia and limited support for joint mobilisations in the treatment of wrist and hand conditions.[12] Intensive passive mobilisation techniques in end-range positions were found to be more effective in improving glenohumeral joint mobility and reducing disability than passive mobilisations performed within the pain-free range for clients with adhesive capsulitis.[13] In a study evaluating therapy interventions for improving range of motion in the upper limb, joint mobilisation along with a supervised exercise program and splinting were found to be effective.[14]

The use of joint mobilisation in the treatment of unstable joints requires careful focus on restricted motion. In a study by Cruz-Diaz et al,[15] 90 people with a history of recurrent ankle sprain showed improvement in ankle range of motion, postural control, and self-reported instability following sessions of ankle dorsiflexion mobilisation which is often restricted after ankle sprain. The authors concluded that joint mobilisation accompanied by active movement could be a valuable tool for restoring ankle function in clients with a history of recurrent ankle sprain.

ASSESSING CLIENTS FOR TREATMENT

A number of assessment procedures are used to determine the suitability of clients for remedial massage, the types of tissue(s) to be treated, and the application of specific techniques (see Chapter 2). Assessing clients' suitability for treatment with joint articulation includes history, passive range of motion (PROM) testing and palpation. Findings from all assessments should be integrated and used to guide the treatment plan.

HISTORY

Case history enables practitioners to identify red flags of potentially serious medical conditions requiring referral including:

- Fractures (history of trauma, history of minor trauma if over 50 years or osteoporotic or taking corticosteroid medication, excessive pain, obvious deformity)
- Cancer (past history of malignancy, age over 50 years, failure to improve with treatment, unexplained weight loss, pain at multiple sites, pain at rest)
- Infections (fever, malaise, risk factors for infection including underlying disease process or immunosuppression)

Ask questions to determine whether the pain is mechanical (e.g. pain aggravated by activity, relieved by rest, associated with morning stiffness). Be vigilant for systemic conditions that may present with joint pain including:

- Ankylosing spondylitis (axial spondyloarthritis): A chronic inflammatory disorder that mainly affects the sacroiliac joints and spine and leads to ankylosis. It usually begins between 15 and 35 years of age and is four times more common in men than women. Symptoms are worse after periods of inactivity. Night pain may be present.
- Fibromyalgia: A chronic pain condition characterised by generalised pain and muscle stiffness. Clients with fibromyalgia often complain of extreme fatigue and difficulty sleeping. The whole body becomes hypersensitive to pain. It is thought to be related to biochemical changes in the central nervous system, abnormal central processing of nociceptive pain or central sensitisation. It is sometimes confused with polymyalgia rheumatica, a type of arthritis with associated muscle symptoms.
- Gout: A group of metabolic conditions associated with urate crystal deposits leading to acute arthritis. The client is usually between 30 and 60 years; the ratio of males to females is 20 to 1. The most common presentation is an acutely inflamed joint, usually the first metatarsophalangeal joint.
- Psoriatic arthritis: An autoimmune disease associated with psoriasis and polyarthritis. The usual age of onset is 35 to 55 years. It is slightly more common in females than males. Digits of the hands and feet may be affected first. Between 2% and 10% of people with psoriasis develop psoriatic arthritis.
- Reiter's syndrome: A polyarthropathy with three main symptoms: conjunctivitis, urethritis and polyarthritis. The age of onset is 20 to 60 years, often following venereal acquired infection. The ratio of males to females is 15 to 1.

- Rheumatoid arthritis: This chronic autoimmune inflammatory disease usually begins in the proximal interphalangeal and metacarpophalangeal joints bilaterally and is characterised by symmetrical joint pain and swelling. Women are three times as likely to have rheumatoid arthritis than men and the usual age of onset is between 20 and 40 years of age.
- Systemic lupus erythematosus: A chronic autoimmune inflammatory disease that can affect every organ system of the body. The ratio of females to males is 20 to 1. It can occur at any age but most commonly between 30 and 50 years. It is associated with pleurisy, pericarditis, oral ulcers, arthritis, blood disorders, seizures and a malar (butterfly) rash over the cheeks and nose.[16]

Joint articulation is commonly used to manage joint pain and improve restricted range of motion in chronic phases of the above conditions.

FUNCTIONAL TESTS

Passive range of motion testing is the most important functional test for assessing joint function. Passive range of motion testing should always follow active range of motion testing which provides information about the client's functional movement and level of impairment (the See-Move-Touch principle described in Chapter 2). Ranges of motion are determined by the anatomical structure of the joint. When a joint becomes injured certain ranges of motion may become limited. If the joint capsule is tightened the limitation of movement is sometimes referred to as a capsular pattern (see Table 7.1). Capsular patterns are thought to indicate joint degeneration and may be associated with hard and leathery end-feels, although studies have questioned the validity of capsular patterns for the diagnosis of osteoarthritis.[17] A survey of UK physiotherapists found that the capsular pattern concept was commonly used in the diagnosis of contracted (frozen) shoulder although many respondents understood that to be restricted external rotation alone.[18]

PALPATION

Palpation is used to identify different types of end-feel including:

Hard end-feel

Hard end-feel describes the practitioner's palpatory sensation when a joint is stopped within its normal range by bony approximation, such as a foreign object inside the joint. This could be a piece of floating bone or cartilage or bony block which can occur with osteoarthritic changes in the joint.

Soft end-feel

Soft end-feel is palpated when joint range of motion is limited by inflammation, pain, excessive muscle mass or a soft tissue tumour.

Leathery end-feel

This is felt when joint range of motion is limited by ligament tightness or shortening.

Sometimes crackling sounds (crepitus) are associated with joint movement. It may be audible or felt as a grating

Table 7.1 Capsular patterns of major joints of the body

Joint	Capsular pattern of limitation of joint range of motion
Cervical spine	lateral flexion = rotation, extension
Lumbar spine	lateral flexion = rotation, extension
Shoulder joint	external rotation > abduction > flexion > internal rotation
Elbow joint	flexion > extension; pronation = supination
Wrist joint	flexion = extension
Metacarpophalangeal and interphalangeal joints	flexion > extension
Hip joint	flexion > internal rotation > abduction (order varies)
Knee joint	flexion > extension
Ankle joint (talotibial joint)	dorsiflexion = plantarflexion
Subtalar joint	inversion > eversion
Metatarsophalangeal joints (2nd–5th)	flexion > extension
Metatarsophalangeal joint (1st)	extension > flexion

sensation. It often occurs in osteoarthritis. It can be caused by approximation of bony surfaces and by loose particles or debris (e.g. small pieces of cartilage) in the joint. Crepitus may be a signal to discontinue the technique. Discontinue if pain is elicited as the techniques are performed.

TREATING CLIENTS

Relaxing the muscles around the joint is recommended before performing joint articulations. As an introductory procedure apply a general massage around the joint and related areas. Alternatively, the area may be warmed with a heat pack in preparation for joint articulation.

GUIDELINES[19]

- Place the joint in mid-range. In general, mid-range positions are loose-packed, that is the articulating surfaces are maximally separated and the joint has the greatest amount of free play. For example, the resting (loose-packed) position of the glenohumeral joint is 55° to 70° abduction and 30° horizontal adduction.
- Stabilise the body part.
- Your hands should be as close to the joint as possible.
- Usually the proximal bone is stabilised and the distal bone is mobilised.
- Work with gravity where possible.
- Work within the client's pain tolerance.

After treatment advise clients to avoid all aggravating conditions. Wearing shoes with good shock absorption and controlling body weight are advisable, especially for clients with low back or lower limb complaints. Range of motion exercises within pain tolerance should be encouraged and heat therapy may provide pain relief. A program of muscle stretching and strengthening can be introduced to improve muscle function. Refer clients for osseous manipulation, acupuncture and/or herbal/nutritional support as required.

If joint articulation is carried out after adequate warm-up and within the pain-tolerance then adverse effects are unlikely. If joint inflammation does occur after treatment, advise the client to use an ice pack and rest the joint for a day or two. If symptoms persist, refer clients for further investigation.

TECHNIQUES

The following terms are used to describe the practitioner's position with respect to the client.

- Cephalad: Towards the head
- Caudal: Towards the feet
- Ipsilateral: On the same side as the body part
- Contralateral: On the opposite side to the body part
- Primary Contact: The hand used to move a bone
- Secondary Contact: The hand used to stabilise a bone

1. Cervical spine

Articulation of the cervical vertebrae requires particular caution. It should only be performed after a full assessment of the cervical spine has been carried out (See-Move-Touch principle). Perform all articulations slowly and gently and stop immediately if the client experiences symptoms.

CERVICAL LATERAL FLEXION

This technique is contraindicated if active cervical lateral flexion produces symptoms or if there is a history of disc lesions or neurological symptoms.

With the client supine, stand at the head of the table. Place one hand on the client's shoulder; the other hand is placed horizontally under the occiput. Apply gentle pressure to anchor the shoulder and slowly laterally flex the client's neck towards the opposite shoulder. This is best achieved if you lunge to the opposite side and keep knuckles in contact with the table to avoid cervical flexion. Hold for 5 seconds and repeat on the other side (see Figure 7.2).

CERVICAL ROTATION

This technique is contraindicated if active cervical rotation produces symptoms or if there is a history of disc lesions or neurological symptoms.

With the client supine, stand or sit at the head of the table. Hold the side of the client's head with one hand and slowly and gently rotate the head and neck as far as the client can move comfortably to one side. Hold the rotation for 5 seconds and then repeat on the other side (Figure 7.3).

CERVICAL EXTENSION

The client is supine. Sit at the head of the table. Begin at the lower cervical spine. Using index fingers of both hands placed either side of the spinous processes, gently and slowly lift

Fig. 7.2 Cervical lateral flexion

Fig. 7.3 Cervical rotation

fingers anteriorly so that the head and neck extend over the practitioner's contact. Hold for 3 to 5 seconds and release. Move the fingers to the next cervical vertebra and repeat the technique. Continue moving the fingers up the cervical spine and extending the cervical spine at each level up to the occiput (see Figure 7.4).

When this technique is applied at the occiput/C1 articulation it is sometimes referred to as the occipital release or cranial base release. Some practitioners prefer to use fingertips spread across the base of the occiput. Extension of the suboccipital area is then achieved by extending the interphalangeal joints and sometimes also the metacarpophalangeal joints.

CERVICAL HORIZONTAL TRACTION

This technique is contraindicated if cervical distraction causes symptoms. Sit at the head of the table or stand with one foot forward and the other back to maintain balance. Cup one hand horizontally under the occiput and place the other under the client's chin. Ask the client to hold onto the sides of the table to anchor their shoulders. Gently and slowly apply horizontal traction with the hand contacting the occiput. Hold for 5 seconds and slowly release. No pressure is applied to the contact under the client's chin. Be careful not to apply pressure to the client's throat (see Figure 7.5).

Fig. 7.4 Cervical extension

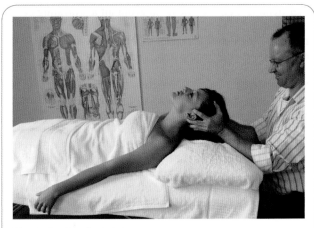

Fig. 7.6 Cervical stair-step manoeuvre

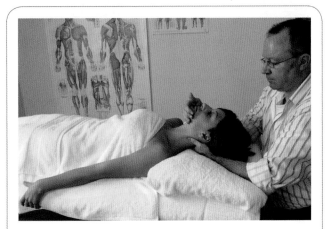

Fig. 7.5 Cervical horizontal traction

CERVICAL STAIR-STEP MANOEUVRE

This technique is contraindicated if the client's symptoms increase with cervical compression or if the client has a history of cervical disc lesion or neurological symptoms.

With the client lying supine, sit at the head of the table. Slowly and gently apply pressure with both palms over the client's parietal bones in inferoanterior direction. Feel for the *steps* as the head moves downward and forward. Rock the head forward and backward over segments that feel restricted or if the head jolts forward too quickly. Consider each cervical segment in turn (see Figure 7.6).

CERVICAL FACET ARTICULATION

Cervical facet articulations are contraindicated if active range of motion produces symptoms or if the client has a history of cervical disc lesion or neurological symptoms. For both facet rotation and lateral flexion the client lies supine and the practitioner is seated at the head of the table.

i. Rotation

Place the palms of the hands over the client's ears. The fingers contact the facet joints and laminae of C6 or C7. Gently and

Fig. 7.7 Cervical facet rotation

slowly rotate the head in small movements (< 10°) about the point of contact in the facet joints. After several rotations to each side, move the fingers up the spine and repeat the small rotations at C5 or C4. When restrictions are located, continue gently rocking and rotating the facet joints several times to improve their range of motion. Continue moving up the cervical spine, repeating the small rotations at each level (see Figure 7.7).

Fig. 7.8 Cervical facet lateral flexion

Fig. 7.9 Thoracic longitudinal mobilisation

ii. Lateral flexion

Place the hands in the same position as above but this time move the fingertips more laterally. Gently rock the client's head in small movements from side to side at the level of the point of contact on the facet joints. If restrictions in the movement are palpated, continue gently rocking the facet joints several times to improve their range of motion. Move up the cervical spine, laterally flexing the facets at each level (see Figure 7.8).

2. Thoracic spine and rib cage

The following mobilisations are designed to reduce thoracic hypomobility. All thoracic and rib cage techniques are contraindicated if the client is osteoporotic.

THORACIC LONGITUDINAL MOBILISATION

The client is prone. If the client is covered with a towel, extra folds of towel are placed in the lumbar area so that the movement is not restricted. Hook the heel of one hand over the sacral base, fingers pointing towards the feet. The heel of the other hand contacts the spinous process of one of the lower thoracic vertebrae. Your arms are crossed. As the client exhales, apply pressure on the body contacts to slowly separate your hands. Hold for 5 seconds and release the stretch slowly. Move the thoracic hand to a new position contacting a spinous process in the mid thoracic spine and repeat the stretch as the client exhales. Repeat again with the thoracic hand contacting the spinous process of one of the upper thoracic vertebrae (see Figure 7.9).

THORACIC DIAGONAL MOBILISATION

Similar to the longitudinal mobilisation above, except that the heel of one hand contacts the iliac crest and the heel of the other hand contacts the rib angles in the lower thoracic area on the opposite side. As the client exhales, your hands are moved apart to create a diagonal stretch of the lower thoracic region. Hold for 5 seconds. Repeat the technique on the middle and upper rib angles and on the other side (see Figure 7.10).

Fig. 7.10 Thoracic diagonal mobilisation

THORACIC ROCKING

The client is prone. Stand facing across the client. Using the heels of both hands in unison, contact the contralateral rib angles and gently push laterally in a rhythmical fashion to create a rocking motion through the rib cage. The rib cage recoils passively between lateral pushes. Contacts move up and down the rib angles. Repeat on the other side (see Figure 7.11).

ARM OVERHEAD RIB MOBILISATION

The client lies supine.

i. Upper ribs. (The technique is described here for the client's left upper ribs. Reverse the contacts for the right upper ribs.) Stand at the head of the table. The client's arm is abducted as far as possible. Hold the client's left arm at the elbow with your left hand. Your right palm contacts the client's upper pectoral area lateral to the sternum, fingers pointed laterally. In this position rib mobilisation is achieved by gentle pressure on the upper ribs as the client exhales. Repeat three times maintaining some pressure between exhalations.

ii. Lower ribs. Stand at the side of the table between the client's arm and the table. Hold the client's left arm at the elbow with your right hand, abduct the arm as far as possible and face towards the client's feet. Use a lunge position to stand low. With your left hand, contact the client's lower ribs in the mid-axillary line. Stretch is achieved by gentle pressure inferiomedially as the client

exhales. Repeat three times, maintaining some pressure between exhalations. Repeat on the other side (see Figure 7.12).

RIB ROTATION

This technique is contraindicated if the client experiences symptoms on thoracic and/or lumbar rotation or during the technique.

The client is seated and places their interlocked fingers behind their neck. Stand behind the client and place one hand through the loop of one elbow from anterior to posterior and place it on top of the client's hands. The heel of the other hand contacts the lower rib angles on the opposite side. As the client exhales, use both hands to rotate the client away from the rib contact hand. Hold the stretch for 5 seconds then repeat to the other side (see Figure 7.13 on p 101).

3. Lumbar spine and pelvis

The following mobilisation may be beneficial for clients with lumbar facet syndrome. Lumbar mobilisations are contraindicated if the client is osteoporotic or has a history of disc lesion or neurological symptoms.

Fig. 7.11 Thoracic rocking

Fig. 7.12 Arm overhead upper and lower rib mobilisation

Fig. 7.13 Sitting rib rotation

Fig. 7.14 Lumbar longitudinal mobilisation

Fig. 7.15 Lumbar rotational mobilisation

LUMBAR LONGITUDINAL MOBILISATION

The client is prone. If the client is covered with a towel, extra folds of towel are made in the lumbar area so that the towel does not restrict movement. Stand at the side of the table facing across the client. Hook the heel of the cephalad hand on the sacral base. The heel of the caudal hand contacts the spinous process of one of the lower lumbar vertebrae, fingers pointing superiorly. Your arms are crossed. As the client exhales, apply pressure to the bony contacts and slowly separate your hands. Hold the stretch for 5 seconds before releasing slowly. Repeat with the cephalad hand contacting the spinous processes of an upper lumbar vertebra (see Figure 7.14).

LUMBAR ROTATIONAL MOBILISATION

This technique may be helpful for restricted sidebend coupling of the facet joints. It is contraindicated for clients with hyperlordosis, spondylolisthesis or pain on lumbar rotation.

The client lies prone. Stand facing across the patient. Fold a towel in quarters and drape it across the client's pelvis. Place the heel of the cephalad hand along the contralateral paravertebral muscles in the lumbar area. The caudal hand is placed over the towel and under the contralateral anterior superior iliac spine. As the client exhales, gently apply pressure towards the floor to the lumbar paravertebral muscles. Maintain the pressure and gently lift the pelvis with the caudal hand. This creates a slight rotation of the lumbar spine. Hold for 5 seconds. Release gently. Repeat on the other side (see Figure 7.15).

SI JOINT MOBILISATION

This technique is contraindicated if sacroiliac ligaments are sprained. The client lies prone, covered with a towel. Stand level with the pelvis facing across the client. Place your caudal hand over the client's sacrum, fingers pointing superiorly. The cephalad hand contacts the gluteal area on one side, fingers pointing inferiorly. Your arms are crossed. Apply gentle pressure inferiorly with the caudal hand and superiorly with the cephalad hand and hold for 5 seconds. Repeat on the other side. This technique applies a slight rotational force through the sacroiliac joint. (Note: the inferior pressure on the ilium makes the leg on that side appear to lengthen during this technique.) Repeat with hands reversed (see Figure 7.16).

4. Shoulder joint

SHOULDER ROTATION

With the client supine, lying close to the side of the table, stand at the side of the table in lunge position facing towards the client's head. Hold the client's elbow with the lateral hand, and place your other hand over the shoulder. Using both hands in unison, rotate the glenohumeral joint. Use your body weight by alternately bending and straightening your knees to perform the shoulder rotation. You can also slowly abduct the client's

Fig. 7.16 SI joint mobilisation

Fig. 7.17 Shoulder rotation

arm while continuing to rotate the shoulder joint. Care must be taken if abduction is painful (as is the case in many shoulder conditions) (see Figure 7.17).

SHOULDER TRACTIONS

The glenohumeral joint is gently tractioned in five ranges of motion. The client is supine.

i.   Inferior traction. Face the client's head and stand in lunge position. Hold the upper limb with both hands (e.g. one proximal to the wrist and the other proximal to the elbow). Gently traction the client's glenohumeral joint in an inferior direction by transferring weight from the front foot to the back foot.

ii. Anterior traction. Hold the upper limb with both hands (e.g. one proximal to the wrist and the other proximal to the elbow). Raise the client's arm to 90° flexion and gently traction the client's arm towards the ceiling.

iii. Superior traction. Stand at the head of the table. Hold the upper limb with both hands, one proximal to the wrist and the other proximal to the elbow. The client's arm is raised overhead to its comfortable limit. (Note that full flexion may be limited in many clients with shoulder problems.) Gently traction the client's glenohumeral joint in a superior direction within the client's pain-free range.

iv. Lateral traction. Stand facing across the client. The client's arm is abducted to 90° (or to its comfortable limit). Hold the upper limb with both hands, one proximal to the wrist and the other proximal to the elbow. Traction the client's glenohumeral joint in a lateral direction.

v.   Medial traction. Stand on the contralateral side. Place the client's arm into adduction by moving the arm across the chest with the elbow flexed. Apply gentle traction to the arm across the body (see Figure 7.18).

SHOULDER PROGRESSIVE CYLINDRICAL ARTICULATION

This technique is designed to circumduct the humeral head at the glenohumeral joint. The client lies supine close to the side of the table. Stand on the ipsilateral side of the client between the client's arm and the table and face cephalad. Place the palm of the medial hand just distal to the shoulder joint. The palm of the other hand holds the client's elbow and stabilises the arm close to your side.

Use both contacts in unison to transcribe a cylinder with the humerus emphasising the posterior pressure. While this motion is maintained, slowly abduct the arm by gradually moving cephalad. The degree of abduction is limited by the

client's mobility but rarely needs to reach more than 120° (see Figure 7.19 on p 104).

SHOULDER PROGRESSIVE HUMERAL EXTERNAL ROTATION

The purpose of this technique is to externally rotate the humeral head at the glenohumeral joint. The client lies supine close to the side of the table, forearm supinated, elbow flexed to approximately 90° and arm abducted to 45°. Stand on the ipsilateral side of the client facing cephalad and hold the client's wrist with the lateral palm on the anterior aspect of the wrist, and the medial hand holding under the client's elbow.

Repeatedly lift and lower the client's elbow with the medial hand while the other hand passively maintains elbow flexion. This repetitive action with the elbow causes the humerus to

Fig. 7.18 Shoulder tractions

Fig. 7.19 Shoulder progressive cylindrical articulation

Fig. 7.21 Shoulder progressive humeral internal rotation

Fig. 7.20 Shoulder progressive humeral external rotation

externally rotate. Continue repetitions of shoulder external rotation as the humerus is slowly abducted to approximately 120° (see Figure 7.20).

SHOULDER PROGRESSIVE HUMERAL INTERNAL ROTATION

This technique is similar to progressive humeral external rotation except that the humerus is internally rotated at the glenohumeral joint. The client's pronated arm is abducted to 45° with the elbow flexed to 90°. Face across the client and hold under the client's elbow with the cephalad hand and over the top of the client's wrist with the caudal hand. Progressively lift and lower the client's elbow with the caudal hand while the other hand passively maintains elbow flexion. This repeated lifting and lowering of the client's elbow causes the humerus to internally rotate. Continue repetitions of shoulder internal rotation while taking small steps backwards to abduct the humerus to approximately 120° (see Figure 7.21).

SHOULDER FIGURE-8

The client is supine, clasping their elbows with their hands. Stand at the head of the table, hold under the client's forearms distal to the elbows and flex the client's shoulders to 90°.

Apply slight traction to the shoulders by gently raising the client's arms towards the ceiling. Create a figure-8 movement by slowly making circles first with one elbow and then the other (see Figure 7.22 on p 105).

5. Elbow joint

ELBOW ARTICULATION

The client is supine lying near the side of the table with their extended arm raised vertically with the palm facing medially. Stand on the ipsilateral side of the client facing across them. Place the palm of your caudal hand on the dorsal aspect of the elbow. Wrap your fingers around the medial aspect of the elbow. Hold the client's wrist with the cephalad hand. Your caudal hand moves the client's elbow in a small anticlockwise circle for the left elbow, or clockwise circle for the right elbow (see Figure 7.23 on p 105).

ELBOW JOINT CAPSULE STRETCH

The client is supine. Hold the client's arm either side of the elbow. Traction is applied in both directions to gently stretch the joint capsule. Hold for 5 seconds (see Figure 7.24 on p 105).

6. Wrist and hand

WRIST PRONATED LONGITUDINAL THENAR KNEADING

This technique is designed to articulate the carpal bones in a sagittal plane. The client lies supine with the arm pronated and elbow extended. Stand on the ipsilateral side of the table and face cephalad. Place the thenar eminences of both hands together on the dorsum of the client's hand over the proximal metacarpal heads. Point your thumbs superiorly along the client's forearm. With the second, third and fourth fingers, apply counterpressure to the palm of the client's hand. The client's arm may be raised to a comfortable position off the table. While maintaining pressure, move your hands alternately up and down in a sagittal plane causing carpal shearing. Repeat several times before moving the contacts proximally by about 1 cm. Repeat the process. The contacts move progressively proximal until they reach the proximal carpal row (see Figure 7.25 on p 105).

Fig. 7.22   Shoulder figure-8

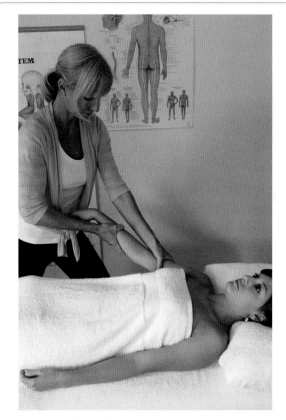

Fig. 7.24   Elbow capsule stretch

Fig. 7.23   Elbow articulation

Fig. 7.25   Wrist pronated longitudinal thenar kneading

WRIST PRONATED TRACTION AND CIRCUMDUCTION

This technique is designed to articulate the carpal bones under traction. The client is supine with the arm raised to about 20–30° and the forearm pronated. Stand on the ipsilateral side and face cephalad. Place the thenar eminences of both hands together on the dorsum of the client's hand over the wrist. Place your fingertips under the client's wrist either side of the carpal tunnel. Gently traction and circumduct the client's arm keeping the client's hand pronated (see Figure 7.26 on p 106).

Fig. 7.26 Wrist pronated traction and circumduction

Fig. 7.27 Wrist semi-supinated traction and circumduction

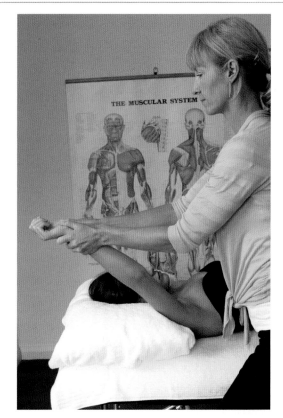

Fig. 7.28 Wrist overhead traction and circumduction

WRIST SEMI-SUPINATED TRACTION AND CIRCUMDUCTION

This technique is similar to the pronated traction and circumduction technique except that the client's hand is semi-supinated (i.e. thumb points towards the ceiling). This technique articulates the carpal bones under traction with emphasis on the radiocarpal and ulnacarpal articulations. Place the thenar eminences of both hands together on the radial side of the client's wrist with thumbs crossed. The fingertips are placed under the wrist. Maintaining pressure with the hands, slowly circumduct the arm, keeping the client's hand semi-supinated (see Figure 7.27).

WRIST OVERHEAD TRACTION AND CIRCUMDUCTION

The client lies supine with the extended arm raised overhead with palms facing the ceiling. Stand ipsilaterally at the level of the client's shoulders and face cephalad. Place the webs of both hands just proximal to the client's trapezium and pisiform. Lunge superiorly to traction the client's carpal bones. With traction maintained, the client's hand is slowly circumducted in both directions (see Figure 7.28).

METACARPOPHALANGEAL AND INTERPHALANGEAL MOBILISATION

The client is seated or lies supine with their arm raised to about 20° flexion. Stand on the ipsilateral side and face towards the client's head. Isolate the joint to be mobilised by placing thumb or finger contacts either side of the joint and close to the joint. A number of mobilisations can be performed including flexion/extension, rotation and traction (see Figure 7.29 on p 107).

METACARPAL SHEARING

The client is supine or seated, forearm pronated. Contact the dorsum of the client's hand with your thenar eminence and your fingers wrapped around the client's palm. Shear each metacarpal individually in an anterior–posterior direction (see Figure 7.30 on p 107).

7. Hip joint

HIP ROTATION

The purpose of this technique is to mobilise the femoral head in the acetabulum. It is useful for stretching the acetabular capsule. The client lies supine near the side of the table with the hip and knee flexed. Stand on the ipsilateral side of the client in lunge position and face towards the client's head. Place your clasped hands over the client's knee. Lie your caudal forearm along the medial aspect of the client's tibia. By transferring weight alternately between your front foot and back foot, make small circles with the client's knee. (Note the

Fig. 7.29 Metacarpophalangeal and interphalangeal mobilisation

Fig. 7.31 Hip rotation

Fig. 7.30 Metacarpal shearing

Fig. 7.32 Hip figure-8

comparatively restricted end-feel of the medial arc of hip rotation.) (see Figure 7.31).

HIP FIGURE-8

The client lies supine with hip and knee flexed to 90°. Face across the client and place one hand over the knee joint and the other under the Achilles tendon. Maintaining the lower leg parallel to the table, alternately trace small circles with the knee and with the foot which creates a figure-8 of the hip joint (see Figure 7.32).

HIP TRACTION

The client is supine and holds the top of the table with both hands overhead. A towel folded into a strap is placed on the posterior aspect of the lower leg under the Achilles tendon. The ends of the towel are crossed over the dorsum of the foot and wrapped under the plantar aspect of the foot. Next the lateral end of the towel is twisted over the medial end. This has the effect of internally rotating the leg. Firmly grip the twisted ends of the towel, further internally rotate the leg and raise it 20° off the table. Slow and gentle traction is applied to the leg. Hold for 5 seconds and slowly release (see Figure 7.33).

Fig. 7.33 Hip traction

HIP ROTATION SIDELYING

This technique aims to mobilise the femoral head anteromedially at the acetabular joint. The client lies on the uninvolved side close to the edge of the table and slightly bends the hip and knee of the lower leg. Stand behind the client facing across the client. The upper leg is straight. The client holds

Fig. 7.34   Hip rotation sidelying

Fig. 7.36   Knee articulation (lateral approach)

Fig. 7.35   Knee rotation (inferior approach)

the edge of the table in front to prevent rolling forward. Rest your caudal knee on the edge of the table for balance. Place your cephalad palm over the lateral aspect of the client's greater trochanter, fingers and thumb pointing anteriorly. With your other palm, reach under the ipsilateral leg and hold the femur just proximal to the knee. The upper leg is extended, abducted and internally rotated and then slowly circumducted while anteromedial pressure is maintained on the greater trochanter with your cephalad hand (see Figure 7.34).

8. Knee joint

KNEE ARTICULATION (INFERIOR APPROACH)

The client lies supine, near the side of the table. Stand on the ipsilateral side of the client just inferior to the knee, and face cephalad. Rest your medial tibia on the table with your flexed knee pointing superomedially. Rest the client's mid calf over your knee. Place your lateral palm over the lateral aspect of the knee joint and the medial palm over the medial aspect of the knee joint. Wrap the fingers of both hands around the sides of the knee, point the thumbs superiorly and contact the sides of the patella. Lie your caudal forearm along the medial edge of the tibia to stabilise the leg. Slowly rotate the client's knee, keeping the lower leg still with your medial forearm (see Figure 7.35).

KNEE ARTICULATION (LATERAL APPROACH)

This technique is contraindicated in clients with medial collateral ligament sprains. The client is supine. Face across the client and place your caudal knee on the table. Place the client's mid calf across your thigh. Place the palm of your cephalad hand over the knee, and your caudal palm over the front of the ankle. In this position, slightly internally rotate the client's leg. Using your hands, alternately make small circles with the knee and ankle in a bicycle-pedalling motion (see Figure 7.36).

9. Ankle and foot

ANKLE PRONE CIRCUMDUCTION

The client lies prone near the side of the table with the knee flexed to 90°. Stand on the ipsilateral side and face across the client. Lie the palm of your cephalad hand over the plantar aspect of the calcaneus. Hold the dorsal aspect of the metatarsophalangeal joints with the palmar aspect of your caudal hand. Circumduct the talotibial joint and its adjacent articulations in both directions (see Figure 7.37 on p 109).

CALCANEUS PRONE ARTICULATION

The client is prone with feet overhanging the end of the table. The client's knee is flexed to 90° or less. Stand at the foot of the table facing cephalad. Place your palms on the lateral and medial aspects of the calcaneus with your fingers interlocked, and take a firm grip on the calcaneus. Articulate the calcaneus in all directions (see Figure 7.38 on p 109).

TARSALS PRONE PLANTARFLEXION

The client lies prone close to the side of the table with the knee flexed to 90°. Stand on the ipsilateral side and face inferomedially. Place the palm of the caudal hand on the dorsum of the foot. With your other hand, hold the plantar surface of the foot just distal to the calcaneus, fingers running transversely across the mid-plantar area. The client's foot is fully plantar flexed and inverted. From this position, *fold* the client's forefoot towards the calcaneus to mobilise the tarsal joints (see Figure 7.39 on p 109).

Fig. 7.37 Ankle prone circumduction

Fig. 7.39 Tarsals prone plantarflexion

Fig. 7.38 Calcaneus prone articulation

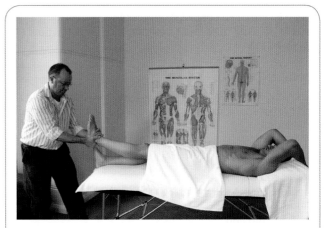

Fig. 7.40 Ankle traction

ANKLE TRACTION

The client is supine and holds the head of the table with both hands. Stand at the foot of the table facing cephalad. Place your medial hand on the client's medial arch, thumb under the sole and fingers wrapping over the dorsum of the foot. Hold the ankle with your lateral hand, the thumb across the front of the ankle and the fingers wrapping around the Achilles tendon. Apply gentle traction in an inferior direction to the client's slightly dorsiflexed foot. Hold the traction for 5 seconds, and slowly release (see Figure 7.40).

Fig. 7.41 Metatarsal shearing

Fig. 7.42 Phalanges mobilisation

METATARSAL SHEARING

The client is supine. Stand at the foot of the table facing cephalad. Place thenar pads of both hands over the dorsal surface of the metatarsal heads, fingers wrapping around to the plantar surface. Slowly shear each metatarsal several times in an anterior–posterior direction (see Figure 7.41).

PHALANGES MOBILISATION

The client is supine. Stand or sit at the foot of the table. Contact either side of the metatarsophalangeal or interphalangeal joint to be mobilised using thumb and index finger contacts. The proximal contact stabilises the joint. Perform a slow rotation in both directions and apply gentle traction (see Figure 7.42).

CONTRAINDICATIONS

Contraindications include all those for Swedish massage as well as contraindications that apply specifically to joint articulation:

- acutely inflamed joints
- recent fracture
- osteoporosis
- malignancy
- joint instability
- rheumatoid collagen necrosis
- joint ankylosis
- vertebrobasilar insufficiency (for cervical articulation)
- infections
- joint replacement
- severe osteoarthritis
- history of disc lesions or radiculopathy.

Caution is required for:

- pregnancy
- hypermobility
- the presence of neurological signs
- spondylolisthesis.

KEY MESSAGES

- Joint articulation is used to treat joint pain and stiffness.
- Assessing clients for joint articulation includes history, functional tests and palpation.
- Capsular pattern refers to limitations of specific ranges of motion that develop when the joint capsule tightens. The concept has not been supported by recent research findings.
- A leathery or hard end-feel may indicate joint degeneration.
- Crepitus is sometimes heard when joints move. It suggests joint degeneration.
- Joint articulations are performed when the surrounding muscles are relaxed and warm. Joints are usually placed in mid-range. Generally the practitioner stabilises the proximal bone and articulates the distal one.
- Joint articulations are performed within the limits of accessory movements of joints and within the client's pain tolerance.
- The usual contraindications of Swedish massage apply to joint articulation as well as joint instability or ankylosis, joint replacement, severe rheumatoid arthritis or osteoarthritis, vertebrobasilar insufficiency (cervical articulation) and history of disc lesions or radiculopathy.

Review questions

1. What is the difference between joint articulation/mobilisation and joint manipulation?
2. Circle true or false:
   a) Physiological movements can be actively performed by clients.　　True/False
   b) Joint play is determined by the laxity of the joint capsule.　　True/False
   c) Joint articulation uses physiological and accessory movement.　　True/False
3. What does the term loose-pack joint position mean?
4. What is the capsular pattern for:
   a) cervical spine?
   b) shoulder?
   c) hip?
   d) knee?
5. List four contraindications for joint articulation.
6. How would you integrate joint articulation into a remedial massage treatment for a 60-year-old male with osteoarthritis of the right hip?
7. What recommendations would you give a client after treatment with joint articulation?
8. What assessments would you carry out to determine the client's suitability for joint articulation?
9. Name three conditions of the shoulder joint that would benefit from joint articulation.
10. A 31-year-old male presents with chronic pain and inflammation that began in the sacroiliac joints four years ago and has spread to the low back, shoulders and hips. He reports pain that wakes him at night and recent night sweats. His pain seems to get worse after periods of inactivity. This history could suggest:
    a) Reiter's syndrome
    b) Anklyosing spondylitis
    c) Fibromyalgia
    d) Psoriatic arthritis

REFERENCES

1. Esposito S, Phillipson S. Spinal adjusting technique: the chiropractic art. Sydney, Australia: Well Adjusted Publishing; 2005.
2. Hengeveld E, Banks K. Maitland's vertebral manipulation. Volume 1. 8th edn. London: Churchill Livingstone; 2013.
3. Bryans R, Descarreaux M, Duranleau M, et al. Evidence-based guidelines for the chiropractic treatment of adults with headache. J Manipulative Physiol Ther 2011;34(5):274–89.
4. Blanpied P, Gross A, Elliott J, et al. Clinical practice guidelines linked to the international classification of functioning, disability and health from the orthopaedic section of the American Physical Therapy Association. J Ortho Sports Phys Ther 2017;47(7):A1–A83.
5. Bussieres A, Stewart G, Al-Zoubi F, et al. Spinal manipulative therapy and other conservative treatments for low back pain: a guideline from the Canadian Chiropractic Guideline Initiative. J Manipulative Physiol Ther 2018;41(4):265–93.
6. Foster NE, Anema JR, Cherkin D, et al. Prevention and treatment of low back pain: evidence, challenges, and promising directions. Lancet 2018;391:2368–83.
7. Ferreira ML, Ferreira PH, Latimer J, et al. Comparison of general exercise, motor control exercise and spinal manipulative therapy for chronic low back pain: a randomized trial. Pain 2007;131:31–7.
8. Cleland JA, Glynn P, Whitman JM, et al. Short-term effects of thrust versus nonthrust mobilization/manipulation, directed at the thoracic spine in patients with neck pain: a randomized clinical trial. Phys Ther 2007;87(4):431–40.
9. Pollack Y, Shashua A, Kalichman L. Manual therapy for plantar heel pain. Foot 2018;34:11–16.
10. Vaillant J, Rouland A, Martigne P, et al. Massage and mobilization of the feet and ankles in elderly adults: effect on clinical balance performance. Man Ther 2009;14:661–4.
11. Jayaseelan D, Scalzitti D, Palmer G. The effects of joint mobilization on individuals with patellofemoral pain: a systematic review. Clin Rehabil 2018; 32(6):722–33.
12. Heiser R, O'Brien V, Schwartz D. The use of joint mobilization to improve clinical outcomes in hand therapy: a systematic review of the literature. J Hand Ther 2013;26(4):297–311.
13. Vermeulen HM, Rozing PM, Obermann WR, et al. Comparison of high-grade and low-grade mobilization techniques in the management of adhesive capsulitis of the shoulder: randomized controlled trial. Phys Ther 2006;86(3):355–68.
14. Michlovitz S, Harris A, Watkins M. Therapy interventions for improving joint range of motion: a systematic review. J Hand Ther 2004;17(2):118–31.
15. Cruz-Diaz D, Lomas Vega R, Osuna-Perez M, et al. Effects of joint mobilization on chronic ankle instability: a randomized controlled trial. Disabil Rehabil 2015;37(7):601–10.
16. Carnes M, Vizniak N. Quick reference evidencebased conditions manual. 3rd edn. Burnaby, BC: Professional Health Systems; 2009.
17. Klassbo M, Harms-Ringdahl K, Larsson G, et al. Examination of passive ROM and capsular patterns in the hip. Physiother Res Int 2003;8(1):1–12.
18. Hanchard NC, Goodchild L, Thompson J, et al. A questionnaire survey of UK physiotherapists on the diagnosis and management of contracted (frozen) shoulder. Physiother 2011; 97(2):115–25.
19. Kessler R. Management of common musculoskeletal disorders. 3rd edn. Philadelphia: Lippincott; 2005.

8

Myofascial release

Learning Outcomes

- Describe the properties and function of fascia and the causes and consequence of myofascial restrictions.
- Assess clients for myofascial restrictions.
- Describe the current evidence for the effectiveness of myofascial releasing techniques.
- Apply myofascial releasing techniques effectively and safely to a range of clients.
- Advise and resource clients who have been assessed and treated with myofascial releasing techniques.

INTRODUCTION

Myofascial release has been used in one form or another for a very long time. Andrew Taylor Still, the father of osteopathy, practised gentle release methods for connective tissue restrictions in the nineteenth century to assist in bringing about three-dimensional functional symmetry to his clients. The term *myofascial release* was coined in 1981 when it was first used to describe courses taught at Michigan State University. Other pioneers working with fascia include Janet Travell, Ida Rolf, Milton Traeger and John Barnes, each of whom developed their own approaches to assessing and treating clients with fascial restrictions.

Myofascial techniques are generally classified as direct (deep) or indirect (gentle). Direct techniques work on deep fascial restrictions. Ida Rolf's work, developed in the 1950s, involved direct myofascial techniques and movement education.[1] Many contemporary myofascial techniques like structural integration, postural integration and deep tissue massage techniques have been developed from Rolf's original work. Indirect techniques, on the other hand, use gentle tractions to generate heat and increase blood flow, thereby releasing fascial restrictions.

John Barnes[2] first developed his myofascial techniques to alleviate long-standing post-operative pain from spinal fusion in a client who had not responded to other techniques. Pain relief is one of the main uses of myofascial release today, including treatment and management of post-operative pain and sporting and other injuries.[3] It is considered a very efficient technique for managing clients with either physical or emotional trauma.[4,5] Gentle myofascial techniques in particular are used by physical therapists for clients with chronic pain who can be treated without adding further mechanical stress to their bodies. The gentleness of indirect myofascial technique is also well suited to treating children, older clients and clients suffering from stress and anxiety-related conditions.

FUNCTIONAL ANATOMY REVIEW

The body is made up of different types of connective tissue including bone, adipose tissue, lymph, blood and fascia that support and protect most structures in the body. Fascia is a three-dimensional web of tough connective tissue that spreads throughout the body as a single structure. It gives the body its form and scaffolding and connects all structures of the body.[6] The analogy that is commonly used to describe fascia is that of a knitted sweater: just as pulling one sleeve affects the whole sweater, fascial distortions or restrictions in any area can affect the whole body.[7] In other words, fascial tissue can be seen as an interconnected tensional network that 'adapts its fiber arrangement and density, according to local tensional demands'.[8] It contains contractile cells, free nerve endings and mechanoreceptors and is likely to play a proprioceptive, nociceptive and mechanically active role.[9]

The main functions of fascia are:

- maintaining normal shape
- maintaining vital organs in their correct position
- resisting mechanical stress (strength, support, elasticity and cushioning)
- nutritive: loose connective tissue contains fluid that serves as a transport medium for cellular elements of other tissues, blood and lymph
- providing an additional surface area for muscle attachments (deep fascia)
- conserving body heat in fat stores (superficial fascia)
- fighting bacterial infection: histiocytes offer defence when infectious substances pass through planes in connective tissue
- healing: fascia deposits collagen fibres (scar tissue) to assist in healing injuries.

Connective tissue is characterised by few cells dispersed in a large extracellular matrix. The extracellular matrix contains a fibrous component made up of elastin and collagen and a non-fibrous component called ground substance. Ground substance contains proteins that attract and bind water. Different structures of the body require collagen and elastin in different proportions depending on their function.[10]

Fascia is a colloid, which means that it is composed of particles of solid matter suspended in fluid.

- The fluid (ground substance) contains glycosaminoglycans (predominantly hyaluronan), proteoglycans, glycoproteins and water. Ground substance is highly viscous. It is hydrophilic (water-loving) which aids lubrication and resists compression like a shock absorber.
- The solid matter (fibrous component) is made up of fibroblasts, chondrocytes, collagen and elastin. Fibroblasts, the major cell type, adapt to mechanical loading according to its strain magnitude, duration and frequency.[11] Collagen provides strength and elastin fibres allow structures to return to their original shape after stretching. The fibres align along lines of stress to absorb tensile forces.

Superficial and deep fascia are dense irregular connective tissue containing thick bundles of collagen arranged irregularly to resist tension applied in many directions. Deep fascia is a coarse sheet of connective tissue that surrounds and infuses with muscles, bones, nerves, blood vessels and organs. It includes fascia surrounding a group of muscles, epimysium surrounding individual muscles, and perimysium surrounding fascicles within muscles (see Figure 8.1). The deepest fascia is the dura of the craniosacral system. Superficial fascia (hypodermis) lies directly below the skin. It contains fat, muscle tissue, cutaneous blood vessels and nerves.

Myers[7] described the fascial system as conveying mechanical information through its response to pushes and pulls. He described a number of myofascial meridians or common pathways for this mechanical communication including (see Figure 8.2 on p 114):

- Superficial back line
- Superficial front line
- Spiral line
- Arm lines
- Functional lines
- Deep front line

As we load and unload fascia the water content of the tissue changes which affects its pliability. Collagen fibres in connective tissue tend to bind together when they are not used or when they are under sustained pressure. The adhesions that are formed can put pressure on sensitive structures like nerves and blood vessels.[10] Borgini et al[12] described a number of theories that could explain the effect of trauma, overuse syndromes, poor postural biomechanics, inactivity or psychological states on connective tissue. These include changes in cell structure and function,[13–15] alterations to collagen fibre composition,[16, 17] transformation of fibroblasts into myofibroblasts,[18–21] and alterations to the ground substance via neurophysiological and biochemical changes.[14, 22]

WHAT IS MYOFASCIAL RELEASE?

Myofascial release is an interactive hands-on technique for evaluating and treating the whole body via its fascial network. The body's connective tissue network responds to mechanical pressure. The aim of myofascial release is to restore the normal physiological state of fascia. In particular, myofascial release aims to:

- lengthen contracted tissue
- reduce fascial adhesions
- increase range of motion
- decrease pressure on sensitive structures like nerves and blood vessels
- restore normal gliding of collagen and elastic fibres within the ground substance

Because of its viscous nature, fascia resists compression forces. Its resistance increases in proportion to the pressure applied to it. This means that gentle sustained pressure is required to affect fascia. Colloids also respond to heat by changing from a gel-like consistency to a more watery state.

Deep myofascial releasing techniques (including rolfing, postural integration, deep connective tissue massage) have

Fig. 8.1 Myofascia

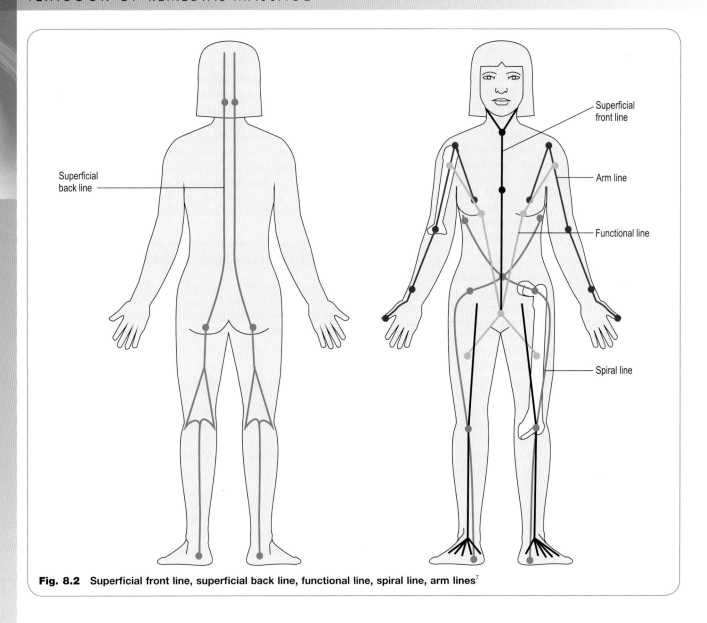

Fig. 8.2 Superficial front line, superficial back line, functional line, spiral line, arm lines[7]

evolved to include the integration of controlled breathing techniques and specific body positioning so that practitioners can reach deep myofascial layers within the client's pain tolerance. Deep myofascial release works by breaking adhesions, elongating and stretching fascia. The deeper forms of myofascial release have been associated with a psychological or emotional response. Rolf[1] proposed that releasing muscle tension also released associated emotional trauma. However, even gentle applications of myofascial release can arouse an emotional response in susceptible clients. Refer clients to a psychologist, counsellor or medical practitioner when dealing with emotional responses that are beyond the scope of remedial massage therapy.

ASSESSING CLIENTS

Assessment procedures for all remedial massage clients includes case history, postural analysis, functional testing and palpation. For myofascial release, palpatory findings are particularly informative.

HISTORY

Myofascial restrictions do not produce referred pain in the same way as trigger points. The effect of the original injury gradually spreads as fascia tightens in many directions producing pain and discomfort. The progression of such symptoms as aching pain, headaches, discomfort, limited range of motion and impaired respiration suggests myofascial restrictions. Clients are often not aware of an original event (e.g. trauma, overuse, jaw clenching, surgery) that may be the cause of their present pain especially if symptoms are felt at a site that is distant from the original injury site. As with all case histories, it is important to identify the presence of red or yellow flags and to refer clients where appropriate (see Chapter 2).

POSTURAL ANALYSIS

Myofascial restrictions influence the way the body moves and adapts and may be evident in postural analysis. For example, internal or external hip rotation, pelvic tilt, leg length discrepancy, forward head carriage, shoulder protraction, hyperkyphosis and hyperlordosis may be associated with myofascial restrictions. The fascial lines of the body are observed and compared (e.g. left lateral line compared to the right, left spiral line compared to the right). Figure 8.3 shows two examples of postural analysis using fascial lines. Treatment plans can then be developed for stretching restricted fascial lines.[7]

FUNCTIONAL TESTS

Clients with myofascial restrictions usually develop compensatory muscle patterns that become evident during functional testing (active, passive and resisted range of motion) (see Chapter 2). Findings from functional testing direct practitioners to target tissues.

PALPATION

Palpatory assessments provide further information including temperature, dryness and tissue adhesions. Fascial restrictions often palpate as cold and dry and with reduced fascial glide. Practitioners need to be mindful that they are palpating myofascial restrictions, not specific muscles. Fascia tend to run in straight lines.[7, 23] The superficial back line, for example, runs from the plantar fascia to the gastrocnemius, hamstrings, sacrotuberous ligament, erector spinae and then to the fascia of the scalp. Fascial lines also run at a consistent depth. They are tied to underlying tissues at muscle and ligament attachments.

Some practitioners describe a myofascial end-feel, that is the practitioner's perception of barriers to movement. Myofascial end-feel is described as soft and rubbery.

TREATING CLIENTS

Myofascial release techniques are interactive in that the practitioner monitors feedback from the client's body which determines the direction, force and duration of the techniques. The direction of the movement does not depend on the direction of specific muscles. Fascia is an extensive three-dimensional network and treatments applied to one area can affect the entire network. A leg traction, for instance, can facilitate a fascial release in the neck.

Myofascial release is performed in a step-by-step progression as each restriction responds to treatment. As the release occurs the practitioner usually palpates a relaxation and elongation of tissues and may observe other involuntary physiological reactions like tonic muscular activity and eye movements.[24] The client may report a sensation of heat, cold or tingling. Changes to the client's posture do not normally happen quickly. The central nervous system takes time to be re-educated to maintain more energy-efficient postures.

Through the combined effect of the client's responses to myofascial release and the therapist's ability to *listen with their hands*, normal functioning may be restored to tissues. This is achieved by removing pressure from nerves, blood vessels, organs and joints and promoting normal function in body tissues.

EVIDENCE FOR THE EFFECTIVENESS OF FASCIAL RELEASING TECHNIQUES

Myofascial release has become increasingly popular in the treatment of musculoskeletal disorders. One systematic review set out to provide evidence for six of Myer's[7] 12 proposed myofascial meridians based on anatomical dissection studies.[9] The researchers found extensive structural continuity for three of the six examined meridians (superficial back line, back functional line, front functional line). The authors confirmed the implications of this research: first, support for the phenomenon of referred pain in non-specific disorders; second,

Fig. 8.3 Postural analysis using fascial lines

support for diagnosis and therapy that is directed beyond a single anatomic structure.

A systematic review evaluating the effectiveness of myofascial release for relieving chronic musculoskeletal pain and improving joint mobility, function and quality of life found eight relevant papers: two trials on lateral epicondylitis (N = 95), two on fibromyalgia (N = 145), three on low back pain (N = 152), and one on heel pain (N = 65).[3] Treatment duration ranged from 30–90 minutes 4 to 24 times during 2–20 weeks. The authors concluded that there was insufficient evidence to support the use of myofascial release therapy in the treatment in chronic musculoskeletal pain.

Other systematic reviews have found limited evidence with low risk of bias for the effectiveness of soft-tissue therapy for the management of musculoskeletal disorders and injuries in the upper and lower extremities. For example, Piper[25] concluded that myofascial release and movement re-education (muscle energy technique) may benefit patients with persistent lateral epicondylitis. In addition, myofascial release to the gastrocnemius, soleus and plantar fascia was found to be effective in improving foot function in patients with plantar heel pain. No studies were found examining the effectiveness of soft tissue therapy for other musculoskeletal disorders or injuries of the lower extremity.

A large number of small trials have shown promising results. For example:

- Meltzer et al[26] conducted an in vitro study to potentially explain the immediate clinical outcomes associated with myofascial release. The authors concluded that treating with myofascial release following modelled repetitive motion strain resulted in normalisation in apoptic (cell death) rate and cell morphology. This could reflect tissue texture changes and increased myofascial elasticity.
- Martin[27] performed 20 sessions of myofascial release on one client with diffuse systemic sclerosis and found remodelling of the connective tissue affected by diffuse systemic sclerosis. The client was found to have increased range of motion in joints, reduced effects of Raynaud's phenomenon and reduced pain.
- Arroyo-Morales et al[28] studied 62 healthy individuals for the usefulness of massage as a recovery method after high-intensity exercise and concluded that myofascial release favoured the recovery of heart ventilation and diastolic blood pressure after high-intensity exercise.

APPLYING THE TECHNIQUES

Myofascial release can be used as a modality in its own right or in combination with other manual therapies including other remedial massage techniques, sports massage and craniosacral therapy. Myofascial techniques are usually performed without oil or lubricant to prevent sliding over tissues.

Good ergonomics are required, whether applying deep or gentle techniques, to minimise stress on the practitioner's body. Massage therapists are prone to musculoskeletal injuries, especially of the low back, wrists and thumbs.[29] All massage techniques should be based on sound biomechanical principles and adapted to suit the needs of individual therapists and clients. Correct table height and stance are fundamental. Awkward and prolonged techniques, particularly those using thumbs or extended wrists, should be replaced by the correct use of forearms, knuckles and fists.

Myofascial Release (MFR) techniques

1. DEEP TECHNIQUES

Deep connective tissue release focuses on the deeper tissue structures of the muscle and fascia to provide physiological release of tension or adhesions in tissues and psychological release from stored emotional memories.[2] Deep myofascial release involves the use of slow, deep pressure applied with fingers, knuckles, fists, forearms or elbows (see Figure 8.4 on p 117).

Technique

- Lower the table height so that body weight can be used efficiently.
- Do not use oil so that the superficial layers of skin and fascia are moved. (Note: a small quantity of cream or lotion may be used if the client has very dry or fragile skin.)
- Warm up the area using compressions or other dry warm-up techniques.
- Use body supports (e.g. thoracic roll) and body positioning to stretch tissues before applying the techniques.
- Work with the client's breathing. Work through superficial tissues to locate deep layers and advance the contact as the client exhales.
- Work within the client's pain range and ask for regular feedback.
- Apply slow short strokes over small areas.
- Always maintain correct posture and use body weight to reduce pressure on joints (e.g. transferring weight from the back leg to the front) and use a variety of body parts including knuckles, fist, forearm and elbow. Avoid hyperextending thumbs and wrists. Elbows should be kept straight but not locked.
- Use larger contacts (e.g. forearms) before smaller contacts (e.g. thumb and fingers).
- After applying the technique, stretch the muscle and/or take the joint slowly through its full range of motion.
- Instruct the client to drink plenty of water.

Techniques can be applied to specific regions of the body or along fascial lines. For example, techniques applied to the superficial back line could include:

- knuckles to plantar fascia
- knuckles around lateral malleoli
- thumb frictions across the lateral ligaments
- knuckles around calcaneus
- knuckles/forearm to gastrocnemius
- thumbs or fingertips to separate gastrocnemius and soleus
- forearms and fists to hamstrings
- knuckles around ischial tuberosity (flex and externally rotate the hip for better access)
- fists to gluteals (face across the client and glide from sacrum inferolaterally)
- thumb/knuckles to sacrotuberous ligament
- forearms/knuckles along erector spinae
- fists/knuckles to posterior cervical muscles
- fingers to scalp fascia.

2. GENTLE TECHNIQUES

The style of myofascial release described in this section is based on the work of John Barnes.[2] This style uses gentle open-handed touch to maximise the contact area (except

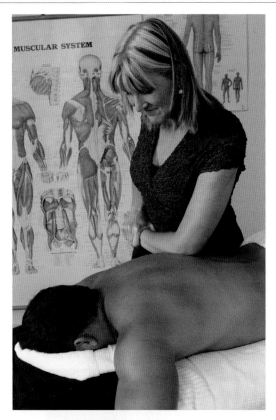

Fig. 8.4   Deep myofascial release

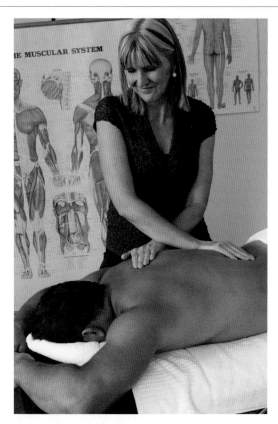

Fig. 8.5   Cross-hand technique

for small children where finger contact may be more appropriate). The technique is progressively applied to one area and after a softening and elongation of affected tissues has been achieved, then to another restricted area. Myofascial release is a very safe technique. Appropriate monitoring of clients' responses prevents inadvertently overstretching the soft tissues of the body.

Key features of gentle myofascial releasing techniques are:

- Light
- Sustained
- Interactive
- Progressive.

Applying gentle techniques involves:

- locating the restriction (e.g. palpate for cold, dry, tight tissue)
- applying gentle pressure to engage the elastic component of the myofascia which has a springy feel (if your hands are not allowed to sink into the first barrier before proceeding, the client may experience a burning sensation as the skin is overstretched)
- gently stretching target tissue between your contacts until a resistance to further stretch is felt – this stretch realigns the elastin and collagen fibres and is maintained until the hands stop at another firm (collagen) barrier
- holding until the soft tissues relax or elongate ('calm sensation of relaxation'[30]) for usually 3–5 minutes. After the initial release, further releases may occur without any change in contact (Bertolucci[24] described a 'singular

springy sensation that causes the force of the practitioner to rebound', and then further suggested that this 'sense of firmness' is a hallmark of MFR and should increase in intensity as the technique is applied)

- from this new (elongated) position, further stretching the tissues between your hands to take up the tissue slack until another barrier is felt[2]
- repeating the process until the tissues are fully elongated.

Gentle pressure is required to overcome barriers because of the viscous nature of fascia. A low load applied slowly and gently facilitates more flow in a viscous medium than a high load applied quickly or with heavy pressure. Thermotherapy may also be beneficial.

Techniques

1. Cross-hand technique

One commonly used technique, the cross-handed technique, can be applied all over the body on areas of fascial restriction. The hands are placed lightly onto an area of fascial restriction and allowed to sink into the tissues until a barrier is perceived. This is sometimes called the depth barrier. Next, the hands separate slowly until another barrier is felt. This is called the elastic and muscular barrier. Your hands now follow the tissues in whatever direction they move until a release or softening and elongation of the tissue is achieved. This usually takes from 3 to 5 minutes. Fascial release may be felt between 90 and 120 seconds but it may be premature to release the technique at this point. Maintaining the technique for at least 3 minutes may achieve longer-lasting results (see Figure 8.5).

A study by Borgini et al[12] correlated perceptions of discomfort in 40 subjects with low back pain with the duration of a fascial release technique. The mean time to reduce perceived pain to half was 3.24 minutes. In subjects who had been experiencing symptoms for less than 3 months the mean time was 2.58 minutes.

To minimise stress on your own body, place your hands on the area being treated and lean forward so that depth is achieved with your own body weight. The arms are kept flexed at the elbows, ensuring that you follow the tissues as they release rather than pushing through them.

2. Traction techniques

When performing traction techniques (i.e. leg and arm pulls, (see Figures 8.6 and 8.7 on page p 118–119) both the client and the practitioner sense the elongation in the treated limb. Apply a gentle, slow, sustained traction to the whole limb, holding at each restriction before moving onto the next. The limbs move through an arc into abduction and then across the body into adduction. When a myofascial release has taken place the limb feels heavy and loose.[30] Traction techniques can increase the range of motion of the extremity. These

techniques take time. Rushing the movements will not provide any long-lasting changes. The results of waiting and working with the tissues are worth the effort.

Try to keep your upper trapezius muscles relaxed and your knees flexed while performing this technique. Contacts for the arm pull are usually two hands around the wrist, or one hand at the wrist and the other at the elbow. For the leg pull, the contacts are either two hands at the ankle, or one hand at the knee and one at the ankle. Be careful not to hold the limb too tightly. Change hand contacts as often as is required for the client's comfort and to minimise the stress on you.

3. Transverse holds

Fascia in the body is predominantly vertically oriented. However, there are very important transverse planes. These can be found at the areas of transitional spinal curves (i.e. C7–T1, T12–L1 and L5–S1) and at each joint. The hyoid bone and cranial base can also be regarded as a transverse plane.

Myofascial release for the thoracic inlet and the respiratory and pelvic diaphragms are usually performed with clients in the supine position. (However, if the client is unable to lie supine, the techniques can be performed with the client prone

Fig. 8.6 Arm pull

Fig. 8.7   Leg pull

or in a sidelying position.) Sit or stand at the side of the table level with the transverse structure being treated. Place the cephalad hand under the client's back, and the caudal hand on the anterior aspect of the body at the level of the transverse plane. Light anteroposterior pressure is applied with the caudal hand until a barrier is felt. After 90 to 120 seconds you may feel a movement in the tissues. Follow this movement with your caudal hand and repeat the process if another tissue restriction is palpated. When the release is complete remove both hands slowly.

C7–T1 Thoracic inlet/anterior chest wall   For the thoracic inlet the anterior hand is placed just under the clavicles at the sternoclavicular joint. The thoracic inlet release is often used before myofascial releasing techniques for the neck, shoulder or cranium. It is considered beneficial for clients with breathing problems, musculoskeletal problems of the neck, shoulder and upper limb, and to promote lymph drainage (see Figure 8.8).

T12–L1 Respiratory diaphragm release   For the respiratory diaphragm release, the anterior hand is placed over the xiphoid process and on the upper part of the abdomen. This technique is useful for low back pain because iliopsoas and quadratus lumborum muscles communicate with this diaphragm. The quadratus lumborum is also involved in breath-

Fig. 8.8   Thoracic inlet release

ing. The respiratory diaphragm and thoracic inlet release can be used to open the chest for more efficient breathing (see Figure 8.9 on p 120).

L5–S1 Pelvic diaphragm release   For the pelvic diaphragm release, the anterior hand is placed on the abdomen with the hypothenar eminence at the superior border of the

Fig. 8.9 Respiratory diaphragm release

Fig. 8.11 Cranial base release

Fig. 8.10 Pelvic diaphragm release

pubic ramus and the rest of the hand over the suprapubic region. The pelvic diaphragm release may be beneficial for low back pain, sacral pain and lower abdominal discomfort (see Figure 8.10).

4. Cranial base release

Sit at the head of the table with the client lying supine. Cup the client's occiput in both hands and let your hands rest on the table. Spreading fingers of both hands, place your fingertips under the occiput and appy slow gentle pressure with the fingertips in an anterior direction. As the tissues relax and elongate, the client's head extends over your fingertips. This is a very useful technique for the treatment of neck pain, stress and headache (see Figure 8.11).

INTEGRATING MYOFASCIAL RELEASING TECHNIQUES WITH REMEDIAL MASSAGE

Myofascial techniques are often used at the beginning of a remedial massage before oil has been applied, or at the end of the treatment after the oil has been removed. The use of myofascial release before any other remedial techniques may

enhance the efficacy of the entire treatment and may also reduce your workload. Table 8.1 presents some of the key considerations associated with the integration of myofascial release into a remedial massage treatment.

CONTRAINDICATIONS AND PRECAUTIONS

Contraindications for myofascial release are similar to those for other forms of manual therapies including:

- any red flag (indication of serious underlying medical condition)
- acute inflammation
- lumps and tissue changes
- rashes and hyperaemia
- obstructive oedema
- mood alterations (e.g. depression, anxiety)
- contagious or infectious disease that may be spread by the upper respiratory tract or by direct contact with the skin
- fever
- cellulitis
- osteoporosis (for deep myofascial release)
- the client being unable to give informed consent
- the client being under the influence of alcohol or other substance.

Perform myofascial release with caution when the following conditions are present:

- Hypotension. Myofascial release may lower blood pressure. Instruct the client to lie quietly for a few minutes after treatment and to get up slowly as they may feel light headed.
- Haematoma, open wounds, recent surgery, healing fracture. Do not work directly on these areas.
- Osteoporosis and advanced degenerative changes. Work gently and focus on uninvolved areas.
- Anti-coagulant therapy. Be aware that the client may bruise easily.

KEY MESSAGES

- Myofascial release is an interactive hands-on technique for assessing and treating conditions such as musculoskeletal

Table 8.1 Integrating myofascial release (MFR) into remedial massage treatment

1. MFR initially, augmented by remedial massage techniques	The first session often focuses on reducing or eliminating the client's presenting symptoms. ■ Treat the area of the main presenting condition first. ■ Monitor for signs that may arise in an area distant to the tissues being treated. Signs could include heat, cold, tingling or pain sensations (vasomotor responses) indicating a further area in need of treatment. ■ Treat with transverse plane releases, cross-hand technique or leg or arm pull techniques. In subsequent sessions focus on the underlying cause of the symptoms. This may involve areas of discomfort which may be distant from the site of initial symptoms. ■ Eliminate causative and perpetuating factors where possible. ■ Mechanical stresses cause myofascial restriction. Restrictions occur at the injury site and because of fascia's extensive network, pain and restrictions may migrate in many directions. ■ Work systematically through the body with MFR to release restrictions for long-term relief. Work in the correcting direction according to postural analysis (e.g. moving the superior frontal line superiorly and the superficial back line inferiorly). Work superficial layers before deep ones then work on sites where fascial meridians cross, especially spiral and functional lines.[7] ■ Use a range of remedial techniques (e.g. trigger point therapy, muscle stretching, soft tissue releasing techniques, deep transverse friction) to eliminate mechanical factors such as chronic inefficient postural adaptations or inefficient movement patterns. Use Swedish massage or other relaxation techniques to eliminate systemic factors such as emotional stress.
2. Other remedial techniques initially, augmented by MFR	MFR aims to improve circulation, relieve pressure on pain-sensitive structures, allow for greater cellular nutrition, respiration and elimination, improve range of motion. ■ Upper body treatment using remedial techniques. Include respiratory diaphragm and thoracic inlet release. ■ Lower body treatment with remedial technique. Include respiratory diaphragm and the pelvic diaphragm. ■ Use cross-hand technique on affected areas.
3. Client education	■ Advise the client to drink plenty of water after treatment. ■ Educate the client in ways to minimise mechanical stresses. ■ Eliminate causative factors (e.g. chronic inefficient postural habits) where possible. ■ Encourage the client to be aware of the effects of poor postures and to adopt good postural habits.[23] ■ Heat packs may be beneficial. ■ Suggest exercises such as Pilates, yoga, walking. If stress of any sort is a factor, meditation, tai-chi or Qigong may be beneficial.

pain, tight muscles, limited range of motion and poor posture.

■ Myofascial release techniques fall into two main categories: direct (deep) myofascial release and indirect (gentle) myofascial release.

■ Assessment of clients for myofascial release includes history, postural analysis, functional assessment and palpation.

■ Myofascial postural analysis involves observing distortions in posture in relation to myofascial meridians.

■ Fascial restrictions often palpate as tight, cold and dry.

■ Fascia responds to mechanical approaches that influence its viscous and plastic properties. Deep myofascial release involves working through superficial layers, slowly applying pressure to a deep myofascial layer, working in time with the client's breathing and using a pain scale; gentle myofascial release involves gentle sustained pressure (3–5 minutes).

■ Treatment involves beginning in one area of myofascial restriction, and waiting for release (elongation) of tissues before moving to another area.

■ Treatment can be applied locally or throughout the whole body, usually along myofascial meridians. When working myofascial meridians, begin with superficial lines before deep lines.

■ Myofascial release has been associated with release of stored emotional memory.

■ The gentle nature of indirect myofascial release makes it a popular and safe technique.

Review questions

1. Fascia is a colloid, which means it is made up of:
   a) loose and dense connective tissue
   b) solid matter suspended in a fluid
   c) regular, irregular and elastic connective tissue
   d) areolar and reticular connective tissue
2. The solid matter of fascia includes:
   a) glycosaminoglycans and water
   b) glycosaminoglycans and fibroblasts
   c) fibroblasts and chondrocytes
   d) water and collagen
3. One of the aims of deep myofascial release is to:
   a) loosen adhesions between connective tissue layers
   b) excite nerve endings
   c) sedate nerve endings
   d) facilitate fibroblast production
4. Fascial restrictions are usually palpated as:
   a) red, hot and swollen
   b) cold, moist and tight
   c) cold, moist and painful
   d) cold, dry and tight
5. What influence does temperature have on fascia?
   a) the lower the temperature, the more liquid the ground substance
   b) the higher the temperature, the more solid the ground substance
   c) the lower the temperature, the more solid the ground substance
   d) temperature has no influence on fascia
6. The resistance of a colloid increases in proportion to the pressure applied to it. True / False
7. Thoracic inlet release is suitable for clients with breathing problems. True / False
8. Myofascial release is performed progressively towards the heart. True / False
9. Gentle myofascial release is suitable for most clients. True / False
10. When fascia is immobilised the ground substance gradually liquefies. True / False
11. List five functions of fascia.
12. Some clients experience an emotional release during myofascial release. How would you manage such a response in a client?
13. Fascia is hydrophilic. How does this property influence the application of techniques?
14. List three ways in which the application of deep myofascial release techniques differs from the application of other remedial massage techniques.
15. How can myofascial release be integrated with other remedial techniques?
16. Describe the tissue feel when fascia reaches its maximum release.
17. How does palpation for myofascial restriction differ from palpation for trigger points?

REFERENCES

1. Rolf I. Rolfing: the integration of human structures. Michigan: The University of Michigan; 1977.
2. Barnes JF. Myofascial release: the search for excellence. Padi, Pennsylvania; 1990.
3. Laimi K, Makila A, Barlund E, et al. Effectiveness of myofascial release in treatment of chronic musculoskeletal pain: a systematic review. Clin Rehabil 2018;32(4):440–50.
4. Muniz e Silva D, de Andrade Alexandre DJ, Silva J. Immediate effect of myofascial release on range of motion, pain and biceps and rectus femoris muscle activity after total knee replacement. J Bodyw Mov Ther 2018;22(4):930–6.
5. Marizeiro DF, Florencio AC, Nunes AC, et al. Immediate effects of diaphragmatic myofascial release on the physical and functional outcomes in sedentary women: a randomized placebo-controlled trial. J Bodyw Mov Ther 2018;22(4):924–9.
6. Clay JH, Allen L, Pounds DL. Clay & Pounds' basic clinical massage therapy: integrating anatomy and treatment. 3rd edn. Philadelphia: Wolters Kluwer; 2015.
7. Myers T. Anatomy trains: myofascial meridians for manual and movement therapists. 3rd edn. Edinburgh: Churchill Livingstone; 2014.
8. Schleip R, Jager H, Klinger W. What is 'fascia'? A review of different nomenclatures. J Bodyw Mov Ther 2012;16:496–502.
9. Wilke J, Krause F, Vogt L, et al. What is evidence-based about myofascial chains: a systematic review. Arch Phys Med Rehabil 2016;97(3):454–61.
10. Fritz S. Mosby's essential sciences for therapeutic massage. Anatomy, physiology, biomechanics, and pathology. 5th edn. St Louis, MO: Mosby Elsevier; 2017.
11. Meltzer KR, Cao TV, Schad JF, et al. In vitro modeling of repetitive motion injury and myofascial release. J Bodyw Mov Ther 2010;14(162):e171.
12. Borgini E, Stecco A, Day J, et al. How much time is required to modify fascial fibrosis? J Bodyw Mov Ther 2010; 14:318–25.
13. Chaitow L. Biochemistry and bodywork. J Bodyw Mov Ther 2018;12:95.
14. Hammer WI. Functional soft-tissue examination and treatment by manual methods. 3rd edn. Sudbury: Jones & Barlett Pub; 2007.
15. Masi AT, Hannon JC. Human resting muscle tone (HRMT): narrative introduction and modern concepts. J Bodyw Mov Ther 2008;12: 320–32.
16. De Deyne PG, Meyer R, Paley D, et al. The adaptation of perimuscular connective tissue during distraction osteogenesis. Clin Orthop Relat R 2000;379:259–69.
17. Matsumoto F, Trudel G, Uhthoff HK. High collagen type I and low collagen type III levels in knee joint contracture: an immunohistochemical study with histological correlate. Acta Orthop Scand 2002;73:335–43.
18. Schleip R, Klingler W, Lehmann-Horn F. Active fascial contractility: fascia may be able to contract in a smooth muscle-like manner and thereby influence musculoskeletal dynamics. Med Hypotheses 2005;65:273–7.
19. Schleip R, Naylor IL, Ursu D, et al. Passive muscle stiffness may be influenced by active contractility of intramuscular connective tissue. Med Hypotheses 2006;66:66–71.
20. Chiquet M, Tunc-Civelek V, Sarasa-Renedo A. Gene regulation by mechanotransduction in fibroblasts. Appl Physiol Nutr Me 2007;32:967–73.
21. Grinnell F. Fibroblast mechanics in three-dimensional collagen matrices. J Bodyw Mov Ther 2008;12:191–3.
22. Stecco L, Stecco C. Fascial manipulation: practical part. Padova: Piccin Ed; 2009.
23. Schultz R, Feitis R. The endless web: fascial anatomy and physical reality. Berkeley, CA: North Atlantic Books; 1996.
24. Bertolucci L. Muscle repositioning: a new verifiable approach to neuro-myofascial release? J Bodyw Mov Ther 2008;12(3):213–24.
25. Piper S, Shearer H, Cote P, et al. The effectiveness of soft-tissue therapy for the management of musculoskeletal disorders and injuries of the upper and lower extremities: a systematic review by the Ontario Protocol for Traffic Injury Management (OPTIMa) collaboration. Manual Ther 2016;21:18–34.
26. Meltzer K, Cao T, Schad J, et al. In vitro modeling of repetitive motion injury and myofascial release. J Bodyw Mov Ther 2010;14(2):162–71.
27. Martin M. Effects of the myofascial release in diffuse systemic sclerosis. J Bodyw Mov Ther 2009;13(4):320–7.
28. Arroyo-Morales M, Olea N, Martinez M, et al. Psychophysiological effects of massage-myofascial release after exercise: a randomized sham-control study. J Altern Complement Med 2008;14(10):1223–9.
29. Albert W, Currie-Jackson N, Duncan C. A survey of musculoskeletal injuries amongst Canadian massage therapists. J Bodyw Mov Ther 2008;12(1):86–93.
30. Manheim C. The myofascial release manual. 4th edn. Thorofare, NJ: Slack; 2008.

Lymphatic drainage massage

9

Learning Outcomes

- Describe the reported benefits of lymphatic drainage massage.
- Assess clients' suitability for lymphatic drainage massage.
- Describe the current evidence for the effectiveness of lymphatic drainage massage.
- Apply basic lymphatic drainage massage effectively and safely to a range of clients.
- Advise and resource clients who have been assessed and treated with lymphatic drainage massage.

INTRODUCTION

Lymphatic drainage massage is a gentle, light-touch, non-invasive technique which can be used to treat specific conditions, complement existing healthcare protocols or as a relaxing massage treatment. It is a style of bodywork which is designed to promote the free flow of lymph throughout the body. Lymphatic drainage massage is distinctly different from other types of massage which generally use strokes that manipulate the soft tissues of the body (muscles, tendons, ligaments, fascia, joints or connective tissue) in that it is mainly concerned with the flow of lymph in the superficial lymph vessels just below the surface of the skin. The lymphatic system is responsible for optimum functioning of fluid circulation and plays an important part in maximising our ability to rejuvenate and to establish resistance to stress and disease.[1]

Manual Lymphatic Drainage (MLD) was developed in France by Emil Vodder in the 1930s. Over the years many scientists, doctors and therapists have contributed to Dr Vodder's techniques which has enabled MLD to gain worldwide acceptance and recognition in medicine and physiotherapy. MLD and other forms of lymphatic drainage massage have become popular in contemporary massage therapy, particularly to relieve post-traumatic oedema. Its reported benefits, which arise from mechanical stimulation of the flow of lymph,[2] include:[3–8]

- reducing or preventing lymphoedema
- alleviating fluid congestion (e.g. swollen ankles, puffy eyes)
- stimulating the immune system to reduce frequency of recurring infections (e.g. colds, flu, ear or chest infections)
- promoting healing (e.g. wounds, acute injuries, burns). After traumatic injury lymphatic drainage massage is performed proximal to the injury and not directly over it.
- inducing relaxation and restful sleep
- reducing pain (e.g. in arthritic conditions)
- relaxing hypertonic muscles
- reducing cellulite
- stimulating bowel and bladder movements
- promoting hormone balance (some menstrual conditions and menopause)
- removing metabolic wastes, excess water, toxins, bacteria, large protein molecules and foreign substances from the tissues
- promoting general health and wellbeing
- improving many chronic conditions (e.g. sinusitis, scleroderma, acne and other skin conditions, chronic fatigue)
- assisting in conditions arising from venous insufficiency
- scar treatment (lymphatic drainage massage may soften and improve elasticity of scar tissue)
- assisting treatment of some neurological disorders (e.g. multiple sclerosis, migraine, Parkinson's disease, trigeminal neuralgia).

EVIDENCE FOR THE EFFECTIVENESS OF LYMPHATIC DRAINAGE MASSAGE

Manual lymphatic drainage is part of complex decongestive therapy for breast cancer-related lymphoedema along with compression therapy, skin care and lymph-reducing exercises. More than one in five patients develops breast cancer-related oedema, which has a negative impact on quality of life. This high prevalence has prompted a large number of clinical trials and literature reviews on the effectiveness of manual lymphatic drainage in fluid removal post breast-cancer surgery and/or radiation therapy. As is commonly reported, the quality of the studies varies considerably making conclusions difficult to draw. However, reviews consistently report that complex physical therapy is effective in limb volume reduction.[9] For example, a review of the literature concluded that manual lymphatic drainage was safe and may offer additional benefits to compression bandaging for those with mild-to-moderate breast cancer-related lymphoedema.[10] Another systematic review of four relevant studies reported that manual lymphatic draining in addition to standard conservative therapy for the management of breast cancer-related lymphoedema led to a significant reduction in the volume of lymphoedema, but might not improve subjective symptoms or arm function.[11]

Although most lymphoedema is secondary to cancer treatments (surgery and/or radiotherapy) chronic oedema can also result from prolonged volume overload from various venous diseases like post-thrombotic syndrome or chronic venous insufficiency.[12] Reviews generally have found conflicting results because of the quality and quantity of available trials. However, the body of literature suggests that the greatest improvements in lymphoedema, particularly breast cancer-related lymphoedema, occur when a combined treatment program is used; that is, when manual lymphatic drainage is used in combination with other treatments like compression garments and pumps.[9]

Few studies have focused on the effectiveness of manual lymphatic drainage as a treatment for conditions other than lymphoedema. Practitioners treating patients after trauma or injury are often concerned that oedema will delay recovery. There is moderate evidence to support the use of manual lymphatic draining for improving oedema, range of motion, and activities of daily living in patients with orthopaedic injuries.[13] Yuan et al[14] investigated treatments for fribromyalgia, a chronic pain condition associated with fatigue, sleep disturbance, tenderness, stiffness and mood disturbances. This study focused on non-pharmcological interventions like massage therapy that are frequently recommended by health professionals. The authors found that myofascial release improved fatigue, stiffness and quality of life; connective tissue massage improved depression and quality of life; manual lymphatic drainage was superior to connective tissue massage for stiffness, depression and quality of life; Shiatsu improved pain, pressure pain threshold, fatigue, sleep and quality of life; and Swedish massage did not improve outcomes.

FUNCTIONAL ANATOMY REVIEW[7]

The term *lymph* comes from the Latin *lympha*, which means water. Lymph is a colourless or slightly yellowish fluid, whose composition is similar to blood plasma except that the protein and cholesterol content of lymph are a little lower. Body tissues are bathed in intracellular fluid (i.e. fluid which lies inside the cells and makes up about two-thirds or approximately 25 litres of the body's water) and interstitial fluid (i.e. the remaining one-third of the body's water or approximately 10–12 litres which is located between the cells).

Blood carries oxygen and nutrients to the cells and carries away carbon dioxide and other wastes. Fluid leaks out of the blood capillaries and is reabsorbed again through diffusion. The rate at which fluid leaks from the capillaries is determined by pressures on either side of the capillary walls. These pressures (*Starling forces*) are exerted by fluid and protein on either side of the capillary wall. All body cells are bathed in interstitial fluid. In order to keep the volume of fluid in the interstitial compartment constant, excess interstitial fluid (about 10% or approximately 2 litres) and large proteins must be returned to the bloodstream. This process is carried out almost entirely by the lymphatic system, which forms an elaborate system of drainage vessels (see Figure 9.1).

Excess interstitial fluid first drains into small, thin walled lymphatic capilliaries (initial lymphatics) and then into larger lymphatics. Lymphatic capilliaries have disjunct endothelial cells and a discontinuous basement membrane which allow liquids and macromolecules (proteins) and lymphocytes to be reabsorbed. Larger lymphatics contain valves to ensure that lymph flow is one-way and have muscular walls which can pump the interstitial fluid (now termed *lymph*) towards lymph nodes. Lymphocytes within lymph nodes police all fluid which passes through them and an immune response may be initiated if a foreign body is encountered (this is why our lymph nodes swell when we are unwell).

From the lymph capillaries the fluid passes to pre-collectors, then to collectors and finally to lymphatic trunks, which return the fluid back to the bloodstream at the junction of the venous angle in the neck. The thoracic duct is the largest of the lymphatic vessels and drains lymph from the lower limbs and many internal organs. It opens into the left venous angle, the junction of the subclavian and internal jugular veins. The much smaller right lymphatic duct drains part of the heart, lungs, right arm, right side of the face, head and neck emptying into the right venous angle (see Figure 9.2 on p 125).

Lymph nodes (sometimes called lymph glands) are found throughout the body and are generally located in adipose tissue. These nodes consist of lymphoid tissue, which contains specialised cells that can help fight infection and other diseases such as cancer. Lymph nodes vary greatly in size, some being as small as a pinhead and others up to 3 cm long. There are about 500–700 lymph nodes in the body. The number of nodes varies from person to person and in different parts of the body (see Figure 9.3 on p 125). The branched sinus system

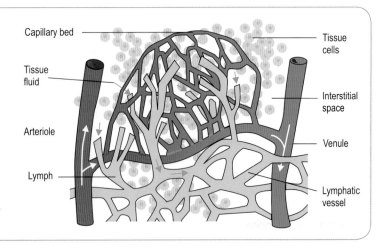

Fig. 9.1 Relationship between a blood capillary and lymphatic capillaries

in the nodes slows the lymph flow allowing macrophages to phagocytose toxins, cell debris, bacteria, infectious organisms or cancer cells. Lymph nodes have more lymph vessels entering them (afferent vessels) than leaving them (efferent vessels). Seventy per cent of the fluid that enters a lymph node is absorbed into the veins of the node (see Figure 9.4 on p 125).

FUNCTION OF THE LYMPHATIC SYSTEM

One of the major functions of the lymphatic system is to remove protein from interstitial fluid. Other functions include the production of small lymphocytes which play a key role in cellular immunity, and the production of large lymphocytes which are capable of synthesising antibodies. It also acts as a drainage system to return interstitial fluid containing dead cells, proteins, bacteria, foreign bodies, pathogenic agents and fats back to the cardiovascular system to be flushed out of the body. Lymph nodes act as filters for debris and infective agents that have gained access to the lymphatic system. The intestinal lymphatic system has two non-communicating lymphatic networks: one that contains the lymphatics that drain the intestine muscular layer, and the other that contains the lymphatic capilliaries (lacteals) that absorb dietary fats in the villi of the small intestine.[15] Absorbed fats are carried to the blood via the thoracic duct so that metabolism of the fats can commence.

The major function of the lymphatic system that concerns massage therapists is the movement of interstitial fluid and protein via the lymph vessels back to the bloodstream. If this protein-rich fluid accumulates, oedema prevents normal tissue function and metabolism.

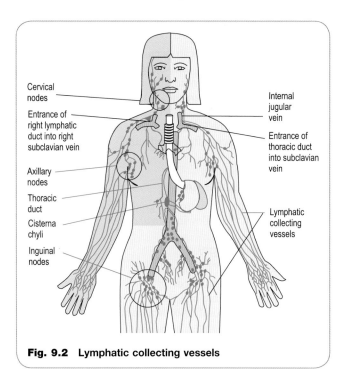

Fig. 9.2   Lymphatic collecting vessels

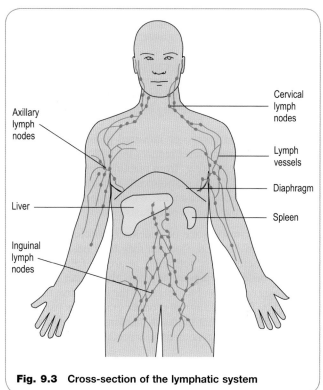

Fig. 9.3   Cross-section of the lymphatic system

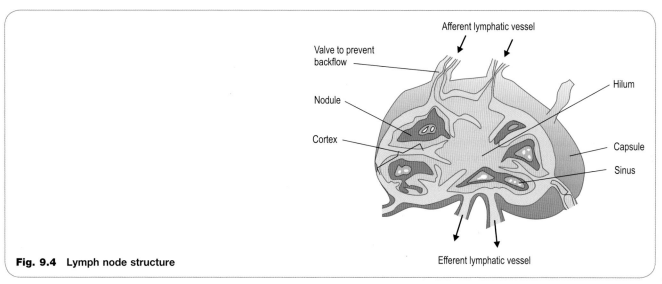

Fig. 9.4   Lymph node structure

OEDEMA

Oedema is a condition where excessive tissue fluid accumulates in the body. Oedema is the result of an imbalance between incoming and outgoing fluid which causes an abnormal amount of water to collect in the tissues. It should never be considered a diagnosis but rather a symptom of an underlying disorder. There are many possible causes of oedema including:

- acute nephritic syndrome
- heart failure
- Hodgkin's lymphoma and non-Hodgkin's lymphoma
- deep vein thrombosis
- pregnancy
- pulmonary oedema
- acute injury or allergic reaction – the hormones histamine and bradykinin act by raising the permeability of the capillary wall which leads to greater filtration of proteins and fluids in the tissues
- sodium excess – oedema can result from excessive table salt which causes water retention and increased protein excretion in the urine (renal oedema – the first visible signs of renal oedema are swelling of the eyelids and oedema in both lower legs)
- reduced protein uptake or impaired protein processing – lower blood protein level reduces the colloid osmotic pressure in the plasma (e.g. from malnutrition, malabsorption or protein loss due to gastrointestinal disease)
- hydrodynamic congestion due to local impediment to blood flow such as thrombosis or fibrosis.

The primary consequence of oedema is mechanical impairment of organ function. Oedema may have been present for some time before it is noticeable in areas of the body. The longer an oedema is present in tissue, the greater the chance that fibrosis can occur. Fibroblasts in the connective tissue are activated by free proteins that produce granulation tissue. This tissue is soft at first but gradually hardens and becomes sclerotic as further collagenous fibre is produced.

Lymphoedema

Lymphoedema refers to localised oedema due to lymphatic obstruction. According to the International Society of Lymphology,[16] lymphoedema is an external (and/or internal) manifestation of lymphatic system insufficiency and deranged lymph transport: 'In its purest form, the central disturbance is a low output failure (mechanical insufficiency) of the lymphvascular system; that is, overall lymphatic transport is reduced … the lymphatic system (whether vessels, nodes, interstitium, etc, or combinations) transport has fallen below the capacity needed to handle the presented load of microvascular filtrate including plasma protein and cells that normally leak from the bloodstream into the interstitium. Swelling is produced by accumulation in the extracellular space of excess water, filtered/ diffused plasma proteins, extravascular blood cells and parenchymal/stromal cell products'. One of the main reasons for the prevalence of lymphoedema is surgical intervention and lymph node dissections as can occur in mastectomy to prevent the spread of breast cancer. It is estimated that 20% of patients treated for melanoma, breast, gynaecological or prostate cancer will experience secondary lymphoedema.[17] Other reasons for lymphoedema are trauma to lymph vessels, deep vein thrombosis, venous insufficiency, filariasis,[a] impaired venous circulation, dysplasia of lymphatic vessels and radiation therapy.

Lymphoedema is classified as primary or secondary.

PRIMARY LYMPHOEDEMA

Primary lymphoedema is not common. It almost exclusively affects the lower extremity and there is usually no family history. Primary lymphoedema originates from a developmental abnormality that is present but not always clinically evident at birth. It may become visible months after birth or many years later in life. A trauma or a simple event such as an insect bite can trigger a lymphoedema to occur. In primary lymphoedema the person may have had defective lymphatic drainage for many years before problems occur. If the lymphoedema is only mild, it may disappear within a few days or may stay and continue to worsen.

SECONDARY LYMPHOEDEMA

Secondary lymphoedema can occur in any part of the body (limbs, joints or viscera) and usually develops as a result of surgery, radiation, chronic venous insufficiency, trauma, paralysis of a limb or parasites. Damage to lymph vessels or nodes always entails the risk of developing lymphoedema which may occur immediately or weeks, months or even years later. It may also occur after an infection, insect bite, aircraft travel or sunburn.

STAGES OF LYMPHOEDEMA

Any lymphoedema left untreated gradually worsens and will progress through the following stages:

Stage 0 (latency stage)

- Subclinical stage of lymphoedema
- Transport capacity reduced
- No visible or palpable oedema
- Complaints of discomfort or heaviness

Stage 1 (mild)

- Visible signs of oedema
- Pitting on pressure
- Reduces on elevation or overnight, returns gradually during the day
- Smooth texture of skin and softness of tissue

Stage 2 (moderate)

- Accumulation of protein-rich oedema
- No longer pits easily
- Connective tissue proliferation causing fibrosis
- Oedema does not reduce overnight or on elevation
- Prone to developing infections

Stage 3 (severe)

- The third stage is known as lymphostatic elephantiasis
- Extreme increase in volume
- The extremity is column-shaped, resembling the limb of an elephant

---

[a]Filariasis is an infectious tropical disease caused by roundworms.

- Natural skin folds are extremely deepened, the dermal tissues progressively harden and the back of the hand or foot is massively swollen
- Non-pitting
- Skin changes (e.g. papillomas, hyperkeratosis)
- Fibrosis and sclerosis

ASSESSING CLIENTS

All potential lymphatic drainage clients need to be screened for red flags for serious conditions and to determine their suitability for the technique. Case history, observation and palpation are particularly useful assessment tools for lymphatic drainage massage clients.

HISTORY

A thorough case history should be taken before commencing lymphatic drainage massage. It is necessary to know about medication, past illness, surgery and any current illness. As lymphatic drainage massage is not appropriate for all conditions, the case history enables you to determine the suitability of the client for treatment. A referral may be necessary to rule out contraindications before treatment can begin.

Clients with lymphoedema may have a history of surgery or radiation therapy. Signs or symptoms of lymphoedema may include:

- transient swelling of a limb after surgery
- infection due to lymph statis
- sensation of heaviness, aching and tightness in the affected part
- limitation of movement
- rings, watches or clothing becoming tight
- swelling aggravated by heat, overuse, sustained positions, prologed inactivity and more obvious at the end of the day
- permanent swelling (> 3 months)
- asymmetrical, especially in the upper limb
- Stemmer's sign (unable to pinch the skin at the base of the second toe)[18]

RED FLAG CONDITIONS FOR OEDEMA[19]

- Sudden onset
- Significant pain
- Shortness of breath
- History of a heart disorder or an abnormal cardiac examination
- Haemoptysis, dyspnoea, or pleural friction rub
- Hepatomegaly, jaundice, ascites, splenomegaly or haematemesis
- Unilateral leg swelling with tenderness

Chronic heart, kidney or liver disorder are suggested by generalised oedema that develops slowly.

POSTURAL ANALYSIS

Postural observation should note the presence of any of the following:

- loss of muscle definition
- swollen appearance (e.g. puffy face, hands, feet and legs)
- swollen joints.

FUNCTIONAL TESTS

- Decreased joint range of motion may result from fluid accumulation.

PALPATION[20]

Palpation can show oedema to be boggy, spongy or soggy and may elicit tenderness. The overlying skin and superficial fascia feel taut. Determining the nature of the oedema (e.g. pitting or non-pitting) helps identify its cause and stage. Pitting refers to the persistence of the indentation after digital pressure has been released. Pitting oedema can occur when any pressure is applied to the limb (e.g. wearing tight socks). In non-pitting oedema the indentation does not persist after the pressure is released. Non-pitting oedema occurs in conditions like lymphoedema and hyperthyroidism.

DIFFERENTIAL DIAGNOSIS

- Small lymph nodes are often detected in the axilla and groin of healthy individuals.
- Localised lymphadenopathy is common and usually the result of local infection.
- In Hodgkin's lymphoma the lymph nodes palpate as rubbery; in tuberculosis they may feel matted; in metastatic carcinoma they feel craggy.
- Tender nodes usually indicate acute infection.
- Nodes which are fixed to deep structures or skin are usually malignant.[21]
- Peripheral causes of oedema include orthostatic oedema, lymphoedema, lipoedema or chronic venous insufficiency (see Table 9.1).

TREATING CLIENTS

It is important to remember that lymphatic drainage massage is a specialist treatment and should be provided by practitioners who are trained in this technique. Practitioners must not provide healthcare of a type that is outside the scope of their training and experience. Lymphatic drainage to breast tissue can only be provided by practitioners who have specialist post-graduate training in complex physical therapy, decongestive therapy or lymphedema management. Remedial massage therapists may perform lymphatic drainage massage to other (non-sensitive) areas of the body and to areas proximal and lateral to breast tissue with appropriate draping across the anterior chest/breast region.

Due to the success of lymphatic drainage massage in treating lymphoedema many hospitals and medical centres to employ lymph drainage therapists to participate in treatment.

BASIC PRINCIPLES

1. Clear the major lymph nodes in the area first. Proximal areas are treated before distal areas and the direction of massage follows lymph flow. The massage sequence is designed to clear an area before directing lymph into it. For example, the upper arm is massaged before the forearm; the thigh before the lower leg; and the abdomen before the legs.
2. Pressure is light. Contact is superficial; that is, only to skin depth, not muscle depth. Firm pressure is only used

Table 9.1 Peripheral causes of oedema[22,23]

Type of oedema	Process	Nature of oedema	Skin thickening	Ulceration	Pigmentation	Foot involvement	Bilateral
Orthostatic	Prolonged standing or sitting	Soft pitting	–	–	–	Yes	Always
Lymphoedema	Lymphatic obstruction	Soft early, later hard and non-pitting	Marked	Rare	–	Yes	Often
Lipoedema	Fatty deposits in legs	Minimal	–	–	–	–	Always
Chronic venous insufficiency	Deep venous obstruction or valvular incompetence	Soft, pitting; later brawny	Occasional	Common	Common	Yes	Occasionally

when fibrosis or hard oedema is present. Lymphatic drainage massage should not cause pain.

3. The massage movements should be done at a moderate pace. This is important as lymphatic drainage massage causes mechanical emptying and filling of the lymphatic vessels. If the massage movements are too fast the vessels are not given the opportunity to fill completely before the next movement is applied, rendering the massage inefficient.

4. Movements should be smooth, rhythmic and repetitious. The object is to stimulate a peristaltic wave-like action within the lymph vessels to stimulate the lymphangions, the functional units of lymph vessels. Smooth muscles in the walls of the lymphatic vessels cause the lymphangions to contract sequentially to aid the flow of lymph.

5. Movements are predominantly circular and performed in a wave-like rhythm which also promotes general relaxation.

6. Movements have a pressure or working phase which promotes the movement of fluid in the desired direction, followed by a relaxation phase to allow lymph capillaries to refill.

7. Each movement should be repeated 5–7 times to stimulate the lymph collectors.

LENGTH OF TREATMENT

General lymphatic drainage massage takes about 60 minutes but treatment time should not be fixed. Shorter treatment times (e.g. 20 minutes) may also be of value to many clients. The treatment time will depend on the age and health of the client and the purpose of treatment. If treatment time is too long the client may develop side effects like mild headache, nausea or fatigue.

EXPLANATION OF TREATMENT

Always explain lymphatic drainage massage to your clients, including the reason for lightness of pressure, the duration of the treatment, recommended treatment frequency and areas to be massaged. Also discuss what to expect from the treatment including how clients may feel after treatment and how they may assist treatment. Recommendations for the immediate period after treatment could include drinking plenty of

water, doing only light exercises and refraining from eating a heavy meal. Other recommendations include epsom salts baths and a diet that is rich in diuretic foods like pineapple, papaya, berries, cucumbers, radishes, celery, aloe vera juice and watermelon.[20]

Pressure

To be most effective the pressure of lymphatic drainage massage needs to be light to avoid compression of the superficial lymph vessels and lymph collectors which would prevent or considerably hamper the flow of lymph during massage. Correct pressure is achieved when the top layer of skin moves against the level immediately beneath, not against muscle which would indicate pressure that is too heavy. A reddening of the skin may also indicate that the pressure is too heavy. Lymphatic drainage massage should not be painful. Firm pressure may be indicated when treating chronic lymphoedema which has become fibrotic. Note that fibrosis occurs in the connective tissue not in the muscle. Pressure should always be applied within the client's pain-free range. Overworking an area or using too much pressure may cause bruising or inflammation.

Lymphatic drainage strokes

There is a small number of specific strokes used in lymphatic drainage.

1. STATIONARY CIRCLES

These strokes are used more frequently than all other strokes. As the name implies the stroke is stationary – it does not generally glide or slide over the skin. The movements may be small or large stationary circles, clockwise or anti-clockwise, using flat fingers or the whole of the palm. The strokes stretch the skin numerous times in the one area before moving to the next area (see Figure 9.5 on p 129).

2. PUMP TECHNIQUE

Pumping is performed with the palm of the hand and fingers. It is an exaggerated movement of the wrist using a hinge action to carry the hand forward over the area being treated (see Figure 9.6 on p 129).

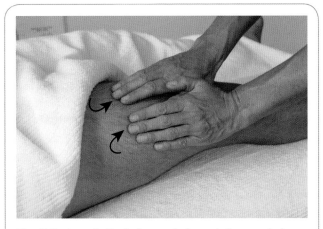

Fig. 9.5 Lymphatic drainage strokes: stationary circles

Fig. 9.7 Lymphatic drainage strokes: scoop technique

Fig. 9.6 Lymphatic drainage strokes: pump technique

Fig. 9.8 Lymphatic drainage strokes: rotary technique

These four movements are combined to produce pressure-on/pressure-off kneading movements that can be circular, oval, deep, shallow, large or small.

Summary

- Massage slowly. Lymph is thicker than blood and moves more slowly. Flow rates of lymph in the skin vary from one area of the body to another (e.g. lymph from the head and neck moves more slowly than lymph in the legs). Strokes should be rhythmical and performed at the rate of one stroke per second but this may vary depending on the individual treatment.
- Use gentle pressure to increase lymph production and lymph flow through stimulation of lymph capillaries and lymph collectors. Heavy pressure may hamper the flow of lymph or cause the delicate lymph vessels to spasm.
- Drain in the correct direction. Knowing the direction of lymph flow is required for effective lymphatic drainage massage.
- Apply pressure smoothly during the working phase and release pressure during the resting phase of each stroke. This allows for filling or refilling of lymph vessels and the stimulation of the lymph collectors during the massage (see Figure 9.9 on p 130).

3. SCOOP TECHNIQUE

The scoop technique involves turning the palms out from the body by rotating the wrists in a corkscrew motion (see Figure 9.7 on p 129).

4. ROTARY TECHNIQUE

This movement uses the palm of the hand and thumb to create sweeping circular movements in the direction of lymph flow. The writs are used to increase and decrease the pressure of the stroke (see Figure 9.8).

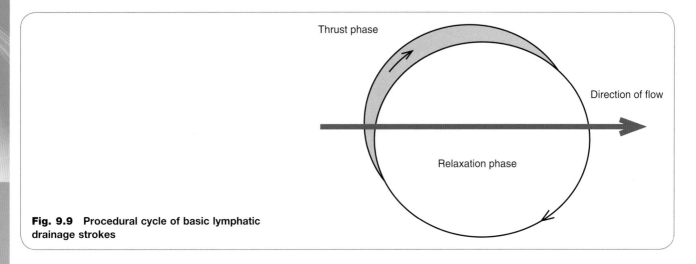

Fig. 9.9 Procedural cycle of basic lymphatic drainage strokes

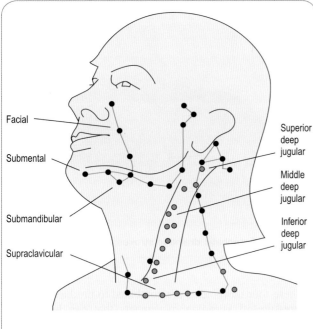

Fig. 9.10 Superficial and deep nodes of the head and neck

- The area closest to the terminus (the triangular area just above the clavicle where lymph returns to the subclavian veins) is treated first so that the peripheral areas can be drained. On the extremities, regional lymph nodes are treated first, then the massage begins proximally and continues distally.

REGIONAL LYMPHATIC DRAINAGE MASSAGE

The following section presents an overview of lymph anatomy, direction of lymph flow and indications for lymph drainage massage for specific regions of the body: the head and neck, upper torso, upper limb, lower torso, lower limb and thorax.

The head and neck

The lymphatics of the neck are arranged in deep and superficial chains (see Figure 9.10):

- The deep jugular chain extends from the base of the skull to the clavicle and consists of superior, middle and inferior groups of lymph nodes. The *superior deep jugular nodes* receive primary drainage from oral cavity tonsils, the larynx, pharynx, pyriform sinus and above the vocal folds. This group of lymph nodes also receives lymph from more superficial nodes in the upper head and neck (retropharyngeal, spinal accessory, parotid, superficial cervical and submandibular nodes).

  The *middle deep jugular nodes* receive primary drainage from the larynx above the vocal folds, lower pyriform sinus (located on each side of the laryngeal orifice) and posterior cricoid. They receive secondary drainage from the deep jugular nodes above them and the lower retropharyngeal nodes. The *inferior deep jugular nodes* receive primary drainage from the thyroid, trachea and cervical oesophagus. They receive secondary drainage from the deep jugular nodes above them and the paratracheal nodes. The retropharyngeal and paratracheal nodes lie posteriorly around the midline viscera. They receive drainage from these viscera and from the deep structures in the midline of the head; that is, the nasopharynx, posterior nasal cavity, paranasal sinuses and posterior oropharynx. They drain towards the deep jugular chain. The superficial nodes tend to drain secondarily, as mentioned, to the deep nodes (see Figure 9.11 on p 131).

- The superficial nodes are the submental, superficial cervical, submandibular, spinal accessory and anterior scalene. The *submental nodes* drain the chin, the middle of the lower lip, tip of the tongue and anterior mouth. These nodes in turn drain to the submandibular nodes. The submandibular nodes drain the upper lip, lateral lower lip, lower nasal cavity, anterior mouth and the skin of the cheek. The *submandibular nodes* in turn drain to the superior deep jugular nodes (see Figure 9.12 on p 131). The *superficial cervical nodes* located along the external jugular vein receive drainage from the cutaneous lymphatics of the face, especially from around the parotid gland, behind the ear, parotid and occipital nodes.

  The superficial cervical nodes then drain into the superior deep jugular nodes. The nodes in the posterior triangle lie along the spinal accessory nerve. These nodes drain the parietal and occipital regions of the scalp. The upper nodes drain to the superior deep jugular nodes while the

Labels on Fig. 9.10: Facial, Submental, Submandibular, Supraclavicular, Superior deep jugular, Middle deep jugular, Inferior deep jugular

Labels on Fig. 9.9: Thrust phase, Direction of flow, Relaxation phase lower nodes drain down to the supraclavicular nodes. The anterior scalene (Virchow's) nodes receive drainage from the thoracic duct and are located at the junction of the thoracic duct and left subclavian vein. The supraclavicular nodes receive drainage from the spinal accessory nodes and from infraclavicular sources. All of these lymphatics eventually drain into the venous system either through or together with the thoracic duct on the left, or the right lymphatic duct (see Figure 9.13).

Indications for lymphatic drainage of the head and neck include:

- acne vulgaris or rosacea
- facial muscle contractures
- puffy eyes
- after root canal surgery and tooth extraction
- sinusitis
- nasal congestion

- syringitis (inflammation of the eustachian tube)
- Bell's palsy

The upper torso

All lymph vessels of the upper torso drain into the axilla (see Figure 9.14 on p 132). The superficial nodes begin in lymphatic plexuses in the skin and end at the axillary lymph nodes. The deep vessels follow the principal vascular and neurovascular bundles and end in the lateral axillary lymph nodes.

Axillary lymph nodes are the regional group for the whole of the upper extremity. There can be 20 to 30 large nodes in this area.

- The lateral group lies medial to and behind the axillary vein. This group receives lymph from the whole upper arm except for the lymph vessels that accompany the cephalic vein.

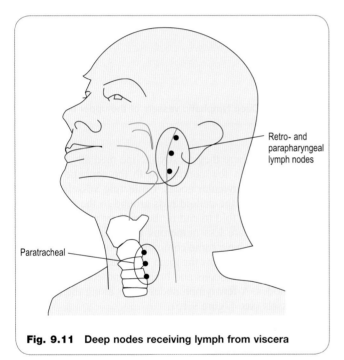

Fig. 9.11 Deep nodes receiving lymph from viscera

Retro- and parapharyngeal lymph nodes

Paratracheal

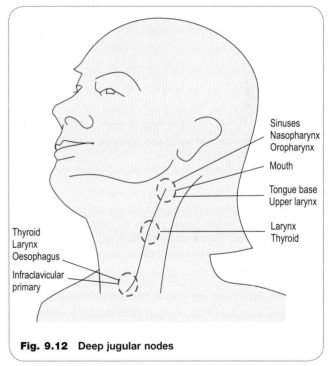

Sinuses
Nasopharynx
Oropharynx

Mouth

Tongue base
Upper larynx

Larynx
Thyroid

Thyroid
Larynx
Oesophagus

Infraclavicular primary

Fig. 9.12 Deep jugular nodes

Fig. 9.13 Direction of lymphatic drainage in the head and neck

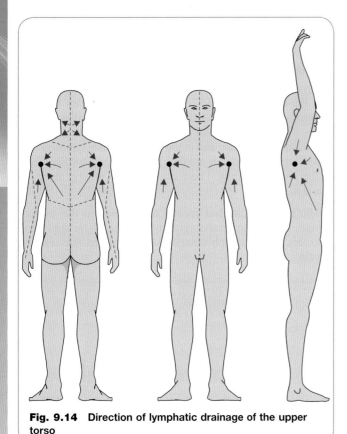

Fig. 9.14 Direction of lymphatic drainage of the upper torso

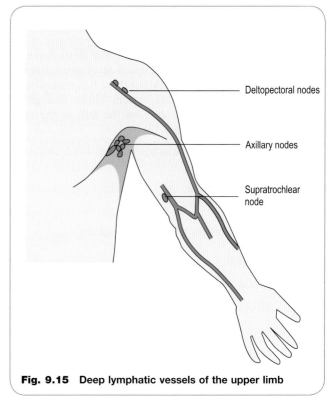

Fig. 9.15 Deep lymphatic vessels of the upper limb

- The anterior (pectoral) group lies along the lower border of the pectoralis minor. Vessels from the skin and muscles of the anterior and lateral walls of the trunk above the umbilicus and the central and lateral areas of the breast drain into these nodes.
- The posterior (subscapular) group lies along the lower margin of the posterior wall of the axilla. Vessels from the skin and muscles of the lower part of the back of the neck and the dorsal aspect of the trunk drain into these nodes.
- The central group is embedded in the fat of the axilla and receives lymph from all the preceding groups of axillary lymph nodes.
- The apical group is situated posterior to the upper border of the pectoralis minor, above its lower border and extends to the apex of the axilla. Lymph vessels that accompany the cephalic vein drain into these nodes as do lymph vessels from part of the breast and all other axillary nodes. The efferent vessels of this group unite to form the subclavian trunk which opens either into the internal jugular and sub-clavian vein or into the jugular lymphatic trunk. On the left side it may end in the thoracic duct.

Superficial vessels on the anterior surface begin in the palm of the hand, draining the fingers towards the wrist. The vessels on the front of the wrist pass into the forearm following the median vein up to the cubital region. From there they follow the medial border of the biceps to pierce the deep fascia at the axillary fold to end at the lateral axillary nodes. On the dorsal surface most of the vessels run parallel upwards finally passing around the borders of the limb to join the vessels on the anterior aspect. Some of the lateral vessels reach the level

of the deltoid where they mostly incline medially to join the anterior vessels; a few continue with the cephalic vein and end in the infraclavicular nodes. Collecting vessels from the front and back of the deltoid pass around to the anterior and posterior axillary fold to end in the axillary nodes.

Deep vessels are less numerous than the superficial ones with which they have some communication at intervals along their course. They follow the main neurovascular bundles, the radial, ulnar, interosseous and brachial and end in the lateral axillary nodes. A few lymph nodes occur along the course of these vessels (see Figure 9.15).

Indications for lymphatic drainage massage of the upper limb include:

- lymphoedema
- acute and chronic conditions of the upper limb (e.g. adhesive capsulitis, tendinitis, lateral epicondylitis, osteoarthritis, repetition strain injury).

The lower torso

Most of the lymph from the lower torso drains into the inguinal lymph nodes located in the groin (see Figure 9.16 on p 133).

The superficial inguinal lymph nodes are arranged in two groups:

- An upper group situated below the inguinal ligament. This group receives lymph from the abdominal wall below the umbilicus, gluteal region and part of the lateral region of the upper thigh. The inferior nodes of the upper group receive vessels from external genitalia, part of the anal canal, the perianal region and uterine lymph vessels.
- A lower group situated along the terminal end of the great saphenous vein. Vessels from the entire lower torso

Fig. 9.16 Direction of lymphatic drainage of the lower torso and lower limb

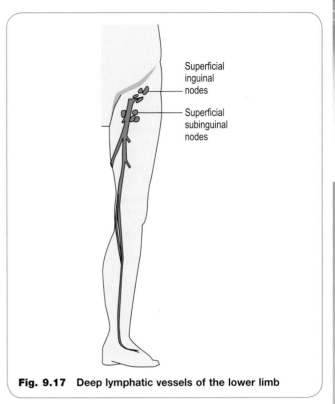

Fig. 9.17 Deep lymphatic vessels of the lower limb

(superficial) except for the back and lateral aspects of the calf drain into these nodes.

The few deep inguinal nodes are located on the medial side of the femoral vein. These nodes receive the lymph vessels that accompany the femoral vessels, vessels from the external genitalia and a few vessels from the superficial nodes. Vessels from the superficial and deep nodes pass through the femoral canal to the external iliac lymph nodes.

The popliteal lymph nodes are embedded in the fat of the popliteal fossa. There are approximately five to seven small lymph nodes which receive vessels from the back and lateral aspects of the calf. The efferent vessels from these nodes ascend with the femoral blood vessels to the deep inguinal nodes.

Superficial vessels begin in the foot: a median set follow the great saphenous vein and a lateral set follow the small saphenous vein. The vessels of the medial group begin on the dorsum of the foot (tibial side), ascend in front of or behind the malleolus and accompany the great saphenous vein to the groin. They end in the lower group of the superficial inguinal nodes. The vessels from the lateral set begin on the dorsum of the foot (fibular side). Some join the medial group; the others accompany the small saphenous vein and end in the popliteal lymph nodes.

The deep vessels accompany the main blood vessels (anterior tibial, peroneal, popliteal and femoral groups) to pass directly to the deep inguinal nodes except where some vessels from the lower leg end at the popliteal nodes (see Figure 9.17).

Indications for lymphatic drainage massage of the lower limb include:

- lymphoedema
- chronic venous conditions
- acute injuries
- chronic injuries and conditions (e.g. arthritis)
- leg ulcers
- restless leg syndrome
- heavy, tired legs
- fluid retention.

The thorax

The groups of vessels and nodes in the thorax are known as the intercostal, diaphragmatic, internal mammary, innominate and tracheo-bronchial, the first three of which are discussed here.

- Intercostal lymph nodes are located near the vertebral end of each intercostal space and receive vessels from the parietal pleura of the posterior abdominal wall. The vessels that accompany the intercostal arteries come from the costovertebral and intervertebral joints and also drain into these nodes. The efferents of the nodes of the upper 6–7 intercostals on both sides run independently of the thoracic duct to empty into the subclavian vein. The lower five join on each side to form a descending intercostal trunk, which passes through the aortic opening to enter the cisterna chyli.
- The diaphragmatic lymph nodes make up three groups: the posterior, anterior and middle. The *posterior* group is situated at the lower part of the oesophagus and receives vessels from the oesophagus, back of the pericardium and diaphragm. Efferents from these nodes empty directly into the thoracic duct or the descending intercostal lymph trunks. The *anterior* group is large and situated on the sternal and costal origins of the diaphragm behind the xiphoid process and the seventh costal cartilages. They receive vessels from the front of the pericardium, anterior intercostal lymph nodes and anterior part of the diaphragm and from the anterior and upper surface of the liver. The *middle* group of vessels from the lateral part of the diaphragm and their efferents pass to the anterior or posterior groups.

133

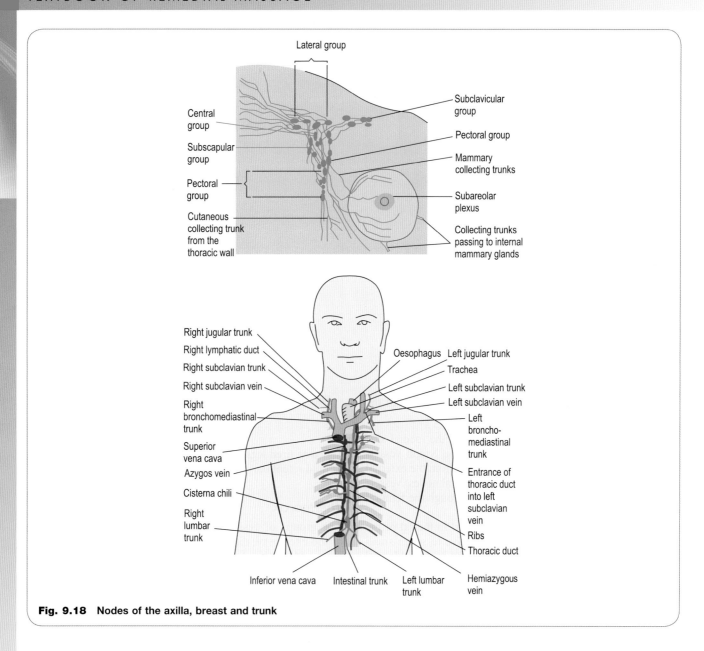

Fig. 9.18 Nodes of the axilla, breast and trunk

■ Internal mammary lymph nodes are situated in the upper four intercostal spaces close to the sternum, where they receive vessels from the anterior (diaphragmatic) nodes and the vessels which accompany the intercostal and branches of the internal mammary arteries. The anterior intercostal afferent vessels of the internal mammary chain drain the parietal pleura almost as far back as the angles of the ribs. Vessels also drain the skin of the breast and the medial part of the stroma (see Figure 9.18).

Superficial lymph drainage of the trunk and back covers the cutaneous area of the trunk extending from the level of the umbilicus to the clavicle in front to halfway up the neck on the back. These vessels originate in the fascia and converge on the axillary lymph nodes. On the back the vessels run downwards from the lower part of the neck, horizontally from the area of the scapula and upward from the iliac crest to converge round the posterior fold of the axilla. The cutaneous

vessels on the front, from the level of the umbilicus to below the breast, run diagonally upward, horizontally over the pectoral area and downward from the clavicle, again to converge on the axillary nodes (see Figure 9.19 on p 135).

Indications for lymphatic drainage massage for the thoracic and lumbar areas include:

■ after surgery (mastectomy, lumpectomy)
■ painful or swollen breasts
■ lower back and neck pain
■ chronic conditions (e.g. osteoarthritis, chronic bronchitis, emphysema).

CONTRAINDICATIONS AND PRECAUTIONS

The new levels of acceptance and high public use of manual lymph drainage calls for high levels of responsibility on the

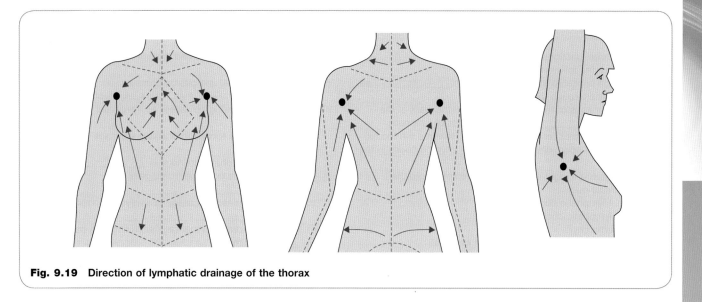

Fig. 9.19 Direction of lymphatic drainage of the thorax

part of practitioners to apply techniques safely and competently. There are only a few absolute contraindications to lymph drainage massage (see below). There are also conditions for which it is advisable to seek clearance from the client's doctor before commencing treatment. Lymph drainage massage is often recommended as a complementary therapy for cancer treatment. Previous thinking that massage could cause the spread of cancer from the primary tumour is being challenged as no evidence has been produced to support this claim. Furthermore the scientific literature cites numerous positive benefits of massage for cancer.[24]

Contraindications for lymphatic drainage massage can be classified as absolute, relative and local.[7]

ABSOLUTE CONTRAINDICATIONS

- Chronic congestive heart failure, untreated heart failure or cardiac oedema, acute renal insufficiency. A load is placed on the venous system when there is an increase in the volume of lymph arriving at the subclavian veins. Significantly increasing the load could place strain on the heart and kidneys.[2]
- Acute infections and fever.
- Acute deep vein thrombosis (known or suspected).
- Unexplained pain.
- After recent surgery.
- After recent trauma (e.g. whiplash, fractures, sprains or dislocations, or when the extent of the injury is not known).
- Severe unstable hypertension (i.e. elevated blood pressure above the normal range for a prolonged period of time).
- Systemic illness (e.g. fever, diarrhoea, vomiting, unexplained oedema).
- Oedema that contributes to joint stability.[18]

RELATIVE CONTRAINDICATIONS

- Malignancies. Advise clients who have active cancer or who are recovering from cancer to get clearance from their doctor before commencing lymphatic drainage massage.[25]

- Recent thrombosis. Older clients, clients with veins in poor condition and past history of thrombosis may be a contraindication.
- Varicose veins. Massage above the involved area.
- Bronchial asthma. Treat clients when the condition is receding, omitting sternum and chest massage. Never treat bronchial asthma in an acute phase. Care should always be taken with asthmatics to keep treatments short as over-treatment can bring on a mild attack of asthma.[4]
- Low blood pressure. A full body lymphatic drainage massage may lower blood pressure. Treatment time should be reduced for the first session and increased in subsequent sessions if no problems occur.[4]
- Moles, beauty spots, burns, fresh scars, bruises or skin problems.
- Renal insufficiency or clients receiving haemodialysis. Care should be taken to keep treatments short as such clients tire and bruise easily.
- Gynaecological cysts and other conditions of the uterus. Avoid deep abdominal massage.

LOCAL CONTRAINDICATIONS

- Varicose veins, thrombosis after inflammation has subsided.
- Local inflammation without fever (e.g. open wound, sprains).
- Sports injuries with oedema or inflammation.

Neck

- Hypersensitivity of the carotid sinus.
- Hyperthyroidism.

Abdomen

- Pregnancy.
- During menstruation.
- After recent abdominal surgery.
- Radiation fibrosis.
- After pelvic deep venous thrombosis.
- Crohn's disease.
- Diverticulosis.

Review questions

1. Name three functions of the lymphatic system.
2. Complete the following:
   a) Lymph is filtered as it passes through _____ as it travels through the body.
   b) Contractions of the smooth muscle in the walls of the _____ (the functional units of lymphatic vessels) stimulates the flow of lymph towards the thorax.
   c) There are approximately _____ lymph nodes in the body.
3. Lymph from the right upper quadrant empties into the
   a) thoracic duct
   b) right lymphatic duct
   c) left lymphatic duct
   d) cisterna chyli
4. What is the primary consequence of oedema?
5. How does lymphoedema differ from oedema?
6. What is the main cause of lymphoedema?
7. Complete the following table:

Primary lymphoedema	Secondary lymphoedema
Mainly affects _____	Occurs in any part of the body
Developmental abnormality. Can be triggered by _____	Usually develops after _____

8. Name three contraindications for lymphatic drainage massage.
9. Select the most correct answer. Orthostatic oedema:
   a) is associated with skin pigmentation, ulceration and pits on pressure
   b) is occasionally bilateral and is sometimes associated with skin thickening
   c) is always bilateral and pits on pressure
   d) is always bilateral and does not usually involve the feet
10. Complete the following guidelines for lymphatic drainage massage.
    a) The pressure of lymphatic drainage massage is _____
    b) The rate of lymphatic drainage is _____
    c) Begin lymphatic drainage massage at the _____
    d) Lymphatic drainage massage is always performed in the direction of _____
    e) In lymphatic drainage massage each stroke is performed _____ times.
    f) Strokes are predominantly _____ and performed in a wave-like rhythm
    g) Each stroke has a working phase and a resting phase to create a variation in _____
11. Which of the following is not an indication for lymphatic drainage massage?
    a) chronic pain
    b) sub-acute inflammation
    c) shortness of breath
    d) slowly developing generalised oedema
    e) lymphoedema
    f) acne vulgaris
    g) severe pain

REFERENCES

1. Chikly B. Silent waves. Lymph, interstitial fluid and primo-vascular system. The theory and practice of lymphatic drainage therapy. 3rd edn. Scotsdale, AZ: International Health & Healing Publishing; 2017.
2. Fritz S. Mosby's essential sciences for therapeutic massage. Anatomy, physiology, biomechanics, and pathology. 5th edn. St Louis, MO: Mosby Elsevier; 2017.
3. Cash M. Sport and remedial massage therapy. New York, NY: Random House; 2012.
4. Wittlinger G, Wittlinger H. Introduction to Dr Vodder's manual lymphatic drainage. Rev edn. Heidelberg: Karl V. Haug: Verlag; 1990.
5. Yates J. A physician's guide to therapeutic massage. 3rd ed. Toronto, ON: Curties–Overzet Publishing; 2004.
6. Fontera WR, Delisa JA, Gans BM, et al. Delisa's physical medicine & rehabilitation: principles and practice. 5th edn. Philadephia, PA: Lippincott Williams & Wilkings; 2010.
7. Foldi M, Foldi E. Foldi's textbook of lymphology for physicians and lymphedema therapists. 3rd revised edn. London: Elsevier Health Sciences; 2012.
8. Piller N, O'Connor M. The lymphoedema handbook: causes, effects and management. Melbourne: Hill of Content; 2006.
9. Finnane A, Janda M, Hayes S. Review of the evidence of lymphedema treatment effect. Am J Phys Med Rehabil 2015;9(6):483–98.
10. Ezzo E, Manheimer M, McNeely D, et al. Manual lymphatic drainage for lymphedema following breast cancer treatment. Cochrane Database Syst Rev 2015; 21(5):CD003475.
11. Shao Y, Zhong D. Manual lymphatic drainage for breast cancer-related lymphoedema. Eur J Cancer Care 2017;26:e12517.
12. Muller M, Klingberg K, Wertli M, et al. Manual lymphatic drainage and quality of life in patients with lymphoedema and mixed oedema: a systematic review of randomised controlled trials. Qual Life Res 2018;27:1403–14.
13. Majewski-Schrage T, Snyder K. The effectiveness of manual lymphatic drainage in patients with orthopedic injuries. J Sport Rehabil 2016;25(1): 91–7.
14. Yuan S, Matsutani A, Marques A. Effectiveness of different styles of massage therapy in fibromyalgia: a systematic review and meta-analysis. Manual Ther 2015;20:257–64.
15. Miller MJ, Newberry RD. Microanatomy of the intestinal lymphatic system. Ann NY Acad Sci 2010;1207(Suppl 1):E21–E28. Doi: 10.1111/j.1749 -6632.2010.05708.x.
16. International Society of Lymphology. The diagnosis and treatment of peripheral lymphedema: 2016 Consensus document of the International Society of Lymphology. Online. Available: https:// www.internationalsocietyoflymphology.org/ wp-content/uploads/2017/12/20106-35060-1-PB.pdf; 2016.
17. Cancer Australia. What is secondary lymphoedema? Australian Government Cancer Australia. Online. Available: https://canceraustralia.gov.au/ clinical-best-practice/lymphoedema; 2019.
18. Australasian Lymphology Association. The importance of early diagnosis of lymphoedema for medical practitioners. Australasian Lymphology Association. Online. Available: http:// www.lymphoedema.org.au/about-lymphoedema/ the-importance-of-early-diagnosis; 2019.
19. Thompson AD, Shea MJ. MSD Manual Professional Version. Edema. Online. Available: https:// msdmanuals.com/en-au/professional/cardiovascular -disorders/symptoms-of-cardiovascular-disorders/ edema; 2019.
20. Fritz S, Chaitow L, Hymel GM. Clinical massage in the healthcare setting. St Louis, MI: Mosby Elsevier; 2008.
21. Douglas G, Nicol F, Robertson C. Macleod's clinical examination. 13th edn. Edinburgh: Churchill Livingstone; 2013.
22. Bickley L. Bates' guide to physical examination and history taking. 11th edn. Philadelphia: Lippincott-Raven; 2013.
23. Vines S. Lymphedema: from diagnosis to treatment. Inter Med J 2017;38(2):97–105.
24. Russell N, Sumier S, Beinhorn C, et al. Role of massage in cancer care. J Altern Complement Med 2008;14(2):209–14.
25. Cancer Research UK. Research into massage and cancer. Online. Available: https:// www.cancerresearchuk.org/about-cancer/ cancer-in-general/treatment/complementary -alternative-therapies/individual-therapies/massage; 2015.

The low back and pelvis

INTRODUCTION

Low back pain is the leading cause of disability in the world[1] but for most people a specific nociceptive cause of the pain cannot be identified.[2] In the period 2014–2015, 1 in 6 Australians (16% or 3.7 million people) reported back problems.[3] Acute episodes of low back pain generally last no more than 6 weeks, but two-thirds of those who suffer acute episodes will still have some pain after 3 months. Recurrence is common and in a small number of people, the pain may become persistent and disabling.[2] Risk factors for developing low back pain include a physically demanding job that involves lifting, bending and being in awkward postures, and lifestyle factors such as smoking, obesity and low levels of physical activity. Increased risk is also associated with previous episodes of low back pain, other chronic conditions like asthma, headache and diabetes, and poor mental health.[2] Serious medical causes of low back pain are rare but it is vital that remedial massage therapists can identify red flags and other conditions that require specific precautions for safe practice.

The vast majority of clients with low back pain will be classified as non-specific, that is, the pathoanatomical cause of the pain cannot be found.

FUNCTIONAL ANATOMY REVIEW

The lumbar spine is designed for both stability and mobility. Five large vertebrae and discs bear the weight of the upper body. Between pairs of vertebral bodies are intervertebral discs which are composed of an annulus fibrosus (concentric rings of fibrocartilage) and a nucleus pulposus (a central mass of pulpy tissue). The discs act as shock absorbers and give the spine its flexibility. When the vertebral column is flexed, extended or bent sideways, the disc distorts as uneven loads are applied. Excessive loads can cause intervertebral discs to bulge or prolapse. Vertebral arches on the posterior aspect of the vertebral bodies provide protection for the spinal cord which passes through the vertebral foramina framed by the vertebral bodies, pedicles and lamina. Spinal nerves enter and exit the spinal cord through the intervertebral foramina (IVF) which are bounded above and below by the pedicles of adjacent vertebrae. Spinal nerves are vulnerable to pressure from bulging or herniated discs (see Figure 10.1 on p 138).

Superior and inferior articular processes form facet joints which prevent excessive movements between vertebrae. The superior facets are concave and face medially and posteriorly; the inferior facets are convex and face laterally and anteriorly. The articular facets of L1–4 lie in the sagittal plane, favouring flexion and extension and limiting rotation. The facets change their orientation from L1 to L5 so that the facets of L5/S1 lie more in the coronal plane (i.e. they are angled more outwards). This orientation counteracts the tremendous anterior shear force that occurs at this level. The pars interarticularis lies between the superior and inferior articular processes (see Figure 10.2 on p 138).

The orientation of the facets permits coupled movements; that is, when movement in one direction is combined with movement in another. In the lumbar spine, lateral flexion appears to be associated with rotation.[4, 5]

The anterior and posterior longitudinal ligaments are firmly attached to the discs and guard against excessive flexion and extension movements of the flexible column. Movement is further limited by joint capsules and other ligaments including the ligamentum flavum, the intertransverse ligaments and the iliolumbar ligaments. The iliolumbar ligaments attach to the transverse processes of L4 and L5, the sacrum and the ilium (see Figure 10.3 on p 138).

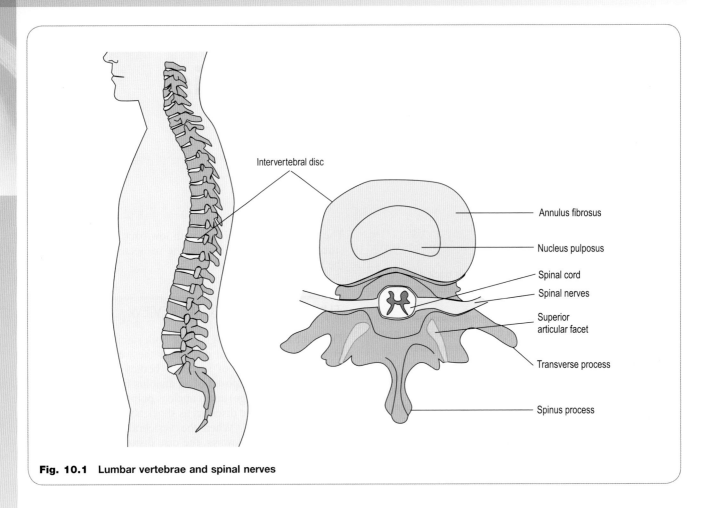

Fig. 10.1   Lumbar vertebrae and spinal nerves

Intervertebral disc

Annulus fibrosus

Nucleus pulposus

Spinal cord

Spinal nerves

Superior articular facet

Transverse process

Spinus process

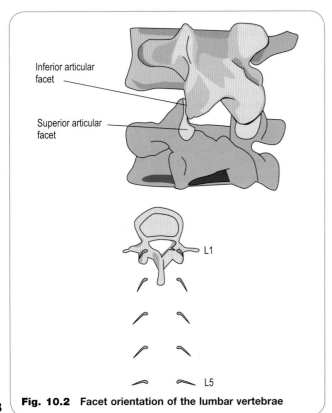

Inferior articular facet

Superior articular facet

L1

L5

Fig. 10.2   Facet orientation of the lumbar vertebrae

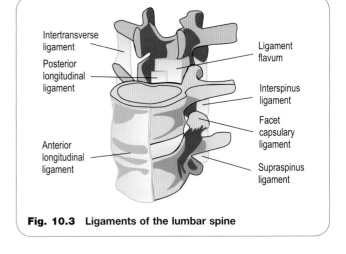

Intertransverse ligament

Posterior longitudinal ligament

Anterior longitudinal ligament

Ligament flavum

Interspinus ligament

Facet capsulary ligament

Supraspinus ligament

Fig. 10.3   Ligaments of the lumbar spine

The lumbosacral angle (the angle between the sacral base and the horizontal) is approximately 41° in the average adult.[6] The pelvic girdle is made up of the iliac bones and the sacrum. The two sacroiliac joints posteriorly and the symphysis pubis anteriorly are held together by strong ligaments (e.g. anterior and posterior sacroiliac ligament, interosseous ligaments, sacrotuberous and sacrospinous ligaments). There are no muscles that attach directly to the sacroiliac joints. The sacroiliac joint has a self-locking or close pack position; that is, the most congruent position that helps to stabilise the pelvis as weight is transferred from one leg to the other during the push-off phase of the gait cycle. Lumbar motion and sacral motion are coupled: when the lumbar spine is flexed, the sacral base tilts posteriorly (sacral counternutation); when the lumbar spine is extended, the sacral base tilts anteriorly (sacral nutation). The ilia can tilt forwards and back on the sacrum (both left and right moving together or separately). The sacrum can also move on the ilium. There is more movement in sacroiliac joints in women than in men because the pelvis is wider and flatter.

Normal biomechanics of the lumbosacral spine require the support of muscles of the lower back, abdomen and pelvic floor. (see Table 10.1 on p 140 and Figure 10.4 on p 141). When these muscles become weak or injured, loads that are normally counteracted by muscle contraction may be transmitted to deeper structures like vertebrae and discs. Moreover, the orientation of the pelvis and spinal curvature may be affected by imbalances in muscles attaching to the pelvis such as the hamstrings, quadriceps, piriformis, psoas and hip adductors (see Figure 10.5 on p 142).

ASSESSMENT OF THE LUMBAR AND SACROILIAC REGION

It is often not possible or necessary to establish definitive diagnoses for many musculoskeletal problems. It is essential, however, that clients requiring referral to other healthcare practitioners are identified. The first task of remedial massage therapists is to identify clients' suitability for remedial massage by identifying red and yellow flags. For those clients for whom remedial massage is suitable, assessments help identify the duration and severity of their conditions and the most likely tissue types involved. In some cases clients' signs and symptoms will fit patterns of common conditions but even when this is the case, it is important to remember that correlations between clinical presentations and definitive diagnoses are often low. Assess all clients, even those who come with previous medical diagnoses, not only to confirm their diagnoses but also to gather such important information as clients' preferences for treatment types and styles and the need for modification of techniques for safe and competent practice.

Assessment procedures for remedial massage clients are discussed in detail in Chapter 2. A biopsychosocial model is required to understand the complexity of low back pain disability.[2]

CASE HISTORY

- Ask clients to point to the site of pain as they may have different understandings of anatomical terms. For example 'hip' could mean iliac crest, sacroiliac joint, buttock, greater trochanter or the actual hip joint.
- Clients with low back pain, especially those with disc herniations, may prefer to stand rather than sit during the case history.
- Identify any red flags that require referral for further investigation (see Table 10.2 on p 142).
- Determine if the pain is likely to have a mechanical cause. (Is the pain associated with rest or activity, certain postures or time of day?) Ask clients to show you movements and positions that aggravate or relieve the pain and to

Assessment of the low back and pelvis

1. Case history
2. Outcome measures
3. Postural analysis
4. Gait assessment
5. Functional tests
   Active range of motion tests
   flexion, extension, lateral flexion, rotation
   Passive range of motion tests
   flexion, extension, lateral flexion, rotation
   Resisted range of motion tests
   flexion, extension, lateral flexion, rotation
   Resisted and length tests for specific muscle tests including
   Piriformis
   Iliopsoas
   Quadratus lumborum
   Erector spinae
   Gluteus maximus
   Hamstrings
   Quadriceps
   Abdominal muscles
   Special tests including
   Kemp's quadrant test
   Valsalva
   SLR
   Centralisation/peripheralisation
   Patrick's test
   Sacroiliac compression
   Sacroiliac distraction
   Sacral springing
   Leg length test
6. Palpation

be specific with descriptions of aggravating or relieving activities.

- Mechanical pain is usually highly reactive to changes in posture, position or activity.
- Morning pain relieved with daily activity is often associated with arthritis.
- Current research suggests that client reports of numbness, weakness, tingling or burning do not appear to be very helpful in identifying lumbar radiculopathy.[8]
- Pain that is not relieved by lying down, back pain at night and morning stiffness lasting more than half an hour may be helpful in identifying ankylosing spondylitis[a] (axial spondyloarthritis).[8]
- A report of 'no pain when seated' appears to be the most useful information for the diagnosis of lumbar spinal stenosis[b],[8]
- Pain relieved by standing may be useful for identifying SI joint pain.[8]
- Determine if the pain is likely to be associated with visceral function, neurogenic, vascular or psychosocial issues (yellow flags).

---

[a]Ankylosing spondylitis is an autoimmune disease characterised by chronic inflammation of the back and sacroiliac joints. Pain and stiffness are the main symptoms.
[b]Spinal stenosis is a narrowing of the spinal canal which causes the spinal cord and nerves to be compressed. It occurs most commonly from the degenerative changes of ageing but is also caused by disc herniation, osteoporosis or tumour.

Table 10.1 Major muscles of the low back and pelvis[7]

Muscle	Origin	Insertion	Action
Erector spinae Superficial muscles of the spinal column	Strong aponeurosis from posterior sacrum and adjacent iliac crest	Fibres ascend and divide into three columns 1. Iliocostalis – lateral column, inserts into angles of ribs 2. Longissimus – middle column, inserts into thoracic and cervical transverse processes and mastoid process 3. Spinalis – medial column, confined to the thoracic region, inserts into spinous processes	Extend the spine, laterally flex the spine
Deep muscles of the spinal column Multifidus	Sacrum, ilium, transverse processes of lumbar, thoracic and inferior four cervical vertebrae	Spinous process of vertebra above	Extend spine, laterally flex spine, stabilise vertebrae in local movements of vertebral column
Rotators	Transverse process of all vertebrae The rotators form the deepest layer in the lumbar and thoracic region	Spinous process of vertebra above	
Quadratus lumborum	Iliac crest	12th rib, L1–L4/5	Extends lower back, laterally flexes trunk
Iliopsoas	Psoas major and minor originate from T12 to L4/5 Iliacus originates from the superior iliac fossa	Lesser trochanter of the femur	Flexes hip Trunk flexor Assists in lateral flexion of the trunk and internal rotation of hip
Piriformis	Anterior surface of sacrum	Greater trochanter of femur	Laterally rotates and abducts hip
Gluteus maximus	Medial iliac crest and posterior inferior sacrum	Iliotibial band of the tensor fasciae latae and gluteal tuberosity of the femur	Extends and laterally rotates the hip joint
Hamstring muscles	Ischial tuberosity	Tibial condyle, pes anserine tendon, fibula head and deep fascia of the leg	Flex the knee; extend and laterally rotate the hip joint
Quadriceps femoris	Anterior inferior iliac spine, linea aspera, greater trochanter, gluteal tuberosity	Tibial tuberosity via the patella ligament	Flexes the hip joint and extends the knee
Rectus abdominis	Pubic crest and pubic symphysis	Cartilage of ribs 5–7, xiphoid process	Flexes lumbar spine, compresses abdomen
External oblique	Inferior 8 ribs	Iliac crest and linea alba	Laterally flexes spine, rotates spine, compresses abdomen, flexes spine
Internal oblique	Iliac crest, inguinal ligament and thoracolumbar fascia	Cartilage of last 3 or 4 ribs and linea alba	Laterally flexes spine, rotates spine, compresses abdomen, flexes spine
Transversus abdominis	Iliac crest, inguinal ligament, lumbar fascia, cartilages of inferior 6 ribs	Xiphoid process, linea alba and pubis	Compresses abdomen
Pelvic floor muscles Levator ani ■ Pubococcygeus ■ Iliococcygeus	Pubis Ischial spine	Coccyx, urethra, anal canal, perineum Coccyx	Supports and maintains position of pelvic viscera, resists increased intra-abdominal pressure
Coccygeus	Ischial spine	Lower sacrum and upper coccyx	Supports and maintains position of pelvic viscera, resists increased intra-abdominal pressure

(Note: Gluteus medius, gluteus minimus, obturator internus and externus, gemellus superior and inferior and quadratus femoris are discussed in Chapter 18).

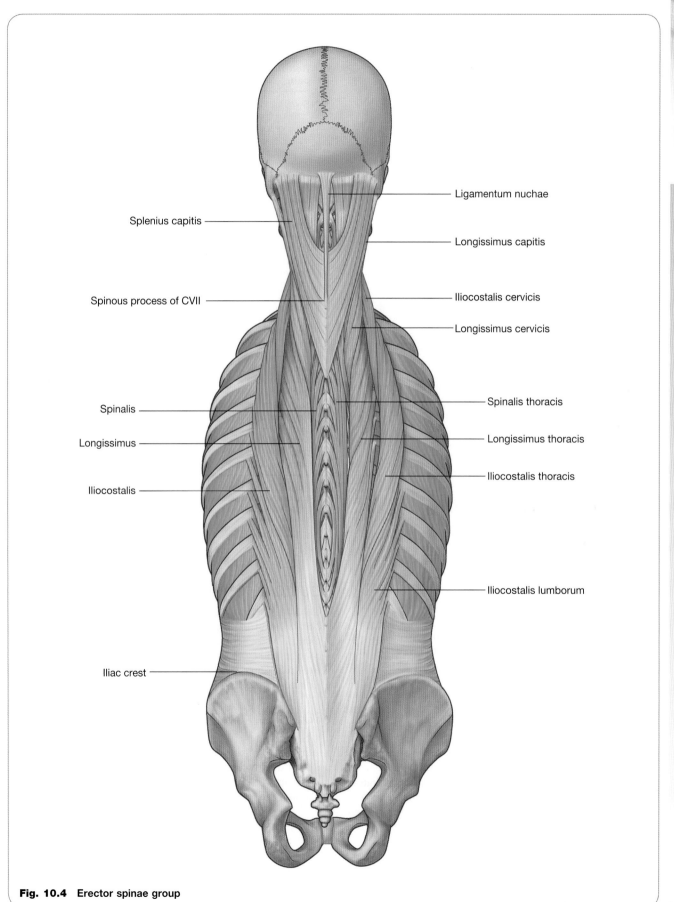

Ligamentum nuchae

Splenius capitis

Longissimus capitis

Spinous process of CVII

Iliocostalis cervicis

Longissimus cervicis

Spinalis

Spinalis thoracis

Longissimus

Longissimus thoracis

Iliocostalis

Iliocostalis thoracis

Iliocostalis lumborum

Iliac crest

Fig. 10.4 Erector spinae group

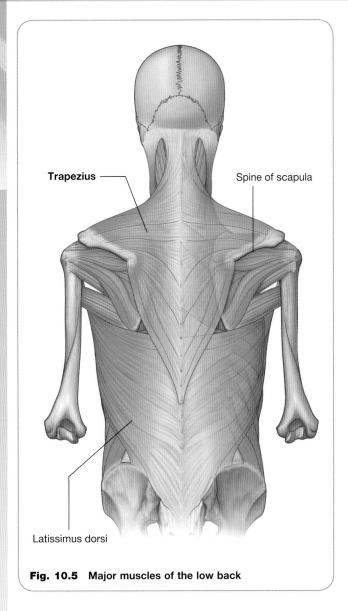

Trapezius

Spine of scapula

Latissimus dorsi

Fig. 10.5 Major muscles of the low back

Table 10.2 Red flags for serious conditions associated with acute low back pain

Red flags for acute low back pain	Possible condition
Symptoms and signs of infection (e.g. fever) Risk factors for infection (e.g. underlying disease, immunosuppression, penetrating wound)	Infection
History of trauma Minor trauma (if >50 years, history of osteoporosis, taking corticosteroids)	Fracture
Past history of malignancy Age >50 years Failure to improve with treatment Unexplained weight loss Pain at multiple sites Pain at rest	Cancer
Absence of aggravating factors	Aortic aneurysm Other serious condition
Widespread neurological symptoms and signs in the lower limb (e.g. gait abnormality, saddle area numbness) ± urinary retention, faecal incontinence	Cauda equina syndrome (a medical emergency and requires urgent hospital referral)
Morning stiffness in the lower back that improves with exercise and worsens with rest	Axial spondyloarthritis (anklyosing spondylitis)

Adapted from the Acute Musculoskeletal Pain Guidelines Group[4] and the New Zealand Guidelines Group[9] and Hartvigsen et al.[2]
Note that acute pain in this context refers to pain of less than three months' duration.

- Pain from the kidney, gall bladder or prostate is not usually aggravated by activity or relieved by rest, whereas mechanical back pain may be relieved by lying down.
- Neurogenic back pain from a spinal cord tumour or from a primary or secondary vertebral bone tumour is generally constant and remains unchanged by postural position.
- Symptoms of vascular claudication are aggravated by walking and relieved by standing still or resting.
- Sacroiliac joint sprain causes local pain that may radiate to the low back and buttock. The pain can be sharp and stabbing, aggravated by movement and relieved by lying down. It may be difficult to differentiate sacroiliac joint sprain from a condition originating in the lumbar spine. Clients with sacroiliac joint dysfunctions experience pain most intensely around one or both sacroiliac joints with or without referral to the lateral thigh. Focal tenderness on palpation of the sacroiliac joints and positive special tests can also help differentiate.

OUTCOME MEASURES

Outcome measures are questionnaires that are used to assess clients' level of impairment and to define benefits of treatment. The benefit is assessed in terms of client-perceived changes to health status. Common outcome measures for low back pain and disability are the Oswestry Disability Index and Roland-Morris Low Back Pain and Disability Questionnaire.

POSTURAL ANALYSIS

- Scoliosis and hyperlordosis are common conditions affecting the lumbar spine and pelvis and should not be missed.
- Soft doughy lipomata (fatty masses) appearing as lumps in the area of the low back may be a sign of spina bifida (non-union of the vertebral arch at the spinous process).
- A hairy patch (faun's beard) in conjunction with a lipoma further suggests an underlying bony pathology.
- Birth marks or excessive port wine marks should be carefully investigated since they suggest underlying bony pathology (spina bifida).
- A step defect is a visible or palpable step from one spinous process to the next. This most commonly occurs at L5/S1 and suggests spondylolisthesis.

Fig. 10.6 Performing PROM of the lumbar spine. A: Flexion; **B:** Extension; **C:** Lateral flexion; **D:** Rotation.

GAIT ASSESSMENT

Many conditions of the lumbosacral spine and sacroiliac joints will affect the symmetry and rhythm of gait (see Chapter 2). In lower-crossed syndrome, for example, changes in movement patterns with hip extension, hip abduction and trunk flexion are often observed.[10]

FUNCTIONAL TESTS

Thoracolumbar range of motion tests have repeatedly been shown to be very reliable although their diagnostic accuracy[c] remains unclear.[8] Findings of functional tests should be correlated with case history, postural and gait analysis and other functional assessments and interpreted in this context.

Active range of motion (AROM)

FLEXION (60°)[d]

- Trunk flexion mostly occurs in the hip joints with only a very small amount occurring in the lumbar spine.
- The lumbar spine flattens but does not reverse to a kyphosis as it does in the cervical spine.
- Instruct clients to return to the erect position if they experience any pain. Special care is required with disc clients as flexion may aggravate symptoms. Ask all clients to bend forward slowly and only as far as they can without pain.

EXTENSION (25°)

- Extension will produce increased pain for a range of clients including those with spondylolisthesis or hyperlordosis and may also be painful for disc clients.

LATERAL FLEXION (SIDEBEND) (25°)

- Stabilise the iliac crest with one hand and gently guide the client with the other hand on their shoulder.

- Compare both sides and observe the coupling of the lumbar spine facet joints (lateral flexion associated with slight vertebral rotation).

ROTATION (30°)

- Stabilise the pelvis by placing one hand on each side. Ask the client to turn their shoulders to the left and then the right as far as they comfortably can. Alternatively, ask clients to stand with their thighs against the treatment table or sit on the table and then to turn their shoulders left and right as far as they comfortably can.

Passive range of motion (PROM)

PROM of the lumbar spine is difficult to perform because of the weight of the trunk, and as a result many remedial massage therapists do not routinely perform PROM tests of the lumbar spine. However, PROM can be performed with the client seated and the practitioner placing their forearm across the top of the shoulders to guide the movements. The other hand rests on the lumbar spine to palpate the movement (see Figure 10.6).

Resisted range of motion (RROM)

Ask the client to sit and then try to bend forward, backwards, to the side and to rotate their trunk against your resistance. Use the same contacts described for PROM.

Tests for specific muscles associated with low back conditions[12, 13]

Test the major muscles of the lumbar spine and pelvis for length and strength. Make bilateral comparisons where possible and always consider other reasons for apparent muscle imbalances such as age, underlying pathology and lifestyle.

1. PIRIFORMIS

Resisted test

Resisted external (lateral) rotation of the hip can be performed in a variety of positions to suit the comfort of the client and practitioner. One option is for the client to sit on the treatment table with their knees bent over the side. Kneel beside the

---

[c]Diagnostic accuracy refers to the degree of agreement between a clinical test and a reference standard. It is usually expressed in terms of sensitivity, specificity and likelihood ratios (see Chapter 2).[8]
[d]Reese and Bandy (2010) reviewed published data on joint ranges of motion and suggest that the normative values for the lumbar spine are 60° flexion, 30° extension, 30° lateral flexion and 6° rotation.[11]

client. One hand contacts the medial lower leg above the ankle; the other contacts the lateral aspect of the knee. Tap the medial lower leg and ask the client to push against that hand; that is, to externally rotate their hip against your resistance. Figure 10.7 shows the test in the prone position.

Length test

A tight piriformis muscle holds the hip in lateral rotation. Clients may have a *toe out* gait and on postural analysis stand with their foot excessively turned outwards. A test for piriformis contracture is to ask the client to lie prone, knee flexed to 90°, and to let their foot drop to the side. A tight piriformis will limit medial rotation which is suggested if the foot fails to drop to 30–40° (see Figure 10.8).

Clinical significance

The sciatic nerve exits the sciatic notch and runs underneath the piriformis muscle. In 15% of the population the sciatic nerve passes through the piriformis[14] and muscle spasm or contracture can press on the nerve and cause sciatic neuritis (piriformis syndrome) (see Figure 10.9). If straight leg raising has produced pain, numbness or tingling in the low back, posterior thigh and/or lower leg, straight leg raising is performed a second time with the hip externally rotated (i.e. foot turned out). If the posterior thigh and leg pain is relieved in the second test, piriformis syndrome is suggested. Although not a common cause of posterior thigh and leg pain compared with nerve compression originating from the lumbosacral spine, piriformis syndrome can usually be simply and effectively treated when identified.

2. ILIOPSOAS

Resisted test

The client lies supine. Stand contralaterally. Place one hand on the contralateral ASIS to stabilise the pelvis. With the other hand, slightly abduct and externally rotate the client's leg and raise it to 40° flexion. Ask the client to hold their leg in this position. Tap the client's medial tibia and ask the client to push up against your hand as if they were lifting their leg towards their opposite shoulder against your resistance (see Figure 10.10).

Length test

The Thomas test is used to test the length of the iliopsoas. The client should be wearing a gown or loose clothing and the technique requires appropriate draping. The client sits on the edge of the foot of the table and rolls back bringing both knees to their chest in the process. Ask the client to hold their knees to their chest with their arms. The client slowly releases

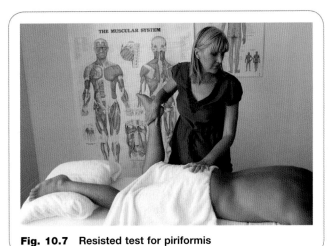

Fig. 10.7 **Resisted test for piriformis**

Fig. 10.8 **Piriformis length test**

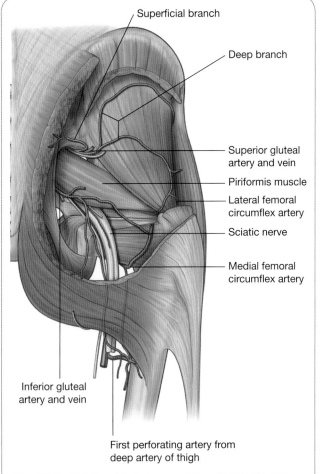

Superficial branch

Deep branch

Superior gluteal artery and vein

Piriformis muscle

Lateral femoral circumflex artery

Sciatic nerve

Medial femoral circumflex artery

Inferior gluteal artery and vein

First perforating artery from deep artery of thigh

Fig. 10.9 **Relationship between piriformis muscle and the sciatic nerve**

Fig. 10.10 Resisted test for iliopsoas

Fig. 10.11 Thomas test for iliopsoas contracture

Fig. 10.12 Resisted test for quadratus lumborum

one leg and lets it fall over the end of the table, while maintaining the original degree of hip flexion on the other leg (see Figure 10.11). A shortened iliopsoas will prevent the thigh dropping to the level of the table.

The following variation of the Thomas test is easier for the client because it can be performed in the usual supine position and therefore minimises the position changes required during assessment. The client flexes the hip and knee on the opposite side to the one being tested and holds their knee against their chest. The test is positive if the straight leg lifts off the table during this manoeuvre indicating a flexion contracture of the iliopsoas muscle.

Clinical significance

A unilateral contracted iliopsoas may contribute to scoliosis; a bilaterally contracted iliopsoas may contribute to hyperlordosis – two very common postural observations in remedial massage.

3. QUADRATUS LUMBORUM
Strength test

The client lies on their side with their arms crossed across the chest. Hold the client's feet to prevent them from lifting off the table. Ask the client to raise their shoulders and trunk off the table (sidebend the trunk) without using their arms (see Figure 10.12).

Length test

Postural observation may reveal a pelvic tilt (i.e. elevated iliac crest/hip hike) and a concave scoliosis on the side of the shortened quadratus lumborum.[15] Contracture restricts trunk sidebending towards the opposite side.

Clinical significance

A unilateral contracted quadratus lumborum may contribute to scoliosis: the pelvis is normally elevated on the contracted side. Bilaterally contracted quadratus lumborum may contribute to hyperlordosis.

4. ERECTOR SPINAE
Strength test

The client lies prone and clasps their hands behind their back. Ask the client to lift their head and shoulders off the table (see Figure 10.13 on p 146).

Length test

The client sits with legs extended and the pelvis vertical and flexes forward towards the knees. In the normally flexible adult the distance between their forehead and their knees will be about 10 cm. Next, the client sits on the table with their legs bent over the side. If trunk flexion is greater in the sitting position then short hamstrings are suggested (see Figure 10.14). (Note: Clients with a history of disc problems may not be able to flex their lumbar spine without pain. Use the See-Move-Touch principle in all testing procedures).

Fig. 10.13   Strength test for erector spinae

Fig. 10.15   Resisted test for gluteus maximus

Fig. 10.14   Erector spinae length test

Clinical significance

Erector spinae muscles are usually short and tight on the concave side of a scoliosis. Bilateral erector spinae muscles may be contracted in clients with hyperlordosis.

5. GLUTEUS MAXIMUS

Resisted test

The client lies prone, flexes one knee to 90° and tries to raise the thigh (on the same side) off the table against resistance (see Figure 10.15).

Length test

The client lies supine and takes their knee towards the opposite shoulder. Normally, adult clients should be able to flex their hips to 110–120°. (Note: sign of the buttock: Elevate the client's straight leg until restriction is encountered and then flex the knee and increase hip flexion. Cases where passive hip flexion with the knee flexed is more limited or painful than straight leg raising is a red flag and requires referral for further examination to eliminate such pathologies as infection, osteomyelitis of the upper femur, septic sacroiliac arthritis, ischiorectal abscess and fractured sacrum).[16, 17]

Clinical significance

The gluteus maximus muscle is an important stabiliser of the lumbo-pelvic region, especially of the sacroiliac joint. For example, severe weakness is associated with hip extensor gait (when the hip is thrust forward and the trunk extended after heel strike). Gluteus maximus weakness has been associated with overuse of hamstring muscles in abnormal hip extension firing patterns.[18] Iliotibial band syndrome is also associated with imbalances between gluteus maximus, tensor fasciae latae, hamstring and quadriceps muscles.

6. HAMSTRINGS

Resisted test

Resisted knee flexion can be tested prone, sitting or supine. In the prone position, the client flexes their knee to 90°. Place one hand on the client's gluteal region and the other on the calf just proximal to the ankle. Instruct the client to bring their heel to their buttock against your resistance (see Figure 10.16).

Length test

The Sit and Reach Test is used to test the length of the hamstrings. The client sits with their legs straight out in front of them and reaches forward towards their toes. Normal hamstring length enables the client to touch their toes. Note that the Sit and Reach test also tests the flexibility of the lumbar spine (see Figure 10.17).

Straight leg raising also tests the length of the hamstrings. Clients with normal length hamstrings can usually achieve 80° elevation.

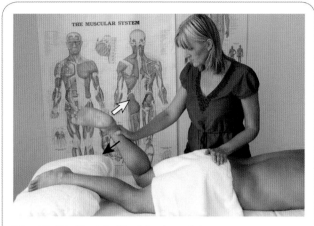

Fig. 10.16 Resisted test for hamstrings

Fig. 10.18 Resisted test for quadriceps

Fig. 10.17 Length test for hamstrings: Sit and Reach test

Clinical significance

Variations from normal hamstring strength or length alter the biomechanics of the hips, sacroiliac joints, spine and knees. Hamstring muscles may be weak compared to quadriceps muscles in hyperlordosis. Weak hamstrings may also cause heavy heel strike when walking. Tight hamstrings have been associated with posterior pelvic tilt and abnormal hip extension firing patterns.[18, 19] Imbalance between hamstring, tensor fasciae latae, gluteus maximus and quadriceps is implicated in iliotibial band syndrome.

7. QUADRICEPS

Resisted test

Resisted knee extension can be tested supine, sitting or prone. In the sitting position, the client flexes their knee to 90°. Place one hand on the client's tibia just proximal to the knee and the other just proximal to the ankle. Instruct the client to try to straighten their leg against your resistance (see Figure 10.18).

Length test

The client lies prone and flexes their knee. Normally, the client's heel will reach their buttocks (see Figure 10.19).

Fig. 10.19 Length test for quadriceps femoris

Clinical significance

Variations from normal quadriceps strength or length alter the biomechanics of the hips, sacroiliac joints, spine and knees. Quadriceps muscles may be short and tight compared with hamstrings in clients with hyperlordosis. Weak quadriceps may be associated with hypolordosis. Weak quadriceps can cause abnormal hip rotation in the acceleration phase of gait or back knee gait (manually pushing the knee into extension in stance phase).

Fig. 10.20 Strength tests for abdominal muscles. **A:** Rectus abdominis; **B:** Oblique muscles.

8. ABDOMINAL MUSCLES

RECTUS ABDOMINIS

Strength test

The client lies supine and tilts their pelvis posteriorly or performs a partial sit-up with knees bent and feet on the floor.

INTERNAL AND EXTERNAL OBLIQUES

Strength test

The client lies supine and tilts their pelvis posteriorly or performs a partial diagonal sit-up (i.e. elbow reaches towards opposite knee) with knees bent and feet on the floor (see Figure 10.20).

TRANSVERSUS ABDOMINIS

Transversus abdominis compresses the abdomen wall. To test its strength, instruct the client to draw in their navel to flatten their abdomen.

Length test

Although unlikely to be encountered in clinic, shortened abdominal muscle would restrict trunk extension.

Clinical significance

Weakness of any part of the core may predispose to low back injury. Weakness of rectus abdominis is often observed in hyperlordotic postures.

PELVIC FLOOR MUSCLES

Pelvic floor muscles are part of the core muscles that stabilise the lumbar spine during movement. A test for pelvic floor muscle strength that is often used is the ability to stop the flow of urine completely and rapidly. Refer clients with pelvic floor muscle weakness to a physiotherapist or exercise therapist.

Special tests

Special tests aim to isolate and identify the client's condition and in so doing often reproduce symptoms. Clients should be instructed to perform tests within their pain tolerance. Ask clients to indicate the exact location of symptoms and confirm that they are the same as those described in the case history. Special tests should be interpreted cautiously and confirmed by other clinical indicators.

KEMP'S QUADRANT TEST

The client is standing and extends and laterally flexes their trunk (ask the client to run their hand down the back of their thigh). This manoeuvre compresses the posterolateral elements of the spine; that is, the facet joints and the posterolateral disc (see Figure 10.21 on p 149).

VALSALVA

The client is seated. Ask the client to close their mouth, pinch their nostrils closed and forcibly exhale. (Demonstrate this manoeuvre for the client). The Valsalva manoeuvre raises the intrathecal pressure. Pain in the low back or pain radiating down the leg(s) suggests pathology such as disc derangement. (Note: this test is not recommended for people with uncontrolled or acute hypertension or for diabetics with potential retinopathy).

STRAIGHT LEG RAISE (SLR)

This test is designed to reproduce back and/or leg pain. The client is supine and draped appropriately. Slowly raise the client's leg with one hand supporting the calcaneus and the other hand placed on top of the knee or on the ipsilateral anterior superior iliac spine (see Figure 10.22 on p 149). Ask the client to report any pain as soon as it is felt and when this occurs note the degree of elevation (normally hip flexion is approximately 80°). Pain usually arises from hamstring tightness or pressure on the sciatic nerve. To distinguish between these two possibilities, lower the leg a few degrees and dorsiflex the foot. Pain on dorsiflexion indicates sciatica. Pain on SLR that is experienced in the opposite leg could suggest a space-occupying lesion in the back (e.g. disc herniation, infection or tumour).

CENTRALISATION/PERIPHERALISATION

Centralisation (the movement of symptoms from distal or lateral regions to more central regions) is useful in identifying painful lumbar discs.[8] Instruct the client to extend their back

Fig. 10.21 Kemp's test

Fig. 10.22 Straight Leg Raise

Fig. 10.23 Patrick's test

tenderness and swelling in the calf. Bilateral supine gastrocnemius stretch may reproduce local vein pain but the test is not definitive. History of recent surgery or travel may be the best indicator. Compartment syndrome should also be considered if there is unexplained or unidentified calf pain. Refer clients with calf pain which seems out of proportion for that which is expected, paraesthesia or muscle weakness and/or signs of loss of blood flow to the leg and foot.

PATRICK'S TEST

The client is supine with the leg on the involved side in the figure 4 position (i.e. hip flexed, abducted and externally rotated and the foot placed across the opposite leg). Stand ipsilaterally. Pain in the inguinal area suggests hip pathology. With the palm of the cephalad hand on the contralateral anterior superior iliac spine, gently apply pressure on the flexed knee with the palm of the other hand (see Figure 10.23). Increased pain on this manoeuvre may suggest SI pathology.

Note that all sacroiliac pain provocation tests demonstrate fair to moderate reliability and moderate diagnostic utility for identifying sacroiliac joint pain.[8]

SACROILIAC COMPRESSION

The client lies on their side. Place one hand on top of the other over the uppermost aspect of the lateral ilium and apply pressure towards the floor to compress the sacroiliac joints (see Figure 10.24). If the client experiences increased pain on this manoeuvre, SI pathology may be indicated.

as far as possible, return to neutral and then repeat the movement up to 10 times. If pain centralises (e.g. changes from pain in the low back, buttock, posterior thigh and calf to pain in the low back and buttock) a bulging lumbar disc is indicated. Stop the movement if the pain peripheralises. (Note: A small group of clients tend to centralise with lateral flexion; a minority with flexion).

Note: If a client has calf pain it is important to eliminate deep venous thrombosis (DVT). Symptoms may include pain,

Fig. 10.24 Sacroiliac joint compression

Fig. 10.25 Sacroiliac joint distraction

SACROILIAC DISTRACTION

The client lies supine. Face the client and place the palm of each hand on the contralateral anterior superior iliac spine. If pain is reported when gentle lateral pressure is applied, sacroiliac pathology is suggested (see Figure 10.25).

SACRAL SPRING TEST

Springing directly over the sacrum (sometimes called the *sacral thrust test*) and over both sacroiliac joints may reproduce symptoms in sacroiliac joint lesions. A positive spring test along with positive sacral compression and distraction tests demonstrates good diagnostic utility for detecting sacroiliac lesions (see Figure 10.26).[8]

LEG LENGTH

With the client standing, the practitioner measures the distance from the anterior superior iliac spine to the most inferior point of the medial malleolus and compares with the other side (see Figure 10.27 and box on p 151). If clinical symptoms are present, referral for a standing scanogram (an X-ray of the hips, knees and ankles when the client is standing) may be required for a more accurate measurement.

PALPATION

In the prone position:

- Palpate the space between the spinous processes of L4 and L5 which is at the level of the L4/5 disc and also level with

Fig. 10.26 Sacral spring test

the top of the iliac crests. The spinous processes mark the level of the actual vertebral body as spinous processes extend directly posteriorly in the lumbars (compare the thoracic spinous processes which extend inferiorly and posteriorly).

- Palpate the spinous process of L5/S1.
- Palpate the smaller spinous processes of the sacrum. S2 spinous process is level with the PSISs.

Fig. 10.27 Measuring leg length

- Gaps between the lumbar or sacral spinous processes or absence of spinous processes may indicate spina bifida.
- A step defect may be observed from one spinous process to the next. This most commonly occurs at L5/S1 and suggests spondylolisthesis.
- Palpate the iliac crests.
- Palpate the supraspinous ligaments. The interspinous ligaments located underneath the supraspinous ligaments are not directly palpable.
- Feel for muscle spasm in the erector spinae muscles either side of the spinous processes.
- Look for muscle spasm and fatty nodules in the gluteal muscles.
- Palpate the sacral triangle from the posterior superior iliac spines to the top of the gluteal cleft. Pain may be due to ligamentous sprain at the posterior superior iliac spine or the sacrotuberous or sacrospinous ligaments.
- The sciatic nerve runs under or through the piriformis muscle approximately midway between the ischial tuberosity and greater trochanter. The sciatic nerve may be more easily palpated when the client is lying on their side with their hip flexed. (Caution with hip flexion in clients with a history of disc pathology).

In the supine position:

- Palpate abdominal muscles. To observe the abdominal muscles ask the client to cross their arms over their chest and perform a partial sit-up. (Caution: do not ask a client to perform this action if it is likely to induce back pain).
- Palpate the inguinal area. Sources of pain in this region include inflamed inguinal nodes, the hip joint, a psoas spasm or a psoas abscess.

REMEDIAL MASSAGE TREATMENT

Assessment of the low back provides essential information for developing and negotiating treatment plans, including:

- client's suitability for remedial massage therapy
- duration of the condition (i.e. acute or chronic)
- severity of the condition (i.e. grade of injury; mild, moderate or severe pain)
- type(s) of tissues involved
- priorities for treatment if more than one injury or condition is present
- whether the signs and symptoms suggest a common condition of the low back
- special considerations for individual clients (e.g. client's preference for treatment types and styles, specific population considerations).

Treatment options must always be considered in the context of the best available evidence for treatment effectiveness. Use clinical practice guidelines where they exist (see Chapter 3). Further research is required to prove effectiveness of many low back treatments. Clinical guidelines from Denmark,[20] the USA[21] and the UK[22] recommend self-management and psychological therapies as first line treatment. That means recommending to patients with non-specific low back pain that they stay active, do appropriate exercises and undertake a psychological program to help manage their pain. Exercises like Tai Chi, yoga, motor control (to restore strength,

Leg length inequality

1. Anatomical (true) shortness
Causes include:
- growth asymmetry
- fracture (tibia, fibula, calcaneus, femur)
- epiphyseal injury
- hip disorder (e.g. Perthes' disease, slipped capital femoral epiphysis)
- osteoarthritis of the hip, knee or ankle
- neuromuscular (e.g. cerebral palsy, poliomyelitis)
- flat foot (usually pronating) on the same side
- osteomyelitis

2. Functional (apparent) shortness
Causes include:
- imbalance of pelvic and lumbar musculature, ligaments and fascia (e.g. posterior iliac rotation on the same side/anterior iliac rotation on the opposite side, forward sacral torsion to the same side/backward sacral iliac rotation on the opposite side, forward sacral torsion to the same side/backward sacral torsion to the opposite side, lumbar convexity to the opposite side, short hamstrings or tensor fasciae latae).

Short leg tests
Client standing: measure from the ASIS to the most inferior point of the medial malleolus.

Table 10.3 Recommendations for treating and managing low back pain[23]

Recommendations	Acute low back pain (less than six weeks duration)	Chronic low back pain (more than 12 weeks' duration)
First line treatments	Advice to stay active; patient education	Advice to stay active; patient education; exercise therapy; cognitive behavioural therapy
Second line treatments	Spinal manipulation; massage; acupuncture, superficial heat	Spinal manipulation; massage; acupuncture; yoga; mindfulness-based stress reduction; interdisciplinary rehabilitation
If the above treatments fail	Non-steroidal anti-inflammatory drugs	Non-steroidal anti-inflammatory drugs; selective norepinephrine reuptake inhibitors; surgery

co-ordination and control of the deep core stabilising muscles supporting the spine), aerobic exercises like walking, swimming, cycling and general muscle reconditioning exercises are recommended.

If those therapies fail or stop working, then manual and physical therapies such as spinal manipulation (guidelines from Denmark, UK, US), massage (guidelines from UK and US), yoga and acupuncture (guidelines from US) are recommended.[24] Physical and manual treatments include a graded activity or exercise program that targets improvements in function and prevents worsening disability and some form of manual therapy. A summary of key messages from clinical guidelines is summarised in Table 10.3.

Despite its long tradition, massage therapy remains grossly under-researched. A systematic review by Kumar et al[25] included nine studies, the overall quality of which was considered low. The authors concluded that massage may be an effective treatment compared to placebo and some active treatment options (such as relaxation), especially in the short term. Evidence for the effectiveness of massage therapy for non-specific low back pain was conflicting and contradictory when compared to other manual therapies like mobilisation, standard medical care, and acupuncture.

MUSCLE STRAIN

Muscle strains can occur from traumas including falls, car accidents and sports injuries. They also occur from overuse and repetitive microtrauma as can occur after long periods of unaccustomed activity. Strains can occur in the paraspinal muscles which support the spine in all its movements.

Assessment

HISTORY

The client complains of low back pain after a fall, accident or sports injury or after a period of unaccustomed activity (e.g. shovelling, horse riding). Pain can be experienced immediately or within the next 24–48 hours (delayed onset muscle soreness). Pain is associated with activity and generally relieved with rest.

POSTURAL ANALYSIS

Muscle spasm in the lumbar paravertebral muscles and functional scoliosis may be evident.

Key assessment findings for muscle strain

- History of trauma or repetitive overuse
- Functional tests
  - AROM positive
  - RROM positive for affected muscle(s)
  - Resisted and length tests positive for affected muscle(s)
- Palpation positive for pain, spasm, myofibril tears/scar tissue

---

GAIT ANALYSIS

Gait may be guarded.

FUNCTIONAL TESTS

AROM: limited in one or more directions.
PROM: mild to no pain except at end of range when muscle is stretched.
RROM: painful.
Resisted and length tests positive for involved muscles.
Special tests: negative.

PALPATION

Muscle spasm is usually evident. The client reports tenderness or pain on palpation of the affected muscle.

Overview of treatment of muscle strains

A typical remedial massage treatment for mild to moderate muscle strains of the low back includes:

- Swedish massage to the back, pelvis, posterior and anterior lower limbs.
- Remedial techniques, including:
  - deep gliding frictions along the muscle fibres (see Figure 10.28 on p 153)
  - cross-fibre frictions (see Figure 10.28 on p 153)
  - soft-tissue releasing techniques
  - deep transverse friction at the site of muscle injury
  - heat therapy (see Chapter 3)
  - trigger point therapy (see Chapter 6)
  - myofascial release (see Chapter 8).

Fig. 10.28 (a) Deep gliding frictions and (b) cross-fibre frictions of lumbar erector spinae: (c) deep gliding frictions and (d) cross-fibre frictions of quadratus lumborum

A range of remedial massage techniques for muscles of the low back and pelvis is illustrated in Table 10.4.

- Address any underlying conditions or predisposing factors (e.g. scoliosis or thoracic hyperkyphosis).

CLIENT EDUCATION

Educate clients about the importance of maintaining a physical fitness program and of developing appropriate levels of fitness before activities are commenced. Where possible, clients should take an increasingly active role in their treatment through rehabilitation and health promotion activities.

Home exercise program

A program of progressive rehabilitation should accompany remedial massage treatment. Aim for maximum strength and full length of all major muscles. Unresolved strains can contribute to recurrence and to the development of more serious back injuries. Introduce stretching exercises as soon as possible and progress to isometric exercises within the client's pain tolerance. Clients may be referred for manipulation of the lower back.

NON-SPECIFIC LOW BACK PAIN

Non-specific low back pain refers to low back pain that is not associated with a specific condition for which a pathoanatomical cause can be found. It accounts for most low back pain and could include strains (described above), sprains and low back pain originating from the facet (zygapophyseal) joint and/or joint capsule.[2] Non-specific low back pain may originate from trauma, overuse or unaccustomed exercise leading to muscle strain and facet joint ligamentous sprain. Psychosocial factors and co-morbidities can also contribute. There is often no radiation of pain.

Assessment

HISTORY

Clients report a history of direct trauma, overuse, fatigue or repetitive microtrauma over hours or days. The pain is often described as dull and aching although it may be sharp. The

---

Key assessment findings for non-specific low back pain

- Client is often a young adult; history of trauma or repetitive overuse.
- Functional tests
  - AROM positive
  - PROM positive for ligamentous sprains
  - RROM positive for muscle strains
  - Resisted test and muscle length tests positive for affected muscles
  - Special tests – Kemp's positive in lumbar facet syndrome
- Palpation positive for tenderness ± pain at site of strain, sprain or subluxation

---

pain is usually easily localised. The onset of pain is immediate or shortly after injury. Clients also describe decreased mobility and muscle spasm. Clients are often young adults and often describe having recently undertaken an unaccustomed activity (e.g. playing social cricket).

FUNCTIONAL TESTS

AROM: limited and painful in one or more directions (pain in one direction suggests muscle strain; pain in many directions suggests joint capsule injury or a combination of muscle and joint injury). More pain on extension suggests lumbar facet syndrome.

PROM: painful when sprained ligaments are stretched. Ligamentous sprain is suggested when AROM tests are painful and RROM tests are negative.

RROM: painful for affected muscles.

Resisted and length tests: positive for affected muscles.

Special tests: are often negative except for Kemp's test which may be positive for lumbar facet syndrome.

PALPATION

Clients report tenderness on palpation at the site of muscle strain or ligament sprain.

Table 10.4 Remedial massage techniques for major muscles of the low back and pelvis

Muscle	Soft tissue release	Trigger point	Stretch	Client education[15]	Home stretch
Piriformis	The client lies prone. Apply pressure into ipsilateral piriformis with thumb, fingers, elbow or palm. Flex the client's knee to 90°. Passive release: hold the client's foot or hold the client's foot or hold the medial aspect of the calf with forearm and slowly move the client's leg medially and laterally to the client's full range of motion (internally and externally rotating the hip) while pressure is maintained on the piriformis. Active release: contact the ipsilateral piriformis as above while the client performs the same movement unassisted.		The client lies in the prone position, knee flexed to 90° and foot dropped out to the side. Stabilise the middle of piriformis with the cephalad palm, fingers pointing towards the sacrum. The other hand holds the medial aspect of the lower leg proximal to the ankle. CRAC: The client tries to bring their foot back to the middle of the table against your resistance for 7 seconds and then takes their foot as far laterally as possible. The client should stretch to their comfortable tolerance. Knee injury clients are contraindicated.	Place a pillow between the thighs when sleeping on the side, take regular breaks to stretch piriformis when driving long distances, change positions often if sitting for prolonged periods.	Lying supine, flex the hip to 90° and place the foot on the floor laterally to the other leg which remains straight. With one hand on the pelvis on the flexed leg side push down towards the floor; the other hand pulls the bent leg towards the floor until a stretch is felt in the piriformis muscle.

Table 10.4 Remedial massage techniques for major muscles of the low back and pelvis—cont'd

Muscle	Soft tissue release	Trigger point	Stretch	Client education[15]	Home stretch
Iliopsoas	Active release: Client lies supine with knee flexed and foot on the table. Apply pressure to ipsilateral psoas with fingers. (Caution is required in locating psoas which is deep to abdominal organs). The technique should only be performed if the client can tolerate it (i.e. no more than 7 out of 10 on a pain scale). Ask client to slowly slide their heel along the table while pressure is maintained on the muscle.	Trigger points are inaccessible. Remedial massage treatment focuses on stretching techniques only.	i) Use contracture testing position with buttock close to the edge of the table. The client flexes the contralateral knee and holds it with their hands. Use one hand to assist the client to hold this position. The other hand contacts the ipsilateral thigh proximal to the knee. The client tries to lift their knee against your resistance for 7 seconds, after which they try to stretch the iliopsoas by lowering their leg towards the floor. ii) The client is supine, close to the side of the table. The client flexes the contralateral knee and places their foot on the table. Face caudally and stand with the lateral thigh against the table. Contact the opposite ASIS to stabilise the pelvis. The client holds the sides of the table and drops their ipsilateral leg over the side of the table (the client has to be close enough to the side of the table so that the hip can extend). Your other hand contacts the ipsilateral thigh just proximal to the knee. The client tries to lift their knee against your resistance for 7 seconds, after which you try to stretch the iliopsoas by lowering their leg towards the floor. iii) The client is prone and flexes their knee to 90°. (If the psoas is tight the lumbar spine will dip towards the table). Stand ipsilaterally and place one hand on the client's sacrum, the other under the knee, approaching from the medial side and stabilising the calf and foot with their forearm. Elevate the knee until the muscle stretch is felt, making sure that the pelvis remains on the table. The client tries to take their thigh to the table against your resistance for 7 seconds and then tries to elevate the thigh as far as possible to stretch the muscle.	Avoid prolonged sitting with knees flexed to 90°. Sit on a seat that slants forward to avoid holding iliopsoas in a sustained contracted position.	The client kneels on the floor with one knee bent and the leg to be stretched behind. The client gently lunges forward until a stretch is felt in the front of their hip. Hold for 30 seconds.

Continued

Table 10.4 Remedial massage techniques for major muscles of the low back and pelvis—cont'd

Muscle	Soft tissue release	Trigger point	Stretch	Client education[15]	Home stretch
Quadratus lumborum	Apply pressure with palms or fingers to the quadratus lumborum muscles and ask client to breathe in slowly against resistance. This can be performed in the prone position or sitting.		i) Any movement that flexes or laterally flexes the trunk stretches the quadratus lumborum. For example, lying on one side over 3 or 4 pillows will stretch the quadratus lumborum.[13] ii) The client is supine holding onto the sides of the table. Cross one leg over the other at the ankles, keeping both legs extended. Holding the crossed ankles with both hands, slowly walk the client's feet in an arc towards the lower foot side. PNF stretch can be performed in this position with the client trying to bring their crossed legs back to the middle of the table against the practitioner's resistance (arms or hip). iii) The client is supine with one knee crossed over the other. Drop both knees to the side of the top knee.	Shock-absorbing and supportive footwear for good foot and ankle biomechanics, a heel lift in cases of true short leg, a firm mattress, placing a pillow under the thighs when sleeping supine.	Trunk flexion and sidebend stretches.

Table 10.4 Remedial massage techniques for major muscles of the low back and pelvis—cont'd

Muscle	Soft tissue release	Trigger point	Stretch	Client education[15]	Home stretch
Erector spinae	Active release: with the client sitting on the table and their feet on the floor, place the proximal phalanges of the fingers on the erector spinae either side of the spine at the thoracolumbar junction or above. The client slowly bends forward (may hold the side of the table) as your knuckles strip inferiorly along the erector spinae. (Do not use this technique on clients whose symptoms increase with lumbar flexion).		Trunk flexion stretches are usually performed actively. i) Sitting with legs extended and leaning forward until the stretch is felt. ii) Lying supine, client brings their knees to their chest as far as possible. iii) Kneeling on the floor, sitting back on their feet, the client takes their head towards the floor until the stretch is felt.	Use shock-absorbing and supportive footwear, avoid high-heeled shoes, correct lifting techniques.	Same as treatment stretches.

Continued

Table 10.4 Remedial massage techniques for major muscles of the low back and pelvis—cont'd

Muscle	Soft tissue release	Trigger point	Stretch	Client education[15]	Home stretch
Gluteus maximus	Active release: the client is sidelying and flexes and extends their bent upper leg while pressure is applied to the gluteus maximus.		The client is supine and takes their knee to the opposite shoulder (contraindicated for disc clients or any client who experiences pain on the movement). Provide resistance for 7 seconds as the client's knee moves back to the starting position. The knee is then actively or passively taken further towards the opposite shoulder.	Avoid prolonged sitting, use a small pillow behind the knees when sleeping supine.	i) The client is supine and takes one knee to the opposite shoulder. ii) The client lies supine with knees flexed and feet flat on the floor and places one foot across the other knee. They interlock their fingers around the thigh of the uncrossed leg and use their arms to draw their thigh towards their chest.

Table 10.4 Remedial massage techniques for major muscles of the low back and pelvis—cont'd

Muscle	Soft tissue release	Trigger point	Stretch	Client education[15]	Home stretch
Hamstring	The client lies in the prone position. Passive: using elbows/knuckles of one hand, glide along the muscle fibres or apply pressure at the site of the muscle lesion while the other hand holds the ankle and flexes and extends the client's leg. Active: as above but the client flexes and extends their leg unassisted.	Semi-tendinosus / Semi-membranosus / Biceps femoris	The client lies supine and raises their leg until they feel the muscle stretch. Using hands or shoulder, the practitioner resists the client as they attempt to return their leg to the table. Hold the resistance for 7 seconds after which the client tries to raise their leg further within the pain-free range. Repeat three times.	Use chairs that match the client's leg length and have a well-rounded and padded edge. Use a foot stool when seated. Take frequent breaks during long-distance driving.	There are a number of ways to stretch the hamstrings including: i) The client sits with their legs straight out in front of them or with one leg bent. The foot of the bent leg is placed on the floor alongside the thigh of the other leg and the knee rests on the floor. The client reaches forward towards their toes. ii) The client kneels with one leg straight out in front. The client leans forward from their hips towards their toes.
Quadriceps	Active: The client sits with their legs over the side of the table. Ask the client to slowly straighten and bend their leg as you apply pressure to the muscle lesion with fingers, thumbs or knuckles to glide along the muscle fibres.		Client prone. Ask client to bend one knee towards their buttocks as far as they can comfortably. At that point apply resistance while the client tries to straighten their leg for 7 seconds (the client performs an isometric contraction of the quadriceps muscle). After the contraction the client tries to take their heel to their buttocks again. Repeat three times.	Avoid shortening and/or prolonged immobilisation of the quadriceps muscles, avoid deep knee bends and complete squats, avoid prolonged sitting with hips at 90°, avoid full flexion of the hip when sleeping on the side.	Lying prone or standing, take the heel towards the buttocks.

Fig. 10.29 Longitudinal (A) and rotational (B) tractions of the lumbar spine

Differential diagnosis

Rule out non-mechanical causes of back pain including hae-matoma, abdominal aortic aneurysm and visceral referred pain (appendicitis, peritonitis, kidney pathology).[26]

Overview of treatment and management

Current evidence recommends prioritising self-management approaches, including staying active and staying at work.[24]

A typical remedial massage treatment for mild or moderate non-specific low back pain includes:

- Swedish massage therapy to the back, pelvis, posterior and anterior lower limbs.
- Remedial massage therapy, which includes techniques for muscle injury/muscle imbalances such as deep gliding frictions along the muscle fibres, cross-fibre frictions, active and passive soft tissue releasing techniques, deep transverse friction, trigger point therapy and muscle stretches (see Table 10.4).
  - Apply myofascial releasing techniques for myofascial restrictions. Thermotherapy may be beneficial. Techniques such as longitudinal and rotational tractions of the lumbar spine (see Figure 10.29) may be beneficial for facet joint lesions (described in detail in Chapter 7).
  - Multifidus and rotators release are also useful for improving mobility of facet joints (see Figure 10.30). Work ipsilaterally. Use both thumbs together or one on top of the other. Slowly apply downward (anterior) pressure to engage muscles in the paravertebral gutter. Release muscle tightness by performing three or four small superior/inferior movements over a distance of about 1 cm, then three or four small lateral movements (i.e. deep gliding and cross-fibre frictions). Release pressure slowly and slide to a new location. Note: deep anterior pressure over the lumbar spine is contraindicated in clients with spondylolisthesis and hyperlordosis. Use with caution in clients with osteoarthritis or history of lumbar disc herniation.

CLIENT EDUCATION

It is important that clients with low back pain stay active within their pain tolerance. Advise clients to avoid strenuous unaccustomed activities and of the musculoskeletal benefits

Fig. 10.30 Multifidus and rotators release

of regular and varied physical activity. Lifting and posture advice could help prevent future back problems. Referral to a chiropractor, osteopath or manipulative physiotherapist may be warranted for treatment of joint dysfunctions that do not resolve spontaneously. A full neurological examination is indicated in the presence of lower limb pain or other neurological symptoms.

Home exercise program

A program to stretch shortened muscles and strengthen weak ones should be instigated as soon as possible within the client's pain-free range.

Many clients with non-specific low back pain will recover within days or weeks, depending on the type of tissue injured, severity of injury and presence of complicating factors. Long-term treatment is designed to address any underlying conditions or predisposing factors to future back problems and to reinforce the importance of regular and varied exercise.

OSTEOARTHRITIS

Osteoarthritis is a painful condition that typically affects knees, hips or hands. It is the most common reason a person

Fig. 10.31 Radiograph of osteoarthritis of the lumbar spine

FUNCTIONAL TESTS

AROM: limitation ± pain in some ranges depending on the structures involved (e.g. extension may be painful and/or limited by facet degeneration or IVF encroachment, flexion may be painful and/or limited by disc degeneration).
PROM: limited ± painful in lateral flexion, rotation and extension.
RROM: negative unless there is associated muscle spasm. Specific muscle tests may be positive for associated muscle spasm.
Special tests are usually negative unless osteoarthritis is causing neural compression.

PALPATION

Palpation of the lumbar spine usually reveals tenderness over the affected joints.

Differential diagnosis

- Ankylosing spondylitis (axial spondyloarthritis): A key difference between ankylosing spondylitis and osteoarthritis is age of onset – the former usually begins between 15 and 35 years of age. Clients with ankylosing spondylitis complain of progressive morning pain and stiffness which is worse after periods of inactivity. Pain in osteoarthritis is usually relieved by rest.
- Psoriatic arthritis: psoriasis is a chronic autoimmune disease that causes red, scaly patches of inflammation and excessive skin production. Plaques frequently occur on the skin of the elbows and knees, but can affect any area including the scalp, palms of hands and soles of feet, and genitals. Between 10% and 30% of people with psoriasis develop psoriatic arthritis about 10 years after the onset of skin symptoms (i.e. typically between 30 and 50 years of age).
- Rheumatoid arthrosis (RA): Key differences between RA and osteoarthritis are age of onset (RA 30–60 years at time of onset), symmetrical involvement of joints (RA begins in bilateral proximal interphalangeal joints and metacarpophalangeal joints), associated prodrome (fever, malaise, night sweats), and ratio of females to males (3 to 1 in RA).[26]

Overview of treatment and management

Many patients with osteoarthritis may be receiving inappropriate care. According to Hunter,[27] the focus of care needs to shift from drugs and surgery to exercise, weight loss and self-management. Exercises to strengthen the muscles either side of the joint are recommended to improve joint stability. Low impact aerobic exercise like swimming, cycling, Tai Chi,

develops lower limb disability. Structural changes occur within the bone, the synovium and the cartilage.[27] Osteoarthritis pathology involves subchondral bone remodelling, synovial inflammation and loss of articular cartilage.[28] Inflammatory cytokines perpetuate disease progression via catabolic pathways.[29] Radiographs show asymmetrical joint space narrowing, osteophytes, subchondral bone sclerosis and subluxation[30] (see Figure 10.31). There is usually a long history of low back pain, stiffness and limited range of motion by the time the client is diagnosed. Osteoarthritis is most common in weight-bearing joints. In the lumbar spine it occurs most often at L4–L5.

Assessment

HISTORY

Clients are often over 50 years old, although the prevalence of osteoarthritis in younger people is likely to be under-estimated. Pain is described as slowly developing, dull and aching, aggravated by activity and relieved by rest. Clients often describe stiffness, especially in the morning. Pain can vary from a dull ache to severe, sharp pain and there may be nerve pinching and radiation of pain. Osteoarthritis is most common in weight-bearing joints that have been subjected to abnormal stresses (e.g. from overuse or obesity).[27]

rowing and paddling sports may also be helpful, particularly if they assist with weight loss. Exacerbations will occur but usually no more than 2–3 days/month. Self-management refers to learning how to manage those exacerbations (e.g. with topical anti-inflammatories or ice). Research into the role of diet and nutrition in managing osteoarthritis recommended reducing dietary cholesterol and ensuring that patients meet recommended intakes for micronutrients such as vitamin K.[31]

Most osteoarthritis clients respond positively to Swedish massage, heat and gentle stretches. Use light pressure for the initial treatment and consider restricting treatment options to Swedish massage until the client's response to massage therapy has been assessed. Heavy pressure and rigorous or long application of techniques can sometimes inflame arthritic joints.

Determine the type of tissue involved to guide selection of appropriate treatment techniques. Osteoarthritis is often accompanied by myofascial adhesions and muscle contracture.

A typical remedial massage treatment for osteoarthritis of the lumbar spine includes:

- Swedish massage therapy to the back, pelvis and posterior lower limbs.
- Remedial massage therapy, including thermotherapy and lumbar stretches (e.g. longitudinal and rotational tractions of the lumbar spine, bilateral leg traction. Caution: use the See-Move-Touch principle, especially before applying rotational tractions) (see Figure 10.29 on p 160). Apply specific muscle techniques including trigger point therapy and muscle stretches (see Table 10.4) to treat muscle spasm/imbalance. (Caution: proceed gently with older clients and regularly check their pain levels to avoid an acute exacerbation). Myofascial release may be beneficial for treating fascial restrictions.

CLIENT EDUCATION

Educate patients about osteoarthritis – that it is now considered a condition that can improve with weight loss and exercise. Encourage strengthening exercises for the muscles around the joint and low impact aerobic exercises. Footwear with shock-absorbing soles lessens jarring impacts when walking. Lifting and posture advice is important. A good supportive mattress and pillow may be beneficial. Investigate work ergonomics and recommend measures to minimise mechanical overload caused or aggravated by occupational tasks (e.g. avoiding repetitive tasks that overload the joints). Consider referral to a naturopath for specific dietary, herbal and nutritional support. Heat packs on affected joints may bring pain relief.

Home exercise program

Encourage clients to do strengthening exercises for muscles either side of the joint and to find an aerobic exercise that they enjoy. Clients appear to respond well to low-impact activities like aquarobics, swimming, Tai Chi or walking with appropriately cushioned footwear.

Address any underlying conditions or predisposing factors such as scoliosis or muscle weaknesses and contractures.

LOWER CROSSED SYNDROME

Lower crossed syndrome is a commonly observed back condition that results from a lower kinetic chain reaction of the lumbopelvis, hip, knee and ankle in which the hip flexors and back extensors shorten and tighten and the abdominal and gluteal

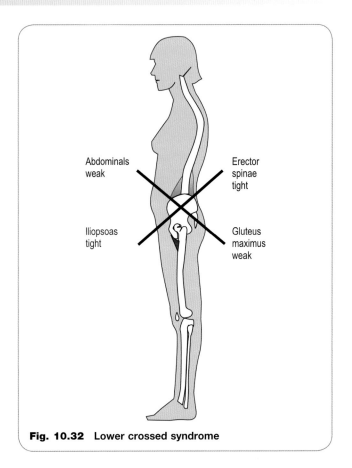

Fig. 10.32 Lower crossed syndrome

muscles weaken (see Figure 10.32).[10] Clients may complain of chronic low back pain that is aggravated by extension and relieved by forward flexion. The pain is also aggravated by prolonged standing, wearing high-heeled shoes and activities that hyperextend the spine. There is usually no radiation of pain, although lower crossed syndrome is also associated with piriformis syndrome which may cause pressure on the sciatic nerve. The condition may result from repetitive action as may occur in gymnastics and water polo, immobilisation including sitting for prolonged periods or poorly rehabilitated previous injuries.

Key assessment findings for lower crossed syndrome

- History can include repetitive activity, poorly rehabilitated previous injury, prolonged immobilisation. Pain after prolonged standing, bending backwards; pain relieved by lumbar flexion; usually no radiation of pain.
- Postural analysis: Hyperlordotic lumbar spine.
- Functional tests:
  - AROM positive in extension
  - PROM usually negative
  - RROM may be positive for affected muscles
  - Resisted and length tests positive for affected muscles including short iliopsoas, rectus femoris, erector spinae, quadratus lumborum, tensor fasciae latae, hip adductors; weak abdominal muscles, gluteal muscles
  - Special tests negative except for Kemp's.
- Palpation positive for tenderness ± pain on anterior pressure of the lumbar spine; tightness palpable in affected muscles.

Assessment

HISTORY

Clients with lower crossed syndrome/hyperlordosis usually describe a dull aching pain that can be localised at the lower back. The pain is aggravated by extension or prolonged standing and relieved by flexion. There is usually no radiation of pain and no neurological symptoms except in cases of associated piriformis syndrome where clients may experience sciatic pain. The patient often has difficulty lying supine with legs extended and prefers to lie with knees bent.

POSTURAL ANALYSIS

Lumbar hyperlordosis is evident and may be accompanied by compensatory thoracic kyphosis.

FUNCTIONAL TESTS

AROM: lumbar extension increases pain and trunk flexion relieves it.
PROM: usually negative.
RROM: may be positive for affected muscles.
Resisted and length tests may indicate muscle weakness (e.g. abdominal muscles, gluteal muscles) and shortness (e.g. iliopsoas, erector spinae, quadratus lumborum, rectus femoris) respectively.
Special tests: Kemp's test is usually positive and all other special tests negative.

PALPATION

Anterior pressure over L3 area often reproduces the pain. Tightness of affected muscles is usually palpable.

Differential diagnosis

Lower crossed syndrome is not difficult to identify. However, it is important to identify those clients with the possible presence of spondylolisthesis. Spondylolisthesis clients may experience bilateral sciatica and/or other neurological symptoms. Some also present with a hairy tuft over the lumbosacral area and a palpable step defect.

Overview of treatment and management

Remedial massage therapy focuses on the identification and correction of muscle imbalances associated with hyperlordosis. Check for relative imbalances between abdominal muscles and lumbar extensor muscles (erector spinae and quadratus lumborum), hip flexors (iliopsoas and rectus femoris) and gluteal muscles. In most cases abdominals, gluteal muscles and hamstrings will need to be strengthened in a home exercise program and erector spinae, iliopsoas, rectus femoris and quadratus lumborum need to be stretched during treatment and at home.

A typical treatment for lower crossed syndrome includes the following:

- Swedish massage to the back, buttocks and anterior thighs. Place a pillow in front of the client's waist during prone massage to reduce the lordosis and avoid undue anterior pressure on the spine. When the client lies supine, place a pillow under their thighs.
- Remedial massage is directed to addressing muscle imbalances found during assessment. Tight muscles require

stretching. Trigger point therapy and soft-tissue releasing techniques are usually beneficial (see Table 10.4). Tight muscles may respond to thermotherapy. Treat fascial restrictions with myofascial releasing techniques (see Chapter 8).

CLIENT EDUCATION

Client education includes avoiding all postures and activities that exacerbate lumbar lordosis. For example, advise the client to bend their knees when lying on their back or on their side. Advise the client to use a footstool when sitting or place a pillow under the thighs so that their knees are higher than their hips. When standing, they should use a footstool for one leg. Thermotherapy may be beneficial. Referral for osseous manipulation may be helpful.

Home exercise program

Many clients respond well to an exercise program. Muscle stretches performed during treatment (e.g. erector spinae, quadratus lumborum, iliopsoas and rectus femoris) should be continued at home. A program to strengthen weak muscles (e.g. abdominal muscles, gluteal muscles and hamstrings) may be progressively introduced for long-term biomechanical improvements. If pelvic floor muscles are weak, refer the client to a physiotherapist for specific exercises.

Address any underlying conditions or predisposing factors such as scoliosis, overtraining or obesity. Refer for a full neurological examination if the client has lower limb pain or other neurological symptoms.

LUMBAR DISC SYNDROME

Lumbar disc syndrome is a rare presenting condition, accounting for 1–3% of clients with low back pain. A herniated disc is a fragment of the nucleus pulposus which protrudes through tears or ruptures in the annulus fibrosus. The displaced disc fragment may press on spinal nerves, often producing pain which can be severe. L4–L5 and L5–S1 account for 95% of all disc herniations.[26] A herniated disc can result from a single excessive strain or injury or from chronic overloading of the disc (see Figure 10.33 on p 164).

Assessment

HISTORY

Lumbar disc herniation occurs most commonly in 25–45-year-olds. Clients may describe a recent trauma, heavy or awkward

---

Key assessment findings for lumbar disc syndrome

- Client usually 25–45 years old; history of recent trauma, heavy lifting, or niggling low back pain; pain may be severe; dermatomal radiation of pain.
- Functional tests:
  - AROM positive, particularly for flexion
  - PROM positive, particularly in flexion
  - RROM negative unless associated muscle strain
  - Resisted and length tests usually negative unless associated muscle strain
  - Special tests: positive Valsalva, SLR, centralisation.
- Palpation positive for tenderness ± pain at the level of the lesion.

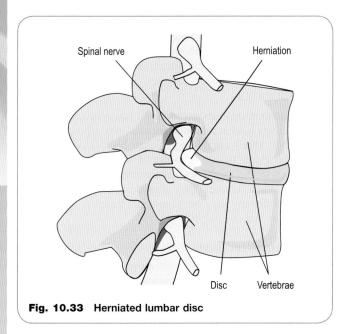

Fig. 10.33 Herniated lumbar disc

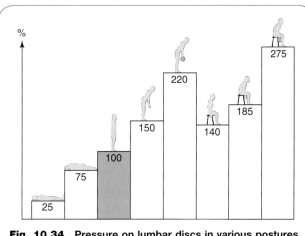

Fig. 10.34 Pressure on lumbar discs in various postures

lifting or repetitive stress trauma. Alternatively, the client may simply have leaned forward, usually to one side, when the injury occurred. These clients typically have a history of niggling low back pain. Unilateral sciatica commonly results from a herniated disc in the low back. Pain is often described as sharp and shooting and radiates in a dermatomal pattern. Symptoms include pain radiating from the buttock to the back of the leg and sometimes to the foot, burning, paraesthesia (tingling, numbness, pins and needles), sharp electric-shock pain and muscle weakness. Pain may be felt immediately or over a day or so after an episode of heavy or awkward lifting. Pain is aggravated by sitting, bending forward, coughing, sneezing or straining and is usually relieved by lying down (see Figure 10.34).

Features that are suggestive of lumbar disc syndrome include:

1. Severity of pain.
2. Dermatomal radiation of pain (e.g. L5/S1 disc herniation may impinge on the sciatic nerve root causing pain in the posterolateral leg and lateral foot).

3. Pain on Valsalva, SLR; pain centralises with repeated lumbar extension.[e]

POSTURAL ANALYSIS

The client may adopt an antalgic posture (i.e. the client leans away from the side of injury).

GAIT ANALYSIS

Clients with lumbar disc symptoms will move slowly and cautiously. In acute cases, clients may adopt an antalgic lean.

FUNCTIONAL TESTS

AROM: positive in flexion and/or any direction that increases neural compression.
PROM: positive in flexion and/or any direction that increases neural compression.
RROM: negative unless associated muscle strain.
Note: PROM and RROM tests may not be performed because of the potential to put further pressure on the disc. Special tests: Valsalva, SLR and centralisation are often positive. A positive SLR in conjunction with changes in reflexes, muscular strength and sensation suggest that lumbar radiculopathy is highly likely.[8] If pain centralises during repeated lumbar extension a bulging lumbar disc is indicated.[8]

PALPATION

The client commonly reports tenderness to palpation at the level of the lesion (usually over L4–S1). Spasm is usually palpated in muscles associated with adaptive contracture to guard against further pressure on the disc.

Differential diagnosis

- Cauda equina syndrome can result when a large central disc herniation presses on the cauda equina with effects on bowel and bladder function. It is a very rare (less than 1% of low back pain clients) but serious condition that requires urgent medical attention. The most significant finding leading to diagnosis is urinary retention. (Ask all disc clients if they have had any recent difficulty with urination or defecation.[26])
- Central or lateral canal stenosis refers to narrowing of the spinal canal caused by bone and/or soft tissue encroachment (e.g. congenital defects, spondylosis, thickening of the ligamentum flavum). Narrowing of the spinal canal can lead to compression of the spinal cord. Clients present with an inconsistent pattern of back and leg pain that is increased by activity and relieved by rest. Symptoms may be relieved by extension and flexion of the lumbar spine.
- Piriformis syndrome refers to sciatic neuritis caused when mechanical or chemical irritants infiltrate the epineurium of the nerve as a result of piriformis contracture. Although not a common cause of posterior thigh and leg pain, the piriformis is easily assessed and treated. It may be caused by trauma to the gluteal region or excessively tight external hip rotators. A positive SLR test with hip neutral and a negative SLR with hip in external rotation suggest piriformis syndrome.

---

[e]In a small number of clients, pain centralised in a direction other than extension.

Overview of treatment and management

Because of its severity most clients with acute lumbar disc herniation immediately consult a medical practitioner, chiropractor, osteopath or physiotherapist. All clients with severe pain (i.e. pain above 7 or 8 out of 10 on a pain scale) should be referred for further investigation and treatment. The aim of treatment in the acute phase is usually to control pain, reduce nerve compression, prevent any further nerve compression and to teach clients how to protect and stabilise their lower back. Clients are advised to stay as active as possible within their pain-free range. Gentle intermittent mobility such as pottering around the house is encouraged. In the acute phase many clients adopt an antalgic posture (usually trunk flexed and sidebent). As soon as the client can achieve lumbar lordosis without pain it should be encouraged (e.g. by using lumbar supports). Clients may be able to tolerate the Mackenzie back exercises if, when lying prone, extending a straight leg decreases or centralises their pain (see Appendix 10.1). Clients should avoid any movement that peripheralises pain both during treatment and in home exercise programs.

Typical remedial massage treatments for acutely inflamed lumbar discs include cryotherapy, acupressure, Reiki and reflexology. Note that anti-inflammatory or analgesic medication and muscle relaxants are prescribed. However, clinical guidelines now recommend non-steroidal anti-inflammatory drugs (NSAIDs) as a second-line or adjunctive treatment option. Paracetamol and systemic glucocorticoids are not recommended. Muscle relaxants may have limited use in selected patients.[24] Instruct clients to contact their medical practitioner should they require urgent care.

Most clients seek remedial massage for treatment of subacute or chronic back pain. However, even a history of disc herniation in the absence of presenting symptoms is sufficient to require modificaton of remedial massage techniques because of the recurrent nature of the condition. A typical treatment for subacute lumbar disc herniation includes:

- Swedish massage to the back, buttocks and posterior thighs. Pillows should be arranged to maintain pain-free lumbar lordosis if possible. (Caution: even Swedish massage strokes aggravate symptoms in some clients). Initial treatments should be short until the client's tolerance to massage in the prone position has been ascertained.
- Remedial massage therapy includes gentle bilateral leg traction within the client's painfree range. Remedial massage therapy for muscle strains/muscle imbalance includes deep gliding frictions along the muscle fibres, cross-fibre frictions and soft-tissue releasing techniques. Use the See-Move-Touch principle (see Chapter 2) and avoid techniques that could produce symptoms or aggravate the condition, particularly when performing trigger point therapy and muscle stretches. Incorrect or inappropriate stretches (especially into flexion) may aggravate the condition. For example, caution should be applied when performing a hamstring muscle stretch on a client with a recent history of pain on lumbar flexion. Note also that some practitioners suggest that spasm in the quadratus lumborum and lumbar erector spinae muscles creates a positive splinting for the lower back and therefore should not be completely released in the case of acute disc clients or clients with a history of disc damage. For example, focusing on deep tissue techniques to erector spinae on the side of the

lesion and leaving some protective splinting in the erector spinae on the contralateral side and bilateral quadratus lumborum may stabilise the low back in the acute stage. Thermotherapy and fascial releasing techniques are often used.

CLIENT EDUCATION

Posture and lifting advice may be helpful. Encourage clients to maintain good lumbar ergonomics at work, at home, while driving and undertaking all activities of daily living. Advise clients to get in and out of bed by rolling onto their side without twisting their lumbar spine, bending knees and using their arms to push their trunk upright, making sure their pelvis remains perpendicular to the spine. Clients should avoid sitting, forward bending particularly with a twist, lifting and any activities or positions that aggravate symptoms. If clients do lift, they must use appropriate lifting techniques (e.g. tighten core muscles when lifting, bend their knees, hold the load close to their body). Advise clients about the use of shock-absorbing soles when walking, about supportive mattresses and about weight loss if appropriate.

Refer clients to a chiropractor, osteopath or manipulative physiotherapist for spinal manipulation. Refer clients to an appropriate healthcare practitioner for identified yellow flags. Clients may also be referred for nutritional advice, for acupuncture and for exercise therapy. Always refer clients at six weeks post injury who have muscle weakness or who fail to respond to treatment.

Home exercise program

Erector spinae strengthening (e.g. prone alternating upper and lower limb raises) and core strengthening exercises are recommended as soon as they can be performed within the client's pain-free range and without aggravating symptoms. Erector spinae strengthening exercises can be performed slowly to fatigue then at speed to fatigue and repeated three times. (Encourage the client to count the number of repetitions to fatigue so they can monitor their progress.) As the client recovers, conditioning and proprioceptive training for the trunk and lower limbs can be progressively introduced. Pilates core strengthening programs (e.g. 'table top'[f] exercise, or the 'plank'[g] for fit people) and swimming could be useful for long-term prevention of pain and relapse.

The long-term aim of treatment of lumbar disc herniation is to educate and encourage clients to resume full normal activities. Remedial techniques are designed to maintain or improve good biomechanics. Most cases of acute lumbar disc herniation resolve spontaneously as the herniated material is reabsorbed. However, recurrences are not uncommon and have been associated with the presence of yellow flags.[2] Early assessment and intervention of yellow flags is essential.

SPONDYLOLISTHESIS

Spondylolisthesis is the forward slipping of a vertebra on the vertebra below. The term derives from the Greek words

---

[f]Lie on your back and bends both hip until they are perpendicular to the floor, keeping you knees bent and shins parallel to the floor. Gently curl your head and shoulders off the floor.

[g]From a hands and knees position on the floor, lower your forearms to the floor with elbows directly under your shoulders and hands shoulder-width apart. Move your feet backwards one at a time and maintain a straight line from your heels to your head.

Fig. 10.35 Radiograph of spondylolisthesis

Fig. 10.36 Grades of spondylolisthesis

Assessment

HISTORY

Clinical presentations vary and clients are often asymptomatic. Clients may complain of low back pain, sciatica and other neurological symptoms. Note that spondylolisthesis is the most common cause of bilateral sciatica. The pain may be sharp and severe. Severe symptoms or neurological symptoms differentiate spondylolisthesis from an uncomplicated hyper-lordotic posture.

Key assessment findings for spondylolisthesis

- History of pain after prolonged standing, bending backwards; pain relieved by lumbar flexion; ± bilateral sciatica or other neurological symptoms.
- Postural observation: hyperlordosis ± hairy tuft over lumbosacral area.
- Functional tests:
  - AROM positive in extension; pain reduced in flexion
  - PROM positive in extension; pain reduced in flexion
  - RROM usually negative
  - Special tests negative except for Kemp's test.
- Palpation; anterior pressure over L5/S1 is positive; ± step defect.

POSTURAL ANALYSIS

A hyperlordotic lumbar spine is commonly observed. There may be a hairy tuft (faun's beard) over the lumbosacral area.

FUNCTIONAL TESTS

AROM: Pain and neurological symptoms usually increase with extension and decrease with flexion.
PROM: Pain and neurological symptoms usually increase with extension and decrease with flexion.
RROM: Usually negative.
Special tests: Kemp's test is usually positive.

PALPATION

Clients report tenderness and/or pain over L5–S1 (or region of slippage) and caution is required when applying anterior pressure to the area. Sometimes a 'step deformity' is palpable (i.e. the anteriority of the spinous process above palpates as a hollow or dip in the spine).

Differential diagnosis

A less common cause of low back pain with bilateral sciatica is a central disc bulge exerting pressure on both sciatic nerves.

---

spondylos for vertebra and *olisthesis* for slippage or displacement. The slippage is most commonly due to a pars interarticularis defect (a separation of the vertebral body and the arch). Ninety per cent occur at L5. The cause of the condition is unclear although structural forces are involved. One widely accepted theory is that mechanical stresses cause a stress fracture of the pars interarticularis. The prevalence of spondylolisthesis is 5–7% in Caucasians and 40% in Inuit populations (possibly due to the vertical papoose fashion of carrying infants). For this reason, clients are sometimes advised to avoid vertical pouches or upright walkers for infants. Onset can occur after walking begins although the most common age is between 10 and 15 years. It is more common in people who have high levels of physical activity such as diving, gymnastics, weight lifting or pole vaulting where hyperextension and jarring stresses can occur.

Radiographs of spondylolisthesis show:

- anterior slippage of the vertebrae
- discontinuation of the posterior longitudinal ligament line
- oblique views have a 'collar on the Scotty dog' (see Figure 10.35).

Grading of spondylolisthesis is based on the percentage of forward slip of one vertebra (usually L5) compared to the vertebra below (usually S1) (see Figure 10.36). The higher the grade, the greater the instability.

- Grade 1: up to 25%
- Grade 2: up to 50%
- Grade 3: up to 75%
- Grade 4: up to 100%.

Spondylolisthesis may be distinguished from lower crossed/hyperlordosis syndrome by the presence of neurological symptoms, a palpable step-defect and a hairy tuft over the lumbosacral spine.

Overview of treatment and management

All clients with spondylolisthesis should be assessed by a medical practitioner, chiropractor, osteopath or physiotherapist. In most cases, remedial massage treatment will be provided in conjunction with other treatment (e.g. spinal manipulation, exercise therapy). This is potentially a very serious condition. Great attention is required to avoid lumbar extension in all phases of treatment. For example, incorrect pillow placement when the client is prone could increase lumbar lordosis and exert anterior pressure on the displaced vertebra. When the client is supine, ensure that the client lies with their knees flexed or place pillows under their knees to increase lumbar flexion. Posture and exercise advice for managing spondylolisthesis is similar to that for hyperlordotic (lower crossed posture), including avoiding all activities that extend the spine and cultivating flexion activities such as bringing knees to chest.

A typical treatment for spondylolisthesis includes the following:

- Swedish massage therapy to the low back and buttocks (pillow under the client's waist when prone: pillow under their thighs when supine). Avoid any strokes that place anterior pressure on the area of slippage.
- Remedial massage techniques include deep gliding friction, cross-fibre friction, trigger point, or active and passive release for affected muscles. Use only those techniques that can be performed without inducing lumbar extension (e.g. avoid deep massage on the multifidus and rotator muscles). Fascial releasing techniques for fascial restrictions are commonly used. Stretching techniques that flex the lumbar spine are beneficial (e.g. client supine, bilateral knees to chest). Thermotherapy may be beneficial.

CLIENT EDUCATION

Advise the client to avoid lumbar extension: consider sleeping position and mattress, workstation ergonomics, sitting with knees higher than hips, when standing for a long time putting one foot on a foot rail. Provide lifting advice (disc degeneration occurs at the level of the spondylolisthesis more rapidly than at any other level of the spine). Advise clients to avoid high-heeled shoes, use shock-absorbing soles and discuss weight loss if appropriate. Refer clients to a chiropractor, osteopath or manipulative physiotherapist for vertebral and sacral manipulation. Clients with spondylolisthesis should always be co-managed with a general medical practitioner, chiropractor, osteopath or physiotherapist. Some clients have reported benefit with acupuncture.

Home exercise program

Clients with spondylolisthesis may benefit from isometric strengthening of core stabilisers, and stretching low back extensor and hip flexor muscles, conditioning and proprioceptive training for the trunk and lower limbs, and painfree range of motion exercises.

Remedial massage therapy should continue with increasing reliance on home exercise programs and client self-help. Any underlying conditions, predisposing or complicating factors like scoliosis or sports and training programs that emphasise hyperextension should be addressed.

SACROILIAC SYNDROME

The sacroiliac joint is subject to mechanical lesions, including sprains and movement dysfunctions. Normally the sacroiliac joints have very little movement. Ligamentous laxity is a contributing factor during pregnancy when sacroiliac movements are enhanced by the action of the hormone relaxin, producing a 4 mm increase in the width of the symphysis pubis. Pain of mechanical origin is usually unilateral and can be aggravated by movements that stress the joint. There are usually no neurological symptoms. Note that pain in this area can also be referred from the lower lumbar spine or hip joint. It is also a common site for secondary malignant deposits or Paget's disease.

Assessment

HISTORY

The client usually describes a dull ache, although occasionally sacroiliac sprains can produce sharp stabbing pain. The most intense pain is reported over the sacroiliac joint itself but pain may refer to the buttock, groin or posterior thigh although it rarely extends below the knee. In clients with inflammatory sacroiliitis there is often a history of buttock pain that alternates from one side to the other. It is usually not relieved by lying down, is worse at night and is associated with stiffness in the back. Pain relieved by standing appears to be a useful indicator for sacroiliac joint sprain.[8]

Key assessment findings for sacroiliac syndrome

- History of recent trauma, repetitive overuse or stress of the low back and pelvis, pregnancy; unilateral SI pain ± radiation to buttock, groin, posterior thigh. Pain relieved by standing.
- Functional tests:
  - AROM: positive, especially flexion and extension of the pelvis
  - PROM: may be positive, especially flexion and extension of the pelvis
  - RROM: usually negative
  - Special tests: Patrick, SI compression and distraction, leg length, sacral springing may be positive.
- Palpation positive for tenderness ± pain over SI joint.

POSTURAL ANALYSIS

Mechanical sacroiliac lesions may be associated with scoliosis, leg length inequality and musculoskeletal compensations that may be identified during postural observation.

FUNCTIONAL TESTS

AROM: positive when weight bearing, moving from sitting to standing, walking, flexion or extension of the pelvis.
PROM: may be positive with flexion or extension of the pelvis.

ASISs–level

Left ASIS lower than right

ASIS–equal
flaring

ASIS–umbilicus distance
greater on left than right

Fig. 10.37 Assessing pelvic symmetry

PRONE SACROILIAC JOINT MOBILISATIONS

The client is prone and the pelvis is covered with a towel. Stabilise the sacrum with your caudal hand, fingers pointed superiorly; the cephalad palm contacts over the gluteal area on one side, fingers pointing inferiorly so that your hands are either side of the sacroiliac joint. Apply gentle pressure inferiorly with the caudal hand. Reverse the hand positions and apply gentle pressure with the caudal hand in a superior direction. Repeat both movements on the other sacroiliac joint (see Figure 10.38 on p 169).

SUPINE PELVIC ROCKING

The client is supine, pelvis and lower limbs covered with a towel. Face towards the head of the table and contact the client's anterior superior iliac spines with each hand. Apply gentle posterior pressure to the anterior superior iliac spine on one side, release the pressure, and then apply posterior pressure on the other. Pressure can also be applied one side at a time superiorly and inferiorly and medially and laterally (see Figure 10.39 on p 169).

- Tapotement can be applied directly over the sacrum and SI joints.
- Cross-fibre frictions to iliolumbar ligaments and sacrotuberous ligament (see Figure 10.40 on p 170).
- Thermotherapy may be beneficial.
- Treat any muscle imbalance with specific muscle techniques such as trigger point therapy, soft-tissue releasing techniques and stretches to specific muscles, including piriformis, quadratus lumborum, gluteus maximus, hamstrings and hip adductors (see Table 10.4). Myofascial releasing techniques may be beneficial for treating fascial restrictions. Hip joint articulation and a lymphatic pump from the feet may indirectly mobilise the sacroiliac joints.

LYMPHATIC PUMP

The client lies supine, legs extended. Hold the ankle of one leg and apply gentle pulsing pressure towards the client's head. (The leg acts as a lever to gently rock the pelvis posteriorly on one side). Repeat seven times, at a rate of one pulse a second. Next apply gentle pulsing tractions to the leg so that the pelvis gently rocks anteriorly on that side. Repeat the whole sequence (seven pushes and seven tractions) on the other leg and then repeat the sequence holding both legs at once (see Figure 10.41).

CLIENT EDUCATION

Refer for osseous manipulation and for a heel lift in cases of anatomical short leg. Advise clients to avoid cross-legged sitting. Minimise impacts caused or aggravated by occupation (e.g. avoiding repetitive tasks that overload the joints). Using footwear with shock-absorbing soles lessens jarring impacts when walking, and losing weight can reduce symptoms. A home exercise program should be introduced to strengthen and stretch muscles as indicated.

Address any underlying conditions or predisposing factors (e.g. scoliosis or hyperlordosis).

RROM: usually negative unless there are associated muscle imbalances.

Specific muscle tests: resisted tests and muscle length tests may be useful for identifying associated muscle imbalances.

Special tests: Pain provocation tests such as the Patrick test, compression and distraction tests and sacral springing demonstrate fair to moderate reliability; some have moderate diagnostic usefulness.[8]

PALPATION

With the client supine, place the palms of the hands on the anterior superior iliac spines and palpate for the distances between the anterior superior iliac spines and the umbilicus, and the height of the anterior superior iliac spines from the table (see Figure 10.37).

In the prone position, gently rock the sacrum from side to side and up and down. Palpate the sacroiliac joints for tenderness.

Overview of treatment and management

A typical remedial massage treatment for SI sprain includes the following:

- Swedish massage to the lumbosacral area (including the gluteal muscles and piriformis muscle) and posterior thighs.
- Remedial massage therapy, which includes prone sacroiliac joint mobilisations and supine pelvic rocking (anterior/posterior, superior/inferior and medial/lateral) within the client's pain-free range (to avoid stretching sprained ligaments).

Fig. 10.38 Prone sacroiliac mobilisation

Fig. 10.39 Supine pelvic rocking

Fig. 10.40 **Cross-fibre frictions to A:** iliolumbar ligaments and **B:** sacrotuberous ligaments

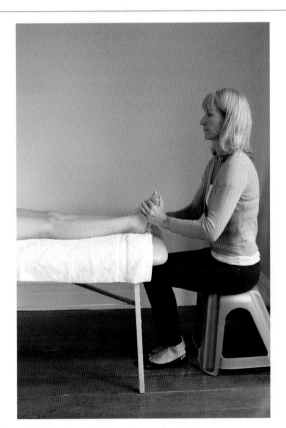

Fig. 10.41 **Lymphatic pump**

KEY MESSAGES

- Low back pain has a high prevalence in the community and is a common presenting condition to remedial massage clinics.

- Most (85–95%) low back pain is non-specific; that is, a specific pathoanatomical cause cannot be located.
- Assessment of clients with low back conditions involves history, outcome measures, postural analysis, gait analysis, functional tests (including resisted tests and muscle length tests for specific muscles of the low back and lower limbs) and special tests for the low back.
- Assessment findings may indicate the type of tissue involved (contractile or inert), duration of condition (acute or chronic) and severity.
- Assessment findings may indicate a common presenting condition such as
  - muscle strains
  - non-specific low back pain
  - osteoarthritis
  - lower crossed syndrome
  - lumbar disc herniation
  - spondylolisthesis
  - sacroiliac syndrome.
- Although serious conditions of the low back are rare, clients with such conditions will present for remedial massage from time to time. Caution is required when treating all clients with low back pain, especially when there are indications of lumbar disc herniation and spondylolisthesis. Be conservative in treatment: if in doubt, refer.
- Incorporate the best available evidence in therapy planning. Current evidence for non-specific low back pain recommends advice to stay active, an exercise program and psychological support as first-line treatments.
- Short-term treatments tend to focus on presenting symptoms; long-term treatments tend to focus on potential contributing factors (e.g. lifestyle factors, underlying structural features or underlying disease processes).
- Educating clients about likely causal and predisposing factors is an essential part of remedial massage therapy, particularly for potentially catastrophic and incapacitating conditions of the low back like disc herniation and spondylolisthesis.

APPENDIX 10.1
McKenzie self-treatments for sciatica[32]

'If your problem is worse with bending forward, after sitting, or in the morning, a few exercises originally developed by a physical therapist Robin McKenzie from New Zealand, may also be helpful — the sphinx, cobra, and standing back extension. The sphinx and cobra can be performed a few times a day. Carry out 10–12 repetitions slowly. If it hurts in your low back, but not in your leg that is fine. If however, leg pain increases then stop the exercise. The standing back extension manoeuvre can be performed a few times every 20 minutes when you have been sitting.

Fig. 2 Sphinx

Fig. 1 Rest position for cold pack

Since your nerves are behind your disc bending forward usually squeezes the bulging disc into the spinal nerve roots. Therefore, it is important to avoid slouching or slumping forward when sitting, standing or bending for things. McKenzie realized that it is also helpful to 'milk' the disc forward of the nerve roots by performing a variety of back bending or extension exercises. These may be uncomfortable in your back, BUT after a few repetitions you should feel that your leg symptoms are lessening. Scientific studies have proven that this is a good sign and means the exercises are right for you. If however, you feel your leg symptoms worsening then you are not ready for these movements yet.'

Review questions

1. A 20-year-old man has played a social game of cricket on the weekend, his first game since he left school. He woke the next day with low back pain that was very uncomfortable and made it hard for him to sit at his desk at work. On examination, Valsalva, SLR and compression are negative. His postural observation is unremarkable. A provisional assessment could be:
   a) Non-specific low back pain
   b) Hyperlordosis of the lumbar spine
   c) Spondylolisthesis
   d) Lumbar disc syndrome
2. A 23-year-old client has low back pain that is worse at the end of the day after she has been standing at work. She gets most relief when she lies on her back and brings her knees up to her chest. The pain does not refer beyond the low back and there are no neurological symptoms. A provisional assessment could be:
   a) Non-specific low back pain
   b) Lower crossed/hyperlordosis syndrome
   c) Spondylolisthesis
   d) Osteoarthritis
3. Straight leg raising (SLR) test is used to distinguish between:
   a) Lumbar disc and osteoarthritis
   b) Sciatica and hip flexor tightness
   c) Sciatica and hamstring tightness
   d) Osteoarthritis and sciatica
4. The most common level for a lumbar disc herniation to occur is:
   a) L4/L5   b) L3/L4
   c) L1/L2   d) L5/S1

5. The Valsalva test of the lumbar spine is used to indicate the presence of:
   a) a space-occupying lesion such as a disc prolapse
   b) paravertebral muscle strain
   c) lumbar facet syndrome
   d) spondylolisthesis
6. A client has low back pain that is aggravated by lumbar extension and relieved by forward flexion. He has a hairy tuft over the lumbosacral spine. He describes radiating pain down the back of both thighs. A likely assessment is:
   a) lumbar facet syndrome
   b) spondylolisthesis
   c) lower crossed/hyperlordosis syndrome
   d) lumbar disc syndrome
7. Name three signs and symptoms that could suggest a lumbar disc prolapse.
8. Briefly describe the precautions you would take when treating a client with spondylolisthesis.
9. A patient is observed to have a hyperlordotic spine. List three muscles that may be short and tight.
10. a) What is the clinical significance of a tight piriformis muscle?
    b) Draw or describe a test for piriformis muscle length.
11. Draw or describe a home stretch for the following muscles:
    a) iliopsoas
    b) quadratus lumborum
    c) quadriceps femoris
12. List three red flags for acute lumbar pain.

REFERENCES

1. Buchbinder R, van Tulder M, Oberg B, et al. Low back pain: a call for action. Lancet 2018;391:2384–8.

2. Hartvigsen J, Hancock MJ, Kongsted A, et al. What low back pain is and why we need to pay attention. Lancet 2018;391:2356–67.

3. Australian Institute of Health and Welfare. Back problems snapshot. Australian Government Australian Institute of Health and Welfare. Online. Available: https://www.aihw.gov.au/reports/chronic-musculoskeletal-conditions/back-problems/contents/what-are-back-problems; 2018.

4. Legaspi O, Edmond S. Does the evidence support the existence of lumbar spine coupled motion? A critical review of the literature. J Orthop Sports Phys Ther 2007;37(4):169–78.

5. Ha T-H, Saber-Sheikh K, Moore AP, et al. Measurement of lumbar spine range of movement and coupled motion using inertial sensors: a protocol validity study. Manual Ther 2013;18: 87–91.

6. Fritz S. Mosby's essential sciences for therapeutic massage. Anatomy, physiology, biomechanics, and pathology. 5th edn. St Louis, MO: Mosby Elsevier; 2017.

7. Tortora GJ, Derrickson BH. Principles of anatomy and physiology. 15th edn. Stafford, Qld: Wiley; 2016.

8. Cleland J, Koppenhaver S, Su J. Netter's orthopaedic clinical examination: an evidence-based approach. 3rd edn. Philadelphia: Saunders; 2015.

9. New Zealand Guidelines Group. New Zealand Acute Low Back Pain Guide. Online. Available: www.nzgg.org.nz/guidelines/0072/acc1038_col.pdf; 2004.

10. Chaitow L. Muscle energy techniques. 4th edn. Edinburgh: Churchill Livingstone; 2013.

11. Reese N, Bandy W. Joint range of motion and muscle length testing. 2nd edn. St Louis, MO: W.B. Saunders; 2010.

12. Kendall FP, McCreary EK, Provance PG, et al. Muscles, testing and function, with posture and pain. 5th edn. Philadelphia PA: Lippincott Williams and Wilkins; 2005.

13. Avers D, Brown M. Daniels and Worthingham's muscle testing: techniques of manual examination and performance testing. Philadephia, PA: Saunders; 2018.

14. Brukner P, Khan K. Clinical sports medicine. 4th edn. North Ryde, NSW: McGraw-Hill; 2012.

15. Simons D, Travell J, Simons L. Myofascial pain and dysfunction: the trigger point manual. *Vol 1*: upper half of body. 2nd edn. Philadelphia: Williams and Wilkins; 1999.

16. Vizniak N. Physical assessment. Burnaby, BC: Professional Health Systems; 2008.

17. Goodman C, Heick J, Lazaro R. Differential diagnosis for physical therapists: screening for referral. 6th ed. St Louise, MO: Elsevier; 2018.

18. Fritz S, Chaitow L, Hymel GM. Clinical massage in the healthcare setting. St Louis, MI: Mosby Elsevier; 2008.

19. Braman M. The effect of hamstring lengthening on pelvic tilt and lumbar lordosis. Tennessee: University of Tennessee; 2016.

20. Stochkendahl MJ, Kjaer P, Hartvigsen J, et al. National clinical guidelines for non-surgical treatment of patients with recent onset low back pain or lumbar radiculopathy. Eur Spine J 2018;27:60–75.

21. Qaseem A, Wilt TJ, McLean RM, et al. Noninvasive treatments for acute, subacute, and chronic low back pain: a clinical practice guideline from the American College of Physicians. Ann Intern Med 2017;166(7):515–34.

22. UK National Institute for Health and Care Excellence. Low back pain and sciatica in over 16s: assessment and management. National Institute for Health and Care Excellence; 2017.

23. Grace S, Engel R, Vemulpad S. The guidelines on low back pain are clear: drugs and surgery should be the last resort. Sydney: The Conversation; 2018. Online. Available: https://theconversation.com/the-guidelines-on-low-back-pain-are-clear-drugs-and-surgery-should-be-the-last-resort-94746.

24. Foster NE, Anema JR, Cherkin D, et al. Prevention and treatment of low back pain: evidence, challenges, and promising directions. Lancet 2018;391: 2368–83.

25. Kumar S, Beaton K, Hughes T. The effectiveness of massage therapy for the treatment of nonspecific low back pain: a systematic review of systematic reviews. Int J Gen Med 2013;6:733–41.

26. Carnes M, Vizniak N. Quick reference evidencebased conditions manual. 3rd edn. Burnaby, BC: Professional Health Systems; 2009.

27. Hunter D. Everything you ever wanted to know about osteoarthritis. The Health Report 2017. Online. Available: https://www.abc.net.au/radionational/programs/healthreport/everything-you-ever-wanted-to-know-about-osteoarthritis/8664218#transcript; 2017.

28. Goldring S. Alterations in periarticular bone and cross talk between subchondral bone and articular cartilage in osteoarthritis. Ther Adv Musculoskelet Dis 2012;4:249–58.

29. Abramson SB, Attur M. Developments in the scientific understanding of osteoarthritis. Arthritis Res Ther 2009;11:227.

30. Braun H, Gold G. Diagnosis of osteoarthritis: imaging. Bone. 2012;51(2):278–88.

31. Thomas S, Browne H, Mobasheri A. What is the evidence for a role for diet and nutrition in osteoarthritis? Rheumatology 2018;57:iv61–iv74.

32. Liebenson C. McKenzie self-treatments for sciatica. J Bodyw Mov Ther 2005;9:40–2.

The thoracic region

INTRODUCTION

Conditions of the thoracic spine are a less common presenting condition in remedial massage clinics than conditions of the lumbar or cervical spine. They are characterised by hypomobility and consequently play an important role in other conditions including those of the shoulder, neck and chest. For example, clients with neck pain of more than 30 days' duration have been observed to have a high probability of rapid improvement if treated with thoracic manipulation.[1] It is reasonable to expect that remedial massage techniques that improve the mobility of the thoracic spine will also be beneficial in the treatment of chronic neck and shoulder pain. Ageing also results in hypomobility and hyperkyphosis of the thoracic spine, mainly in the T6–T12 region.[2]

FUNCTIONAL ANATOMY REVIEW

There are 12 vertebrae in the thoracic spine with 12 pairs of ribs extending laterally from the vertebral column. Thoracic intervertebral discs are typically thin. The facet joints are small and flat and lie in the coronal plane allowing only slight movement at each segment. The rib cage and sternum provide added stability for the thoracic spine during movement. During load-bearing tasks, increased thoracic pressure from contractions of the diaphragm and deep abdominal and intercostal muscles adds further stability.

TYPICAL VERTEBRAE – T2–T8

The body of a typical thoracic vertebra is bean-shaped. Each rib head attaches to two contiguous vertebral bodies and the intervertebral fibrocartilage between them. The tubercles of the ribs attach to the transverse processes of the lower vertebrae. The spinous processes are long, slender and pointed and project inferiorly so that their tips are located at the level of the intervertebral discs below (see Figure 11.1 on p 174).

SPECIAL FEATURES OF T1 AND T9–12

T1 resembles cervical vertebrae with its horizontal and prominent spinous process. T9 may have no demi-facets; T10 usually has an entire articular facet on either side, partly on the pedicles. The shape and size of the vertebral bodies of T11 and T12 are more like lumbar vertebrae. Their rib facets are large and lie mainly on the pedicles.

Thoracic spine mobility is significantly limited by the rib cage. Movements in one plane are invariably accompanied by one or more coupled movements because of the structural and anatomical features of the thoracic spine. Coupled motion is most evident during lateral flexion and axial rotation. Lateral flexion is associated with axial rotation to the ipsilateral (same) side.[2]

There are three layers of muscles in the thoracic region (see Figure 11.2 on p 175). The superficial layer consists of middle and lower trapezius, rhomboids and latissimus dorsi muscles. The strap-like *erector spinae* form the middle layer of muscles. Muscles of the deep layer connect vertebra to vertebra and rib to rib. Major muscles of the mid and upper back are described in Table 11.1.

ASSESSMENT

The aims of remedial massage assessment of the thoracic region are:

- determining the suitability of clients for massage (screening for red flags)
- determining duration (acute or chronic) and severity of injury, and types of tissues involved
- determining if symptoms fit patterns of common conditions.

Assessment procedures for remedial massage clients are discussed in detail in Chapter 2.

Assessment of the thoracic region

1. Case history
2. Outcome measures
3. Postural analysis
4. Gait analysis
5. Functional tests
   Active range of motion tests
   flexion, extension, lateral flexion, rotation
   Passive range of motion tests
   flexion, extension, lateral flexion, rotation
   Resisted range of motion tests
   flexion, extension, lateral flexion, rotation
   Specific muscle tests including
   Erector spinae
   Latissimus dorsi
   Rhomboids
   Middle and lower trapezius
   Serratus anterior
   Special tests including
   Adam's test
   Deep breathing
   Elevated arm stress test (Roo's test)
   Springing
6. Palpation

CASE HISTORY

- Identify any red flags that require referral for further investigation (see Table 11.2 on p 176).
- Ask clients to point to the site of pain as they may have different understandings of anatomical terms. For example *shoulder pain* could mean pain in the rhomboid region, scapula, upper trapezius, deltoid (anterior, middle or posterior) or shoulder joint pain.
- Determine if the pain is likely to have a mechanical cause. (Is the pain associated with rest or activity, certain postures or time of day?) Ask clients to demonstrate movements and positions that aggravate or relieve pain and to be specific with descriptions of aggravating or relieving activities.

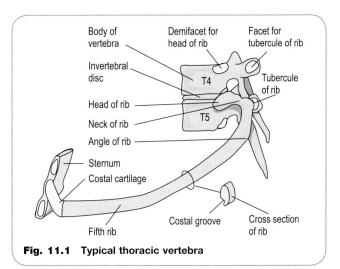

Fig. 11.1 Typical thoracic vertebra

Table 11.1 Muscles of the mid and upper back

Muscle	Origin	Insertion	Action
Erector spinae			As a group, extend the vertebral column
Iliocostalis thoracics	Angles of ribs 7–12	Angles of ribs 1–6, transverse process of C7	
Longissimus thoracic	Transverse and accessory processes of L1–5, anterior layer of thoracolumbar fascia	Transverse processes of T1–12, and lower nine or 10 ribs	
Spinalis thoracics	Spinous processes of L1–2, T11–T12	Spinous processes of T1–4/8	
Latissimus dorsi	An aponeurosis from T6–T12, all lumbar vertebrae and the posterior half of the iliac crest	Floor of biceps groove of humerus	Internally rotates, adducts and extends the humerus
Rhomboid major	T2–T5	Medial border of scapula between spine and inferior angle	Adducts and elevates the scapula
Rhomboid minor	C7 and T1	Medial border at spine of scapula	
Middle trapezius	Spinous processes of T1–T5	Acromion and spine of scapula	Adducts the scapula
Lower trapezius	Spinous processes of T6–T12	Spine of scapula	Rotates the scapula (along with upper fibres)
Serratus anterior	Outer ribs 1–8 or 9	Anterior surface of medial border of scapula	Abducts the scapula

(Note: Upper trapezius and levator scapulae are discussed in Chapter 12; intercostal muscles are discussed in Chapter 14.)

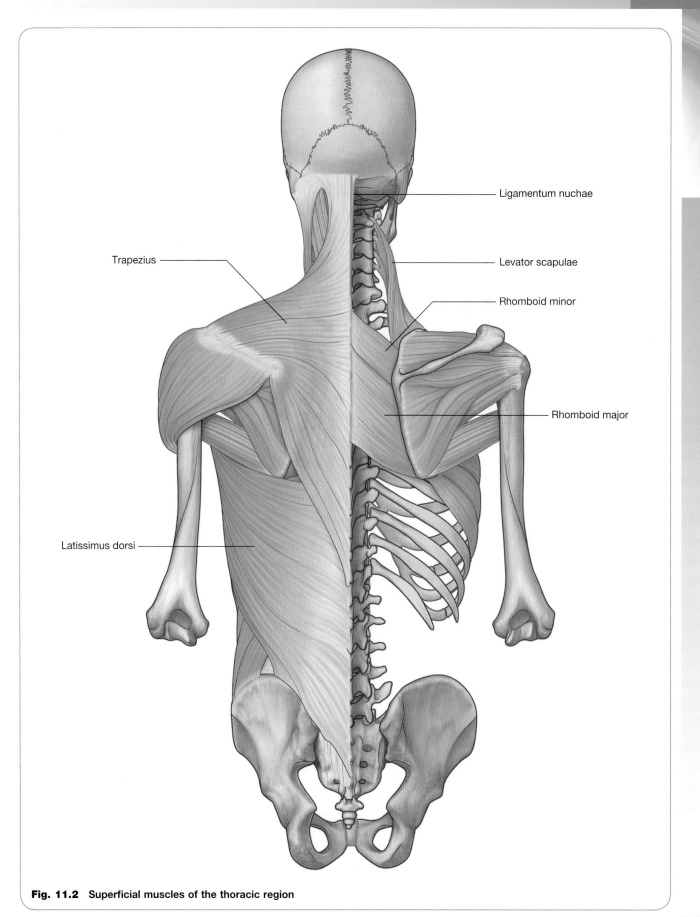

Ligamentum nuchae

Levator scapulae

Rhomboid minor

Rhomboid major

Trapezius

Latissimus dorsi

Fig. 11.2 Superficial muscles of the thoracic region

Table 11.2 Red flags for serious conditions associated with acute thoracic spine

Red flags for acute thoracic pain	Possible condition
Minor trauma (if >50 years, history of osteoporosis and taking corticosteroids) Major trauma	Fracture
Fever Night sweats Risk factors for infection (e.g. underlying disease process, immunosuppression, prolonged use of corticosteroids)	Infection
Past history of malignancy Age >50 years Failure to improve with treatment Unexplained weight loss Pain at multiple sites Pain at rest Night pain	Cancer
Chest pain or heaviness Movement, change in posture have no effect on pain Abdominal pain Shortness of breath, cough	Other serious condition

Adapted from the New Zealand Guidelines Group[3]
Note that acute pain in this context refers to pain of less than three months' duration.

- Mechanical pain is usually highly reactive to changes in posture, positions or activity.
- Morning pain relieved with daily activity is often associated with arthritis.
- Determine if the pain is likely to be associated with visceral, neurogenic, vascular or psychosocial functions (yellow flags).
- Pain from the gallbladder, liver or stomach is not usually aggravated by activity or relieved by rest, whereas mechanical back pain may be relieved by lying down.
- Neurogenic back pain from a spinal cord tumour or from a primary or secondary vertebral bone tumour is generally constant and remains unchanged by postural position.

OUTCOME MEASURES

Outcome measures are questionnaires that are used to assess clients' levels of impairment and to define benefits of treatment. The benefit is assessed in terms of client-perceived changes to health status. The Patient Specific Functional Scale is an example of outcome measures that could be used to assess conditions affecting the thoracic region.

POSTURAL ANALYSIS

Common conditions of the thoracic spine include:

- scoliosis
- hyperkyphosis: look for postural hyperkyphosis (e.g. upper crossed syndrome), lower cervical/upper thoracic region (dowager's hump) and Scheuermann's disease

- flattened thoracic curvature (*dishing*) usually between the scapulae (T2 to T7).

GAIT ANALYSIS

Conditions of the thoracic region are less likely to affect the symmetry and rhythm of normal gait than those affecting the lumbar and pelvic regions or the weight-bearing lower limbs. However, changes in the centre of gravity and other adaptations to unlevel shoulders and forward or tilted head position will be evident.

FUNCTIONAL TESTS

Thoracic range of motion is tested with the client seated on the massage table, arms crossed in front of the body. This stabilises the pelvis, enabling thoracic movement to be more accurately assessed. Active, passive and resisted range of motion are often tested in one plane before moving to the next; however they are dealt with discretely here for illustrative purposes. For example active, passive and resisted thoracic flexion can be tested first, followed by active, passive and resisted thoracic extension tests.

Active range of motion (AROM)

Standing thoracic range of motion is greatest during axial rotation (40°), then lateral bending (26°), flexion (21°) and extension (13°).[2]

FLEXION

- Stand behind the client.
- Instruct the client to bend forward slowly as far as they can without pain.

EXTENSION

- Stand at the side of the client and place a hand on the spine at T12 level. Ask the client to bend backwards from the contact point as far as they comfortably can.

LATERAL FLEXION (SIDEBEND)

- Ask the client to take their shoulder towards the hip on the same side. Stabilise the iliac crest with one hand and gently guide the client with the other hand on their shoulder as they laterally flex the trunk.
- Compare both sides and observe the coupling of the thoracic spine facet joints and posterior ribs.

ROTATION

Ask the client to turn their shoulders to the left and then the right as far as they comfortably can.

Passive range of motion (PROM)

Passive range of motion of the thoracic spine can be performed with the client seated. Place your forearm across the top of the client's shoulders to guide the movements. Your other hand rests on the middle thoracic spine as the client's trunk is flexed, extended, laterally flexed and rotated. Next your spinal contact is moved to the upper thoracic spine and the movements are repeated (see Figure 11.3).

Fig. 11.3   PROM tests of the thoracic spine

Resisted range of motion (RROM)

The six ranges of motion of the thoracic spine tested in AROM are also tested against resistance. Resisted range of motion tests are best performed with the client sitting on the treatment table to minimise extraneous muscle recruitment (see Figure 11.4 on p 178).

Resisted and length tests for specific muscles

Tests for specific muscles usually follow positive resisted range of motion tests or indications from other assessments including postural analysis where muscle imbalances may be identified. Muscle imbalances arise from muscle contractures and weaknesses. Mobilisers (e.g. upper trapezius) tend to

Fig. 11.4 RROM tests of the thoracic spine

Fig. 11.5 Erector spinae strength test

Fig. 11.6 Erector spinae length test

tighten and shorten; stabilisers (e.g. lower trapezius, serratus anterior) tend to weaken and lengthen.[4]

ERECTOR SPINAE

Strength test

Resisted trunk extension. The client lies prone and is instructed to raise their chest off the table without using their arms (see Figure 11.5).

Length test

Lumbar and thoracic erector spinae can be tested by having the client sit on the end of the table, feet flat on the floor, and bend their trunk forward towards the floor. Normally there should be 10 cm or less between the client's head and their knees[6] (see Figure 11.6). (Note: posterior tilting of the pelvis during trunk flexion suggests short hamstrings.)

Clinical significance

Ererctor spinae may be relatively weak in the thoracic spine in hyperkyphotic postures. Unilateral contractures are common in scoliosis.

LATISSIMUS DORSI

Resisted test

Stand behind the client whose extended arm is adducted and internally rotated. Instruct the client to hold this position as you try to move the arm diagonally forward (into flexion and abduction). Alternatively, clients reproduce the action of performing a 'lat pull-down' at the gym. The elbow is flexed and the upper arm raised up to 90° and abducted to 45°. Apply resistance as the client tries to bring their elbow downwards and backwards (see Figure 11.7).

Length test

The client lies supine and brings their arms into full flexion. Clients with shortened latissimus dorsi will not be able to rest their arms on the table above their heads. The length of latissimus dorsi can also be tested in the same position by observing the client's low back when their arm is raised overhead.

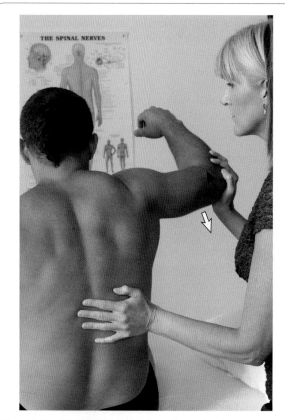

Fig. 11.7 Resisted tests for latissimus dorsi

Fig. 11.8 Length test for latissimus dorsi

Fig. 11.9 Resisted test for rhomboid muscles

An increased arch in the low back suggests latissimus dorsi shortening (see Figure 11.8).

Clinical significance

Bilateral shortening brings the shoulders forward and increases thoracic kyphosis.

RHOMBOID MAJOR AND MINOR

Resisted test

Stand behind the client. The client takes their flexed elbow behind their back and adducts it as far as possible. Instruct the client to hold this position. Apply downward pressure with one hand on the client's shoulder. At the same time, with the other hand, try to push the elbow into flexion and abduction (see Figure 11.9).

Length test

Shortened rhomboid muscles will adduct and elevate the scapula. This presentation is rarely observed in clinical practice.

Clinical significance

Lengthened and weakened rhomboids are commonly observed in upper crossed syndrome and in clients who spend frequent hours working at a desk, particularly sitting at a computer. There may be little reason in clinical practice to stretch the rhomboids. A more common need is to strengthen the rhomboids, lower trapezius and serratus anterior muscles in order to depress and adduct the scapula and counteract a rounded shoulder posture.

MIDDLE AND LOWER TRAPEZIUS

Resisted test

To test the middle fibres the client is prone and instructed to abduct their straight arm to 90°, thumbs pointed up to the ceiling. Place one hand on the client's forearm and the other on the client's back over the trapezius muscle. Instruct the client to hold this position as you apply pressure towards the floor. Repeat this procedure with the client's arm abducted to 135° to test the lower fibres (see Figure 11.10 on p 181).

Length test

Middle and lower trapezius contracture is rarely observed in clinical practice. Shortened middle trapezius muscles adduct and depress the scapula.

Clinical significance

Lengthened and weakened middle and lower trapezius are commonly observed in upper crossed syndrome.

SERRATUS ANTERIOR

Resisted test

Ask the client to lie supine, raise their straight arm vertically in front of them (so that the shoulder is flexed to 90°) and to thrust their arm upward to lift their scapula off the table. The client resists as you apply downward pressure to the client's fist (see Figure 11.11 on p 181).

Note that the appearance of winging of the scapula in postural observation or when the client attempts a wall push-up also indicates serratus anterior weakness.

Length test

Serratus anterior contracture is rarely observed in clinical practice.

Clinical significance

Serratus anterior weakness is commonly observed in upper crossed syndrome.

Fig. 11.10 Resisted tests for middle and lower trapezius

Fig. 11.11 Resisted test for serratus anterior

Special tests

Instruct clients to perform tests within their own pain tolerance. If clients experience pain while performing a special test, ask them for the exact location of the pain and confirm that it is the same pain as the one described in the case history.

Adam's test

The client stands and slowly bends forward to touch their toes. Stand behind and observe the symmetry of the ribs during trunk flexion. An abnormal rib hump on one side observed during trunk flexion indicates structural scoliosis (see Figure 11.12 on p 182).

Deep breathing

Instruct the client to remain still while taking a few deep breaths. Pain on deep breathing suggests a rib subluxation or fracture, intercostal or other respiratory muscle strain or a respiratory condition.

Elevated arm stress test (roo's test)

The patient is seated with their arms abducted to 90° and their elbow flexed to 90° (the stop sign position). Ask the client to open and close their fists for 3 minutes at a rate of twice a second. Resulting numbness, tingling or weakness may indicate thoracic outlet syndrome. (Note: these effects may occur in less than 3 minutes.)

Springing

Springing over different regions of the thoracic spine indicates tender or painful areas. It may be useful in identifying

Fig. 11.12 Adam's test

regions of hypomobility, for example in Scheuermann's disease. Springing in the thoracic region involves applying gentle pressure to the spinous processes, facet joints and rib heads. Begin with springing over the spinous processes of the thoracic spine, starting at T12 and moving up to T1. Next spring over the facet joints bilaterally. (Note that thoracic spinous processes project posteriorly and inferiorly so that the tip of each spinous process is level with the facet joints of the vertebra below. For example, the spinous process of T1 is level with the facet joints of T2. It is also important to remember that the most prominent vertebra below the neck is C7 not T1.) The head of each rib inserts anteriorly to the facet joints at that level. This means that the rib head of right rib 4 inserts anteriorly to the right facet joints of T4. This makes direct palpation of the rib heads impossible. Instead, spring the rib angles bilaterally. The rib angles are the most posterior section of each rib, or the highest part of the rib when the client is prone. Move laterally from the spinous processes to the highest part of the rib to spring each rib angle.

PALPATION

Pain produced on palpation helps determine the type of tissue involved in the lesion. Palpate the borders of the scapulae and compare the orientation of the scapulae bilaterally. Note any asymmetry in scapula winging, the levels of the inferior angle or the distances of the medial border from the spine.

To palpate rib alignment place four fingertips in four consecutive intercostal spaces and slide from the spine laterally as far as possible. Start at the floating ribs and work up the rib cage. If the space between two consecutive ribs narrows

considerably the intercostal muscles at that location may be typically contracted.

To palpate erector spinae place eight consecutive finger tips lateral to the lower thoracic spine. Palpate each section of the erector spinae muscle by moving the fingertips laterally across the strap of muscle and then return to the medial edge of the muscle. Continue palpating sections of the erector spinae muscles from the lower to the upper thoracic spine. Repeat on the other side.

Palpate middle and lower trapezius muscles from the lower thoracic spinal insertion using the fingertip sectioned approach described above. Palpate the fibres laterally and superiorly from the lower thoracic spine to the spine of the scapulae. Deep to the trapezius muscle palpate the rhomboids moving from the spine to the medial border of the scapulae.

Palpate infraspinatus in the infraspinatus fossa moving from the medial border laterally. Palpate the supraspinatus belly in the supraspinatus fossa, moving from the medial border of the scapula above the spine of the scapula, across to the medial aspect of the acromium. The levator scapulae insertion is palpable at the medial border of the scapula above its spine. Compare both sides. Latissimus dorsi forms the posterior wall of the axilla where it is easily palpated.

REMEDIAL MASSAGE TREATMENT

Assessment of the thorax provides information for development and negotiation of treatment plans, including:

- client's suitability for remedial massage therapy
- duration of the condition (i.e. acute or chronic)
- severity of the condition (i.e. grade of injury: mild, moderate or severe pain)
- type(s) of tissues involved
- priorities for treatment if more than one injury or condition is present
- whether the signs and symptoms suggest a common condition of the thoracic region
- special considerations for individual clients (e.g. clients' preferences for treatment types and styles, specific population considerations).

Treatment options must always be considered in the context of the best available evidence for treatment effectiveness and clinical practice guidelines where they exist. There is minimal quality evidence on the management of musculoskeletal thoracic pain. The effectiveness of massage and exercise on thoracic pain is not currently known. There is evidence that manipulation may lead to a small although clinically unimportant reduction in pain intensity when compared to placebo and acupuncture.[5] Considering the prevalence of thoracic pain, good quality clinical trials are certainly needed.

MUSCLE STRAIN

Muscle strains usually result from trauma such as accidents, falls and sports injuries. They are not common in the thoracic region because the stability provided by the rib cage protects thoracic muscles from sudden and excessive overload. Strains can also occur as a result of overuse or unaccustomed activity, such as may occur when starting an upper body weights program.

Assessment

HISTORY

The client complains of pain occurring after a trauma (e.g. accident, fall or sports injury) or after a period of unaccustomed activity like pruning a hedge. Pain is related to activity and is relieved by rest.

POSTURAL ANALYSIS

Muscle spasm may be evident on postural observation.

FUNCTIONAL TESTS

AROM: limited and painful usually.
PROM: may be painful at end of range of motion due to passive muscle stretching.
RROM: positive.
Resisted tests and length tests are painful for affected muscle(s).
Special tests: usually negative.

PALPATION

Tenderness and/or pain may be elicited over the affected muscle. Spasm or myofibrial tear may be palpable.

Overview of treatment and management of muscle strain

A typical remedial massage treatment for mild or moderate thoracic muscle strain includes:

- Swedish massage to the back, neck, shoulders and chest.
- Remedial massage techniques for muscle strains including:
  - deep gliding frictions along the muscle fibres
  - cross-fibre frictions
  - soft tissue releasing techniques
  - deep transverse friction
  - trigger point therapy
  - thermotherapy (see Chapter 3).
  - myofascial release (see Chapter 8).

Remedial massage techniques for muscles of the thoracic spine are illustrated in Table 11.3.

Note: Muscles of the thoracic spine are often tight and lengthened (e.g. rhomboid muscles in clients who spend excessive hours working at a desk). For such muscles, avoid techniques that work along the line of the fibre, which could encourage further muscle lengthening. Cross-fibre techniques

are recommended to reduce muscle tightness without lengthening the muscle.

CLIENT EDUCATION

Advise clients to avoid aggravating activities in the early phases of healing. Educate the client about likely causative and predisposing factors and ways to avoid recurrence, including maintaining a physical fitness program and developing appropriate levels of fitness before activities are commenced. Referral for osseous manipulation may be beneficial. Longer-term treatment should be designed to address any underlying conditions or predisposing factors to future musculoskeletal problems.

Home exercise program

As soon as the client can tolerate movement they should begin stretching the muscle and progressively introduce isometric strengthening exercises and a weights program. The aim is to achieve maximum strength and full length of the injured muscle and to restore optimal muscle function in the body.

THORACIC FACET SYNDROME

The facet (zygapophyseal) joint capsule and surrounding structures have nociceptive nerve fibres that respond to compression and distraction forces. Dysfunction of the facet joint involving reversible restriction of facet joint movements and degenerative changes of facet joints may cause back pain. Clients are often young adults who develop acute pain in the region of the facet or rib attachment following unaccustomed exercise or trauma. In older clients there may be an underlying hypomobility of the thoracic spine.

Assessment

HISTORY

The client complains of pain which may be experienced locally and in the region of the rib head attachments to the spine. If referral exists it is typically along the curve of the ribs inferiorly and laterally. Referred pain may also be experienced in the costochondral junctions. The pain may be sharp and aggravated by movement, coughing and deep breathing. There is often a history of a recent episode of thoracic twisting, such as may occur during a boxing session at the gym. Conditions characterised by hypomobility of the thoracic spine may

Table 11.3   Remedial massage techniques for muscles of the thoracic region

Muscle	Soft tissue release	Trigger point	Stretch	Client education[7]	Home exercise
Erector spinae	Active release: with the client sitting on the table and their feet on the floor, place knuckles of both hands either side of the spine on the erector spinae at the thoracolumbar junction or above. The client slowly bends forward, holding the side of the table, as your knuckles glide deeply inferiorly along the erector spinae. (Do not use this technique on clients whose symptoms increase with lumbar flexion.)	A: Iliocostalis thoracis B: Iliocostalis thoracis C: Iliocostalis lumborum D: Longissimus thoracis	Trunk flexion stretches: i) Sitting and leaning forward until the stretch is felt ii) Kneeling on all fours and arching the thoracic spine (cat posture in yoga) (Note: thoracic erector spinae may be long and weak and require strengthening)	Posture correction (e.g. lumbar support when sitting), correct ergonomics at workstation	Stretching: same as in treatment stretches Strengthening: Instruct the client to lie prone with their head in neutral. Ask the client to bring their arms straight up above their head in the fully abducted position. Keeping elbows and knees straight, gently raise one leg and the opposite arm slightly off the ground to activate the erector spinae muscles. Hold for 3 seconds then lower. Raise the alternate arm and leg. Hold for 3 seconds and lower. Repeat up to 5 times.

Table 11.3 Remedial massage techniques for muscles of the thoracic region—cont'd

Muscle	Soft tissue release	Trigger point	Stretch	Client education[7]	Home exercise
Latissimus dorsi	**One option for an active release:** The client sits on the table, feet on the floor, and adducts one arm to 90° and flexes the elbow to 90° (stop sign position). Grasp the posterior border of the axilla as the client slowly extends and adducts their upper arm.		Kneeling and sitting on feet, lean forward towards the floor, stretching both arms overhead	Use a footstool to avoid reaching high for heavy objects	The Mouth Wrap-around test. Turn head 45°. Reach around back of head to corner of mouth. Arms overhead and sidebending the trunk stretches the latissimus dorsi muscle.

Continued

185

Table 11.3 Remedial massage techniques for muscles of the thoracic region—cont'd

Muscle	Soft tissue release	Trigger point	Stretch	Client education[7]	Home exercise
Rhomboids	Active release techniques should not be used to lengthen an already long muscle. Use cross-fibre and diagonal fibre techniques only. The client is seated, feet on the floor. The client slowly protracts and retracts the scapula as you apply cross-fibre or diagonal fibre strokes to the rhomboids.		Rhomboid muscles present more commonly as lengthened and weakened than overcontracted. Consequently there is little need to stretch the muscle. Should a stretch be required, protraction and depression of the scapula would be required. The 'cat posture' (i.e. kneeling on all fours and arching the back) stretches the rhomboids.	Correct rounded shoulder posture	Strengthen the rhomboids by pulling the scapulae together. This exercise is often combined with the doorway stretch for pectoralis major.

Table 11.3 Remedial massage techniques for muscles of the thoracic region—cont'd

Muscle	Soft tissue release	Trigger point	Stretch	Client education[7]	Home exercise
Middle and lower trapezius	Active release techniques should not be used to lengthen an already long muscle. Use cross-fibre and diagonal fibre techniques only.		Middle and lower trapezius muscles present more commonly as lengthened and weakened than overcontracted. Consequently there is little need to stretch the muscle. The 'cat posture' stretches the middle and lower trapezius. The lower trapezius is also stretched by kneeling and sitting on feet, lean forward towards the floor, stretching both arms overhead.	Using an elbow rest if arms need to be held out in front of the body for prolonged periods; adjust workstation so that the chair is pulled close to the table and the client can lean back on the chair.	The middle trapezius stretch stretches middle and lower fibres of trapezius. Strengthening exercises can be performed prone, with the arms horizontally for middle trapezius and overhead for lower trapezius, and then using the back muscles to elevate the arms, head and trunk.

Continued

Table 11.3 Remedial massage techniques for muscles of the thoracic region—cont'd

Muscle	Soft tissue release	Trigger point	Stretch	Client education[7]	Home exercise
Serratus anterior	Active release techniques should not be used to lengthen an already long muscle. Use cross-fibre and diagonal fibre techniques only.		There is little need to stretch serratus anterior in clinical practice. To stretch serratus anterior (e.g. after ischaemic pressure to release a trigger point) the client lies on their side, rests their upper hand on their hip and lets their elbow drop behind their back.	Avoid overuse (e.g. paradoxical breathing, push-ups, chin-ups)[6]	Wall push-ups with the scapula retracted strengthen serratus anterior. Also lying supine, arm raised to 90° flexion, holding weight, protract the scapula.

increase susceptibility to facet syndrome from trauma, repetitive overuse or unaccustomed or prolonged activity.

FUNCTIONAL TESTS

AROM: limited and painful, especially on extension. Pain in more than one direction suggests joint capsule injury.
PROM: limited and painful, especially on extension.
RROM may be painful if there is an associated muscle strain.
Resisted tests and length tests may be painful for local muscle strain.
Special tests are negative except that associated rib subluxation may cause pain on coughing and deep breathing.

PALPATION

Tenderness ± pain may be elicited over the affected facet joint or rib head. There is often a palpable intercostal contracture between adjacent ribs. This can occur posteriorly, laterally or anteriorly.

Differential diagnosis

The most important condition to rule out is rib fracture. A history of trauma and slow resolution of the symptoms suggests this diagnosis. X-rays are required to confirm the presence of a fracture. Lung pathology must also be ruled out. Any history of smoking, fever, weight loss or intractable pain that is not relieved by rest requires medical referral.

Overview of treatment and management

A typical remedial massage treatment for thoracic facet syndrome/rib subluxation includes:

- Swedish massage therapy to the back and chest.
- Remedial massage therapy. The remedial massage technique that is most appropriate at the primary ligamentous site is deep transverse friction applied to the rib head attachment or costochondral joint. Work within the client's pain tolerance, instructing the client to breathe deeply. Work intermittently and alternate with other techniques.
  - Associated intercostal contractures should be located and treated, usually with fingertip deep transverse friction between the approximated ribs. The goal is to release the contracture and to restore normal function to muscle function. Other techniques for muscle contractures include deep gliding frictions along the muscle fibres, cross-fibre frictions, active and passive soft tissue releasing techniques, trigger point therapy and muscle stretches. Massage to the chest may be beneficial. Apply myofascial releasing techniques for myofascial restrictions. Thermotherapy may be beneficial.
- Thoracic mobilisation techniques are recommended for facet joint lesions (see Chapter 7):
  - thoracic longitudinal mobilisation
  - thoracic diagonal mobilisation
  - thoracic rocking
  - arm overhead rib mobilisation
  - rib rotation.

CLIENT EDUCATION

Advise clients to avoid such aggravating activities as extension or rotation, particularly in the early phases of healing.

Fig. 11.13 Strengthening exercise for erector spinae

Referral for osseous manipulation may be beneficial. Longer-term treatment should be designed to address any underlying conditions or predisposing factors to future musculoskeletal problems.

Home exercise program

As soon as the client can tolerate movement they should begin stretching exercises, including trunk lateral flexion away from the side of injury. Progressively introduce strengthening exercises including the erector spinae muscles (see Figure 11.13).

ERECTOR SPINAE STRENGTHENING EXERCISES

Instruct the client to lie prone with their head in neutral and bring their arms straight up above their head in the fully abducted position. Keeping their elbows and knees straight, the client gently raises one leg and the opposite arm slightly off the ground to activate the erector spinae muscles. This position is held for 3 seconds and then released. The client raises the other arm and leg and holds for 3 seconds before lowering to the ground. This sequence is repeated up to 5 times.

OSTEOARTHRITIS

Osteoarthritis represents a range of conditions characterised by loss of articular cartilage and reactive changes in subchondral bone. By the time osteoarthritis is evident in the thoracic spine it is usually also present in the lower lumbar spine, lower cervical spine and weight-bearing joints. In younger clients osteoarthritis may develop after a previous significant trauma.

Assessment

HISTORY

The client is typically middle aged, elderly or has a history of a previous significant trauma. The condition is chronic with episodes of acute exacerbation. The pain may be worse on rising, during periods of inactivity or excessive activity due to the presence of low-grade inflammation. There is generalised reduction in thoracic range of motion with the client reporting stiffness and occasional sharp pain. Clients often report an increase in the severity of symptoms in cold weather.

Key assessment findings for thoracic osteoarthritis

- Client usually over 50 years old; history of dull, aching pain, morning stiffness, pain that worsens with activity and improves with rest
- Functional tests:
  - AROM positive
  - PROM positive
  - RROM usually negative
  - Special tests usually negative
- Palpation positive for tenderness ± pain

Fig. 11.14 Doorway stretch

FUNCTIONAL TESTS

AROM: limited ± painful in some directions.
PROM: limited ± painful in some directions.
RROM: usually negative.
Resisted and length tests for specific muscles usually negative.
Special tests: usually negative (springing may reveal reduced mobilitiy and a hard end-feel).

PALPATION

The client may report tenderness and/or pain on palpation of the affected joints.

Differential diagnosis

Osteoporosis may occur independently although it is often concurrent with osteoarthritis. Further tests such as bone density scans may be required.

Overview of treatment and management

Osteoarthritis is a dynamic condition that can improve with lifestyle modifications like exercise.[8] Acute exacerbations may require anti-inflammatory medications or gels or cryotherapy for pain relief. Treatment often includes gentle thoracic range of motion stretches, especially extension stretches, within the client's pain threshold. Thoracic extension exercises such as the doorway stretch (see Figure 11.14) can be recommended to arrest the progression of hyperflexion. (Note: Variations on the doorway stretch are also used to stretch pectoralis major and biceps brachii. It is recommended here primarily to extend the thoracic spine.)

Although osteoarthritis mainly affects spinal cartilage, the surrounding ligaments and muscles often become contracted and hypertonic. Typical remedial massage treatment for mild or moderate thoracic osteoarthritis includes:

- Swedish massage therapy to the back, neck, shoulders and chest.
- Remedial massage therapy. Apply friction techniques (transverse and longitudinal) to the ligamentous structures. Muscular hypertonicity can be reduced with a range of remedial massage techniques including (see Table 11.3):
  - deep gliding frictions along the muscle fibres
  - cross-fibre frictions
  - active and passive soft-tissue releasing techniques
  - trigger point therapy
  - muscle stretches.

- Thermotherapy may be beneficial in the absence of an acute episode.
- Gentle thoracic mobilising techniques are recommended (see Chapter 7). Be careful to not overwork the area with sustained or overly deep techniques to avoid inflaming the area:
  - compression
  - rhythmic compressions
  - thoracic rocking
  - thoracic longitudinal mobilisation
  - thoracic diagonal mobilisation.
- Myofascial release techniques are reportedly very successful for the thoracic region (see Chapter 8).

CLIENT EDUCATION

Clients should avoid any activity that has a high impact on the spine. For example, it is better to go for a brisk walk than for a run. Wearing shock-absorbing footwear is also advisable. Encourage clients to remain active within their pain threshold. Diets which include long chain omega 3 fatty acids and vitamin K may help reduce pain and improve function in clients with spinal osteoarthritis.[9] Reducing cholesterol if raised may also be beneficial.

Home exercise program

Generalised thoracic range of motion stretches with particular emphasis on thoracic extension should be performed within the client's pain-free range. Progressively introduce strengthening exercises for the erector spinae muscles (see Figure 11.13) and other thoracic muscles as indicated.

HYPERKYPHOSIS OF THE UPPER THORACIC SPINE (DOWAGER'S HUMP)

Dowager's hump is a spinal deformity characterised by hyperkyphosis of the upper thoracic spine (see Figure 11.15). Historically it was most frequently observed in post-menopausal women (hence its name) and associated with osteoporotic bone loss. The demographics for hyperkyphosis appears to be broadening and the prevalence increasing. This may be due to

Normal   Dowager's hump

Fig. 11.15 Hyperkyphosis of the upper thoracic spine

RROM: may be positive for associated muscle strain. Resisted tests and length tests may be positive for affected muscles.

Special tests: negative. (Note: A perpendicular measure of at least 6.5 cm between the bony prominence of C7 or occiput and the wall in a standing position (the Occiput-Wall Distance) is a valid and reliable measure of thoracic kyphosis.[10])

PALPATION

Palpation may reveal contractures of associated muscles, particularly the upper trapezius muscles.

Differential diagnosis

An osteoporotic compression fracture of the anterior body of a thoracic vertebra would be associated with significant pain. Scheuermann's disease, which is also characterised by hyperkyphosis, most commonly affects the lower thoracic spine.

Overview of treatment and management

A typical remedial massage treatment for hyperkyphosis of the upper thoracic spine includes:

- Swedish massage therapy to the back, neck, shoulders and chest.
- Remedial massage therapy. Techniques designed to reduce fibrotic muscles of the upper thoracic region (specifically upper trapezius muscles, erector spinae, levator scapulae, and supraspinatus muscles) and chest (pectoralis major and minor) form the basis of the remedial massage approach (see Table 11.3):
  - deep gliding frictions along the muscle fibres
  - cross-fibre frictions
  - active and passive soft tissue releasing techniques
  - deep transverse friction
  - trigger point therapy
  - muscle stretches.
- Apply myofascial releasing techniques for myofascial restrictions.
- Thermotherapy may be beneficial.

CLIENT EDUCATION

Advise clients to use heat packs nightly draped over the upper thoracic spine and upper trapezius muscle. Refer clients for

sustained flexed posture while using computers and electronic devices and an ageing population.[10]

Assessment

HISTORY

There are usually no symptoms unless a fracture has occurred. Clients typically express concern at their increasing kyphosis. There may be a family history of osteoporosis or early menopause and there may be a history of working at computers, laptops and electronic devices.

POSTURAL ANALYSIS

The most significant indicator is the presence of increased thoracic kyphosis from C7 to the upper thoracic spine.

FUNCTIONAL TESTS

AROM: limited, especially in extension.
PROM: limited, especially in extension.

osseous manipulation of the upper thoracic spine and for hormone assessment where appropriate.

Home exercise program

The doorway stretch (see Figure 11.14) is recommended to extend the upper thoracic spine and open the chest. Another useful stretch is to roll a towel and place it lengthways along the spine just below the kyphotic curve. The client lies supine on the rolled towel for at least 10 minutes a day. Erector spinae strengthening exercises may also be useful (see Figure 11.13). Modest improvements in posture have been noted in clients who have undertaken erector spinae/back extension strengthening when overseen by a physical therapist.[11]

SCHEUERMANN'S DISEASE (VERTEBRAL EPIPHYSITIS)

Scheuermann's disease is a hyperkyphotic thoracic deformity due to anterior wedging of at least three vertebral bodies.[12] Localised pain occurs with activity and prolonged sitting or standing.[12] It affects males and females equally although some studies report a higher incidence in males.[12] Pain peaks during adolescence although patients with a greater degree of hyperkyphosis may experience ongoing pain into adulthood. Those with severe hyperkyphosis (>85°) experience reduced inspiratory capacity.[13] The cause of the condition is unclear although a hereditary component and mechanical factors play a role.[12]

Although physical therapy is not often mentioned in the literature as an effective treatment for Scheuermann's disease, it is often the initial clinical choice and may reduce pain.[12, 14] Brace treatment may be helpful if diagnosed early. Surgery would only be indicated if the hyperkyphosis is large (>70°). Patients who do proceed with surgical management tend to be older, have larger BMI and higher pain scores.[13]

Assessment

HISTORY

Scheuermann's disease affects adolescents between 12 to 15 years of age although clients can present at any age.

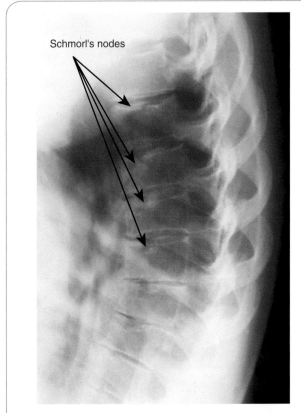

Fig. 11.16 Radiographs of Scheuermann's disease

Clinical presentations vary. There may be no symptoms or the client may experience dull, aching pain and/or tiredness in the mid back. Pain is usually aggravated by activity and relieved by rest. X-rays are required to confirm the diagnosis of Scheuermann's disease. Affected vertebral bodies are wedged anteriorly and endplates are sclerotic and irregular (Schmorl's nodes) (see Figure 11.16). Clients with Scheuermann's disease have an increased incidence of osteoarthritis and spondylolisthesis in the lumbar spine. Disc spaces are also decreased.

POSTURAL ANALYSIS

Hyperkyphotic deformity of the thoracic spine, especially the lower thoracic spine, is evident (see Figure 11.17 on p 193). Scoliosis may also be present. Anterior head carriage and rounded shoulders are commonly observed.

FUNCTIONAL TESTS

AROM: limited ± pain, especially in extension.
PROM: limited ± pain, especially in extension.
RROM: usually negative unless there is associated muscle strain.
Resisted tests and length tests may be positive for affected muscles.
Special tests: Springing positive for hypomobility and hard end-feel.

Key assessment findings for Scheuermann's disease

- The disease onset may occur from late preschoolers to 16 years of age, although most typically between 12 to 15 years of age
- Postural analysis: hyperkyphosis usually in the mid or low thoracic spine
- Functional tests:
  - AROM: limited especially in extension
  - PROM: limited especially in extension
  - RROM usually negative unless associated muscle strain
  - Resisted tests and length tests may be positive for affected muscles
  - Special tests: springing over affected vertebrae reveals limited mobility
- Palpation: The affected area may be rigid. There may be tenderness above and below the hyperkyphotic area

Normal bone density

Osteoporotic (porous) bone density

Fig. 11.18 Osteoporotic bone

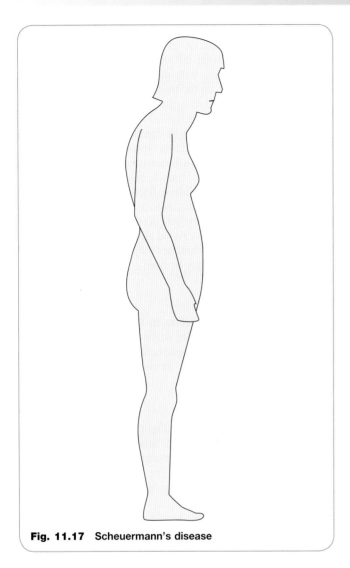

Fig. 11.17 Scheuermann's disease

PALPATION

There may be rigidity in the affected area. Tenderness may be elicited by palpating the vertebrae directly above or below the hyperkyphotic area. Associated muscles may be fibrotic.

Differential diagnosis

Exclude gibbus spine (interruption of normal thoracic kyphosis from previous osteoporotic fracture).

Overview of treatment and management

A typical remedial massage treatment for Scheuermann's disease includes:

- Swedish massage therapy to the back, neck, shoulders and chest.
- Remedial massage therapy. Muscle spasm/overload is addressed using (see Table 11.3):
  - deep gliding frictions along the muscle fibres
  - cross-fibre frictions
  - active and passive soft tissue releasing techniques
  - deep transverse friction
  - trigger point therapy
  - muscle stretches.

- Thoracic spine mobilisation to encourage flexibility in the region (see Chapter 7):
  - compression
  - rhythmic compressions
  - thoracic rocking
  - thoracic longitudinal mobilisation
  - thoracic diagonal mobilisation.
- Apply myofascial releasing techniques for myofascial restrictions.
- Thermotherapy may be beneficial. Heat increases the blood supply to the region and helps relax the ligamentous and muscular contractures. Heat packs also assist pain relief.

CLIENT EDUCATION

Advise clients to be vigilant with posture (avoid slouching in flexion). Practise thoracic extension activities (e.g. the doorway stretch, backstroke swimming) as much as possible. Advise clients about correct lifting techniques. Clients should be referred for spinal manipulation.

Home exercise program

Place a rolled towel along the entire length of the thoracic spine. Lie on the towel for at least 10 minutes per day in order to oppose the increased kyphosis.

Daily extension exercises of the thoracic spine are recommended to increase the mobility of the affected area and to strengthen the back extensor muscles (see Figure 11.13). Low-impact sports and activities may be helpful to maintain strength and mobility.

OSTEOPOROSIS

Osteoporosis involves an imbalance between bone formation and reabsorption that results in loss of bone density (see Figure 11.18). Its cause probably lies in the complex interactions among local and systemic regulators of bone cell function. Oestrogen deficiency, calcium and vitamin D deficiencies and secondary hyperparathyroidism all contribute. Cytokines that influence remodelling have also been identified. As bones become fragile, the risk of fracture increases. Osteoporosis is most prevalent in the axial skeleton, pelvis and proximal long

> **Key assessment findings for osteoporosis**
>
> - Clients are usually women over 50 years old; asymptomatic unless fracture present
> - Postural observation may reveal increased thoracic kyphosis
> - Functional tests:
>   - AROM: limited especially in extension
>   - PROM: limited especially in extension
>   - RROM: usually negative
>   - Special tests: negative (if no fracture present)
> - Palpation: no specific palpatory findings (severe pain and muscle guarding if fracture present)

bones. It occurs predominantly in post-menopausal women or older clients. The primary risk factors for osteoporosis are high alcohol intake, use of corticosteroids, and vitamin D deficiency.[15] Corticosteroids are used for inflammatory conditions such as asthma and rheumatoid arthritis. Lack of sun exposure can lead to low levels of vitamin D. Osteoporosis is of particular relevance for remedial massage therapists because of the increased risk of fracture: deep massage to the spine and ribs is contraindicated.

Assessment

HISTORY

Osteoporosis typically affects elderly females. They are usually asymptomatic. If compression fracture has occurred, clients complain of sharp pain.

POSTURAL ANALYSIS

An increased thoracic kyphosis may be present.

FUNCTIONAL TESTS

AROM: limited, especially in extension.
PROM: limited, especially in extension.
RROM: usually negative.
Special tests: only positive if fracture present.

PALPATION

There are no specific palpatory findings associated with osteoporosis. However, a reactive splinting response and pain may be elicited if a compression fracture is present.

Note that osteoporosis may be associated with other conditions such as Cushing's syndrome, hyperthyroidism, rheumatoid arthritis, disuse and medication use (e.g. glucocorticosteroids, anti-convulsives). Refer clients with associated symptoms for further investigation.

Overview of treatment of a client with a history of osteoporosis

The primary concern when treating osteoporotic clients is the risk of fracture, especially of the ribs. The pressure of all techniques should be light.

A typical remedial massage treatment for an osteoporotic client includes the following:

- Swedish massage therapy to the thoracic region, in particular the erector spinae. It is crucial to massage without putting undue strain on the skeleton. Always massage the muscles in accordance with the client's pain threshold but no anterior pressure on the thorax should be applied. Anterior pressure may inadvertently cause a fragile spine or ribs to spontaneously fracture.
- Remedial massage therapy is directed to reactive contractures within the surrounding muscle and ligamentous tissues. For example, remedial massage for erector spinae, intercostals and rhomboid muscle contracture could include gentle applications of gliding frictions along the muscle fibres, cross-fibre frictions, active and passive soft tissue releasing techniques, trigger point therapy and muscle stretches (see Table 11.3). Avoid all deep techniques. Gentle myofascial releasing techniques may be particularly beneficial and heat therapy may be used.

CLIENT EDUCATION

Osteoporosis requires monitoring by the client's medical practitioner. Periodic bone density scans are required, as well as advice regarding mineral supplements and hormone replacement medication. Clients may choose to consult a naturopath for nutritional support.

Home exercise program

Gentle doorway stretches (see Figure 11.14) are helpful to counteract the thoracic kyphosis. Strengthening exercises for the back and leg muscles are particularly important to reduce the risk of falls and fractures. For example, erector spinae strengthening exercises may be prescribed (see Figure 11.5).

SCOLIOSIS

Scoliosis refers to a lateral curvature of the spine.[a] The prevalence of adolescent idiopathic scoliosis is currently estimated at approximately 0.5–5% globally. The female to male ratio is 2:1 with females also at a greater risk of increased progression of the curve.[16] The two major types of scoliosis are:

1. **Structural (idiopathic) scoliosis.** This is a 3-dimensional deformity characterised by lateral curvature greater than 10° with resultant axial rotation. It is relatively fixed and does not straighten on forward bending of the trunk (Adam's test is positive if the client's rib hump does not straighten on lumbar flexion). It is often associated with vertebral and rib abnormalities and can be so severe as to require bracing and surgery. Adolescent scoliosis (i.e. scoliosis appearing between 10 years and skeletal maturity) accounts for 90% of scoliosis cases. The prevalence of adolescent idiopathic scoliosis is currently estimated at approximately 0.5–5% globally. The female to male ratio is 2:1 with females also at a greater risk of increased progression of the curve.[16] A recent systematic review found in favour of reintroducing school screening in Australian schools in order to identify curves at an early

---

[a]Scoliosis affects all spinal curves (not only thoracic curves). Discussion of scoliosis is included in the thoracic chapter because presence of a left thoracic curve (the majority of thoracic curves are to the right) is a red flag for referral for further examination.

Upper vertebra

Lower vertebra

angle a = angle b

A

B

Fig. 11.19 Structural scoliosis

treatable stage. The definitive cause for structural scoliosis is unknown in the majority of cases, although current thinking suggests multiple factors including biomechanical, neurological, hormonal and environmental.[16] As with many conditions, the earlier and more severe the onset, the poorer the prognosis. Idiopathic scoliosis, even if mild, will impact pulmonary and functional capacity.[17] Curves are measured on radiographs and these measurements have been used to determine those clients requiring bracing and to monitor the progression of the scoliosis (see Figure 11.19). Medical intervention may be required in some cases. Management options take a number of factors into consideration including age of onset. For congenital scoliosis surgery may be indicated if the curve is rapidly progressing. Bracing is not recommended.[17] Medical treatment for infantile (< 3 years of age) and juvenile (4–9 years) idiopathic scoliosis may include casting or 'growth friendly' surgical measures. Medical management of adolescent idiopathic scoliosis (>10 years to skeletal maturity) includes bracing once the Cobb angle (see Figure 11.20) reaches 25° degrees and surgery for a curve greater than 45° or rapidly progressing. Current studies suggest that spinal manipulation may benefit adolescent idiopathic scoliosis, although further high quality studies are needed for verification.[18] To help manage pain and increase core strength the Scoliosis Research Society suggests physical therapy, yoga and chiropractic.[19]

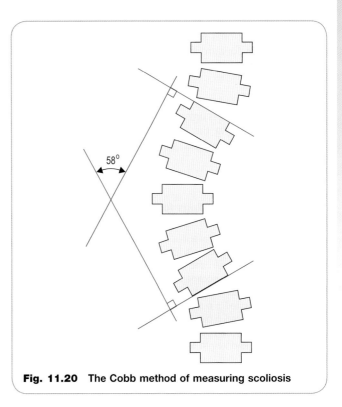

58°

Fig. 11.20 The Cobb method of measuring scoliosis

2. **Functional scoliosis.** This is a temporary curvature that may be associated with pelvic tilt and muscle imbalance due to work, sport or other activity. This type of scoliosis (i.e. non-structural) straightens on forward bending of the trunk (Adam's test is negative). It is correctable with massage, spinal manipulation, exercises and in some cases orthotics.

Assessment

HISTORY

In structural scoliosis, the client initially presents as an adolescent or young adult. There may be mild back pain that does not usually refer. Scoliosis may not be associated with symptoms in the early stages but over time stiffness and pain in the spine are common. Clients may also present with neck pain and headache. Functional scoliosis can occur at any stage and is associated with muscular pain and spasm.

POSTURAL ANALYSIS

Scoliosis is identified on postural observation. Scolioses are often described by the direction of curvature. For example, a left thoracic scoliosis describes a thoracic spine that curves to the left (i.e. the thoracic spine is convex on the left). Curves may be C-shaped or S-shaped. Note that the majority of adolescent idiopathic thoracic curves are right-convex.[20]

FUNCTIONAL TESTS

AROM: limited in some directions.
PROM: limited in some directions.
RROM: may be positive for affected muscle groups.
Resisted muscle tests and length test may be positive for affected muscles.
Special tests: Adam's test helps differentiate between structural and functional scoliosis. Structural scoliosis does not straighten on forward flexion whereas functional scoliosis does. Leg length inequality may be present.

PALPATION

The muscles on the convex side of the curve are usually hypertonic. Palpating the spinous processes from T1 to L5 traces the lateral curvatures.

Key assessment findings for scoliosis

- Structural scoliosis: client is usually an adolescent or young adult; functional scoliosis can present at any age: mild to moderate back pain and associated muscle pain
- Postural analysis: scoliosis present
- Functional tests:
  - AROM: limited ± pain in some directions
  - PROM: limited ± pain in some directions
  - RROM: may be positive for affected muscles
  - Resisted and length tests may be positive for affected muscles
  - Special tests: Adam's test is positive in structural scoliosis
- Palpation: muscle hypertonicity is usually present on the convex side of the curve

---

Differential diagnosis

The onset of scoliosis is usually insidious and progressive. However, it is important to identify red flags in cases where a scoliosis may be secondary to a serious underlying medical condition. Symptoms that require referral to a medical practitioner include severe pain, particularly at night, asymmetric abdominal reflexes, rigidity, deviation to one side during Adam's test, sudden or rapid curve progression or progression after skeletal maturity and abnormal neurologic findings.[21]

Overview of treatment and management

In cases of idiopathic scoliosis, radiographic assessment determines treatment. One way of measuring scoliosis is by the Cobb method: lines are drawn from the top of the most tilted vertebra above the apex of the curve and from the bottom of the most tilted vertebra below the apex. Two lines are drawn perpendicular to these lines. The angle between the intersection of the perpendicular lines is the Cobb angle. Clients with curves that are greater than 35° require referral (see Figure 11.20).

A typical remedial massage treatment for structural or functional scoliosis includes:

- Swedish massage therapy to the back, neck, lower limbs and chest.
- Remedial massage therapy to correct muscle imbalances where possible, reduce pain and increase range of motion. For muscle contractures remedial massage therapy includes (see Table 11.3):
  - deep gliding frictions along the muscle fibres, especially on the concave side
  - cross-fibre frictions, especially on muscles on the convex side
  - active and passive soft tissue releasing techniques
  - deep transverse friction
  - trigger point therapy
  - muscle stretches.
- Manual traction of the spine (e.g. using leg traction techniques) may be beneficial. Apply myofascial releasing techniques for myofascial restrictions. Thermotherapy may be beneficial.
- The scoliosis technique may be useful for structural (idiopathic) scoliosis. The technique is performed in two parts. The aim of the first part is to exaggerate the curvature and to stimulate neural input to the central nervous system. In the second part, the curvature is reversed and muscle-lengthening techniques are applied.

SCOLIOSIS TECHNIQUE:

i) C-shaped curve

1. The client lies prone. The client is instructed to exaggerate the curve by flexing the knee on the side of concavity, stretching the arm overhead on the side of convexity, and turning the head towards the concavity (see Figure 11.21). In this position, massage the paraspinal muscles on the side of concavity. Use cross-fibre techniques only for approximately 3–5 minutes.
2. Reverse the arm and leg positions to the opposite sides to minimise the curve. Continue massaging the same muscle groups using longitudinal gliding (lengthening the fibres) for approximately 5 minutes. (Massage the

Fig. 11.21 The Scoliosis technique: exaggerating the C-curve

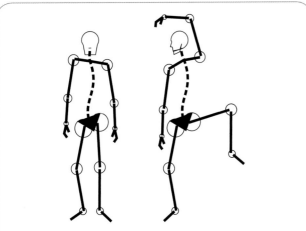

Fig. 11.22 The Scoliosis technique: exaggerating the S-curve

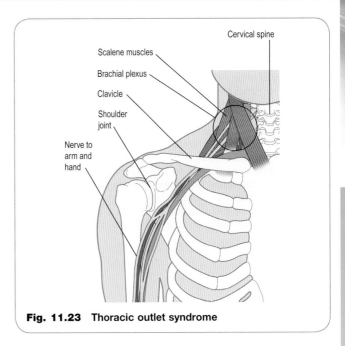

Fig. 11.23 Thoracic outlet syndrome

same muscles as in the previous step on the concave side of the curve only.)

ii) S-shaped curve

1. The client lies prone. Instruct the client to exaggerate the curves by flexing the knee on the side of lumbar concavity, stretching the arm overhead on the side of thoracic convexity and turning the head towards the thoracic concavity (see Figure 11.22). Use cross-fibre techniques for approximately 3–5 minutes massaging muscles on the concave side of the curves only.
2. Reverse arm and leg positions to the opposite sides to minimise the curve. Continue massaging the same muscle groups but using longitudinal gliding (lengthening the fibres) for about 5 minutes. Massage the same muscles as in the previous step.

CLIENT EDUCATION

Advise clients about the importance of maintaining and improving range of motion and of avoiding any activities

that are likely to add excessive load to the spine such as heavy lifting or wearing hard-soled shoes on hard surfaces. Ensure that clients with structural scoliosis who have not reached skeletal maturity or who have not been previously assessed are referred to their medical practitioner for assessment and management. Refer to a podiatrist, chiropractor, osteopath or physiotherapist for consideration of a heel lift if true leg length inequality is suspected. If the client has a leg length discrepancy there is evidence that heel lifts reduce pain and improve function in patients with common musculoskeletal conditions. However, the quality of the evidence is low and further rigorous studies are warranted.[22]

Home exercise program

It is important that all clients with scoliosis undertake an exercise program to help maintain optimum muscle function. Stretching exercises for contracted muscles (concave side) and strengthening exercises for weak muscles (convex side) are recommended. Breathing exercises will help maintain maximum chest expansion. Spinal traction exercises may be considered. Although the quality of evidence is currently low, improvement in function and small curvature reductions have been documented in adolescent clients who undertake scoliosis-specific exercise.[23] For clients with non-structural (functional) scoliosis prescription of Pilates exercises may be of benefit.[24]

THORACIC OUTLET SYNDROME (ANTERIOR SCALENE SYNDROME)

Thoracic outlet syndrome refers to compression on the neurovascular bundle at the thoracic outlet (see Figure 11.23). Symptoms include numbness or paraesthesia in the upper limb. The condition may arise as a consequence of previous shoulder or lower cervical trauma, the presence of a cervical

Key assessment findings for thoracic outlet syndrome

- History of unilateral numbness/paraesthesia in the upper limb; nocturnal pain often wakes clients from sleep
- Postural analysis: head forward position, rounded shoulders
- Functional tests
  - Cervical, thoracic and shoulder AROM and PROM may cause further neurovascular compression and reproduce or aggravate symptoms
  - RROM may be positive for affected muscles
  - Resisted tests and length tests may be positive for specific muscles
  - Special tests: Elevated arm stress test is positive
- Palpation: tenderness and hypertonia in scalenes, pectoralis minor

rib or anomalous or excessively toned or contracted scalene, pectoralis minor and/or subclavian muscles. Sleeping with the arm overhead and having a rounded shoulder posture may predispose people to this syndrome.

Assessment

HISTORY

The client commonly reports constant numbness and/or paraesthesia on the medial side of the arm and hand on the affected side. Pain may occur at night and wake the client from sleep. Thoracic outlet syndrome is also associated with occipital headache. Venous causes are less common and, if present, can lead to swelling in the upper limb. Arterial compression can lead to pallor and sensitivity to cold.

POSTURAL ANALYSIS

The client often has head forward carriage and rounded shoulders.

FUNCTIONAL TESTS

- AROM and PROM of the lower cervical, upper thoracic or shoulder may reproduce or aggravate symptoms.
- RROM tests may be positive in affected muscles.
- Resisted and length tests may be positive in affected muscles.
- Special tests: Elevation arm stress test (Roo's test) is positive.

PALPATION

The anterior scalene and pectoralis minor muscles may be hypertonic and tender to palpation.

Differential diagnosis

Cervical radiculopathy can also mimic the neurological symptoms of thoracic outlet syndrome. Refer all clients with suspected thoracic outlet syndrome to a chiropractor, osteopath or physiotherapist for assessment before commencing massage therapy.

Overview of treatment and management

Remedial massage may be used as an adjunct to other physical therapies. Eight remedial massage treatments over a period of 35 days was found to help manage neurogenic thoracic outlet symptoms and improve mobility.[25] A typical remedial massage treatment for thoracic outlet syndrome includes:

- Swedish massage therapy to the upper back, neck, chest and upper limb.
- Remedial massage techniques, which are designed to address muscle imbalance that could be causing or aggravating the condition. For example, remedial massage therapy for hypertonic anterior scalene, pectoralis minor and other tight cervical muscles could include (see Table 12.4):
  - deep gliding frictions along the muscle fibres
  - cross-fibre frictions
  - active and passive soft tissue releasing techniques
  - deep transverse friction
  - trigger point therapy
  - muscle stretches.
- Apply myofascial releasing techniques for myofascial restrictions.
- Thermotherapy may be beneficial.

CLIENT EDUCATION

Advise clients about postural corrections for forward head carriage and rounded shoulders and to avoid sleeping with arms overhead.

Home exercise program

An exercise program to stretch contracted muscles (e.g. anterior scalenes, pectoralis minor and various cervical muscles) and to strengthen upper trapezius and rhomboids will help correct posture and may relieve neurovascular compression at the thoracic outlet.

KEY MESSAGES

- Assessment of clients with conditions of the thoracic region involves history, outcome measures, postural analysis, gait analysis, functional tests (including resisted tests and length tests for specific muscles) and special tests for the thoracic region (e.g. Adam's test, deep breathing, Roo's test).
- Assessment findings may indicate the type of tissue involved (contractile or inert), duration of condition (acute or chronic) and severity.
- Assessment findings may indicate a common presenting condition (thoracic facet syndrome, osteoarthritis, dowager's hump, Scheuermann's disease, scoliosis and thoracic outlet syndrome).
- Assessment findings also indicate client perception of injury and preferences for treatment.
- Consider Clinical Guidelines, available evidence, clinical efficacy and client preferences when planning therapy.
- Although serious conditions of the thoracic region are rare, clients with such conditions will present for remedial massage from time to time. Caution is required when

treating all clients with pain in the thoracic region, especially when there is a history of trauma, previous malignancy or other indications of potentially serious disease, including fever and chest pain.

- Educating clients about likely causal and predisposing factors is an essential part of remedial massage therapy.

Over time, increase the client self-help component of treatment wherever possible to reduce likelihood of recurrence and/or to promote health maintenance and illness prevention.

Review questions

1. The term *idiopathic* means:
   a) induced by treatment
   b) congenital
   c) unknown cause
   d) of genetic origin
2. A dowager's hump refers to:
   a) an increased kyphosis at the C7 to T3 level
   b) an increased kyphosis at the T9 to L2 level
   c) a flattened kyphosis between the shoulder blades
   d) a hairy tuft over the lower lumbar spine
3. A patient presents with lower right rib cage pain three days after being injured in a game of football. The pain is sharp, localised and continuing to be very painful. He is unable to take a deep breath without pain. Palpation of the injury site is very tender and there is evidence of reflex muscle guarding. A provisional diagnosis would be:
   a) subluxated rib
   b) fractured rib
   c) herniated thoracic disc
   d) intercostal muscle strain
4. An adolescent client is observed to have a moderate to severe scoliosis. An appropriate treatment would be:
   a) Swedish massage, trigger point therapy, muscle stretches and the scoliosis technique
   b) referral to a medical practitioner for further assessment
   c) Swedish massage only
   d) Swedish massage and a weights program
5. Schmorl's nodes on an X-ray are often associated with:
   a) Scheuermann's disease
   b) structural scoliosis
   c) osteoarthritis of the thoracic spine
   d) Tietze's syndrome
6. Describe a test that would help differentiate between structural and functional scoliosis.
7. a) What is Scheuermann's disease?
   b) What group of the population does it most affect?
   c) Name one test or observation that would make you suspect Scheuermann's disease.
   d) What recommendations would you make to a client with Scheuermann's disease?
8. Describe or draw a resisted muscle test for each of the following muscles:
   a) pectoralis major
   b) rhomboid muscles
   c) serratus anterior
   d) middle trapezius

9. A client presents with a history of numbness and pins and needles on the inside of her left arm. During the night she is often woken from sleep with arm pain. The arm elevated stress test brings pins and needles to her arm and hand. The client could have:
   a) dowager's hump
   b) thoracic outlet syndrome
   c) a fractured rib secondary to osteoporosis
   d) osteoarthritis in the upper thoracic spine
10. Osteoarthritis in the thoracic spine is associated with:
   a) osteophytic lipping
   b) disc degeneration
   c) muscle spasm
   d) all of the above
11. In assessing rib pain how would you differentiate a rib fracture from an intercostal muscle strain?
12. The following diagram represents a stretch for which muscle(s)?
   a) middle trapezius
   b) pectoralis major
   c) latissimus dorsi
   d) serratus anterior

REFERENCES

1. Cleland J, Koppenhaver S, Su J. Netter's orthopaedic clinical examination: an evidence-based approach. 3rd edn. Philadelphia: Saunders; 2015.
2. Pan F, Firouzabadi A, Reitmaier S, et al. The shape and mobility of the thoracic spine in asymptomatic adults: a systematic review of in vivo studies. J Biomechanics 2018;78:21–35.
3. New Zealand Guidelines Group. New Zealand acute low back pain guide. Online. Available: www.nzgg.org.nz/guidelines/0072/acc1038_col.pdf; 2004.
4. Chaitow L. Muscle energy techniques. 4th edn. Edinburgh: Churchill Livingstone; 2013.
5. Southerst D, Marchand A-A, Côté P, et al. The effectiveness of non-invasive interventions for musculoskeletal thoracic spine and chest wall pain: a systematic review by the Ontario Protocol

for Traffic Injury Management (OPTIMa) Collaboration. J Manipulative Physiol Ther 2015;38(7):521–31.

6. Reiman MP, Manske R. Functional testing in human performance. Champaign, IL: Human Kinetics; 2009.

7. Simons D, Travell J, Simons L. Myofascial pain and dysfunction: The trigger point manual. Volume 1 Upper half of body. 2nd edn. Philadelphia: Williams & Wilkins; 1999.

8. Hunter D. Everything you ever wanted to know about osteoarthritis. The Health Report 2017. Online. Available: https://www.abc.net.au/radionational/programs/healthreport/everything-you-ever-wanted-to-know-about-osteoarthritis/8664218#transcript; 2017.

9. Thomas S, Browne H, Mobasheri A. What is the evidence for a role for diet and nutrition in osteoarthritis? Rheumatology 2018;57: iv61–iv74.

10. Wiyanad A, Chokphukiao P, Suwannarat P, et al. Is the occiput-wall distance valid and reliable to determine the presence of thoracic hyperkyphosis? Musculoskelet Sci Prac 2018;38:63–8.

11. Bansal S, Katzman WB, Giangregoria LM. Exercise for improving age-related hyperkyphotic posture: a systematic review. Arch Phys Med Rehabil 2014;95:129–40.

12. Loughenbury PR, Tsirikos AI. Scheuermann's kyphosis: diagnosis, presentation and treatment. J Orthop Trauma 2017;31(6):388–94.

13. Polly DW, Ledonio CG, Diamond B, et al. What are the indications for spinal fusion surgery in Scheuermann kyphosis? J Pediatr Orthop 2017. Doi: 10.1097/BPO.0000000000000931.

14. Bezalel T, Carmeli E, Been E, et al. Scheuermann's disease: current diagnosis and treatment approach. J Back Musculoskeletal Rehabil 2014;27(4):383–90. Doi: 10.3233/BMR-140483.

15. Ramirez J, Nieto-Gonzalez JC, Rodriguez RC, et al. Prevalence and risk factors for osteoporosis and fractures in axial spondyloarthritis: a systematic review and meta-analysis. Semin Arthri Rheum 2018;48(1):44–52.

16. Blevins K, Battenberg A, Beck A. Management of scoliosis. Adv Pediatr 2018;65(1):249–66.

17. Abdelaal AA, El Kafy EM, Elayat MS, et al. Changes in pulmonary function and functional capacity in adolescents with mild idiopathic scoliosis: observational cohort study. J Int Med Res 2018;46(1):381–91.

18. Theroux DC, Stomski N, Losco CD, et al. Spinal manipulative therapy for adolescent idiopathic scoliosis: A systematic review. J Manipulative Physiol Ther 2017;40(6): 452–8.

19. Scoliosis Research Society. Treating scoliosis. Milwaukee, WI: Scoliosis Research Society; 2019. Available from: https://www.srs.org/patients-and-families/conditions-and-treatments/adolescents/diagnosing-scoliosis.

20. Hefti F. Pathogenesis and biomechanics of adolescent idiopathic scoliosis (AIS). J Child Orthop 2013;7(1):17–24.

21. Choudhry MN, Ahmad Z, Verma R. Adolescent idiopathic scoliosis. Open Orthop J 2016;10:143–54. Doi: 10.2174/1874325001610010143.

22. Campbell TM, Ghaedi BB, Ghogomu ET, et al. Shoe lifts for leg length discrepancy in adults with common painful muscuolskeletal conditions: a systematic review of the literature. Arch Phys Med Rehabil 2018;99(5):981–93.

23. Thompson J, Williamson E, Williams M, et al. The effectiveness of scoliosis-specific exercises for adolescent idiopathic scoliosis: a systematic review and meta-analysis. Physiotherapy 2017;103(S1):e138.

24. Byrnes K, Wu P-J, Whillier S. Is Pilates an effective rehabilitation tool? A systematic review. J Bodyw Mov Ther 2018;22(1):192–202.

25. Striet R. NTOS symptoms and mobility: a case study on neurogenic thoracic outlet syndrome involving massage therapy. J Bodyw Mov Ther 2014;18(1):42–8.

The cervical region

12

Learning Outcomes

- Assess clients with conditions of the cervical region for remedial massage, including identification of red and yellow flags.
- Assess clients for signs and symptoms associated with common neck conditions and treat and/or manage these conditions with appropriate remedial massage therapy.
- Develop treatment plans for clients with neck conditions, taking assessment findings, duration and severity of the condition, likely tissue types, clinical guidelines, best available evidence and client preferences into account.
- Develop short- and long-term treatment plans to address presenting symptoms, underlying conditions and predisposing factors, and to progressively increase the self-help component of therapy.
- Adapt remedial massage therapy to suit individual client's needs based on duration and severity of injury, the client's age and gender, the presence of underlying conditions and co-morbidities, and other considerations for specific population groups.

INTRODUCTION

Neck pain is common and can be disabling. Currently one in two adults will experience neck pain at some time in their lives.[1] Globally, neck pain is the sixth leading cause of years lived with disability. It is the fifth leading cause in middle to high income socio-demographic regions.

The prevalence of chronic neck pain is rising significantly. Over the past 10 years, chronic neck pain of more than 3 months' duration has increased globally by 21%.[2] Factors contributing to this increase include increasing life expectancy and reduction in mobility due the obesity epidemic. Compounding this, people are less likely to be active if they are experiencing neck pain.[3]

Serious causes of spinal injury, particularly cervical spine injury, although uncommon can have a devastating impact on a client. For example, fractures can be the result of a high-impact trauma in a healthy spine or low-impact movement if the spine is already compromised, such as in the case of

osteoporosis.[4] If spinal instability is suspected the patient should be immediately referred for medical assessment.

An evidence base for the effectiveness of remedial massage in the treatment of neck pain is emerging. For example, one study found that people who have massage therapy for neck pain have a more immediate reduction in pain than those who do not.[5] Neck complaints are common presenting conditions in remedial massage clinics and they frequently recur. A sound knowledge of the underlying anatomical structures and their relationships is required for safe and competent practice.

FUNCTIONAL ANATOMY REVIEW

The biomechanics of the cervical spine are complex, involving three-dimensional spinal coupling movements (i.e. movement in one plane of motion accompanied by movements in other planes) and unequal movements from one vertebra to the next in any range. The pattern of movements is dictated by the orientation of the facet joints.[4] The proximity of vital structures such as the spinal cord, cranial nerves and arteries means that changes in cervical biomechanics can potentially influence their function. The cervical vertebrae are characterised by transverse foramina which transmit the vertebral arteries, veins and sympathetic plexus in the transverse processes of C1–C7 (the vertebral foramen of C7 is small and sometimes absent). C1 and C2 are specialised vertebrae. There is little or no rotation at the atlanto-occipital junction and little to no lateral flexion at C1/C2. C1 (the atlas) is a ring of bone which supports the skull. Its superior articular facets are elliptical and concave and articulate with the occipital condyles to create the nodding movement of the head. Its transverse processes are large and wide and palpable behind the mandible just below the ear. The vertebral foramen is divided by the transverse ligament into a posterior compartment which houses the spinal cord and an anterior compartment containing the dens of the C2 (the axis).The axis with its large dens or odontoid process forms a pivot around which the atlas and head rotate. The weight of the head is transferred to the cervical spine through the lateral atlanto-axial articulations of C2 (see Figure 12.1 on p 202). The spinous processes of C2–C6 are bifid. C2 spinous process is palpated immediately below the external occipital protuberance.

The first of the eight cervical nerves emerges between the skull and the atlas and except for the eighth each nerve emerges above the corresponding vertebra (i.e. C3 spinal nerve exits above C3). The eighth nerve emerges below C7 and thereafter spinal nerves emerge below their corresponding vertebrae (see Figure 12.2). C7 with its long spinous process is known as the vertebra prominens.

Major muscles of the cervical region are summarised in Table 12.1 (see also Figure 12.3 on p 204). Muscle function

in the cervical region can be affected by traumas and stresses applied directly to the head and neck and habitual postures like forward head carriage. Cervical musculature also reflects musculoskeletal adaptations to conditions of the thoracolumbar spine, pelvis and lower limbs including scoliosis or leg length inequality.

ASSESSMENT

Chapter 2 presents details of assessment procedures for remedial massage therapy clients. Assessment procedures are designed to:

- determine the suitability of clients for massage (red flags)
- determine the duration (acute or chronic) and severity of the condition, and the types of tissues that could be involved
- determine if the client's symptoms fit patterns of common conditions.

CASE HISTORY

Identify any red flags that require referral for further investigation (see Table 12.2). For example, a client involved in a recent car accident should be referred for further assessment as symptoms may not appear immediately.

- Features that alert practitioners to the possible presence of serious underlying conditions include the nature and mode of pain onset and its intensity.

Fig. 12.1 Cervical vertebrae

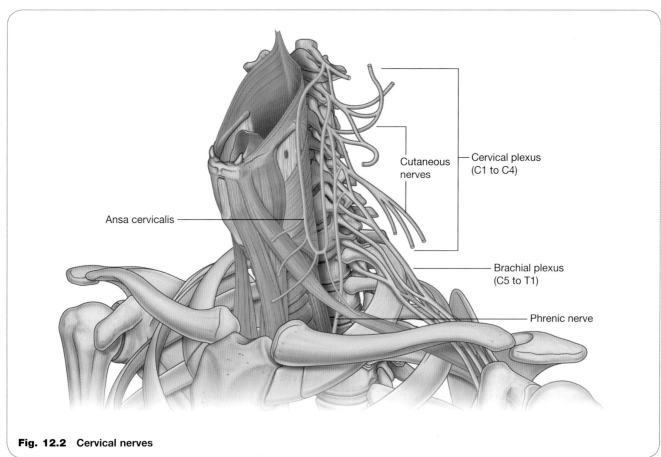

Fig. 12.2 Cervical nerves

Table 12.1 Muscles of the neck

Muscle	Origin	Insertion	Action
Upper trapezius	External occipital protuberance, superior nuchal line, nuchal ligament and spinous process of C7	Acromion process, lateral clavicle, spine of scapula	Ipsilateral lateral flexion and contralateral rotation of the neck and head, elevates scapula
Sternocleidomastoid	Mastoid process and lateral half of superior nuchal line	Anterior manubrium and medial third of the clavicle	Ipsilaterally lateral flexion and contralateral rotation of the head and neck
Levator scapulae	Transverse processes of C1–C4	Superomedial border of scapula	Elevation and retraction of the scapula; ipsilateral lateral flexion and rotation of the neck
Sub-occipital muscles			
Inferior oblique	C2 spinous process	C1 transverse process	Rotation of atlas (turns head ipsilaterally)
Superior oblique	C1 transverse process	Occipital bone	Extension and lateral flexion of the head
Rectus capitis posterior major	C2 spinous process	Occipital bone	Extension of head, ipsilateral rotation of head
Rectus capitis posterior minor	Posterior tubercle of C2	Occipital bone	Extension of the head. As a group, they act to stabilise the head. They also extend and rotate the head at the atlanto-occipital joint to make small, precise head movements.
Posterior cervical muscles			Mainly rotation of the head and neck by the deeper more diagonal muscles and extension of the head and neck by the longer and more vertical muscles.
Splenius capitis	Nuchal ligament, spinous processes of C7–T3/4	Mastoid process	
Spenius cervicis	Spinous processes of T3–T6	Transverse processes of C1–2/3	
Longissimus capitis	Articular processes of C4/5–C7, transverse processes of T1–T4/5	Mastoid process	
Longissimus cervicis	Transverse processes of T1–T5	Transverse processes of C2–C6	
Iliocostalis cervicis	Angles of ribs 3–6	Transverse processes of C4–C6	
Spinalis cervicis (spinalis capitis, is medial part of semispinalis capitis)	Nuchal ligament, spinous process of C7	Spinous process C2	
Semispinalis cervicis	Transverse processes of T1–T5/6	Spinous processes C2–C5	
Semispinalis capitis	(Overlies semispinalis cervicis) Articular processes of C4–C6, transverse processes of T1–T6	Between the nuchal lines	
Multifidus	Articular processes of C4–C7 (cross two to four vertebrae)	Spinous processes of C2–C5	
Scalenus anterior	Transverse processes of C4–C6	Scalene tubercle and superior border rib 1	Ipsilateral lateral flexion and contralateral rotation of the neck; elevates rib 1
Scalenus medius	Transverse processes of C2–C7	Superior surface of rib 1	
Scalenus posterior	Transverse processes of C5–C6	Outer surface of rib 2	Lateral flexes neck ipsilaterally and contralaterally rotates the neck; elevates rib 2

- Severe neck pain, regardless of its cause, is an important risk factor for chronicity. Risk factors for chronicity also include high levels of self-rated disability and pain-related catastrophising, post-traumatic stress symptoms and an increased sensitivity to cold.[6]
- According to the Canadian C-Spine Rule (see Figure 12.4 on p 205), all high-risk clients should be referred for radiographic examination. Clients are considered high risk if they are more than 65 years of age, if the mechanism of injury was dangerous (e.g. head injuries from diving, falls from a height greater than 1 metre or falls down five or more stairs) or if the client reports paraesthesia in the extremities. Correct use of the Canadian C-Spine Rule prevents a serious neck injury from being overlooked and reduces unnecessary imaging.[7] Patients who do not present with sensorimotor deficits or red flag symptoms typically do not require radiography.[8]
- Ask clients to point to the site of pain as they may have different understandings of anatomical terms.
- Determine if the pain is likely to have a mechanical cause. (Is the pain associated with rest or activity, certain postures or time of day?) Ask clients to demonstrate movements and

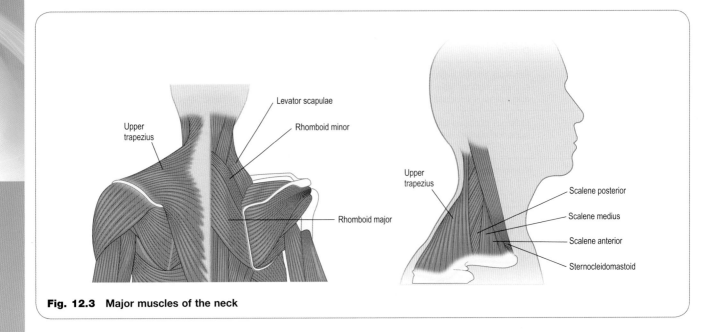

Fig. 12.3 Major muscles of the neck

Assessment of the cervical region

1. Case history
2. Outcome measures
3. Postural analysis
4. Functional tests
   Active range of motion tests
   Flexion, extension, lateral flexion, rotation
   Passive range of motion tests
   Flexion, extension, lateral flexion, rotation
   Resisted range of motion tests
   Flexion, extension, lateral flexion, rotation
   Resisted and length test for specific muscles including
   Upper trapezius
   Sternocleidomastoid
   Levator scapulae
   Suboccipital muscles
   Posterior cervical muscles
   Scalene muscles
   Special tests including
   Cervical compression
   Cervical distraction
   Valsalva
5. Palpation

Table 12.2 Red flags for serious conditions associated with acute neck pain[6, 8, 9]

Red flags for acute neck pain	Possible condition
Fever, night sweats, neck stiffness	Infection including meningitis and osteomyelitis
History of trauma Loss of bone integrity/osteoporosis Systemic steroid use	Cervical fracture
Trauma, Down's syndrome Rheumatoid arthritis	Cervical dislocation Upper cervical ligament insufficiency
Past history of malignancy Age >50 years Failure to improve with treatment Unexplained weight loss Dysphagia, headache, vomiting	Cancer; metastatic, primary
Radiculopathy; neurological symptoms in the limbs Unexplained cranial nerve dysfunction Myelopathy: cervical cord compression	Neurological condition
Cerebrovascular symptoms or signs: Sudden onset, tearing nature, recurrent thunderclap headache, unilateral weakness, vertigo anticoagulant use	Cerebrovascular haemorrhage (blood vessel dissection, stroke, TIA)
Cardiovascular risk factors	Cardiac involvement

positions that aggravate or relieve their pain and to be specific with descriptions of aggravating or relieving activities.

■ Mechanical pain is usually highly reactive to changes in posture, positions or activity.

■ Morning pain relieved with daily activity is often associated with arthritis.

■ Determine if the pain is likely to be associated with visceral function, neurogenic, vascular or psychosocial causes (yellow flags).

■ Pain from glandular fever, rheumatoid arthritis or neurogenic pain from a cancer, for example, are not usually aggravated by activity or relieved by rest, whereas mechanical neck pain may be relieved by lying down.

OUTCOME MEASURES

Outcome measures are questionnaires that are specifically designed to assess clients' level of impairment and to define benefits of treatment. The benefit is assessed in terms of client-perceived changes to health status. The Vernon-Mior

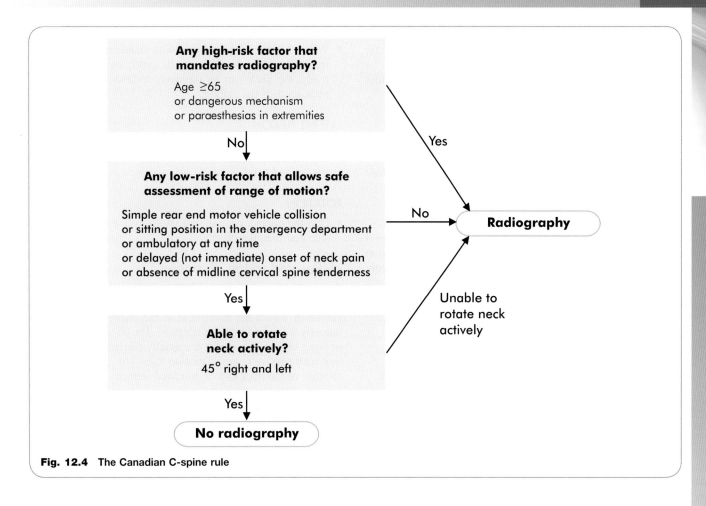

Fig. 12.4 The Canadian C-spine rule

Neck Disability Questionnaire is frequently used to assess clients' perceptions of neck pain.

POSTURAL ANALYSIS

- Viewed laterally, the ear should be in line with the shoulder. A protruding chin could indicate compensation to balance the body's centre of gravity, short occipital muscles and weak deep neck flexors in upper crossed syndrome. Is the chin retracted (military posture)?
- View the client from behind and observe head tilt or rotation. (Note that approximately 50% of cervical flexion and extension takes place between the occiput and C1; approximately 50% of rotation occurs in the C1–C2 spinal segment.) When the client is observed anteriorly the chin should be in line with the sternum.
- Habitual posture deviations may result from postural compensations (e.g. scoliosis, lumbar hyperlordosis or thoracic hyperkyphosis), hearing and visual adaptations.

FUNCTIONAL TESTS

A physical examination adds diagnostic value to the history when identifying cervical conditions. Many clinical tests lack validity and reliability. However, physical examination, including functional tests, may alert practitioners to potentially serious conditions and help determine whether symptoms are of local or referred origin. For example, if neck lateral flexion reproduces the client's arm pain this may indicate that the arm pain is referred from the neck (i.e. radiculopathy).[10] Functional tests also provide information about clients' perceptions of their conditions and their preferences for assessment and treatment styles.

a) Active range of motion

Cervical range of motion varies considerably between individuals and decreases with age, although not at a continuous rate. Women generally have a greater range of motion than men except for lateral flexion.[8]

FLEXION (50°)

- Good quality evidence indicates that clients with neck pain have a significantly decreased active range of motion when compared to clients without neck pain. Thus active range of motion is an important diagnostic indicator.[11] Stand in front of the client and ask them to take their chin towards their chest as far as they comfortably can.
- The client should be able to touch their chin to their chest.

EXTENSION (60°)

- Ask the client to look up to the ceiling as far as they comfortably can.
- The client should be able to extend their neck so that their face is parallel to the ceiling.

LATERAL FLEXION (SIDEBEND) (45°)

- Ask the client to take their ear towards their shoulder as far as they comfortably can.
- The client should be able to tilt their ear to their shoulder approximately 45°.

ROTATION (80°)

- Ask the client to look over their shoulder as far as they comfortably can.
- The client should be able to rotate their neck so that their chin is almost in line with their shoulder.

b) Passive range of motion

Lie the client supine to relax the neck muscles. Great care is needed when performing cervical passive range of motion tests. Perform all neck movements slowly and gently and only ever after you have observed the client's ability to perform active ranges of motion (the See-Move-Touch principle discussed in Chapter 2). Note the end-feel at the end of each range of motion (see Figure 12.5).

FLEXION

- Cup the client's occiput and gently flex the client's neck.

EXTENSION

- When the client is positioned with shoulders level with the top of the table, the neck can be gently extended. Alternatively, the neck can be passively extended by lifting the neck towards the ceiling.

LATERAL FLEXION

- Place one hand on the client's shoulder and with the other cup the occiput. Gently laterally flex the client's neck with the cupped hand.

ROTATION

- Cup the client's occiput and gently rotate the neck to one side and then the other.

c) Resisted range of motion

Resisted range of motion (RROM) tests are designed to identify muscle groups that may be contributing to the client's condition. Resist the movement as the client flexes, extends, laterally flexes and rotates their head. The client may be seated or lying supine. These tests are usually carried out in conjunction with passive range of motion tests. For example, passive rotation of the neck can be followed immediately by resisted

Fig. 12.5 Passive range of motion of the cervical spine

rotation before testing another movement in another plane. If any RROM tests are positive, resisted tests for specific muscle tests are required to identify individual muscles.

d) Tests for specific muscles associated with neck conditions

For any tests involving joint movements remember to take into account individual anatomical variation and the influence of age, lifestyle and underlying pathology on movement. Comparing both sides provides important information about individual clients.

1. UPPER TRAPEZIUS
Resisted test

Test upper trapezius by resisting extension or lateral flexion of the head and neck. The tests can be performed with the client sitting or standing. One possible test is described here.

With the client seated, place one hand on the client's shoulder and the other on the ipsilateral side of their head. Ask the client to take their ear towards their shoulder against your resistance (apply sufficient pressure so that the contraction is isometric, i.e. no head movement actually occurs) (see Figure 12.6).

Length test

Clients with shortened upper trapezius muscles will be unable to take their chin to their chest or to laterally flex their neck to 45° (see Figure 12.7). Rotating the head ipsilaterally helps

isolate upper trapezius from other posterolateral extensors of the neck.

Clinical significance

Shortening of upper trapezius may occur as a result of habitual rounded shoulder posture or chin protraction, as a compensation for hyperkyphotic postures and in chronic stress. Upper trapezius strains are commonly associated with other conditions of the cervical spine, such as cervical osteoarthritis or facet syndrome.

2. STERNOCLEIDOMASTOID
Resisted test

Sternocleidomastoid can be assessed by resisting flexion, ipsilateral lateral flexion or contralateral rotation of the head and neck. The tests can be performed with the client sitting, standing or supine. One test is described here.

The client lies supine with their head turned slightly to one side. Place one hand across the client's forehead and ask the client to try to take their chin to their chest. Resist this movement by applying gentle pressure to the client's forehead. Adjust the pressure so that the contraction is isometric; that is, no head movement actually occurs (see Figure 12.8).

Length test

Clients with shortening of bilateral sternocleidomastoid muscles will have limited extension of the head and neck. Unilateral contraction of sternocleidomastoid limits contralateral lateral flexion and ipsilateral rotation.

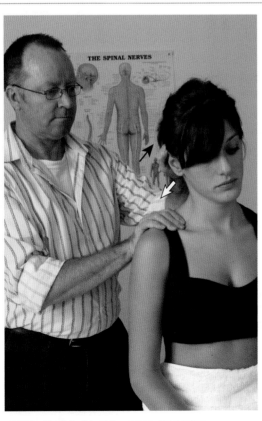

Fig. 12.6 Resisted test for upper trapezius

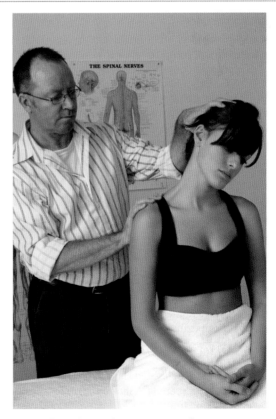

Fig. 12.7 Length test for upper trapezius

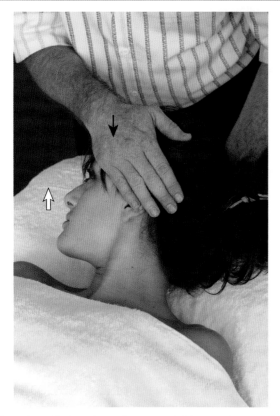

Fig. 12.8 Resisted test for sternocleidomastoid

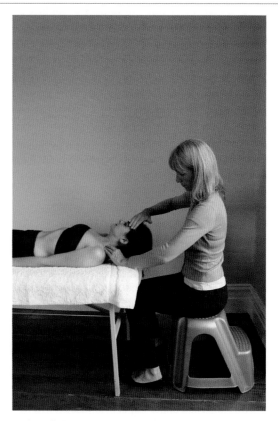

Fig. 12.9 Palpating the attachment of anterior scalene

Clinical significance

Sternocleidomastoid is often implicated in whiplash injuries and in torticollis. Caution is always required when treating injuries of sternocleidomastoid because of its proximity to the carotid artery. Sternocleidomastoid muscle also overlies the cervical lymphatic chain and may be affected by lymph adenopathy such as can occur in upper respiratory tract infections and glandular fever.

Note: Anterior scalene is also tested with sternocleidomastoid during resisted flexion and lateral flexion of the neck. It is distinguished from sternocleidomastoid by palpation to its attachment at the first rib (see Figure 12.9).

3. LEVATOR SCAPULAE

Resisted test

Levator scapulae can be assessed by resisting scapulae elevation, neck extension, lateral flexion or rotation of the neck. One method involves standing behind the seated client, placing hands on the client's shoulders and resisting as they try to shrug their shoulders (see Figure 12.10). (This test will also test upper trapezius.)

Length test

Clients with habitually elevated shoulders could have chronic contracture of levator scapulae. Shortening of levator scapulae could also result in limited neck flexion, lateral flexion or rotation. The client reaches behind their back to the opposite hip, laterally flexes and rotates their neck to the opposite side,

Fig. 12.10 Resisted test for levator scapulae

and then flexes their neck as far as they comfortably can (see Figure 12.11).

Clinical significance

Levator scapulae is commonly tight and short in upper crossed syndrome.

4. SUBOCCIPITAL MUSCLES

It is difficult to isolate the suboccipital muscles in functional tests. Their strength is assessed along with other muscles by resisting extension, lateral flexion or ipsilateral rotation

Fig. 12.11 Length test for levator scapulae

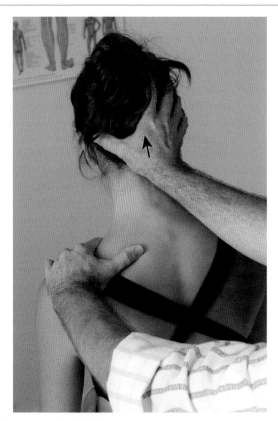

Fig. 12.13 Resisted test for posterolateral neck extensors

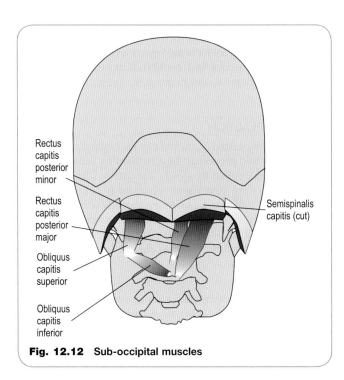

Rectus capitis posterior minor

Rectus capitis posterior major

Obliquus capitis superior

Obliquus capitis inferior

Semispinalis capitis (cut)

Fig. 12.12 Sub-occipital muscles

of the head at the atlanto-occipital joint. Contractures of suboccipital muscles could limit neck flexion, and contra-lateral lateral flexion or rotation. Suboccipital muscles are commonly associated with cervicogenic headache (see Figure 12.12).

5. POSTERIOR CERVICAL MUSCLES

Resisted test

The posterior cervical muscles (i.e. splenius capitis and cervicis, longus colli and capitis, iliocostalis cervicis, longissimus cervicis and capitis, spinalis cervicis and capitis, semispinalis cervicis and capitis, and multifidus) are not distinguishable on resisted tests. Resisted posterolateral neck extension tests splenius capitis and cervicis, semispinalis capitis and cervicis and cervical erector spinae muscles (see Figure 12.13). Note upper trapezius, also a posterolateral neck extensor, is distinguished by turning the client's face away from the side being tested. Palpation may also distinguish individual muscles (e.g. upper trapezius is superficial; fibres of splenius capitis and cervicis are diagonal compared to the more vertical fibres of the erector spinae).

Length test

Contractures of posterior cervical muscles could limit neck flexion and contralateral lateral flexion or rotation.

Clinical significance

Shortened posterior cervical muscles are commonly observed in upper crossed syndrome and may be implicated in cervicogenic headache. It has been postulated that semispinalis capitis plays a role in cervicogenic and muscle tension headaches, whiplash and work-related and chronic neck pain.[12]

Fig. 12.14 Resisted test for scalene muscles

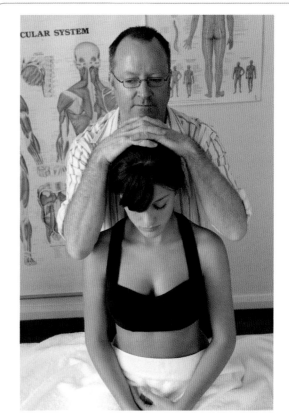

Fig. 12.15 Cervical compression test

6. SCALENE GROUP

Resisted test

The scalene muscles are difficult to isolate by resisted test. They are generally tested by resisting ipsilateral lateral flexion (± contralateral rotation) (see Figure 12.14). Anterior scalenus also flexes the neck and can be tested by resisting anterolateral neck flexion although this also tests sternocleidomastoid.

Length test

Clients with contracture of one or more of the scalene muscles will have limited contralateral lateral flexion and ipsilateral rotation of the neck.

e) Special tests

Special tests are designed to reproduce the client's pain and/or other symptoms. They are always performed within the client's pain tolerance and stopped as soon as symptoms appear. If symptoms are experienced while performing a special test, ask the client for the exact location of the symptom and confirm that it is the same symptom described in the case history.

CERVICAL COMPRESSION

With the client seated, interlock your fingers or place one hand over the other on top of the client's head and slowly and gently apply downward pressure (see Figure 12.15). (Stop immediately the onset or aggravation of symptoms is reported.) Pain may be felt locally or referred to the upper extremity according to the neurological level of the pathology. A positive compression test could indicate narrowing of the intervertebral foramen and nerve root compression or facet joint lesion.

CERVICAL DISTRACTION

Stand behind the seated client and cup the occiput in the palms under the mastoid processes, fingers pointing superiorly. Vertical traction is applied by slowly and gently lifting the head towards the ceiling (see Figure 12.16 on p 211). A positive distraction test indicates ligamentous damage (e.g. after whiplash injury or facet joint sprain). Distraction may also relieve pressure on a nerve root or facet joint. (Note: avoid covering hearing aids with palms. Earrings should be removed.)

VALSALVA

Ask clients if they experience pain or symptoms when they cough, sneeze or laugh. Alternatively, ask clients to hold their breath and bear down. Valsalva raises intrathecal pressure and may elicit local or referred pain for a particular neurological level if a space-occupying lesion such as a herniated disc or tumour is present in the canal. (Note: Valsalva is not recommended for clients with uncontrolled or acute hypertension or with diabetics with potential retinopathy.)

Note: In order to determine if a client needs to be referred for X-rays the Canadian C Spine Rule or NEXUS low risk criteria must be applied.[6] They are simple guidelines for determining clients requiring referral.

under the trapezius muscle. Trace the muscle fibres from the scapula to the transverse processes of C1–C4. Palpate the paraspinal muscles in the space between the spinous and transverse processes.

Supine

The sternocleidomastoid attaches with the trapezius across the base of the occiput to the mastoid processes. With the client supine and head turned to the opposite side, the muscle is easily palpated. A chain of lymph nodes lies along the medial border of the sternocleidomastoid. Lymph nodes are usually not palpable unless they become enlarged and tender (e.g. if the client has an upper respiratory tract infection). The carotid pulse can be palpated in the carotid artery on the anterior border of the sternocleidomastoid muscle above the hyoid bone and lateral to the thyroid cartilage. (Caution: do not palpate both carotid pulses at the same time.) Parotid glands partially cover the angles of the mandible. They are normally only palpable when they are swollen.

With the client supine, use the fingertips of both hands to palpate the spinous processes of C2–C7 in the midline. Palpate the deep posterior cervical muscles and note the diagonal fibres of splenius capitis and cervicis. Palpate multifidi from the articular processes of the last four cervical vertebrae to the spinous processes of the vertebrae two to four levels above. Turn the head slightly to palpate the suboccipital muscles between the inferior nuchal line and the C1 transverse process and spinous processes of C1 and C2.

REMEDIAL MASSAGE TREATMENT

Assessment of the cervical region provides essential information for development and negotiation of treatment plans, including:

- client's suitability for remedial massage therapy
- duration of the condition (i.e. acute or chronic)
- severity of the condition (i.e. grade of injury; mild, moderate or severe pain)
- type(s) of tissues involved
- priorities for treatment if more than one injury or condition is present
- whether the signs and symptoms suggest a common condition of the cervical region
- special considerations for individual clients (e.g. client's preference for treatment types and styles, specific population considerations).

Treatment options must always be considered in the context of the best available evidence for treatment effectiveness and clinical practice guidelines where they exist. Findings of current research are summarised in Table 12.3.

MUSCLE STRAIN

Muscle strains (*pulled muscles*) can occur from traumas including falls, motor vehicle accidents and sports injuries. They are usually the result of extreme stretching that causes myofibrils to tear. Strains also occur from overuse, fatigue and repetitive microtrauma; for instance when the neck is held in an awkward position for long periods. Exposure to a draught has also been implicated. Pain is associated with activity and relieved by rest.

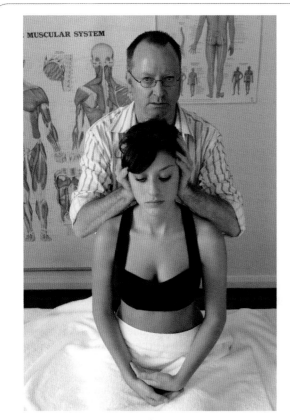

Fig. 12.16 Cervical distraction test

NEXUS LOW-RISK CRITERIA

Cervical spine radiography is indicated for patients with trauma unless they meet all of the following criteria:

1. No posterior midline cervical spine tenderness
2. No evidence of intoxication
3. Normal level of alertness
4. No focal neurological deficit
5. No painful distracting injuries

PALPATION

Pain produced on palpation helps confirm the location of the lesion and determine the type of tissue(s) involved. The neck is best palpated with the client supine or prone to relax the cervical musculature.

Prone

Palpate the mastoid processes, superior nuchal line and external occipital protuberance of the occiput. The spinous processes of C2–C7 are palpable in the midline. C7 and T1 spinous processes are larger than the others. C1 transverse processes are palpable inferior and slightly anterior to the mastoid processes. Transverse processes of C2–C7 are palpable if the neck muscles are relaxed. Facet joints, which lie about 2.5 cm from the midline, are sometimes palpable under the trapezius and paraspinal muscles.

Trace the upper trapezius muscle from its proximal attachments to its insertion at the acromion. Palpate the levator scapulae attachment at the superomedial aspect of the scapula

Table 12.3 Evidence for complementary medicine treatments for neck pain (adapted from Cohen[13])

Treatment	Evidence
Massage therapy	Superior to no treatment and equivalent to other active treatments
Spinal adjustment/ manipulation	Superior to no treatment in the short term. Weak evidence for intermediate-term benefit and for superiority over pharmacotherapy and other therapies
Acupuncture	Weak evidence that acupuncture is superior to no treatment in the short term
Exercise therapy	Strong evidence for intermediate-term relief for non-specific neck pain and whiplash-type injuries. No clear evidence supporting one technique over another or that exercise can prevent the development of neck pain
Traction	There is low-quality evidence that traction is not superior to placebo treatments for neck pain with or without radiculopathy
Soft cervical collar	There is low-quality evidence that a cervical collar is no more effective than physical therapy or other active therapies for cervical radiculopathy and whiplash
Electrotherapy	There is low-quality evidence that various forms of electrotherapy (e.g. transcutaneous electrical nerve stimulation, pulsed electromagnetic field therapy) are better than placebo but not other treatments
Yoga	There is weak evidence that yoga is more effective than home-based exercise treatment

Assessment

HISTORY

The client complains of neck pain after a fall, motor vehicle accident or sports injury or after holding the neck in an awkward position for a long time (e.g. reading in bed, falling asleep in an awkward position, straining to read a monitor). Pain can be experienced immediately or within the next 24–48 hours (delayed onset muscle soreness). Pain is associated with activity and generally relieved with rest.

POSTURAL ANALYSIS

The neck may be held in an antalgic position and movements may be guarded.

Key assessment findings for muscle strain

- History of trauma or prolonged awkward position
- Functional tests
  - AROM positive in one or more directions
  - PROM may be positive at end of range due to passive muscle stretching
  - RROM positive for affected muscle(s)
  - Resisted and length tests positive for affected muscle(s)
- Palpation elicits pain; spasm ± myofibril tears palpable

FUNCTIONAL TESTS

AROM: limited in one or more directions.
PROM: mild to no pain except at end of range when the muscle is passively stretched.
RROM: painful.
Resisted and length tests positive for involved muscles.
Special tests: negative.

PALPATION

Muscle spasm is usually evident. The client reports tenderness or pain on palpation of the affected muscle.

Overview of treatment of muscle strains

A typical remedial massage treatment for mild to moderate muscle strains of the neck includes:

- Swedish massage to the neck, upper back, shoulders, head (± chest).
- Remedial techniques including:
  - deep gliding frictions along the muscle fibres
  - cross-fibre frictions
  - soft tissue releasing techniques
  - deep transverse friction at the site of muscle injury
  - heat therapy (see Chapter 3)
  - trigger point therapy (see Chapter 6).
    (A range of remedial massage techniques for muscles of the cervical region are illustrated in Table 12.4.)
- Myofascial release (see Chapter 8).

Address any underlying conditions or predisposing factors (e.g. scoliosis or thoracic hyperkyphosis).

CLIENT EDUCATION

Advise clients to avoid aggravating activities. For example, using a headset will leave the client's hands free for other tasks when talking on the phone. Clients should avoid sleeping in the prone position. Pillows should support the neck without distorting the normal lordotic cervical curve.

Home exercise program

Exercise on its own can produce a small clinical improvement in neck pain. The degree of improvement may be similar to the effect of manipulation, mobilisation and soft tissue massage or use of pharmaceutical medication.[14] A program of progressive rehabilitation exercises within the client's pain threshold can support remedial massage treatment. Aim for maximum strength and full length of all major muscles. Unresolved strains can contribute to recurrence and to the development of compensatory muscle imbalance. Introduce stretching exercises as soon as possible and progress to isometric exercises within the client's pain tolerance.

Manipulation and multi-modal programs

Grade I and II muscle strains affect activities of daily living but do not exhibit neurological signs. Clients may be referred to a chiropractor, osteopath or manipulative physiotherapist for spinal manipulation.[15] However, the benefit of combining exercise and manual therapy (manipulation, mobilisation and massage) over exercise alone for grades I and II neck muscle strains is unconfirmed.[16]

Table 12.4 Remedial massage techniques for muscles of the cervical region

Muscle	Soft tissue release	Trigger point	Stretch	Client education[24]	Home stretch
Upper trapezius	Passive: the client lies supine. Cup the occiput in one hand. Using knuckles, fingers or thumb of the other hand glide from occiput to acromion as the client's head is laterally flexed with the other hand. Active: The client is seated and the practitioner uses a pincer grip to hold the upper trapezius muscle between the acromion and C7. Maintaining this contact, ask the client to take their head slowly towards their shoulder.		With the client supine, the practitioner places one hand on the ipsilateral shoulder and the other hand cups the occiput. The client's head is rotated slightly to the ipsilateral side. Slowly and gently take the client's head towards the contralateral side.	Avoid carrying a heavy shoulder bag, build up arm rests on chairs if upper limbs are short compared with the torso, avoid foam pillows, take regular breaks from prolonged periods of deskwork and lower the keyboard. Address any underlying conditions or predisposing factors such as high stress levels.	The client sits in a chair and holds the side of the seat with one hand to anchor the shoulder. Next the client laterally flexes their neck to the opposite side and rotates their head towards the same side.
Sternocleidomastoid	A number of variations are possible, including the following passive release: The client is supine. Cup the occiput with the contralateral hand. The fingers of the other hand contact the ipsilateral sternocleidomastoid. Glide down the muscle as the head is laterally flexed with the other hand.		With the client supine or seated, gently laterally flex their neck to the opposite side or rotate their neck to the same side.	Avoid prolonged neck flexion, use a lumbar support to correct slumping in a chair with head forward, avoid lying in bed reading with the head turned towards one side, use a headset.	Laterally flexing away from the affected muscle or rotating the neck towards it will stretch the sternocleidomastoid muscle.

Continued

Table 12.4 Remedial massage techniques for muscles of the cervical region—cont'd

Muscle	Soft tissue release	Trigger point	Stretch	Client education[24]	Home stretch
Levator scapulae	A number of variations can be performed including the following: The practitioner stands behind the seated client and holds the scapula attachment of the muscle as the client slowly moves their head towards their opposite axilla. 		With the client supine, the practitioner anchors the ipsilateral shoulder with one hand and gently takes the client's head towards the opposite axilla. 	Use a document or book stand when reading to reduce neck flexion, for deskwork lower the keyboard or elevate the chair, use a headset.	The client sits, holding the bottom of the seat of the chair or sitting on their hand to stabilise the shoulder. The muscle is stretched by contralateral lateral flexion and ipsilateral rotation of the neck (i.e. the client takes their head towards the axilla on the unaffected side).
Suboccipital muscles	A number of variations can be performed, including the following: With the client seated, the practitioner places both thumbs under the occiput and instructs the client to slowly flex and extend their head. Repeat with thumbs at different positions under the occiput. 		With the client seated or supine, gently flex their neck. Contralateral rotation can also be used to stretch the more diagonal muscles. 	Avoid forward head posture, keep the neck warm (e.g. wearing scarves or jackets with hoods), avoid prolonged neck extension (e.g. painting a ceiling, working under a hoist), using well-designed workstation.	The client interlocks their fingers behind the head and gently pulls their head forward towards the chest.

Table 12.4 Remedial massage techniques for muscles of the cervical region—cont'd

Muscle	Soft tissue release	Trigger point	Stretch	Client education[24]	Home stretch
Posterior cervical muscles	A number of variants can be performed, including the following: The client lies supine. Facing the client, spread the fingers of one hand on the paraspinal muscles between the transverse and spinous processes of C1 to C7 on the contralateral side. Either passively or actively, the client's head is rotated across the finger contacts.		The posterior cervical muscles can be stretched by flexing the head and neck. The client can be seated or supine. For the supine stretch the practitioner crosses their arms under the client's head and places their hands on the client's shoulders. The client's head is gently flexed when the practitioner slowly raises their crossed arms. Ensure that the head and neck are controlled at all times during the stretch.	Avoid prolonged neck flexion, for deskwork use a well-designed work station (e.g. elevating the monitor just below eye level) sit upright on an exercise bike (i.e. avoid holding low handle bars), use a lumbar support when sitting to improve head and neck posture.	The client interlocks their fingers behind the head and gently pulls their head forward towards the chest.

Continued

Table 12.4 Remedial massage techniques for muscles of the cervical region—cont'd

Muscle	Soft tissue release	Trigger point	Stretch	Client education[24]	Home stretch
Scalene muscles	A number of variations can be performed including the following: With the client seated, the practitioner uses fingers, thumb or knuckle along the scalene as the client laterally flexes their neck to the opposite side.		With the client seated or supine, gently laterally flex their neck. From this position gently rotate their head towards or away from the affected side.	Keep the neck warm, use a supportive pillow when sleeping, use elbow rests when seated and use headphones when working at a desk.	The client laterally flexes their neck to their comfortable limit and holding that position turns their head to look downwards or upwards

NON-SPECIFIC NECK PAIN (INCLUDING CERVICAL SPRAIN, STRAIN AND FACET SYNDROME)

The term non-specific neck pain is employed when a specific cause is unidentified and many factors could contribute to the pain.[17] Non-specific neck pain may arise from minor trauma, unaccustomed exercise, sudden unguarded movement or overuse and is associated with muscle strain, ligament sprain and facet syndrome. Keyboard usage has been identified as one of the risk factors for developing non-specific neck pain in office workers.[18] Facet syndrome is the term used to describe any injury or condition affecting the cervical facet joints (zygapophyseal joints). It can refer pain to the cranium, cervical spine, shoulder and upper back. Non-specific neck pain may resolve spontaneously in days or weeks. However, evidence indicating that the facets play a major role in chronic neck pain is increasing.[19] A two-year study of patients in a private clinic in the US found that facet syndrome accounted for 55% of neck pain cases, compared to discogenic pain which accounted for 16%.[20]

Assessment

HISTORY

Clients are usually young adults who complain of pain, stiffness and limited range of motion following trauma, overuse, fatigue or repetitive microtrauma over hours or days. The pain is usually localised, although an upper cervical lesion may produce headache and lower cervical lesion may radiate pain to the shoulder or upper back. There is usually no neurological involvement.

FUNCTIONAL TESTS

AROM: limited and painful in one or more directions (pain in one direction suggests muscle strain; pain in many directions suggests joint capsule injury or a combination of muscle and joint injury).[21] Increased pain on extension and rotation suggests facet syndrome.

PROM: may be limited and painful if facet joints, ligaments or joint capsule involved. Increased pain on extension suggests facet joint involvement. (Note that ligament sprains are uncommon.)

RROM: may be positive if muscles have been strained.

Resisted and length tests may be positive if muscles have been strained.

Key assessment findings for non-specific neck pain

- Client is usually a young adult; history of trauma or repetitive overuse
- Functional tests:
  - AROM positive in one or more directions
  - PROM positive if facet joints involved
  - RROM positive if muscle strain involved
  - Resisted tests and muscle length tests may be positive for affected muscles
  - Special tests usually negative
- Palpation positive for tenderness ± pain at site of strain, sprain or subluxation

---

Resisted and length tests usually indicate muscle strain. Special tests are usually negative although cervical compression can produce local pain.

PALPATION

Local tenderness is often reported at the site of injury. Muscle spasm is palpable and occasionally local swelling is present.

Differential diagnosis

Rule out cervical disc syndrome and cervical radiculopathy by history and functional tests. Patients with cervical radiculopathy describe pain radiating into the arm which corresponds to the dermatome of the involved nerve root (see Figure 2.3 on p 12). For diagnostic accuracy a number of special tests are recommended. For example, a combination of Spurling's test (increasing symptoms on passive cervical extension, ipsilateral lateral flexion then axial compression), cervical distraction (decreasing symptoms) and an Arm Squeeze test (significantly more pain on squeezing the middle third of upper arm with the thumb on triceps and fingers on biceps than squeezing the upper third and lower third) has been recommended to assist in the clinical diagnosis of cervical disc syndrome.[22] There is weak evidence that Chinese massage (Tui Na) or Chinese massage with neck traction may help reduce cervical radiculopathy symptoms.[23]

Overview of treatment and management

A typical remedial massage treatment for mild or moderate non-specific neck pain includes:

- Swedish massage therapy to the neck, upper back, shoulder and head (± chest).
- Remedial massage techniques depending on the type of tissue(s) involved. For example, remedial massage therapy for muscle tissue injury/muscle imbalances could include (see Table 12.4):
  - deep gliding frictions along the muscle fibres (see Figure 12.17 on p 218)
  - cross-fibre frictions (see Figure 12.17)
  - active and passive soft tissue releasing techniques
  - deep transverse friction
  - trigger point therapy
  - muscle stretches.
- Use myofascial releasing techniques for myofascial restrictions.
- Thermotherapy may be beneficial.

For facet joint lesions passive joint articulation for the cervical spine and deep multifidus work may be beneficial. Joint articulations include cervical lateral flexion, rotation, extension, horizontal traction, stair-step, facet rotation and facet lateral flexion (see Chapter 7). (Note: if ligament sprain is involved cervical distraction is contraindicated.)

MUTIFIDUS RELEASE

With the client lying supine, sit at the head of the table. Place fingertips of both hands either side of the spine between the spinous process and transverse processes of C6 or C7. Apply anterior pressure to contact the multifidus muscles in the deepest muscle layer. Maintain the pressure and apply small frictions (about 1 cm) along the line of the fibres and then

Fig. 12.17 Upper trapezius (A) deep gliding, (B) cross-fibre frictions; levator scapulae (C) deep gliding, (D) cross-fibre frictions

Fig. 12.18 Multifidus release

across the fibres for several seconds. Release the pressure and move to the vertebra above. Repeat the frictions, working the multifidus muscles at each level up the cervical spine. Muscle spasm is palpable around the subluxated facet joints and is often tender. Always work within the client's pain tolerance (see Figure 12.18).

CLIENT EDUCATION

Advise clients about cervical posture including the importance of thoracolumbar posture. Advise clients about lumbar supports, and ways to improve the ergonomics of work stations and activities of daily living including using supports and pillows. Pillows placed behind the neck (not only behind the head) support the cervical spine. Pillows should be malleable enough to take the weight of the head without distorting the normal lordotic cervical spine. Alternatively, a rolled towel may be placed behind the neck and its height adjusted until the position is comfortable. Advise the client of the importance of a regular fitness program and particularly to prepare for sports or demanding physical work. Clients may benefit from referral to a chiropractor, osteopath or physiotherapist for spinal manipulation.

Home exercise program

Home exercises usually begin by stretching the affected muscles within pain tolerance. Progressively introduce strengthening exercises as soon as possible.

OSTEOARTHRITIS

Osteoarthritis is a painful condition that often relates to structural changes that occur within the bone, the lining of the joint, the synovium and cartilage. Every joint has the capacity

Fig. 12.19 Radiograph of cervical osteoarthritis

RROM: negative unless there is associated muscle strain. Special tests are usually within normal limits unless spinal canal stenosis or disc degeneration is present.

PALPATION

Palpation may elicit tenderness or pain at the affected site. Fibrotic muscle tissue is a common accompaniment. Crepitus and hard end-feel may be present.

Differential diagnosis

Neck pain (± neurological symptoms) increasing on flexion suggests disc herniation or damage; pain increasing on extension could suggest facet involvement or IVF encroachment.

Overview of treatment and management

Current evidence suggests a move from reliance on drugs towards exercise and self-management is required.[26] Advise clients on ways to reduce mechanical overload at work or in their activities of daily living. If osteoarthritis is also present in the lower limbs, weight loss is recommended. It is also likely that increasing thoracic mobility is important in the management of cervical conditions, including osteoarthritis.

A typical remedial massage treatment for cervical osteoarthritis includes:

- Swedish massage therapy to the neck, upper and mid back, shoulders, head (± chest).
- Remedial massage therapy. The range of remedial massage techniques and their application will be determined by assessment results (i.e. use the See-Move-Touch principle described in Chapter 2). The most important remedial techniques for osteoarthritis are joint articulation, heat therapy and myofascial release.
- Joint articulation (see Chapter 7): Cervical horizontal traction may be beneficial. Other cervical stretches are indicated but should be performed with caution (especially with side bending, flexion and diagonal flexion).
- Muscle techniques: If tolerated by the client, remedial massage therapy for chronic muscle contracture or fibrositis could include (see Table 12.4):
  - deep gliding frictions along the muscle fibres
  - cross-fibre frictions
  - active and passive soft tissue releasing techniques
  - deep transverse friction
  - trigger point therapy
  - muscle stretches.

for repair. In osteoarthritis the reparative processes are overwhelmed by destructive processes, often as a result of injury, being overweight or other mechanical load factors. Occupation and genetics also play a role.[25] Osteoarthritis is the most common form of joint disease and in the cervical spine most commonly affects C5–C6. It may be the result of sustained muscle spasm, injuries and overuse. Clients are usually over 50 years old or have a history of a previous significant trauma such as a whiplash injury. X-rays show loss of disc height, loss or reversal of cervical lordosis, osteophytes and subchondral bone/endplate sclerosis (see Figure 12.19). However, 45% of radiographic evidence of osteoarthritis is found in asymptomatic adults. Neurological symptoms may occur especially in arms and hands.

Assessment

HISTORY

Clients are usually over 50 years old or have a history of a previous significant trauma. Typically clients report a recurrent dull ache in the neck that developed slowly or after a period of increased activity. Neck ache or pain is aggravated by repetitive use and relieved by rest. Morning stiffness is common.

FUNCTIONAL TESTS

AROM: limitation ± pain in some directions.
PROM: limitation ± pain on lateral flexion and rotation, and then extension (capsular pattern).

Fig. 12.20 Workstation ergonomics

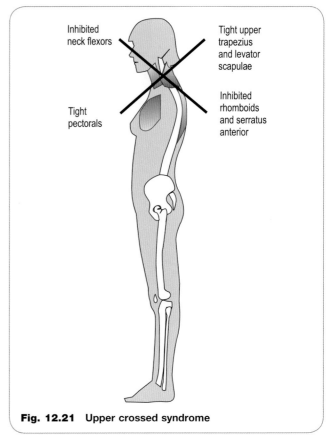

Fig. 12.21 Upper crossed syndrome

CLIENT EDUCATION

Advise clients about neck posture, including using a supportive pillow and mattress. Good ergonomics at work will help prevent repetitive overload of muscles and joints. Desk workers should check the height of their chairs, desks, keyboards and monitors as even small stresses may become significant if sustained for prolonged periods (see Figure 12.20). To reduce pain and improve function clients with osteoarthritis may benefit from diets which include long chain omega 3 fatty acids and vitamin K. Reducing cholesterol if raised is also valuable.[27] A clinical trial of office workers with chronic neck pain found benefit from including black soybeans in their diet. These are rich in essential amino acids and down regulate N-Methyl-D-aspartate receptor levels that plays an important role for maintaining central sensitisation of pain.[28] Advise clients of the importance of shock-absorbing soles to avoid jarring impacts that can be transmitted to the neck when walking. Referral to a chiropractor, osteopath or manipulative physiotherapist may result in an improvement in joint mobility and relieve pain.

Home exercise program

Begin with pain-free range of motion exercises and progressively introduce full-length sustained stretches and pain-free isometric exercises. It is best to exercise after the area has been warmed (e.g. after a warm shower or hot pack).

UPPER CROSSED SYNDROME

A common pattern of myofacial imbalance and postural adaptation which is characterised by forward head carriage, rounded shoulders and hyperextension at the occiput and C1/2 is referred to as upper crossed syndrome. Typically, pectoralis major and minor, upper trapezius, levator scapulae and sternocleidomastoids tighten and shorten, and lower and middle trapezius, serratus anterior and rhomboids tend to weaken (see Figure 12.21).[29] A recent study of female office workers with neck pain found decreased cranio-vertebral angle and stiffness of the upper trapezius muscle in the sitting position.[30] Tightness in the posterior neck muscles differentiates clients

with moderate neck pain and disability from asymptomatic patients.

Assessment

HISTORY

Clients with upper crossed syndrome often describe a dull aching pain in the neck and/or upper back. The pain is

---

Key assessment findings for upper crossed syndrome

- History can include repetitive activity, poorly rehabilitated previous injury, prolonged immobilisation. Pain in the neck and upper back after prolonged sitting/working at a computer; pain relieved by lying down or arching upper thoracic spine backwards; usually no radiation of pain
- Postural analysis: Forward head posture, rounded shoulders and increased thoracic kyphosis
- Functional tests:
  - AROM limited ± painful
  - PROM usually negative
  - Resisted tests and length tests are positive for specific muscles including:
  - short pectoralis major and minor, upper trapezius, levator scapulae, sternocleidomastoid
  - weak lower and middle trapezius, serratus anterior and rhomboids
  - Special tests negative
- Palpation positive for tenderness ± pain at sites of mechanical overload (e.g. mid and upper thoracic spine, mid and upper cervical spine), contractures in affected muscles

aggravated by prolonged periods of neck flexion such as working at a computer, reading or sewing. There is usually no radiation of pain or neurological symptoms, although pain is sometimes reported in the chest, shoulders and arms. Respiratory function may also be compromised. The pain is often relieved by taking breaks from aggravating activities, lying down or extending their upper back.

POSTURAL ANALYSIS

The head is held forward of the centre of gravity line, often with the chin jutting up. Thoracic kyphosis may be exaggerated and the shoulders protracted.

FUNCTIONAL TESTS

AROM: limited ± pain in some ranges of motion (e.g. cervical extension, thoracic extension) may be observed.
PROM: may be limited by muscle shortness.
RROM: positive for affected muscles.
Specific muscle tests may indicate muscle shortness (e.g. pectoralis major and minor, upper trapezius, levator scapulae, sternocleidomastoid) and weakness (e.g. lower and middle trapezius, serratus anterior and rhomboids).
Special tests: usually negative

PALPATION

Muscle contractures are readily palpated. Pressure over areas of mechanical overload (such as the middle and upper cervical spine) may elicit tenderness or pain.

Differential diagnosis

Upper crossed syndrome is usually identified by its characteristic muscle pattern and absence of pain radiation and neurological involvement. However, if accompanied by chest pain, underlying organic disease needs to be eliminated. All clients with neurological symptoms should be referred for further investigation.

Overview of treatment and management

Successful remedial massage treatment depends on identification of appropriate muscles for rehabilitation and client participation in corrective measures. In most cases lower and middle trapezius, serratus anterior and rhomboids will need to be strengthened in a home exercise program. Pectoralis major and minor, upper trapezius, levator scapulae and sternocleidomastoid muscles need to be stretched during treatment and at home.

A typical treatment for upper crossed syndrome includes:

- Swedish massage to the upper back, neck, chest, shoulders and head.
- Remedial massage therapy. The aim of remedial massage is to promote optimal musculoskeletal function. Tight muscles require stretching and specific muscle techniques including (see Table 12.4):
  - deep gliding frictions along the muscle fibres
  - cross-fibre frictions
  - active and passive soft tissue releasing techniques
  - deep transverse friction
  - trigger point therapy.
- Thermotherapy is usually beneficial.

Table 12.5 Effects of impingement on C5–T1 nerves

Nerve	Disc	Muscles affected	Sensation
C5	C4–5	Deltoid, biceps brachii	Lateral upper arm
C6	C5–6	Biceps brachii, wrist extensors	Lateral forearm and hand, thumb, index finger
C7	C6–7	Triceps brachii, wrist flexors	Middle finger
C8	C7–T1	Finger flexors, interossei	Medial forearm and hand, 4th and 5th fingers
T1	T1–2	Interossei	Medial upper arm

- Myofascial releasing techniques are also indicated for myofascial restrictions (see Chapter 8).
- Joint articulation of cervical, and mid and upper thoracic spinal segments may be effective (see Chapter 7).

Address any underlying conditions or predisposing factors such as scoliosis or hypomobile thoracic spine. Refer any client with upper limb pain accompanied by other neurological symptoms for a full neurological assessment.

CLIENT EDUCATION

Posture advice is essential and includes avoidance of all postures and activities that cause the head to be held forward. Advise clients about lumbar supports, good sitting posture and improving the ergonomics of the work area (see Figure 12.20 on p 220). Instruct clients to take regular breaks from activities that aggravate their condition. Clients often respond well to a corrective exercise program, but referral for osseous manipulation may be required.

Home exercise program

Muscle stretches performed during treatment (e.g. pectoralis major and minor, upper trapezius, levator scapulae and sternocleidomastoid) should be continued by the client at home (see Tables 12.5 and 14.3). A program to strengthen weak middle and lower trapezius, rhomboids and serratus anterior should be progressively introduced for long-term biomechanical improvements.

MECHANICAL/ACQUIRED TORTICOLLIS

Mechanical/acquired torticollis or wry neck is occasionally seen in remedial massage clinics. This is an acute episode of muscle spasm and vertebral subluxaton, often brought on by sleeping face down with the neck sustained in flexion and rotation. Many cases resolve spontaneously in 7–10 days.

Assessment

HISTORY

The condition commonly affects people under the age of 30. The client reports sudden onset of severe neck pain which is easily localised and aggravated by movement, especially rotation to the side of injury. Typically, the client reports waking

> ### Key assessment findings for mechanical/acquired torticollis
>
> - The client is a young adult or child. History of acute neck pain following a prolonged period of cervical flexion and rotation. Typically onset on waking after sleeping in prone position. Pain usually aggravated by rotation to affected side. Usually no radiation of pain.
> - Posture adaptations to guard neck movement
> - Functional tests (only performed within client's pain tolerance):
>   - AROM: limited and painful, especially rotation to affected side
>   - PROM: limited and painful, especially rotation to affected side
>   - RROM: limited and painful, especially rotation to side of injury
>   - Resisted tests and length tests positive for specific muscles, especially SCM
>   - Special tests negative
> - Palpation elicits pain at site of injury (usually C4). Muscle spasm evident in the affected SCM and associated muscles

with acute neck pain and being unable to move their neck after sleeping face down. Other histories report onset following activities that involved prolonged cervical flexion and rotation, or after sleeping near an open window or in a room cooled by air conditioning.

POSTURAL ANALYSIS

Clients adopt an antalgic posture, often with their head laterally flexed towards and rotated away from the injured side. Clients turn their whole body to avoid painful neck movements.

FUNCTIONAL TESTS

It may be difficult to perform functional tests in the acute phase. Work only within the client's pain tolerance.

AROM: very limited and painful in one or more directions, usually rotation to the affected side.
PROM: limited and painful in one or more directions.
RROM: limited and painful in one or more directions.
Resisted muscle tests for specific muscles positive (usually for sternocleidomastoid).
Special tests: usually negative.

PALPATION

Palpation at the site of injury (often C4) usually elicits pain.

Differential diagnosis

Special tests (e.g. cervical compression, cervical distraction and Valsalva) usually aggravate symptoms in clients with cervical nerve root compression.

Overview of treatment and management

Clients often present for treatment within hours of the onset. Treatment could include cryotherapy, acupressure, Reiki, reflexology or anti-inflammatory medication. Massage directly

on the sternocleidomastoid or other affected muscles should be brief. Use acupressure and trigger points therapy if it can be tolerated. In the acute phase, clients may benefit from lying on a rolled towel (height adjusted to pain-free position) placed horizontally under their neck for short periods (15–20 minutes). This position helps to restore normal cervical lordosis. Adjust the height of the rolled towel to the client's comfort. Place an ice pack over the rolled towel if required. Introduce corrective exercise therapy, beginning with gentle stretches as soon as they can be tolerated. Myofascial release techniques may be beneficial. Advise clients about sleeping positions, pillows and avoidance of aggravating activities. Refer clients for spinal manipulation. Clients may require daily or second daily treatment for the first week.

After the acute phase, a full assessment should be performed. A typical remedial massage treatment for subacute mechanical torticollis includes:

- Swedish massage therapy to the neck, upper back, shoulders and head (± chest).
- Remedial massage therapy. Remedial massage therapy for sternocleidomastoid and other neck muscles includes (see Table 12.4):
  - deep gliding frictions along the muscle fibres
  - cross-fibre frictions
  - active and passive soft tissue releasing techniques
  - deep transverse friction
  - trigger point therapy
  - muscle stretches.
- Apply myofascial releasing techniques for myofascial restrictions (see Chapter 8).
- Passive joint articulation for the cervical spine may be beneficial for facet joint lesions (see Chapter 7).
- Thermotherapy may be beneficial.

CLIENT EDUCATION

Advise clients to avoid prolonged neck postures, especially flexion and rotation and sudden neck movements. Encourage good sleeping postures (i.e. avoid sleeping prone) and use of pillows that support cervical lordosis. Thermotherapy may be beneficial. Clients may require spinal manipulation by a chiropractor, osteopath or physiotherapist to restore normal biomechanics and prevent relapse.

Home exercise program

Begin with stretches to affected muscles as soon as they can be tolerated and progressively introduce stretches to other cervical muscles and strengthening exercises as indicated. Upper thoracic and shoulder muscles (e.g. arm swings, scapula retraction) may be incorporated as soon as they can be tolerated.

CERVICAL DISC SYNDROME

Acute cervical disc lesions are not commonly seen in remedial massage clinics. Cervical disc lesions account for about 36% of all spinal disc lesions and because of their severity are usually treated initially by medical practitioners, chiropractors, osteopaths and physiotherapists. Almost all cervical disc prolapses occur in the mid to lower cervical spine. Clients with chronic conditions may incorporate remedial massage into their overall treatment and management plans. The prognosis for substantial improvement of a cervical disc prolapse with radiculopathy is 4–6 months. A complete recovery prognosis is 2–3 years.[31] When treating clients with a history of disc prolapse it is important to educate clients of the possibility of relapse and the vulnerability that in many cases persists even years after the initial injury.

Assessment

HISTORY

Clients are usually between 25 and 45 years old. Younger clients usually develop symptoms immediately or shortly after a direct trauma such as a diving or a motor vehicle or sports accident. Older clients may report repetitive overuse or poor posture, which can lead to intervertebral foramen narrowing from osteophyte encroachment, particularly in the presence of congenital osseous variants. Radiographs may show loss (or reversal) of cervical lordosis, osteophyte formation and decreased intervertebral disc space.

Pain and paraesthesia may radiate to the shoulders and upper limbs. Headache and tinnitus are also described. Symptoms can be so severe that clients report being unable to lie down to sleep. Pain can be sharp and shooting. It may also arise insidiously. Table 12.5 illustrates the effects of impingements on the lower cervical and first thoracic nerves.

POSTURAL ANALYSIS

Postural adaptations may be observed. Clients often adopt an antalgic posture and minimise aggravating neck movements.

FUNCTIONAL TESTS

AROM: limited and painful especially towards the affected side.
PROM: limited and painful, especially towards the affected side.
RROM: may be positive for associated muscle weakness or strain.
Resisted and length tests may be positive for affected muscles.
Special tests: usually positive for compression, distraction, Valsalva and any test that challenges the disc.

Key assessment findings for cervical disc syndrome

- The client is usually between 25 and 45 years old with a history of recent trauma, overuse or repetitive microtrauma. Pain may be severe. Pain and paraesthesia may radiate to shoulder and upper limb; headache may be present.
- Postural analysis: Postural adaptations to limit and guard neck movement may be present
- Functional tests
  - AROM limited in most directions, especially flexion
  - PROM limited in most directions
  - RROM may be positive if associated muscle strain or weakness
  - Resisted tests for specific muscles may indicate weakness, or associated muscle strain
  - Special tests (compression, Valsalva) positive
- Palpation may elicit local tenderness; muscle hypotonicity or hypertonicity may be evident

---

PALPATION

Palpation usually elicits tenderness in cervical paraspinal muscles, most often on the affected side. Muscle spasm is also found in areas of compensation.

Differential diagnosis

Clients with severe pain (more than 8 out of 10 on the pain scale), with neurological symptoms or following trauma should be referred for further investigation to rule out fracture, ligament sprain or other serious condition.

Overview of treatment and management

Clients with cervical disc syndrome will have been previously assessed and treated by a medical practitioner, chiropractor, osteopath or physiotherapist. The current standard medication management includes a combination of non-steroidal anti-inflammatories and muscle relaxant, although their use for pain management is not recommended as a first line treatment approach.[32] A recent evidence-based review of non-operative treatment for cervical disc prolapse found evidence for anti-convulsant medication to relieve neuropathic pain and for steroid injections. There was evidence for manipulation and mobilisation and traction may provide short-term pain relief.[33] Remedial massage therapy is usually introduced in the chronic phase and can be a useful adjunct to other forms of treatment. It is important to liaise with other treating practitioners wherever possible so as to deliver the most appropriate care.

A typical remedial massage treatment for cervical disc syndrome after pain and inflammation have been controlled includes:

- Swedish massage therapy to the neck, upper back, shoulders, head (± upper limbs, chest).
- Remedial massage therapy. The selection of remedial massage techniques depends on assessment findings. Muscle strain or spasm invariably accompanies disc syndrome. Remedial massage therapy for muscle tissue injury/overload includes (see Table 12.4):
  - deep gliding frictions along the muscle fibres
  - cross-fibre frictions
  - active and passive soft tissue releasing techniques
  - deep transverse friction
  - trigger point therapy
  - muscle stretches.
- Gentle passive cervical extension stretches may be beneficial (see Chapter 7). Horizontal traction may be beneficial (caution: horizontal traction is contraindicated in cervical ligament sprain). Other passive joint articulation may be beneficial for facet joint lesions, but all techniques must be applied with caution. Use the See-Move-Touch principle described in Chapter 2 to guide treatment.
- Myofascial releasing techniques are useful for myofascial restrictions (see Chapter 8).
- Thermotherapy may be beneficial.

Refer clients for further investigation if no significant improvement has been reported in 6 to 8 weeks, if muscle weakness is progressing or if symptoms worsen (peripheralise). Clients may also be referred for nutritional, herbal or homeopathic support.

CLIENT EDUCATION

Advise clients about cervical posture. Clients should avoid heavy lifting, sudden neck movements, and positions that aggravate their neck condition such as awkward or sustained neck positions. Advise clients about sleeping posture (avoid lying in the prone position or with arms overhead) and to use a supportive pillow and mattress. Referral for osseous manipulation may be beneficial. Thermotherapy may be useful for pain relief and reducing muscle spasm.

Home exercise program

A home exercise program may restore muscle balance and by strengthening the cervical muscles reduce the risk of recurrence. All exercises should be performed within the client's pain-free range. Begin with stretches and/or isometric contractions of affected neck muscles and progressively increase to stretching and strengthening muscles of the neck, upper back, shoulders and upper limbs, and proprioceptive training. Advise clients to discontinue any exercise that aggravates symptoms.

WHIPLASH (ACCELERATION/DECELERATION) ASSOCIATED DISORDERS

Whiplash refers to an acute traumatic acceleration-deceleration injury to the cervical spine, commonly caused by rear end or side-impact motor vehicle collisions. The injury often results in a loss (or reversal) of cervical lordosis. Injuries range from mild to severe and can include ligament sprain, disc injury, vertebral subluxation, fracture and muscle tears. They are classified from Grade 0 (no complaints or physical signs) to Grade 4 (fracture or dislocation).

Whiplash is the most common injury for people involved in a motor vehicle accident. It is a significant cost to the Compulsory Third Party (CTP Greenslip) insurance scheme in Australia and appears to have a large effect on the ongoing health of its sufferers. The degree of initial pain and anxiety are more accurate prognostic indicators than physical factors such as the nature of the collision and standard X-ray and MRI imaging.[34] It appears that the cervical multifidus muscle rapidly and progressively degenerates with fatty infiltration in those with a poor whiplash outcome.[35] Conservative treatment has proved to be of benefit to whiplash clients. As with non-specific neck pain the multi-modal program found to provide the most benefit is one which includes traction, mobilisation and manipulation, exercise and education. Up to 6 treatment sessions in an 8-week time frame appears to produce the optimal effect.[15] The Guidelines for the Management of Acute Whiplash Associated Disorders for Health Drofessionals[36] which are based on currently available evidence makes the following recommendations:

Recommended treatments – evidence of benefit

- Reassure client and advise them to stay active
- Return to usual activity
- Exercise – range of motion exercises, low load isometric, postural endurance and strengthening exercises
- Pharmacology – simple analgesics, non-steroidal anti-inflammatories

Not routinely recommended treatments – limited evidence

- Manual therapy
- Thoracic manipulation
- Acupuncture
- Kinesio taping
- Trigger point needling
- Surgical treatment

Treatments where there is no evidence for or against their use

- Massage
- Traction
- Pilates, Feldenkrais, Alexander technique, homeopathy, cervical pillows, magnetic necklaces, spray and stretch
- Heat or ice
- Electrophysical therapies (e.g. TENS, electrical stimulation, ultrasound, laser, shortwave diathermy)

Treatments not recommended – evidence of no benefit

- Reduction of usual activities
- Immobilisation – collars
- Pharmacology – anti-convulsants, anti-depressants
- Muscle relaxants
- Botulinum toxin type A
- Injections – steroid injections
- Pulsed Electromagnetic Treatment

Assessment

HISTORY

The client usually presents with neck pain ± headache and paraesthesia, and limited neck movement following an acceleration-deceleration trauma to the cervical spine. Pain is felt immediately or shortly after injury. Some clients describe feeling sore immediately after the accident with pain and/or headache increasing over the next few hours or days. Symptoms depend on the nature of the injury and the type(s) of tissue involved. Sixty percent of people with whiplash pain

---

Key assessment findings for whiplash-associated disorders

- History of acceleration-deceleration injury. Neck pain and limitation ± headache. Symptoms depend on grade of injury and structures affected.
- Postural analysis: Posture adaptations to limit and guard neck movement
- Functional tests
  - AROM positive in some directions
  - PROM positive if facets, ligaments, joint capsules involved
  - RROM positive if muscle tissue injured
  - Resisted tests and length tests for specific muscles may indicate weakness, strain or contracture
  - Special tests (including compression, distraction, Valsalva) positive in severe cases (e.g. disc involvement)
- Palpation positive for local tenderness and muscle spasm

have pain from the facet joints.[19] More severe cases involve ligament damage and disc degeneration, especially in the mid cervical spine. In some cases, swelling at the site of injury can make swallowing difficult or painful. Osteoarthritis may follow in a few years.

FUNCTIONAL TESTS

AROM: limited and painful; the greater the limitation, the more severe the injury. Reduction in active range of motion is greater in patients with whiplash than those who have neck pain from a non-traumatic origin.[11]

PROM: limited and painful in some directions.

RROM: limited and painful in some directions – pain in many directions suggest joint capsule damage; pain in a single direction suggests muscle strain.

Resisted and length tests positive for specific muscles. Sternocleidomastoid is commonly involved.

Special tests: may be positive if discs or ligaments involved. Positive compression test suggests disc involvement; pain produced by traction suggests ligamentous sprain; pain relieved by traction suggests cervical disc damage.

POSTURAL ANALYSIS

Clients may adopt an antalgic posture and minimise aggravating neck symptoms.

PALPATION

Local tenderness can be elicited at the site of injury and muscle spasm palpated in affected muscles.

Differential diagnosis

Imaging is not routinely recommended for whiplash injuries, as there is a poor correlation between pain and imaging results.[13] It is important to identify and refer any clients with neurological signs (Grade 3) or muscle guarding or symptoms increasing over time (Grade 4) following whiplash injury.

Overview of treatment and management

The first task is to reassure the client and to advise them to stay as active as they can tolerate. Advise them to stay at work. If acute inflammation is present, treatment usually includes cryotherapy, acupressure, Reiki, reflexology or anti-inflammatory medication. Advise the client to lie with a rolled towel behind their neck to restore cervical lordosis if a comfortable position can be found. Introduce corrective exercise therapy (e.g. gentle stretches, range of motion exercises, stabilisation exercises) as soon as tolerated. Myofascial release may be beneficial. Because of the potential for serious injury, screen all whiplash clients carefully and refer clients with neurological symptoms, increasing pain and muscle guarding for further assessment.

A typical remedial massage treatment for mild or moderate whiplash-associated disorder includes:

- Swedish massage therapy to the neck, upper back, shoulders, head (± upper limbs, chest).
- Remedial massage therapy. The selection of remedial massage techniques depends on assessment results which suggest the type of tissue(s) involved. Use the See-Move-Touch principle to guide treatment (see Chapter 2). Remedial

massage therapy for muscle tissue injury/overload includes (see Table 12.4):

- deep gliding frictions along the muscle fibres
- cross-fibre frictions
- active and passive soft tissue releasing techniques
- deep transverse friction
- trigger point therapy (A study in 2008 found that patients with whiplash showed a distinct pattern of trigger point distribution and that semispinalis capitis was more frequently affected by trigger points in whiplash patients than patients with non-traumatic chronic cervical syndrome or fibromyalgia.[37])
- muscle stretches.
- Gentle joint mobilisation should be introduced when tolerated, particularly extension to restore cervical lordosis (see Chapter 7). Other passive joint articulation may be beneficial for facet joint lesions, but all techniques must be applied with caution. Use the See-Move-Touch principle to guide treatment. Horizontal traction is contraindicated for ligamentous sprains.
- Apply myofascial releasing techniques for myofascial restrictions (see Chapter 8).
- Thermotherapy may be useful.

Refer clients for spinal manipulation to restore normal biomechanics and prevent the onset of osteoarthritis.

CLIENT EDUCATION

Encourage clients to continue their daily activities as usual within pain tolerance. Advise clients about cervical posture for work and activities of daily living. Avoid heavy lifting and sudden neck movements. Activities that require awkward or prolonged neck positions should be avoided. Good sleeping posture (avoid lying in the prone position or with arms overhead) should be maintained. Shock-absorbing shoes help minimise jarring impacts transferred to the neck when walking.

Clients may require education about seat and headrest position to minimise the impact of any subsequent whiplash-associated injuries. The seat should be inclined to less than a 20° angle, the head restraint should be level with the centre of the driver's head and less than 10 cm from the back of the head.

Home exercise program

Introduce range of motion stretches and/or isometric contractions of affected neck muscles as soon as possible.[36] All exercises should be performed within the client's pain-free range. Stretches and strengthening exercises should be progressively increased. The Guidelines for the Management of Acute Whiplash Associated Disorders for Health Professionals[36] contains excellent exercises that could be prescribed for clients. Advise clients to discontinue any exercise/activity that aggravates symptoms.

KEY MESSAGES

- Assessment of clients with conditions of the cervical region involves history, outcome measures, postural analysis, functional tests (including resisted and length tests for specific muscles of the neck) and special tests (e.g. cervical compression, cervical distraction and Valsalva).

- Assessment findings may indicate the type of tissue involved (contractile or inert), duration of condition (acute or chronic), and severity (grade).
- Assessment findings may indicate a common presenting condition such as
  - strain of cervical muscles
  - non-specific neck pain
  - osteoarthritis of the cervical spine
  - upper crossed syndrome
  - mechanical/acquired torticollis
  - cervical disc syndrome
  - whiplash associated disorders.
- Assessment findings indicate the client's perception of injury and preferences for treatment.
- Consider Clinical Guidelines, available evidence, clinical efficacy and client preferences when planning treatment.

- Select the most appropriate remedial massage techniques for the affected tissue(s) (e.g. muscle-specific techniques like trigger point therapy for muscle strains; joint mobilisation for facet lesions). Be conservative in treatment: if in doubt, perform pain-free Swedish massage.
- Although serious conditions of the cervical region are rare, clients with such conditions will present for remedial massage from time to time. Caution is required when treating all clients with neck pain post trauma or with neurological signs.
- Educating clients about likely causal and predisposing factors is an essential part of remedial massage therapy.
- Prioritise self-help component of treatment including exercise, wherever possible to reduce likelihood of recurrence and/or to promote health maintenance and illness prevention.

Review questions

1. A client comes to your clinic with neck pain. She reports being unable to turn her head when she woke up. She is in her late twenties and has had some minor episodes of neck pain in the past but this one is by far the worst. She has had no previous accidents or falls and can't think of anything that could have brought this on. She is in a great deal of pain and is unable to go to work. This history is consistent with:
   a) cervical facet syndrome
   b) cervical disc syndrome
   c) acute torticollis
   d) cervical osteoarthritis
2. In general, traction tests are positive when:
   a) a facet joint is subluxated
   b) a ligament has been sprained
   c) an intervertebral disc has bulged
   d) a muscle has been strained
3. After a whiplash injury, a patient may be suffering with:
   a) a strained sternocleidomastoid muscle
   b) cervical facet syndrome
   c) cervical ligament sprain
   d) all of the above
4. The most common level for a cervical disc herniation to occur is:
   a) C1/C2   b) C3/C4
   c) C5/C6   d) C7/T1

5. Which muscles are usually weakened in upper crossed syndrome? Prescribe a home exercise program to help strengthen these muscles.
6. Draw or describe a home stretch for the following muscles:
   a) upper trapezius
   b) levator scapulae
   c) scalene muscles
7. List three red flags for acute neck pain.
8. The compression test is used to indicate the presence of:
   a) a space-occupying lesion such as a disc prolapse
   b) a muscle strain
   c) upper crossed syndrome
   d) osteoarthritis
9. Osteophytes, loss of disc height and endplate sclerosis may indicate:
   a) osteoarthritis
   b) acute torticollis
   c) a space-occupying lesion such as a disc prolapse
   d) upper crossed syndrome
10. Describe the typical presenting symptoms and signs associated with cervical osteoarthritis.

REFERENCES

1. GBD 2016 Disease and Injury Incidence and Prevalence Colaborators. Global, regional, and national incidence, and years lived with disability for 328 diseases and injuries and for 195 countries, 1990–2016: A systematic analysis for the Global Burden of Disease Study 2016. Lancet 2017; 390(10100):1260–344.
2. Hurwitz EL, Randhawa K, Yu H, et al. The Global Spine Care Initiative: A summary of the global burden of low back and neck pain studies. Eur Spine J 2017;27(S6):796–801.
3. Mansfield M, Thacker M, Spahr N, et al. Factors associated with physical activity participation in

adults with chronic cervical spine pain: a systematic review. Physiotherapy 2018;104(1):54–60.
4. Loughenbury P, Tsirikos AI, Gummerson N. Spinal biomechanics – biomechanical considerations of spinal stability in the context of spinal injury. J Orthop Trauma 2016;30(5):369–77.
5. Cheng YH, Huang GC: Efficacy of massage therapy on pain and dysfunction in patients with neck pain: a systematic review and meta-analysis. Evid-Based Compl Alt Med, Online. Available: http://dx.doi.org/10.1155/2014/204360;2014.
6. Blanpied PR, Gross AR, Elliott JM, et al. Neck Pain: Revision 2017. Clinical Practice Guidelines

linked to the International Classification of Functioning, Disability and Health from the Orthopaedic Section of the American Physical Therapy Association. J Orthop Sports Phys Ther 2017;47(7):A1–A83. Doi:10.2519/jospt.2017.0302.
7. Swartz E, Floyd R, Cendoma M. Cervical spine functional anatomy and the biomechanics of injury due to compressive loading. J Athlet Train 2005; 40(3):155–61.
8. Leichtle UG, Wunschel M, Socci M, et al. Spine radiography in the evaluation of back and neck pain in an orthopaedic emergency clinic. J Back Musculoskel Rehabil 2015;28:43–8.

9. Vijiaratnam N, Williams DR, Bertram KL. Neck pain: what if it is not musculoskeletal? Aust J Gen Pract 2018;47(5):279–82.

10. Cohen SP. Epidemiology, diagnosis and treatment of neck pain. Mayo Clin Prac 2015;90(2):284–99.

11. Stenneberg MS, Rood M, de Bie R, et al. To what degree does active cervical range of motion differ between patients with neck pain, patients with whiplash, and those without neck pain? A systematic review and meta-analysis. Arch Phys Med Rehabil 2017;98:1407–34.

12. Overas CK, Myhrvold BL, Rosok G, et al. Musculoskeletal diagnostic ultrasound imaging for thickness measurements of four principal muscles of the cervical spina. A reliability and agreement study. Chiropr Man Therap 2017;52(2).

13. Cohen SP. Epidemiology, diagnosis, and treatment of neck pain. Mayo Clin Proc 2015;90(2):284–99.

14. Southerst D, Nordin MC, Cote P, et al. Is exercise effective for the management of neck pain and associated disorders or whiplash-associated disorders? A systematic review by the Ontario Protocol for Traffic Injury Management (OPTIMa) Collaboration. Spine J 2016;16:1503–23.

15. Sutton DA, Cote P, Wong JJ, et al. Is multimodal care effective for the management of patients with whiplash-associated disorders or neck pain and associated disorders? A systematic review by the Ontario Protocol for Traffic Injury Management (OPTIMa) Collaboration. Spine J 2016;16:1541–65.

16. Fredlin K, Loras H. Manual therapy, exercise therapy or combined treatment in the management of adult neck pain: a systematic review and meta-analysis. Musculoskelet Sci Pract 2017; 31:62–71.

17. Hidalgo B, Hall T, Cagnie B, et al. The efficacy of manual therapy and exercise for treating non-specific neck pain: an update of systematic reviews. J Back Musculskelet Rehabil 2017;30(6):1149–60.

18. Jun D, Michaleff Z, O'Leary S, et al. Physical risk factors for the development of non-specific neck pain in office workers: a systematic review. Int Arch Occup Environ Health 2017;90(5):373–410.

19. Candido KD, England B. Cervical spine pain related to the facet joints. Tech Reg Anesth Pain Manag 2015;19:109–18.

20. Yin W, Bogduk N. The nature of neck pain in a private pain clinic in the United States. Pain Med 2008;9(2):196–203.

21. Carnes M, Vizniak N. Quick reference evidencebased conditions manual. 3rd edn. Burnaby, BC: Professional Health Systems; 2009.

22. Thoomes EJ, van Geest S, van der Windt DA, et al. Value of physical tests in diagnosing cervical radiculopathy: a systematic review. Spine J 2018;18:179–89.

23. Wei X, Wang S, Zhu L: Clinical evidence of Chinese massage therapy (Tui Na) for cervical radiculopathy: a systematic review and meta-analysis. Evid-Based Compl Alt Med, Online. Available: http://dx.doi.org/10.1155/2017/9519285; 2017.

24. Simons D, Travell J, Simons L. Myofascial pain and dysfunction: the trigger point manual. Vol 1: upper half of body. 2nd edn. Philadelphia: Williams and Wilkins; 1999.

25. Hunter DJ: Everything you ever wanted to know about osteoarthritis. The Health Report 2017. Online. Available: https://www.abc.net.au/radionational/programs/healthreport/everything-you-ever-wanted-to-know-about-osteoarthritis/8664218#transcript; 2017.

26. Hunter DJ. Osteoarthritis management: time to change the deck. J Orthop Sports Phys Ther 2017;47(6):370–2.

27. Thomas S, Browne H, Mobasheri A, et al. What is the evidence for a role for diet and nutrition in osteoarthritis? Rheumatology 2018;57:iv61–iv74. Doi:10.1093/rheumatology/key011.

28. Li X, Tian F, Wang F. The effects of black soybean (Glycine max var.) on chronic cervical pain of sedentary office workers in a northern Chinese population. Food & Function 2015;26:3500–11.

29. Morris CE, Bonnefin D, Darville C. The torsional upper crossed syndrome: a multi-planar update to Janda's model, with a case series introduction of the mid-pectoral fascial lesion as an associated etiological factor. J Bodyw Mov Ther 2015;19: 681–9.

30. Kocur P, Wilski M, Lewandowski J, et al. Female office workers with moderate neck pain have increased anterior positioning of the cervical spine and stiffness of upper trapezius myofascial tissue in sitting posture. PM&R 2018;piiS1934–482. Doi: 10.1016/j.pmrj.2018.07.002

31. Wong JJ, Cote P, Quesnele JJ, et al. The course and prognostic factors of symptomatic cervical disc herniation with radiculopathy: a systematic review of the literature. Spine J 2014:14:1781–9.

32. Foster NE, Anema JR, Cherkin D, et al. Prevention and treatment of low back pain: evidence, challenges, and promising directions. Lancet 2018;391:2368–83.

33. Greis AC, Young GW, Usman-Oyowe I. Nonoperative management of cervical disc herniations: an evidence-based approach. Semin Spine Surg 2016:28:68–74.

34. Sarrami P, Armstrong E, Naylor JM, et al. Factors predicting outcome in whiplash injury: a systematic meta-review of prognostic factors. J Orthopaed Traumatol 2017;18:9–16.

35. Elliott JM, Cornwall J, Kennedy E, et al. Towards defining muscular regions of interest from axial magnetic resonance imaging with anatomical cross-reference: Part II — cervical spine musculature. BMC Musculoskel Dis 2018;19: 171–84.

36. NSW Government State Insurance Regulatory Authority: The guidelines for the management of acute whiplash associated disorders for health professionals. 3rd edn. Online. Available: https://www.sira.nsw.gov.au/resources-library/motor-accident-resources/publications/for-professionals/whiplash-resources/SIRA08104-Whiplash-Guidelines-1117-396479.pdf; 2014.

37. Ettlin T, Schuster C, Stoffel R, et al. A distinct pattern of myofascial findings in patients after whiplash injury. Arch Phys Med Rehabil 2008;89(7):1290–3.

13 The head and face

INTRODUCTION

This chapter is divided into three sections. The first describes assessment and treatment of headache, which is the most common condition of the head and face for which clients seek remedial massage. Two further sections deal with sinusitis and temporomandibular joint (TMJ) disorders which are also commonly treated by remedial massage therapists. Some of the treatments introduced in this chapter have long been used in remedial massage but have rarely been the subject of scientific research. It is important for massage therapists to be acquainted with traditional treatments and to make their own judgments, through experience and research, about their efficacy.

HEADACHE

Headache is a large public health problem, experienced by people living in high and low income regions of the world.

Approximately 2 billion live with migraine and 1 billion with tension-type headache each year. The headaches were most burdensome in women between ages 15 and 49 years.[1] Migraine in particular is among the most disabling disorders worldwide. It is the second largest cause of disability globally.[1] In Australia, 1 in 5 people (4.9 million) live with migraine; 71% of these are women.[2] The total economic costs of migraine in Australia in 2018 was estimated to be $35.7 billion.

Headache is pain in any part of the head, including the scalp, face and interior of the head. Primary headaches (such as migraine, cluster headache and tension-type headache) are those for which no other causative factor can be found. Secondary headaches can have numerous causes including dental disorders, glaucoma, sinusitis, brain cancers, cerebral haemorrhages, viral infections, caffeine withdrawal and dehydration. Headaches arise from activation of pain-sensitive structures including skin and subcutaneous tissue, muscles, extracranial coverings and arteries, periosteum of the skull, intracranial venous sinuses, dura mater at the base of the brain, cranial nerves V, IX and X and the first three cervical nerves. The pathophysiology of migraine involves a hypersensitivity of the brain to triggers which affect the trigeminovascular system, leading to neuropeptide release, local inflammation and an increase in neural activity across certain parts of the brain. Tension-type headaches primarily involve pain mechanisms peripheral to the brain and are influenced by factors including genetic, environmental, head and neck mechanics and co-existing mood disorders.[3]

ASSESSMENT OF THE HEADACHE CLIENT

Assessment of the headache client provides essential information for development and negotiation of treatment plans, including:

- client's suitability for remedial massage therapy
- duration of the condition (i.e. acute or chronic)
- severity of the condition (i.e. mild, moderate or severe pain)
- type(s) of tissues involved and the most appropriate treatment for the condition[4]
- priorities for treatment if more than one injury or condition is present
- whether the signs and symptoms suggest one of the classifications of headache

Assessment of the headache client

1. Case history
2. Outcome measure
3. Postural analysis
4. Functional tests
   AROM cervical spine
   Flexion, extension, lateral flexion, rotation
   PROM cervical spine
   Flexion, extension, lateral flexion, rotation
   RROM cervical spine
   Flexion, extension, lateral flexion, rotation
   Resisted and length tests for specific muscles, including
   Sub-occipital muscles
   Posterior cervical muscles
   Upper trapezius
   Sternocleidomastoid
   Special tests as indicated
   Special tests for the cervical spine (see Chapter 10)
5. Palpation

- special considerations for individual clients (e.g. client's preference for treatment types and styles, specific population considerations).

Although serious causes of headache are rare, headache clients require careful screening to identify those clients who require referral for further investigation.

Case history

A thorough case history with targeted questions is the most important assessment strategy for identifying potentially serious causes of headaches. Practitioners should be vigilant for red flags which suggest such disorders (see Table 13.1). Clients with one or more red flags should be referred for an immediate medical consultation and further investigation.[5]

Note:

- Headaches that have been present for more than 6 months are usually not life threatening.
- Recurring headaches in clients who appear well and have a normal examination are rarely serious. Recurring headaches that began in childhood or early adulthood in clients with a normal examination are usually benign. However, if the type or pattern of the headache changes in clients with a known primary headache disorder, investigation for secondary headache should be carried out.
- Most single symptoms of primary headache disorders other than aura are non-specific.
- Questions are not only designed to identify red and yellow flags but also to suggest the type of headache. Ask about:
  - Location of headache (e.g. headache in the occipital/suboccipital region could indicate cervicogenic headache or stress-induced headache; temporal pain may suggest temporal arteritis, tension-type headache, TMJ dysfunction; orbital headache may suggest eye strain, sinusitis or stress-induced headache; headaches preceded by aura

Table 13.1 Red flags for serious conditions associated with headache

Red flags for headache[6]	Possible condition
Abrupt onset (e.g. thunderclap headache – severe, peaks within a few seconds)	Subarachnoid haemorrhage
New headache after the age of 50	Increased risk of serious cause (e.g. cancer, giant cell arteritis)
New onset headache with history of cancer or immunodeficiency	Brain infection, metastases
Headache with fever, neck stiffness and meningeal signs (Brudzinski's sign: lifting the head off the table in the supine position causes the legs to lift up; Kernig's sign: hip and knee flexed to 90°, knee extension from this position causes pain; nuchal rigidity)	Meningitis, subarachnoid haemorrhage, subdural empyema
Headache with neurological symptoms (e.g. altered mental state, confusion, neurogenic weakness, diplopia, papilloedema, focal neurological deficits) if not previously documented as a migraine with aura	Encephalitis, subdural haematoma, subarachnoid or intracerebral haemorrhage, cancer, other intracranial mass, increased intracranial pressure
Headache following trauma	Epidural, subdural, subarachnoid or intraparenchymal haemorrhage, dissection of carotid or vertebral artery
Headache worsening with Valsalva manoeuvre or recumbency	Intracranial cancers
Progressively worsening headache	Mass lesion, subdural haematoma, medication overuse
Systemic symptoms (e.g. weight loss, fever)	Sepsis, thyrotoxicosis, cancer
Headache during pregnancy or post-partum	Cortical vein/cranial sinus thrombosis, carotid dissection, pituitary apoplexy

may suggest migraine). Ask clients to point to the site of pain as they may have different understandings of anatomical terms.
  - Character and intensity of pain (e.g. throbbing suggests vascular headache; dull aching could suggest cervicogenic headache). Is the pain incapacitating? Ask if the headache wakes the client from sleep. Clients with severe pain require referral.

- Onset and chronicity. Ask how long the client has been experiencing headaches and how quickly the headache reaches a peak. Clients with abrupt onset headaches reaching a peak in 5 or 10 minutes require referral.
- Precipitating and aggravating factors (e.g. headache aggravated by stooping, straining, coughing may suggest hypertension; headache precipitated by bright light, noise, stress or certain foods could be a migraine; headaches aggravated by a head-low position could be vascular or suggest sinusitis; headaches before menstrual periods could be related to hormonal change).
- Frequency and duration (e.g. headache lasting from several hours to 1 or 2 days suggests migraine; intermittently persistent headache several times a days could suggest a brain cancer). It is important to ascertain if the headaches are becoming more frequent and severe over a period of months and if so refer for further investigation.

■ Determine if the pain is likely to have a mechanical cause. Is the pain associated with rest or activity, certain postures or time of day? Cervicogenic headache is caused or aggravated by neck movements and sustained postures.[7] Ask clients to demonstrate movements and positions that aggravate or relieve their pain and to be specific with descriptions of aggravating or relieving activities. Cervicogenic headaches usually present as one-sided neck and occipital pain and may radiate to the forehead, eyes, temples or ears. Morning pain relieved with daily activity is often associated with arthritis.

■ Determine if the headache is likely to be vascular. Migraine is the most common vascular headache. Clients are typically 10 to 40 years of age, are more likely to be female than male and describe episodes of throbbing pain that may last several hours, or up to 3 days.

■ Enquire whether the clients' previous treatments for headache have included massage therapy and if so ask about their response to treatment.

TYPES OF HEADACHE

The following classifications have been adapted from the International Headache Society.[8] The most relevant classifications for remedial massage therapists are discussed here.

Primary headache

Migraine

Migraine is the third leading cause of years lived with a disability globally, with 1 in 10 people currently living with migraine.[1] Women, students, and urban residents are affected more frequently.[9] The term *migraine* is derived from the old French word *migraigne* meaning half head and reminds us that 60% of migraine sufferers experience pain unilaterally. One in five sufferers experience an aura (a group of neurological symptoms, including disturbances of vision that precede head pain). Migraines are often severe. They are episodic and can occur as often as once or twice a week but not daily. The International Headache Society has established the following diagnostic criteria for migraine.

Migraine without aura Diagnostic criteria:

A. At least five attacks fulfilling criteria B–D
B. Headache attacks lasting 4–72 hours (when untreated or unsuccessfully treated)

Classification of headache[8]

Primary headaches
1. Migraine
2. Tension-type headache
3. Trigeminal autonomic cephalalgias
4. Other primary headache disorders including cough headache, exercise headache, sexual activity headache, thunderclap headache, cold headache, external compression headache, external traction headache, stabbing headache, nummular headache, hypnic headache and new daily persistent headache.

Secondary headaches
5. Headache attributed to trauma or injury to the head and/ or neck
6. Headache attributed to cranial and/or cervical vascular disorder
7. Headache attributed to non-vascular intracranial disorder
8. Headache attributed to a substance or its withdrawal
9. Headache attributed to infection
10. Headache attributed to disorder of homoeostasis
11. Headache or facial pain attributed to disorder of the cranium, neck, eyes, ears, nose, sinuses, teeth, mouth or other facial or cervical structure
12. Headache attributed to psychiatric disorder

Painful cranial neuropathies, other facial pain and other headaches
13. Painful lesions of the cranial nerves and other facial pain
14. Headache not elsewhere classified and Headache unspecified

---

C. Headache has at least two of the following four characteristics:
 1. unilateral location
 2. pulsating quality
 3. moderate or severe pain intensity
 4. aggravation by or causing avoidance of routine physical activity (e.g. walking or climbing stairs)
D. During headache at least one of the following:
 1. nausea and/or vomiting
 2. photophobia and phonophobia
E. Not better accounted for by another ICHD-3 diagnosis.[8]

Migraine with aura Diagnostic criteria:

A. At least two attacks fulfilling criteria B and C
B. One or more of the following fully reversible aura symptoms:
 1. visual
 2. sensory
 3. speech and/or language
 4. motor
 5. brainstem
 6. retinal
C. At least three of the following six characteristics:
 1. at least one aura symptom spreads gradually over 5 minutes
 2. two or more aura symptoms occur in succession
 3. each individual aura symptom lasts 5–60 minutes
 4. at least one aura symptom is unilateral

5. at least one aura symptom is positive
6. the aura is accompanied, or followed within 60 minutes, by headache

D. Not better accounted for by another ICHD-3 diagnosis.[8]

Tension-type headache

Historically, tension-type heartache was considered to be of psychogenic origin. Numerous recent studies now indicate a neurobiological basis.[8] They are common with a lifetime general population prevalence ranging from 30–78% in various studies. Clients may go to bed with a headache and wake up with it the next day. The International Headache Society has established the following diagnostic criteria.

A. At least 10 episodes of headache occurring on <1 day/month on average (<12 days/year) and fulfilling criteria B–D
B. Lasting from 30 minutes to 7 days
C. At least two of the following four characteristics:
   1. bilateral location
   2. pressing or tightening (non-pulsating) quality
   3. mild or moderate intensity
   4. not aggravated by routine physical activity such as walking or climbing stairs
D. Both of the following:
   1. no nausea or vomiting
   2. no more than one of photophobia or phonophobia
E. Not better accounted for by another ICHD-3 diagnosis.[8]

Trigeminal autonomic cephalalgias (TACs)

A unilateral headache with cranial parasympathetic autonomic features (e.g. ipsilateral conjunctival injection, lacrimation, nasal congestion, rhinorrhoea, forehead and facial sweating, miosis, ptosis and/or eyelid oedema) on the same side.[8]

Cluster headache is an example of a TAC. The pain is severe, strictly unilateral and is located in the orbital, supraorbital and/or temporal regions. Attacks last 15–180 minutes and occur from once every other day to eight times a day. The pain is associated with ipsilateral conjunctival injection, lacrimation, nasal congestion, rhinorrhoea, forehead and facial sweating, miosis, ptosis and/or eyelid oedema, and/or with restlessness or agitation.

Diagnostic criteria:

A. At least five attacks fulfilling criteria B–D
B. Severe or very severe unilateral orbital, supraorbital and/or temporal pain lasting 15–180 minutes (when untreated)
C. Either or both of the following:
   1. at least one of the following symptoms or signs, ipsilateral to the headache:
      a) conjunctival injection and/or lacrimation
      b) nasal congestion and/or rhinorrhoea
      c) eyelid oedema
      d) forehead and facial sweating
      e) miosis and/or ptosis
   2. a sense of restlessness or agitation
D. Occurring with a frequency between one every other day and eight per day
E. Not better accounted for by another ICHD-3 diagnosis.[8]

Secondary headache

Headache attributable to head and/or neck trauma

Headache is the most common symptom following car accidents, head injuries and falls. The headache can be dull, constant and aching. Other symptoms may accompany the headache, such as faintness, poor memory, inability to concentrate, anxiety, fatigue, insomnia, irritability, depression, tinnitus and vertigo. About 85% of chronic post-traumatic headache sufferers will recover completely but this can take many months or even years. Ensure clients are immediately assessed by a medical practitioner following an injury to the head or neck. The International Headache Society has established subcategories based on wherever the headache is acute or persistent, the degree of severity, and whether the trauma was a result of injury to the head, whiplash or craniotomy.[8] The following is an example of diagnostic criteria for persistent (greater than 3 months) headache attributed to traumatic injury to the head.

A. Any headache fulfilling criteria C and D
B. Traumatic injury to the head has occurred
C. Headache is reported to have developed within 7 days after one of the following:
   1. the injury to the head
   2. regaining of consciousness following the injury to the head
   3. discontinuation of medication(s) impairing ability to sense or report headache following the injury to the head
D. Headache persists for >3 months after its onset
E. Not better accounted for by another ICHD-3 diagnosis.[8]

Headache attributable to a substance or its withdrawal

Headaches can occur from use of or withdrawal from a substance known to be able to cause headache. These substances include alcohol, cocaine, histamine, paracetamol, NSAIDs, opioids, caffeine, oestrogen, nitric oxide, phosphodiesterase, carbon monoxide, calcitonin gene related peptide, ergotamine, triptan and acetylsalicylic acid.[8]

Headache or facial pain attributed to disorder of the cranium, neck, eyes, ears, nose, sinuses, teeth, mouth or other facial or cervical structure

The most common headache in this category is cervicogenic headache. Estimates of prevalence vary widely.[10] One study estimated that cervicogenic headaches account for 14–18% of all chronic headaches.[11] Cervicogenic headaches are also among the most responsive to remedial massage treatment. Treatment with manual therapy or specific exercises or manual therapy plus exercises is significantly more effective at reducing cervicogenic headache frequency and intensity than no specific care.[12]

Cervicogenic headache

The mechanism of cervicogenic headache is convergence between cervical afferents and trigeminal or cervical afferents of the C1–3 segments of the spinal cord. The most common source of pain is the C2/3 facet joint.[12] Pain is typically felt in the suboccipital region, unilaterally or bilaterally, and radiates to the head behind the eyes or into the face. The pain is usually dull and aching and is often worse on rising. The headache usually eases as the day goes on but may be aggravated by neck and head movements or by jolting (e.g. when riding in a bus). The International Headache Society has established the following diagnostic criteria:

A. Any headache fulfilling criterion C
B. Clinical and/or imaging evidence of a disorder or lesion within the cervical spine or soft tissues of the neck, known to be able to cause headache
C. Evidence of causation demonstrated by at least two of the following:
　　1. headache has developed in temporal relation to the onset of the cervical disorder or appearance of the lesion
　　2. headache has significantly improved or resolved in parallel with improvement in or resolution of the cervical disorder or lesion
　　3. cervical range of motion is reduced and headache is made significantly worse by provocative manoeuvres
　　4. headache is abolished following diagnostic blockade of a cervical structure or its nerve supply
D. Not better accounted for by another ICHD-3 diagnosis.[8]

Table 13.2 compares characteristics of common types of headache.

Outcome measures

Outcome measures are specifically designed questionnaires that are used to assess clients' level of impairment and to define benefits of treatment. Outcome measures for headache include the Migraine Disability Assessment Test (MIDAS). MIDAS is a simple five-question survey that measures days lost to headache disability during the last 3 months and headache pain on a 10-point scale (see Appendix 13.1).

Postural analysis

Postural analysis may reveal biomechanical compensations resulting from habitual postures like forward head carriage or structural factors such as idiopathic scoliosis that can contribute to headache (see Chapter 2).

Functional tests

CERVICAL SPINE

a) Active range of motion

Flexion (50°)

- Stand in front of the client and ask them to take their chin towards their chest as far as they comfortably can.
- The client should be able to touch their chin to their chest.

Extension (60°)

- Ask the client to look up to the ceiling as far as they comfortably can.
- The client should be able to extend their neck so that their face is parallel to the ceiling.

Lateral flexion (sidebend) (45°)

- Ask the client to take their ear toward their shoulder as far as they comfortably can.

- The client should be able to tilt their ear to their shoulder approximately 45°.

Rotation (80°)

- Ask the client to look over their shoulder as far as they comfortably can.
- The client should be able to rotate their neck so that their chin is almost in line with their shoulder.

b) Passive range of motion (see Chapter 12)

Lie the client supine to relax the neck muscles. Great care is needed when performing cervical passive range of motion tests. Perform all neck movements slowly and gently and only ever after you have observed the client's ability to perform active ranges of motion (the See-Move-Touch principle discussed in Chapter 2). Note the end-feel at the end of each range of motion. Stop the movement if neurological symptoms such as pain, paraesthesia or numbness are produced.

Flexion

- Cup the client's occiput with both hands and gently flex the client's neck.

Extension

- When the client is positioned with shoulders level with the top of the table, the neck can be gently extended. Alternatively, the neck can be passively extended by lifting the neck towards the ceiling.

Lateral flexion

- Place one hand on the client's shoulder and with the other, cup the occiput. Gently laterally flex the client's neck with the cupped hand.

Rotation

- Cup the client's occiput with both hands and gently rotate the neck to one side and then the other.

c) Resisted range of motion

Resisted range of motion (RROM) tests are designed to identify muscle groups that may be contributing to the client's condition. Resist the movement as the client flexes, extends, laterally flexes and rotates their head. The client may be seated or lying supine. These tests are usually carried out in conjunction with passive range of motion tests. For example, passive rotation of the neck can be followed immediately by resisted rotation before testing another movement in another plane. If any RROM tests are positive, resisted tests for specific muscle tests are required to identify individual muscles.

Tests for specific muscles associated with neck conditions

Muscle tightness is commonly associated with headache. Resisted tests and length tests for specific muscles could include suboccipital muscles, posterior cervical muscles and upper trapezius.

d) Special tests

Special tests for headache clients include cervical special tests such as cervical compression, cervical distraction and

Table 13.2 Types of headache[8, 13]

Typical features	Migraine	Cervicogenic headache	Tension-type headache	Cluster
Age of onset	10–40 years	20–60 years	Any age	Common in adolescence and middle age
Gender	Two to three times more common in females than males[14]	Four times more common in females than males	Slightly more common in females than males	Six to one male to female ratio
Onset	Rapid	Slow	Slow	Rapid
Location	Temporal or frontal	Occipital, behind the eyes, temporal	Front, top and sides of the head	Frontal and one eye
Unilateral/bilateral	Unilateral, bilateral in children, aggravation by routine physical activity	Unilateral	Bilateral	Unilateral
Nature of pain	Throbbing/pulsing	Dull ache	Steady ache	Burning
Severity	Moderate to severe	Mild to moderate	Mild to moderate	Severe
Constancy	Episodic attacks	Constant	Chronic, occur frequently, even daily	1 every other day to 8/day
Duration	4–72 hours	Days	30 minutes to 7 days	Short (15 minutes to 3 hours)
Possible associated symptoms	Nausea, vomiting, photophobia, phonophobia. With or without aura (transient focal neurological symptoms of visual, sensor, speech, language, motor, brainstem &/or retinal disturbance). Prodromal and postdromal symptoms (fatigue, difficulty in concentrating, neck stiffness, blurred vision, yawning, pallor)	Occasional neurological symptoms	None	Inflamed, watery eye
Triggers	Menstruation, menopause, stress, fatigue, bright lights, fasting, hypoglycemia, foods rich in tyramine (e.g. aged cheeses, sour cream, and wine), odours, exercise, weather changes, and high altitude[15]	Trauma, posture, provoked by neck movement	Stress, mental concentration, prolonged postural neck contracture, medication withdrawal, dental malocclusion[15]	Vasodilators such as alcohol, histamine or nitroglycerin (used in angina medication).[16] Stress, cigarettes, short naps, aged foods containing tyramine.[15]
Treatment	Avoid precipitating factors. Massage and other physical therapy, stress reduction. Medication for attacks or prevention (avoid long-term use of analgesics as can lead to overuse headache). Avoid oestrogen contraceptives if experiencing migraine with aura.	Physical therapies including remedial massage therapy (e.g. muscle and joint-specific techniques, heat therapy, myofascial release, posture and exercise rehabilitation)	Physical therapies including remedial massage therapy (e.g. muscle and joint-specific techniques, heat therapy, myofascial release, posture and exercise rehabilitation), stress management including Swedish massage	Avoid precipitating factors. Massage and other physical therapy, high flow oxygen, medication

Valsalva (see Chapter 12) and taking blood pressure. Clients over 50 years of age who present with a new or unaccustomed headache should be referred for blood pressure monitoring.

Palpation

Hypertonic muscles are commonly palpated in headache sufferers. Palpation should be gentle, as heavy palpation of affected tissues (e.g. trigger points in the upper trapezius, sub-occipital or temporalis muscles, or facet joints) may reproduce or aggravate headache. The following guide to palpation of the posterior cervical muscles was suggested by Simons et al:[17]

Slight flexion of the head and neck makes the posterior neck muscles more distinguishable by palpation. Palpate posterior cervical muscles in four layers (see Figure 13.1).

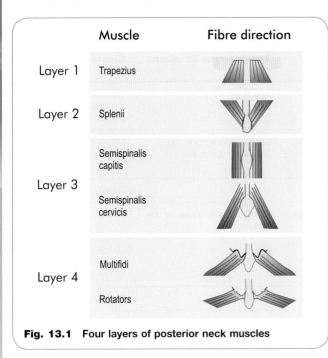

	Muscle	Fibre direction
Layer 1	Trapezius	
Layer 2	Splenii	
Layer 3	Semispinalis capitis	
	Semispinalis cervicis	
Layer 4	Multifidi	
	Rotators	

Fig. 13.1 Four layers of posterior neck muscles

- Most superficial layer: upper trapezius muscle converging to form a roof-top shape.
- Bilateral splenius fibres converge below to form a V shape.
- Semispinalis capitis fibres lie nearly vertical.
- Muscle fibres in the deepest layers converge to form a roof-top (e.g. semispinalis cervicis) and multifidi and rotators (the fourth layer).

Palpate the temporalis muscles. Spread fingertips across the superior aspects of the temporal fossae on either side of the head. Compare the left and right temporalis muscles as the fingertips move inferiorly through the muscle. Palpate the tendon of temporalis just above the zygomatic arch.

REMEDIAL MASSAGE TREATMENT FOR HEADACHE

Cervicogenic headaches are likely to respond well to spinal manipulation, remedial massage techniques for muscle contractures, trigger point therapy, cryotherapy, thermotherapy and ergonomic advice. However, such treatments may also be useful for other types of headache that are associated with cervical joint dysfunction and myospasm of the suboccipital and posterior neck muscles. Clients with headaches arising from non-mechanical causes should be referred for further investigation and treatment. Treatment can include conventional biomedicine, dietary modification, allergy assessment, herbal and nutritional supplements (e.g. magnesium, vitamin B2 (riboflavin) and coenzyme Q10 and possibly vitamin A, calcium and feverfew), homoeopathy, acupuncture and stress management.

Treatment options must always be considered in the context of the best available evidence for treatment effectiveness and clinical practice guidelines where they exist. Reviews investigating the effectiveness of non-invasive physical treatments are only now beginning to support the use of manual therapy for management of migraine, tension-type, cervicogenic, and other headaches.[18–27] Chronic use of analgesic can have a detrimental impact on individuals, including the worsening of primary headache. Pain perception is altered in medication overuse headache, although can be restored by withdrawal from acute pain medication.[28] Medical practitioners may advise medication withdrawal or replacement of analgesic medication with preventative or alternate medications.

Some studies into the benefits of multi-modal care have been published in recent years. For example, remedial massage techniques when used in conjunction with other treatment such as medication review and lifestyle modifications may lead to better patient outcomes.[27] Further research is needed to validate findings and address limitations in current studies. Findings of some current research reviews are summarised in Table 13.3. A review of manual therapies (including myofascial release and trigger point therapy) for tension-type headaches found that clients receiving manual therapies showed better progress than those receiving conventional treatment or placebo.[18]

TREATMENT PROTOCOLS IN REMEDIAL MASSAGE PRACTICE

All remedial massage treatments are adapted to suit the needs of individual clients. Treatment protocols are templates from which individualised treatments can be developed. A typical remedial massage protocol for a cervicogenic headache includes:

- Swedish massage to the neck, upper back, head and face.
- Remedial massage therapy for muscle strains or overload which includes:
  - deep gliding frictions along the muscle fibres
  - cross-fibre frictions
  - active and passive soft tissue releasing techniques
  - deep transverse friction
  - trigger point therapy
  - muscle stretches.

These techniques are described in Chapter 12 (Table 12.4).

- Apply myofascial releasing techniques for myofascial restrictions. The cranial base release is particularly useful for treating headaches (see Chapter 8).
- Cervical passive joint articulation may be beneficial for facet joint lesions (see Chapter 7). Techniques include:
  - cervical lateral flexion
  - cervical rotation
  - cervical extension
  - horizontal traction
  - stair-step technique
  - facet rotation
  - facet lateral flexion.
- Vascular headaches are usually treated with a cold compress to the head and sub-occipital area and heat to lower back, legs or feet. For non-vascular headaches, thermotherapy may be beneficial for hypertonic posterior cervical muscles and upper trapezius.
- Longer-term treatment addresses any underlying conditions or predisposing factors including scoliosis, hyperlordosis, hyperkyphosis, muscle tightness or weakness.

Remedial massage treatments may also include aromatherapy, acupressure, reflexology and Bowen therapy. Although little scientific evidence is available to support their use, these

Table 13.3 Examples of research into the effectiveness of remedial massage therapy for headache

Review	Research design	Review opinion
Chaibi & Russell[20]	Systematic review of six randomised controlled trials for primary chronic headaches (tension-type headaches)	The randomised controlled trials suggest that massage and physiotherapy are effective treatment options in the management of chronic tension-type headaches. Future manual therapy randomised controlled trials are requested addressing the efficacy in chronic migraine with and without medication overuse. Future randomised controlled trials on headache should adhere to the International Headache Society's guidelines for clinical trials (i.e. frequency as primary end-point, while duration and intensity should be secondary end-point, avoid co-intervention, include sufficient sample size and follow-up period for at least 6 months).
Cumplido-Transmonte et al[43]	Systematic review of 10 randomised controlled trials	According to these studies, manual therapy improves symptoms, increasing patients' wellbeing and improving the outcome measures analysed. Manual therapy has positive effects on pain intensity, pain frequency, disability, overall impact, quality of life, and craniocervical range of motion in adults with tension-type headache. None of the techniques was found to be superior to the others; combining different techniques seems to be the most effective approach.
Gerber & Kumbhare[29]	Peer review of Moraska et al[19]	Overall this is the best study so far in assessing the effects of massage therapy in tension-type headache. The study suggests that trigger point release massage therapy may reduce headache frequency. The authors suggest that massage therapy should be considered an adjunct treatment and be combined with medications for the management of chronic tension-type headache. Although the literature supporting massage therapy is not robust, it has no serious adverse effects and may have some positive impact upon central sensitisation.
Lopez et al[21]	Systematic review of 14 randomised control trials	According to our review, patients with tension-type headache receiving manual therapy show more favourable outcomes than patients receiving standard treatment or a placebo. Manual therapy seems to reduce headache frequency and intensity and improve patients' quality of life but does not lead to a decrease in analgesic use. However, our conclusions must be interpreted with caution due to the heterogeneity of study designs, measurement tools, and treatments.
Moore et al[18]	A critical review of 35 papers which met their criteria	The use of manual therapy appears to be the most common non-medical treatment utilised for the management of common recurrent headaches. The authors concluded that there is a need for more rigorous public health and health services research in order to assess the role, safety, utilisation and financial costs associated with manual therapy treatment for headache. For massage therapy, patient self-reporting of partially effective or fully effective headache relief ranged from 33.0–64.5%.

techniques are often used in clinical practice. They are part of the range of techniques available to remedial massage therapists when negotiating treatment plans with clients. They can be integrated into the treatment plan in a number of ways. For example, an essential oil blend may be used as the lubricant in Swedish massage (5 drops in 10 mL of carrier oil) or vapourised in an oil-burner during the treatment. In its traditional form, Bowen is a stand-alone therapy, but a derivative form is presented here which may be integrated with other remedial techniques (although it usually follows Swedish massage). Acupressure is often integrated with Swedish massage.

Aromatherapy

Essential oils that may relieve headaches include roman chamomile, geranium, lavender, sweet marjoram, peppermint, rose rosemary and sage.[30] A study with a small sample size recently found that migraine patients who had aromatherapy had significantly lower pain levels than the migraine control group.[31] Essential oils used for their pharmacological pain management actions are: eucalyptus, lavender, German chamomile, manuka, sweet marjoram, dwarf pine, rosemary and ginger.[32]

Acupressure

Gentle pressure is applied on each acupuncture point for 10 seconds. Points for headache include (see Figure 13.2 on p 236):

- Colon 4 (midway along 2nd metacarpal, thumb side) for tension, headache, sinusitis
- Liver 3 (between first and second toes, 3 fingerbreadths proximal to web on dorsal aspect of foot) for tension, hypertension, urogenital problems
- Facial acupressure headache points (Bladder 1 and 2, Colon 20, Triple Heater 3)
- Suboccipital points (Gall Bladder 20).

Reflexology

Reflexologists use points associated with the head, neck and the underlying cause or predisposing factors of the headache if known (e.g. sinus points for sinusitis or adrenal glands for stress). Techniques include mild pressure directly on the reflex point using fingers, thumbs or knuckles, and *caterpillars* (a stroke involving repeated flexion and extension of the inter-phalangeal joint of the thumb) (see Figure 13.3 on p 237).

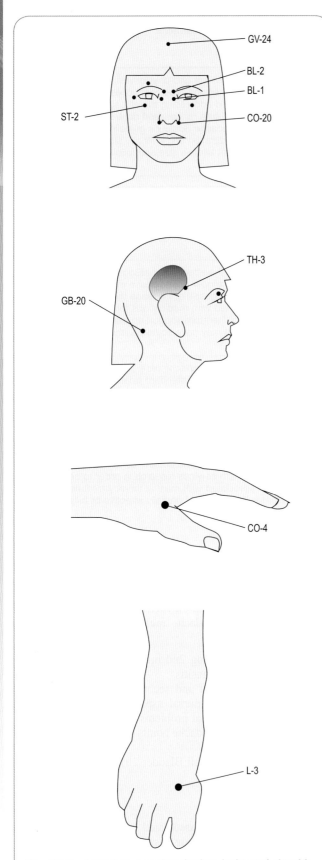

Fig. 13.2 **Acupressure points for headache and sinusitis**

The headache technique (derived from Bowen)

The client lies supine. Sit at the head of the table (see Figure 13.4 on p 237)

1. Using tips of middle fingers, apply light pressure to the inner corner of each eye (Position 1). Avoid any contact with the eye. Hold for 2 seconds. Take up Position 2 before releasing Position 1.
2. Using tips of index fingers, apply light pressure to the inner corner of the eyebrows (Position 2). Hold for 2 seconds. Take up Position 3 before releasing Position 2.
3. Use tips of thumbs, apply light pressure in the middle of the forehead at the hairline (Position 3). Hold for 2 seconds. Take up Position 4 before releasing Position 3.
4. Using the tips of the ring finger or little finger, apply light pressure over the temples (Position 4). Hold for 2 seconds. Take up Position 1 again before releasing Position 4.
   Repeat this procedure (applying light pressure from Position 1, 2, 3 to 4) four times.
5. Apply pressure to Position 4 for 5 seconds using the heels of both hands.

Client education

Client education includes recommendations for self-help such as stress management and avoidance of migraine triggers. Posture advice includes avoiding sustained neck flexion (e.g. when reading or working at a computer) and correcting ergonomics for desk work. The desk should be at elbow height. Office furniture ergonomic design needs to be adjustable to accommodate for individual variance. The top of the screen should be level with or slightly lower than the eyes (see Chapter 12, Figure 12.20).[33]

Home exercises

Lying supine with a rolled towel placed horizontally under the neck may be helpful. Fold a towel in half lengthways and roll it up tightly. Place the rolled towel behind the neck between the head and the shoulders. The height of the roll can be adjusted by unrolling the towel to the most comfortable height. The position should be painless and able to be maintained for 15–20 minutes. A cold compress (for vascular headache) or heat pack (for cervicogenic headache) can be placed over the towel if indicated.

Stretches and strengthening exercises should be prescribed for specific muscles and commenced as soon as possible. Isometric contractions usually begin when full range of motion has been restored. Strengthening exercises can progress to range of motion exercises performed with the chest and neck over the edge of a bench. Such exercises use resistance against gravity to build strong neck muscles that can support and protect the cervical spine in the same way that strong core muscles support the lumbar spine.

SINUSITIS

The paranasal sinuses are air-filled spaces in the bones of the face (frontal, maxillary, ethmoid and sphenoid) (see Figure 13.5 on p 237). They lighten the skull, produce mucus to moisten inspired air and provide a resonance chamber for

Fig. 13.3 Reflexology charts

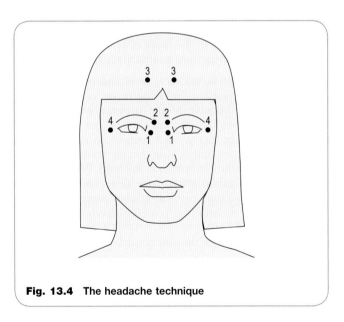

Fig. 13.4 The headache technique

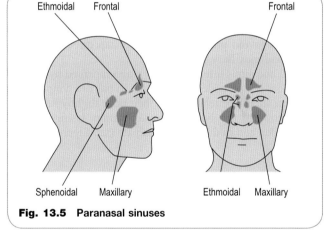

Fig. 13.5 Paranasal sinuses

voice production. Sinusitis refers to inflammation of the paranasal sinuses from over-production of mucus or a swelling of the lining of the sinuses and nose, which causes nasal obstruction and headache. It commonly accompanies a nasal infection but may also be an allergic response to such allergens as pollens or dairy products. It is also associated with cigarette smoking.

ASSESSMENT OF THE CLIENT WITH SINUS PAIN

Assessment of clients for sinusitis focuses on case history, observation and palpation.

Case history

Sinusitis is usually identified by case history. Infection of the frontal sinuses often produces headache that typically reaches a peak within 2 or 3 hours after rising and then subsides through the day. A purulent nasal or postnasal discharge is usually present. Clients describe a feeling of pressure in the head. Infection in the maxillary sinuses may be mistaken for toothache.[34, 35] An allergic rather than microbial cause is suggested if the client reports sneezing and watery rhinorrhoea and has no systemic signs, such as fever or malaise.

Headaches attributed to disorders of the nose or paranasal sinuses or rhinosinusitis headaches were previously known as sinus headaches. Rhinosinusitis headaches may be acute or chronic. The International Headache Society[8] describe the following diagnostic criteria for acute rhinosinusitis headache:

A. Any headache fulfilling criterion C
B. Clinical, nasal endoscopic and/or imaging evidence of acute rhinosinusitis
C. Evidence of causation demonstrated by at least two of the following:
　1. headache has developed in temporal relation to the onset of rhinosinusitis
　2. either or both of the following:
　　a) headache has significantly worsened in parallel with worsening of the rhinosinusitis
　　b) headache has significantly improved or resolved in parallel with improvement in or resolution of the rhinosinusitis
　3. headache is exacerbated by pressure applied over the paranasal sinuses
　4. in the case of a unilateral rhinosinusitis, headache is localised and ipsilateral to it
D. Not better accounted for by another ICHD-3 diagnosis.[8]

Observation

Nasal congestion is often apparent in the client's breathing and speech. Facial signs of allergic responses (atopic facies) such as dark circles under the eyes and watery eyes may be present.

Palpation

Tenderness is often reported on pressure over the affected sinuses. Press in a superior direction on the frontal and maxillary areas (avoid pressure on eyes) or tap directly over the frontal and maxillary sinuses.[36]

Nasal and sinus infection is often accompanied by swollen and tender lymph nodes in the neck. To palpate lymph nodes the client should be relaxed with their neck slightly flexed and rotated towards the side of the examination. Using the pads of the index and middle fingers palpate (see Figure 13.6):

- pre-auricular nodes – in front of the ear
- posterior auricular nodes – superficial to the mastoid process
- occipital nodes – at the base of the skull posteriorly
- tonsillar nodes – at the angle of the mandible
- submaxillary nodes – halfway between the angle and the tip of the mandible
- submental nodes – in the midline behind the tip of the mandible
- superficial cervical nodes – superficial to the sternocleidomastoid muscle
- posterior cervical chain – along the anterior edge of the trapezius
- deep cervical chain – deep to the sternocleidomastoid muscle (often inaccessible). Hook thumb and fingers around either side of the sternocleidomastoid muscle to find them (caution: the carotid artery and internal jugular vein are deep to the sternocleidomastoid muscle)
- supraclavicular – deep in the angle formed by the clavicle and the sternocleidomastoid muscle.

Note that non-tender nodes are frequently found in healthy people. Unexplained enlarged or tender nodes should be referred for further examination.

REMEDIAL MASSAGE TREATMENT FOR SINUSITIS

Remedial massage therapy for sinusitis is designed to help reduce sinus congestion and thereby bring about symptom relief. Eliminating the infection or exposure to allergens is required for resolution of the cause of inflammation.

A typical remedial massage treatment for sinusitis includes:

- Swedish massage to the face, head and neck. Note that sinusitis sufferers often find lying prone very uncomfortable, not only because of the pressure exerted by the massage table on the affected sinuses, but also because Swedish massage therapy that focuses on relaxation and muscle techniques rather than lymph drainage tends to increase lymphatic congestion in the head. Prone neck and head massage should observe the direction of lymphatic drainage; that is, from cervical spinous processes *laterally* and *inferiorly* towards the posterior cervical chains and supraclavicular nodes.
- Remedial massage for sinusitis consists of lymphatic drainage to the neck and head and gentle pressures on the frontal bone and maxilla designed to open the frontal and maxillary sinuses.

Lymphatic drainage of the neck and head

Lymphatic drainage is described in detail in Chapter 9. A modified version of lymphatic drainage for the neck and head is described here. As with all lymphatic drainage the techniques are applied:

- slowly
- lightly
- monotonously (i.e. a high frequency of repetitions)
- with changes in pressure (i.e. pumping lymphatic fluid is achieved by alternating between pressure on and off with the fingers)
- in the direction of lymphatic flow (see Figure 13.7 on p 239).

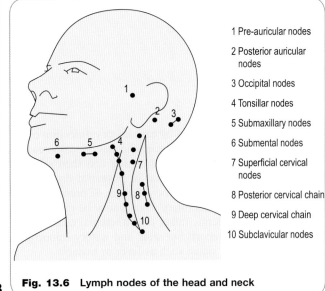

1 Pre-auricular nodes

2 Posterior auricular nodes

3 Occipital nodes

4 Tonsillar nodes

5 Submaxillary nodes

6 Submental nodes

7 Superficial cervical nodes

8 Posterior cervical chain

9 Deep cervical chain

10 Subclavicular nodes

Fig. 13.6 Lymph nodes of the head and neck

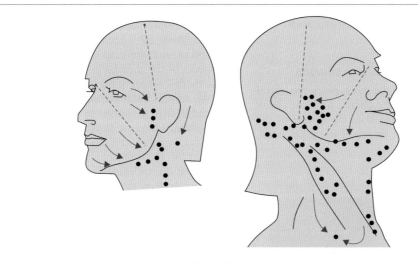

Fig. 13.7 Direction of lymphatic drainage in the neck and head

1. LYMPHATIC PUMP OVER THE STERNUM

Begin and end all lymphatic drainage with a lymphatic pump. The client lies supine. Stand at the head of the table. With one hand on top of the other or side by side, place palms over the sternum or upper chest, fingers pointed inferiorly. Passively move hands up and down with the client's breathing. Ask the client to breathe deeply through the mouth. At the end of one full expiration by the client, maintain enough pressure on the sternum to prevent the rib cage rising as the client inhales. Towards the end of the inhalation, release the pressure as quickly as possible by jumping the hands off the sternum. The client usually makes an involuntary gasping sound as the lungs suddenly expand. Note the difference between a lymphatic pump and the technique used in cardiopulmonary resuscitation: there is no attempt to depress the sternum beyond its natural level at the end of a forced expiration. This technique is contraindicated in clients with osteoporosis.

2. LYMPHATIC DRAINAGE OF THE HEAD AND NECK

The client is supine with slight elevation of the head (use a pillow or adjust the headpiece) to assist lymphatic drainage. Treatment begins with lymphatic drainage of the neck.

- Apply gentle pressure to the supraclavicular nodes for 10–15 seconds.
- Using fingertips, make spiral movements or stationary circles up the cervical chains (via the sternocleidomastoid muscle) towards the mastoid process, breaking contact to move in small increments along the muscle. At each point of contact, repeat the spiral/circular movement 5 to 7 times, making sure the pressure varies with each application (*pressure on–pressure off*).
- Drain the cervical chain towards the suprasternal nodes using a light pumping or stripping movement of the thumb or fingers. Pressure variation is achieved by slightly firmer stripping strokes draining inferiorly, followed by lighter return strokes. To pump the lymph, alternately apply gentle pressure with the fingers and release it moving progressively inferiorly along the sternocleidomastoid.

Repeat this procedure several times. Apply a similar procedure from the mastoid process along the base of the occiput to the midline and drain back towards the posterior auricular nodes.

3. LYMPHATIC DRAINAGE OF THE FACE

- Apply gentle pressure to the pre-auricular nodes for 10–15 seconds.
- Apply spirals or stationary circles away from the pre-auricular nodes in three sections:
    i) towards the midline of the mandible (include tonsillar, submaxillary and submental nodes)
    ii) towards the nose
    iii) towards the midline of the forehead.
- At each point of contact, repeat the spiral/circular movement 5 to 7 times, making sure pressure varies with each application (*pressure on–pressure off*). Break contact to move in small increments towards the midline of the face.
- Drain lymph towards pre-auricular glands using thumb or fingers to strip or pump towards the ears. Use a slightly firmer drainage stroke and a lighter return stroke to vary the pressure when using a stripping technique. To pump the lymph, alternately apply gentle pressure with the fingertips and release it, moving progressively towards the pre-auricular nodes.

Repeat this procedure several times. The technique can also be applied to submaxillary nodes halfway between the chin and angle of the mandible. Lymph is drained from the sides of the nose towards the submaxillary nodes.

4. REPEAT THE LYMPHATIC PUMP DESCRIBED IN 1

Another useful lymphatic drainage technique for the neck is known as the *claw technique*. The client lies supine. Stand at the side of the table facing superiorly. With fingers spread so that the index finger is at C1–2 level and the little finger is at C6–C7 level just lateral to the spinous processes on the contra-lateral side, slowly draw the fingers anteriorly and inferiorly, flattening the fingers as they reach the sternocleidomastoid muscle and draining towards the supraclavicular nodes (see Figure 13.8). Repeat several times.

Opening the frontal and maxillary sinuses

- Standing or sitting at the side of the table, place the lateral aspect of the cephalad thumb on the client's forehead (hook under the supraorbital ridges) and hold the bridge of the nose with the thumb and index finger of the other hand.

Fig. 13.8 Claw technique

Make sure your hand is not covering the client's nose or mouth. Apply superior pressure with the contact on the frontal bone for 5 seconds (Figure 13.9a).
- Stand or sit at the head of the table. Using either the lateral aspects of the thumbs or tips of the fingers, hook around the medial aspect of the zygomatic arches either side of the nose. Apply lateral pressure for 5 seconds (Figure 13.9b).
- Stand or sit at the corner of the top of the table. Using either the lateral aspects of the thumbs or the tips of fingers, hook around the supraorbital ridge with one hand and the medial aspect of the opposite zygomatic arch with the other. Caution: do not contact eyes. Apply diagonal pressure for 5 seconds. Repeat on the other side (see Figures 13.9c).

Other remedial massage techniques for sinusitis include:

Aromatherapy

Essential oils for sinusitis include eucalyptus, clove bud, lavender, organic lemon, pine needle and tea tree.[37] They can be vapourised in an oil burner during the massage, or recommended to the client for use in steam inhalations at home (5 drops of essential oil in a bowl containing 1 litre of steaming water, head covered with a towel, leaning over the bowl with eyes shut and inhaling). Alternatively, 5 drops of essential oil can be added to bath water just before turning off the taps.

Acupressure

Acupressure can be integrated into the massage at any stage. Gently apply digital pressure for 10 seconds to the following

Fig. 13.9 Opening the frontal and maxillary sinuses

acupressure points: Bladder 1, Bladder 2, Colon 20, Triple heater 3, Colon 4, Gall bladder 20 (see Figure 13.2 on p 236). Note that pressure over the sinuses may cause pain if the sinuses are acutely inflamed. Always work within the client's pain tolerance.

Reflexology

Reflexologists use reflex points associated with the head, neck and underlying cause or predisposing factors if known. Mild pressure can be applied directly on the reflex point using fingers, thumbs or knuckles (see Figure 13.3 on p 237).

Client education

Advise clients to address the cause of the sinusitis if possible (e.g. pharmaceutical treatment for bacterial infection, allergy testing, avoiding allergens). Traditional treatments include increased daily water intake and steam inhalations. Where appropriate, refer clients to *Quit Smoking* programs.

HOME EXERCISES

Ocean swimming may help drain the sinuses.

TEMPOROMANDIBULAR JOINT DISORDERS

The temporomandibular joint (TMJ) is the most used joint in the body. It opens and closes approximately 1500–2000 times a day. It is a condylar joint formed between the mandibular fossa of the temporal bone and the condyle of the mandible and covered in white fibrocartilage. The TMJ is surrounded by fibrous capsule lined with synovial membrane. The capsular ligaments lie medially and laterally: the meniscotemporomandibular frenum (retrodiscal pad) lies posteriorly. Further posteriorly and medially are the stylomandibular and sphenomandibular ligaments (Figure 13.10). Three muscles

(temporalis, masseter and medial pterygoid) close the mouth and provide the power to bite and chew; one muscle, lateral pterygoid, opens the mouth (see Table 13.4). Opening is achieved by a combination of rotation and gliding. A disc divides the joint into an upper part for rotation and a lower part for glide. The dual heads of the lateral pterygoid muscle act asynchronously, the upper head hinging the head of the mandible and the lower head pulling the mandible forward.

DISORDERS OF THE TEMPOROMANDIBULAR JOINT

It is estimated that 33% of the population have at least one temporomandibular disorder symptom.[38] Clients are often young adults aged 20–40 years. Females with TMJ dysfunction seek treatment more commonly than males and their symptoms are less likely to improve.[38, 39] Causes of TMJ disorders include trauma, wear and tear, behavioural factors like grinding teeth and regularly chewing gum and malocclusion.

Temporomandibular joint disorders include three main groups:

1. Muscle disorders (the most common TMJ disorder).
2. Derangement disorders (e.g. dislocated jaw, displacement or distortion of the disc). *Clicking jaw* occurs when the condyle of the mandible overrides an anteromedially *displaced disc.* In some cases, the disc may become so distorted that it stops the condyle from translating forwards and locks the jaw closed (see Figure 13.11 on p 242).
3. Conditions like arthritis which causes destruction of cartilage overlaying the TMJ.

ASSESSMENT OF THE CLIENT WITH TMJ DISORDER

Because the biomechanics of the TMJ, cervical spine and cranium are interconnected, assessment of the TMJ also involves assessment of the neck and head.

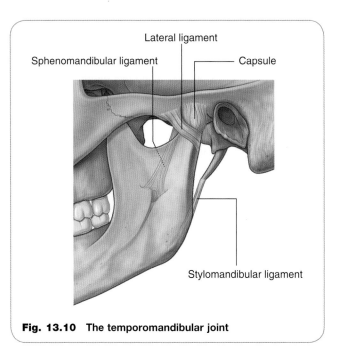

Lateral ligament

Sphenomandibular ligament

Capsule

Stylomandibular ligament

Fig. 13.10 The temporomandibular joint

Table 13.4 Muscles that move the jaw

Muscle	Origin	Insertion	Action
Temporalis	temporal bone	coronoid process of mandible	elevates and retracts mandible
Masseter	maxilla and zygomatic arch	angle and ramus of mandible	elevates mandible
Medial pterygoid	medial surface of lateral pterygoid plate of sphenoid	angle and ramus of mandible	elevates and protrudes mandible, moves mandible from side to side
Lateral pterygoid	greater wing and lateral surface of lateral plate of sphenoid bone	lower head: condyle of mandible Upper head: disc and fibrous capsule	protrudes mandible, opens mouth, moves mandible from side to side

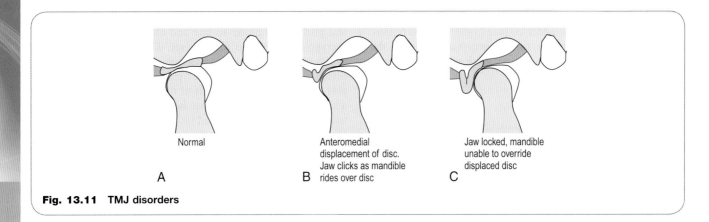

Fig. 13.11 TMJ disorders

Normal

A

Anteromedial displacement of disc. Jaw clicks as mandible rides over disc

B

Jaw locked, mandible unable to override displaced disc

C

Case history

Clients almost always give the diagnosis in the history. Presenting symptoms include sharp unilateral facial pain on movement of the jaw, pain increasing as the mouth is opened, difficulty chewing, clicking jaw and sometimes ear symptoms (pain, impaired hearing, tinnitus), neuralgia and headache. The International Headache Society[8] describes the following characteristics of headache due to TMJ disorder:

A. Any headache fulfilling criterion C
B. Clinical evidence of a painful pathological process affecting elements of the temporomandibular joint(s), muscles of mastication and/or associated structures on one or both sides
C. Evidence of causation demonstrated by at least two of the following:
   1. the headache has developed in temporal relation to the onset of the temporomandibular disorder, or led to its discovery
   2. the headache is aggravated by jaw motion, jaw function (e.g. chewing) and/or jaw parafunction (e.g. bruxism)
   3. the headache is provoked on physical examination by temporalis muscle palpation and/or passive movement of the jaw
D. Not better accounted for by another ICHD-3 diagnosis.[8]

Observation

Observe the mandible in motion and at rest. At rest the teeth are usually not in contact. On closure, teeth are in apposition with the spaces between the upper and lower central incisors aligned.

Postural analysis

TMJ dysfunction may be associated with forward head carriage and myofascial restrictions (e.g. restrictions of the deep front line, superficial back line and spiral line[40]) which may be detected during postural observation.

Functional tests

ACTIVE RANGE OF MOTION TESTS OF THE CERVICAL SPINE (FLEXION, EXTENSION, LATERAL FLEXION, ROTATION)

If any active range of motion tests of the cervical spine are positive, further assessment of the cervical spine is indicated (see Chapter 12).

Table 13.5   Resisted and length tests for muscles of the TMJ

	Resisted test	Test for contracture
Closing the mouth ■ medial pterygoid ■ temporalis ■ masseter	Ask the client to open their mouth. Place the web between your thumb and index finger on the mandible below the level of the teeth. Resist as the client tries to close their mouth.	Limited mouth opening (i.e. unable to place three fingers vertically between upper and lower teeth).
Opening the mouth ■ lateral pterygoid	Hold the client's mandible at the chin and resist mouth opening.	Inability to bring the teeth together.

ACTIVE RANGE OF MOTION OF THE TMJ

- Mandibular depression (opening): clients should be able to open their mouth wide enough for three fingers to be inserted vertically between the incisors.
- Mandibular elevation (closing): the upper and lower teeth should touch.
- Mandibular protrusion: the mandible should protrude far enough for the lower teeth to be placed in front of the upper teeth.
- Mandibular retraction.

RESISTED RANGE OF MOTION OF THE TMJ

It is difficult to isolate muscles of the TMJ because their actions overlap. Consequently, muscles are tested in groups (see Table 13.5).

Palpation

The masseter muscle is easily located in the cheeks when clients clench their teeth. With the muscle relaxed, palpate from the zygomatic arch to the angle of the mandible. Palpating bilaterally enables comparison of the muscles on either side.

Palpate the temporalis muscle in the temporal fossa. Palpate from its superior aspect inferiorly and feel the muscle as it gathers to pass beneath the zygomatic arch. Linear fibrotic tissue may be palpable superiorly to the zygomatic arch, and often anteriorly. To palpate the attachment of temporalis on the coronoid process, have the client open their mouth. Temporalis may be palpable at the coronoid process immediately beneath the zygomatic arch when the client's mouth is open.

Accessibility of lateral pterygoid for palpation is undertaken using the following technique: place a gloved index finger in the client's mouth between the buccal mucosa and the superior gum and point the tip of the finger posteriorly past the last molar to the neck of the mandible. As the client opens their mouth lateral pterygoid is palpable as it tightens against the practitioner's finger.[41]

The following techniques may be used to palpate the TMJ:

i) Place index and middle fingers just anterior to the ears and ask the client to open and close their mouth. Observe the degree of opening, lateral deviation and synchronicity of movement of both temporomandibular joints.

ii) Place gloved index fingers into client's ears and palpate anteriorly as the client opens and closes their mouth.

Fig. 13.12 Myofascial releasing techniques for the temporomandibular joint

REMEDIAL MASSAGE TREATMENTS FOR TMJ DISORDERS

If acute inflammation is present, treatment usually involves cryotherapy or anti-inflammatory medication. There is evidence to suggest that massage and targeted exercises may help provide short-term relief for acute temporomandibular disorders although the evidence is limited.[39, 42] Introduce gentle range of motion exercises as soon as they can be tolerated by the client. A typical remedial massage treatment for a mild or moderate TMJ disorder includes:

- Swedish massage therapy to the upper back, neck, head and face.
- Remedial massage techniques for muscle overload and/or muscle strains, including (see Table 13.6 on p 244):
  - deep gliding frictions along the muscle fibres
  - cross-fibre frictions
  - active and passive soft tissue releasing techniques
  - deep transverse frictions
  - trigger point therapy
  - muscle stretches.
- Myofascial releasing techniques may be beneficial for fascial restrictions (see Figure 13.12).

Client education

Advise clients that most TMJ disorders are temporary and resolve with simple conservative treatment. Avoid hard foods, cut food into small pieces, chew using molars on both sides and avoid chewing gum. Thermotherapy may relieve muscle spasm and pain. Correcting forward head carriage and other posture distortions will improve the biomechanics of the region. Refer to a chiropractor, osteopath or physiotherapist for osseous manipulation. Some clients may require dental splinting. Stress management may be indicated to eliminate teeth clenching and grinding.

HOME EXERCISE PROGRAM

Ask the client to stand in front of a mirror and slowly open and close their mouth making sure the jaw moves in a straight line.

Within pain tolerance they should try to correct any deviations they observe. Specific stretching exercises (see Table 13.6 on p 244) and strengthening exercises (resisting TMJ opening, closing or translating to the side) can be performed as required.

KEY MESSAGES

HEADACHE

- Remedial massage therapy has a key role to play in the treatment and management of headache: in cases of cervicogenic headache and tension-type headache remedial massage may be the primary treatment; in other types of headache remedial massage may be a useful adjunct to other treatments.
- Assessment of clients with headache involves history, outcome measures, postural analysis, functional tests (including resisted tests for specific muscles of the neck and face), special tests for the cervical spine and palpation.
- Case history is particularly important for identifying red flags. There are many different types of headaches, but only rarely are they the result of a serious pathology. Red flags include:[6]
  - Abrupt onset of headache
  - New onset or headache pattern especially when <5 y old or >50 y old
  - Neurologic signs or symptoms
  - Head or neck trauma
  - Fever
  - Weight loss
  - Systemic disease
  - Pregnancy
  - Headaches triggered by exertion, sexual activity, cough, or Valsalva
  - Postural headaches
- Consider Clinical Guidelines, available evidence and client preferences when planning therapy. Current evidence supports the use of manual therapy for migraine, tension-type

Table 13.6 Remedial massage for muscles of the TMJ

Muscle	Soft-tissue releasing techniques	Trigger point	Client education	Stretch
Temporalis	Apply pressure to site of muscle lesion as client slowly opens and closes their mouth.		■ Correct forward head posture. ■ Avoid excessive chewing, clenching and grinding teeth, chewing gum, biting hard food. ■ Reduce stress.	■ Open mouth as far as possible; pull the jaw downward and to the opposite side.
Masseter	As above		As above	As above
Medial pterygoid	As above		As above	■ Open mouth as far as possible. ■ With the web between the thumb and index finger, gently push the chin posteriorly. ■ Move jaw to the side as far as possible.
Lateral pterygoid	As above		■ Avoid excessive chewing, clenching and grinding teeth, chewing gum, biting hard food. ■ Reduce stress. ■ May need occlusal splint.	■ With the web between the thumb and index finger, gently push the chin posteriorly. ■ Move jaw to the side as far as possible.

and cervicogenic headaches as part of a multimodal treatment plan.

■ Be conservative in treatment: if in doubt, refer for further investigation.

■ Remedial massage treatment aims to optimise muscle function, improve facet joint movement, release myofascial restrictions, provide relaxation therapy and educate clients about self-management of headaches.

SINUSITIS

■ Remedial massage therapy may provide symptomatic relief for sinusitis sufferers but does not address causative factors (e.g. infections, allergies).

■ Assessment of clients with sinusitis involves case history, outcome measures, observation and palpation. Be vigilant for red flags, particularly if clients present with headache, although they are unlikely.

- Consider Clinical Guidelines, available evidence and client preferences when planning therapy.
- Remedial massage treatment aims to relieve sinus congestion and to educate clients about self-management of sinusitis.

TEMPOROMANDIBULAR JOINT

- Assessment of clients with TMJ disorders involves history, outcome measures, postural analysis, functional tests (including functional tests of the cervical region and the TMJ) and palpation.
- Consider Clinical Guidelines, available evidence and client preferences when planning therapy.
- Remedial massage may provide symptom relief for mild to moderate TMJ disorders by optimising function in muscles that move the jaw, releasing myofascial restrictions, providing relaxation therapy and educating clients about self-management of TMJ disorders.

Review questions

Headache

1. List five red flags for serious causes of headache.
2. What are the main characteristics of migraine headaches (e.g. location, type of pain, chronicitiy, duration)?
3. What percentage of migraine sufferers experience an aura? What symptoms might they have?
4. How would you distinguish between a vascular and a cervicogenic headache?
5. How can remedial massage assist in the treatment of tension-type headache?
6. Indicate the correct answer by circling True or False:
   i) The most common type of headache is cervicogenic. True/False
   ii) Migraines often strike in the middle of the night. True/False
   iii) Tension-type headaches last no more than 1 or 2 days. True/False
   iv) Rhinosinusitis headache is aggravated by bending forward. True/False
   v) Cervicogenic headaches typically start at the back of the neck and radiate over the head to the forehead. True/False
7. List three important questions that you would include in history taking to help eliminate the possibility of a pathological headache or other headache requiring referral.

Sinusitis

1. Where are the paranasal sinuses located?
2. Name two common causes of sinusitis.

3. What is the role of remedial massage in the treatment of sinusitis?
4. Swedish massage can increase lymphatic congestion in the head. How would you modify your Swedish massage treatment to minimise this effect?
5. What home advice would you give a client with sinusitis?

Temporomandibular joint disorder

1. Describe how lateral pterygoid acts to open the jaw.
2. List four symptoms that can be associated with TMJ dysfunction.
3. A client with normal range of motion of the TMJ should be able to:
   i) Open their mouth wide enough to _____
   ii) Protrude their jaw far enough to _____
4. Draw the pain referral patterns for the following trigger points.

5. What home advice would you give a client with a clicking jaw?

APPENDIX 13.1

MIDAS (The Migraine Disability Assessment Test)[44]

The MIDAS (migraine disability assessment) questionnaire was put together to help you measure the impact your headaches have had on your life over the last 3 months and to communicate this more effectively. The best way to do this is by counting the numbers of days of your life which are affected by headaches. You can do this for yourself as follows:

Please complete questions about ALL your headaches you have had over the last month. Leave the box set to zero if you did not do the activity in the last three months.

For questions 1 and 2, **work or school** means paid work or education if you are a student at school or college. For Questions 3 and 4, **household work** means activities such as housework, home repairs and maintenance, shopping as well as caring for children and relatives.

INSTRUCTIONS • Please answer the following questions about ALL your headaches you have had over the last 3 months. Select your answer in the box next to each question. If a single headache affects more than one area of your life (e.g. work and family life) it is counted more than once. Select zero if you did not have the activity in the last 3 months.

1. On how many days in the last 3 months did you miss work or school because of your headaches? `0`

2. How many days in the last 3 months was your productivity at work or school reduced by half or more because of your headaches?
(Do not include days you counted in question 1 where you missed work or school.) `0`

3. On how many days in the last 3 months did you not do household work because of your headaches? `0`

4. How many days in the last three months was your productivity in household work reduced by half or more because of your headaches?
(Do not include days you counted in question 3 where you did not do household work.) `0`

5. On how many days in the last 3 months did you miss family, social or leisure activities because of your headaches? `0`

What your doctor will need to know about your headache:

A. On how many days in the last 3 months did you have a headache?
(If a headache lasted more than 1 day, count each day.) `0`

B. On a scale of 0 to 10, on average how painful were these headaches?
(where 0 = no pain at all and 10 = pain as bad as it can be.) `0`

Please enter your e-mail address if you would also like an e-mail copy of the results.
(Leave this box blank if you do not need a copy.)

Calculate my Score

REFERENCES

1. GBD 2016 Headache Collaborators. Global, regional, and national burden of migraine and tension-type headache, 1990–2016: A systematic analysis for the Global Burden of Disease Study 2016. Lancet 2018;17:954–76.
2. Deloitte Access Economics. Migraine in Australia Whitepaper. Canberra: Deloitte Access Economics Pty Ltd; 2018.
3. Rizzoli P, Mullally WJ. Headache. Am J Med 2018;131:17–24.
4. Luedtke K, Boissonnault W, Caspersen N, et al. International consensus on the most useful physical examination tests used by physiotherapists for patients with headache: a Delphi study. Manual Ther 2016;23:17–24.
5. Hall T, Briffa K, Hopper D. Clinical evaluation of cervicogenic headache: a clinical perspective. J Man Manip Ther 2008;16(2):73–80.
6. Cady RK. Red flags and comfort signs for ominous secondary headaches. Otolaryngolog Clin 2014;47(2):289–99.
7. Vizniak N. Quick reference evidence-based conditions manual. 3rd edn. Burnaby, BC: Professional Health System; 2009.
8. International Headache Society. The international classification of headache disorders. 3rd edn. Cephalalgia 2018;38(1):1–211.
9. Woldeamanuel YW, Cowan RP. Migraine affects 1 in 10 people worldwide featuring recent rise: a systematic review and meta-analysis of community-based studies involving 6 million participants. J Neurol Sci 2017;372:307–15.

10. Knacktedt H, Bansevicius D, Aaseth K, et al. Cervicogenic headache in the general population: the Akershus study of chronic headache. Cephalalgia. 2010; 30(12):1468–76. https://doi.org/10.1177/0333102410368442.
11. Zito G, Jull G, Story I. Clinical tests of musculoskeletal dysfunction in the diagnosis of cervicogenic headache. Man Ther 2006;11(2):118–29.
12. Bogduk N. The neck and headaches. Neurol Clin 2014;32(2):471–87.
13. Brukner P, Khan K. Brukner & Khan's clinical sports medicine: injuries. Vol. 1. 5th ed. Sydney: McGraw-Hill Education; 2017.
14. Couturier E. Headache, gender and aging. Maturitas 2017;100:95.
15. Seller RH, Symons A. Differential diagnosis of common complaints. Philadelphia, PA: Saunders; 2018.
16. Halker R, Vargas B, Dodick DW. Cluster headache: diagnosis and treatment. Semin Neurol 2010;30(2):175–85.
17. Simons D, Travell J, Simons L. Myofascial pain and dysfunction: the trigger point manual. Vol 1: upper half of body. 2nd edn. Philadelphia: Williams and Wilkins; 1999.
18. Moore CS, Sibbritt DW, Adams J. A critical review of manual therapy use for headache disorders: prevalence, profiles, motivations, communication and self-reported effectiveness. BMC Neurol 2017;17:61. https://doi.org/10.1186/s12883-017-0835-0.

19. Moraska AF, Stenerson L, Butryn N, et al. Myofascial trigger point-focused head and neck massage for recurrent tension-type headache: a randomized, placebo-controlled clinical trial. Pain 2015;31(2):159–68.
20. Chaibi A, Russell MB. Manual therapies for primary chronic headaches: a systematic review of randomized controlled trials. J Headache Pain 2014;15:67. Doi:10.1186/1129-2377-15-67.
21. Lopez CL, Jimenez JM, de la Hoz Aizurua JL, et al. Efficacy of manual therapy in the treatment of tension-type headache. A systematic review from 2000 to 2013. Neurologia 2016;31(6):357–69.
22. Ferragut-Garcias A, Plaza-Manzano G, Rodriguez-Blanco C, et al. Effectiveness of a treatment involving soft tissue techniques and/or neural mobilization techniques in the management of tension-type headache: a randomized controlled trial. Arch Phys Med Rehabil 2017;98:211–19.
23. Kedia S. Complementary and integrative approaches for pediatric headache. Semin Pediatr Neurol 2016;23:44–52.
24. Bevilaqua-Grossi D, Goncalves MC, Carvalho GF, et al. Additional effects of a physical therapy protocol on headache frequency, pressure pain threshold, and improvement perception in patients with migraine and associated neck pain: a randomized controlled trial. Arch Phys Med Rehabil 2016;97:866–94.
25. Malo-Urries M, Tricas-Moreno JM, Estebanez-de-Miguel E, et al. Immediate effects of upper cervical translatoric mobilization on cervical mobility and

pressure pain threshold in patients with cervicogenic headache: a randomized controlled trial. J Manipulative Physiol Ther 2017;40(9):649–58.

26. Jaffari M, Bahrpeyma F, Togha M. Effect of ischemic compression for cervicogenic headache and elastic behavior of active trigger point in the sternocleidomastoid muscle using ultrasound imaging. J Bodyw Mov Ther 2016;21:933–9.

27. Ghanbari A, Askarzadeh S, Petramfar P, et al. 2015 Migraine responds better to a combination of medical therapy and trigger point management than routine medical therapy alone. Neuro Rehabil 2015;37(1):157–63.

28. Munksgaard SG, Jensen RH. Medication overuse headache. Headache. 2014;54(7):1251–7.

29. Gerber NL, Kumbhare D. Physiatry reviews for evidence in practice second-order peer review. Am J Phys Med Rehabil 2018;97(2):141–2. Doi: 10.1097/PHM.0000000000000833.

30. Wright K. A guide to headaches and migraines: symptoms, causes, treatment, prevention. Glasgow: Waverley Books; 2014.

31. Haryanto J, Kusnanto K, Suarllah I, et al. Aromatherapy decreases level of pain among patients who experience migraine. Jurnal Ners.

Online. Available: https://www.neliti.com/publications/115084/aromatherapy-decreases-level-of-pain-among-patients-who-experience-migrain; 2007.

32. Ali B, Al-Wabel NA, Shams S, et al. Essential oils used in aromatherapy: a systematic review. Asian Pac J Trop Biomed 2015;5(8):601–11.

33. Meinert M, Konig M, Jaschinski W. Web-based office ergonomics intervention on work-related complaints: a field study. Ergonomics 2013;56(11): 1658–68.

34. Douglas G, Nicol F, Robertson C. Macleod's clinical examination. 13th edn. Edinburgh: Churchill Livingstone; 2013.

35. Ferguson M. Rhinosinusitis in oral medicine and dentistry. Austral Dent J 2014;59:289–95.

36. Bickley L. Bates' guide to physical examination and history taking. 11th edn. Philadelphia: Lippincott-Raven; 2013.

37. Donato M. How to correctly use essential oils to help prevent flu and other illnesses. Organic Lifestyle Magazine. Online. Available: https://www.organiclifestylemagazine.com/how-to-correctly-use-essential-oils-to-help-prevent-the-flu-and-other-illnesses; 2015.

38. Wright EF. Manual of temporomandibular disorders. 3rd edn. Amos, IA: John Wiley & Sons; 2013.

39. Durham J, Newton-John TR, Zakrzewska JM. Temporomandibular disorders. BMJ 2015;350:h1154. Doi: 10.1136/bmj.h1154.

40. Myers T. Anatomy trains: myofascial meridians for manual and movement therapists. 3rd edn. Edinburgh: Churchill Livingstone; 2014.

41. Stelzenmueller W, Umstadt H, Weber D, et al. Digital palpation of the pterygoideus lateralis muscle. Manuelle Medizin 2016;54:212–18.

42. Amorim CS, Espirito Santo AS, Sommer M, et al. Effect of physical therapy in bruxism treatment: a systematic review. J Manipulative Physiol Ther 2018;41(5):389–404.

43. Cumplido-Trasmonte C, Fernández-González P, Alguacil-Diego I, et al. Manual therapy in adults with tension-type headache: a systematic review. Neurologia 2017; https://doi.org/10.1016/j.nrl.2017.12.004.

44. Stewart WF, Lipton RB, et al. Development and testing of the Migraine Disability Assessment (MIDAS) Questionnaire to assess headache-related disability. Neurology 2001;56(6 Suppl 1):S20–8.

14 The chest

INTRODUCTION

Musculoskeletal chest pain is chest pain that is aggravated by movement. Although chest complaints are an uncommon presenting condition in remedial massage clinics, tight chest muscles are frequently treated in upper crossed syndrome and in any presentation that involves a rounded shoulder posture. Remedial massage therapists are also called upon to assist in management of chronic respiratory conditions like chronic bronchitis and asthma. However, it is important to rule out serious and potentially life-threatening conditions of the cardiac, respiratory and gastrointestinal systems. Chest pain should not be assumed to be musculoskeletal until other causes have been excluded.[1] New chest pain, depending on its cause, may be associated with a high risk of death. A medical assessment may be required which includes a 12-lead electrocardiogram (ECG).[2]

FUNCTIONAL ANATOMY REVIEW

The configuration of the rib cage gives it the flexibility it needs for smooth inspiration and expiration. The sternum is made up of three bony parts: the manubrium, body and xiphoid process to which the diaphragm attaches. Ribs 1 to 10 have both bony and cartilaginous components. The cartilages are located anteriorly and extend approximately 5 to 8 cm from the sternum. The costal cartilages of the first seven pairs (the true ribs) attach directly to the sternum at the sternocostal joints. Ribs 8 to 12 are called false ribs because their costal cartilages attach to the sternum indirectly or not at all. The 11th and 12th ribs are also called floating ribs because they do not attach anteriorly to the sternum (see Figure 14.1 on p 249).

The biomechanics of the sternum and ribs are intimately related to the thoracic vertebrae. All 12 pairs of ribs attach posteriorly to the thoracic vertebrae. The upper ribs 1 to 8 attach to the correspondingly numbered vertebral body and its transverse process and to the vertebral body below. Ribs 9 to 12 attach to the correspondingly numbered vertebrae and transverse processes only.

At each level of the thoracic column, a pair of ribs is connected at two joints (see Figure 14.2 on p 249):

a) costovertebral joint, which is a synovial joint between the head of the rib, the intervertebral disc and the vertebral bodies. The facet on the rib head articulates with a facet of a single vertebra or demifacets of two adjacent vertebrae. An interosseous ligament attaches to the head of the rib between the two articular facets and to the intervertebral disc.

b) costotransverse joint, which is a synovial joint between the rib tubercle and the transverse process of the vertebra below. It is strengthened by three costotransverse ligaments (interosseous, posterior and anterior).

The vertebral bodies are joined by the anterior and posterior longitudinal ligaments. The anterior longitudinal ligament extends along the anterior surfaces of the bodies of the vertebrae; the posterior longitudinal ligament lies within the vertebral canal on the posterior surface of the vertebral bodies.

The ligamenta flava connect the laminae of adjacent vertebrae. These ligaments are thicker in the thoracic spine than in the cervical, and thickest of all in the lumbar spine. The supraspinous ligament connects the spines of C7 to the sacrum. It is thinner and narrower in the thoracic region than in the lumbar. In the cervical region it is replaced by ligamentum nuchae. The intertransverse ligaments are rounded cords that are intimately connected with the deep muscles of the back (see Figure 14.3).

Major muscles of the chest are illustrated in Table 14.1.

When the external intercostal muscles contract, the ribs move in a similar way to a bucket handle, thereby increasing the lateral and anterior dimensions of the rib cage. The vertical dimension of the rib cage increases as the diaphragm contracts and flattens its dome. These muscle contractions, and the increase in chest size that follows, cause a fall in intrapleural pressure and the lungs are forced to expand. Intrapulmonary pressure drops below atmospheric pressure and air moves into the lungs. When the diaphragm and external intercostal muscles relax, the thoracic cavity decreases and the lungs recoil creating an increase in intrapulmonary pressure (above atmospheric pressure), and air leaves the lungs.

Fig. 14.1 **Rib cage**

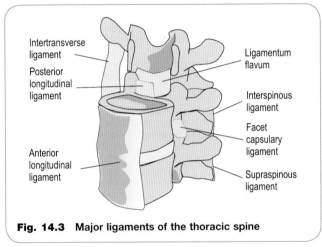

Fig. 14.3 **Major ligaments of the thoracic spine**

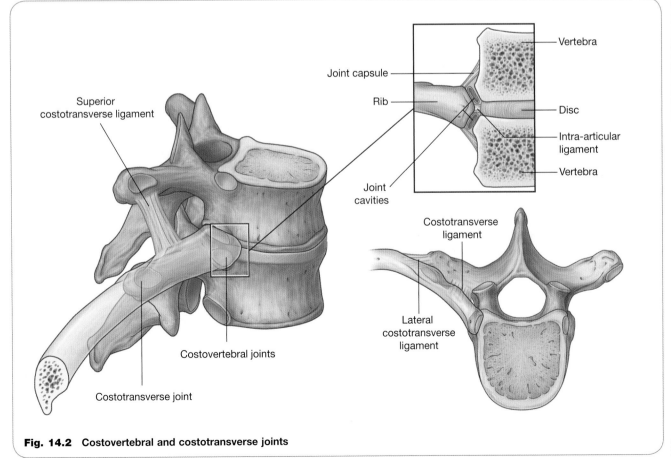

Fig. 14.2 **Costovertebral and costotransverse joints**

Table 14.1   Muscles of the chest

Muscle	Origin	Insertion	Action
Pectoralis major	Clavicular head: clavicle Sternal head: sternum and costal cartilages of ribs 2 to 6	Greater tubercle and intertubercular sulcus of the humerus	Together both parts flex and anteriorly adduct the humerus at the shoulder joint, The sternal part also internally rotates the humerus at the shoulder joint
Pectoralis minor	Ribs 2 to 5 (sometimes ribs 2 to 4 or ribs 3 to 5)	Coracoid process of the scapula	Protracts and abducts the scapula, elevates the ribs to which it attaches when the scapula is fixed as in forced inspiration
Intercostal muscles			
External intercostal	Inferior border of rib	Superior border of rib below	Elevates ribs at the sternocostal and costovertebral joints
Internal intercostal	Inner surface of rib	Inferior border of rib above	Depresses ribs at the sternocostal and costovertebral joints
Diaphragm	Sternal part: two muscular slips from dorsum of xiphoid process Costal part: inner surface of lower 6 costal cartilages and lower 6 ribs Lumbar part: by two muscular crura from bodies of upper lumbar vertebrae, and by arcuate ligaments	Central tendon	Increases volume and decreases pressure of the thoracic cavity

ASSESSMENT

The aim of remedial massage assessment of the chest region includes:

- determining the suitability of clients for massage (red flags)
- determining duration (acute or chronic) and severity of injury, types of tissues involved
- determining if symptoms fit patterns of common conditions.

Assessment procedures for remedial massage clients are discussed in Chapter 2. Any client presenting with chest pain must be assessed for the presence of visceral disease including cardiac disease, peptic ulceration, reflux or malignancies.

The lifetime prevalence of non-cardiac chest pain is approximately 20–33% compared with 6–7% for angina.[3] Findings that may be present in clients with musculoskeletal chest pain include reproducible pain on palpation of the chest wall and chostochondral junctions, or pain on thoracic breathing or breath holding.

CASE HISTORY

- Identify any red flags that require referral for further investigation (see Table 14.2 on p 251).
- Ask clients to point to the site of pain as they may have different understandings of anatomical terms.
- Determine if the pain is likely to have a mechanical cause. (Is the pain associated with rest or activity, certain postures or time of day?) Ask clients to demonstrate movements and positions that aggravate or relieve their pain and be specific with descriptions of aggravating or relieving activities. Any acute trauma must be treated as a medical emergency.

Assessment of the chest

1. Case history
2. Outcome measures
3. Postural analysis
4. Functional tests
   Thoracic spine
   AROM
   flexion, extension, lateral flexion, rotation
   PROM
   flexion, extension, lateral flexion, rotation
   RROM
   flexion, extension, lateral flexion, rotation
   Resisted and length tests for specific muscles including
   Pectoralis major
   Pectoralis minor
   Special tests including
   Deep breathing
5. Palpation

- Mechanical pain is usually highly reactive to changes in posture, positions or activity.
- Chest pain is more common in young athletes than in young people in general. Serious causes need to be ruled out, although the most common causes of chest pain in young athletes are benign.[6]
- History of trauma suggests rib injury.
- Determine if the pain is likely to be associated with visceral function. Pain of cardiac origin, peptic ulceration, gastroesophageal reflux, pneumothorax and pulmonary embolism must be excluded. Look for associated symptoms like

Table 14.2 Red flags for serious conditions associated[4, 5] with acute chest pain

Red flags for acute chest pain	Possible condition
Angina, headache, arm/neck pain, nausea/vomiting), pallor, sweating, dyspnoea, palpitations Presence of risk factors (e.g. previous history of heart disease, hypertension, smoking, diabetes, men >40 years, women >50 years)	Myocardial infarction
Sharp or stabbing chest pain which may refer to lateral neck or shoulder, pain increased by sidelying, relieved by sitting and bending forward Recent or current viral infection, prior pericarditis	Pericarditis
Tearing sensation, pain radiates to back/abdomen, most severe at onset	Aortic dissection
Acute onset dyspnea, sharp chest pain aggravated by inspiration Recent bout of coughing, strenuous exercise or trauma	Pneumothorax
Acute onset dyspnea, chest, shoulder, or upper abdominal pain aggravated by deep breathing, haemoptysis History of risk factors for developing deep venous thrombosis, history of malignancy, unilateral leg swelling, recent surgery, recent long plane or bus trip, female smoker taking contraceptive pill	Pulmonary embolism
Severe sharp stabbing pain with inspiration, history of recent respiratory disorder (e.g. infection, pneumonia, tumour, tuberculosis), dyspnoea	Pleurisy
Pleuritic pain associated with productive cough, pain may refer to shoulder, fever, chills, headaches, malaise, nausea, dyspnea	Pneumonia
History of malignancy, night sweats, older age, tobacco use, weight loss	Malignant pleural effusion
Exposure to tuberculosis, hemoptysis, fever, night sweats, weight loss	Tuberculosis
History of trauma, osteoporosis, prolonged steroid use, age >70, loss of mobility, local tenderness/pain, increased thoracic kyphosis	Fracture

palpitations, shortness of breath, sweating, productive cough or pain relieved with antacid medication.

■ Determine if the pain is likely to be associated with herpes zoster (shingles). Shingles is a unilaterally painful, blistering skin rash that is caused by the varicella-zoster virus, the virus that causes chickenpox. It usually affects adults over 60 years who had chickenpox in their first year of life. A weakened immune system predisposes. The pain and burning sensation can be severe and usually precede the rash which commonly occurs around the trunk from the spine to the front of the chest or abdomen in skin areas supplied by sensory nerves of one or more dorsal root ganglia.[7]

■ Determine if the pain is likely to be associated with psychosocial causes (yellow flags).

A summary of serious symptoms that could require referral includes:[5]

■ abnormal vital signs (bradycardia, tachycardia, tachypnoea, hypertension, hypotension)
■ pallor, sweating, dyspnoea, palpitations
■ fever, chills, headache, malaise, productive cough
■ wheezing, accessory muscle retractions
■ pain intensified with inspiration
■ asymmetric pulses (pulsus paradoxus[a] over 10 mmHg)
■ pain relieved by leaning forward

■ increased pain by lying on the left side
■ symptoms lasting more than 20–30 minutes.

OUTCOME MEASURES

Outcome measures are specifically designed questionnaires that are used to assess clients' level of impairment and to define benefits of treatment. The benefit is assessed in terms of client-perceived changes to health status. The Patient Specific Functional Scale is an example of an outcome measure that could be used to assess conditions affecting the chest.

POSTURAL ANALYSIS[8]

Observe the shape and symmetry of the chest (see Figure 14.4 on p 252). On standing lateral analysis observe head carriage. Severe forward head posture increases contracture of the sternocleidomastoid and anterior scalene muscles, and decreases forced vital lung capacity.[9] Funnel chest (pectus excavatum) is a congenital chest deformity characterised by a depression in the lower sternum. If severe, it can impair cardiac and respiratory function. In pigeon chest (pectus carinatum), which is associated with longstanding early life obstructive airways disease such as chronic bronchitis or asthma, the sternum is displaced anteriorly. Barrel chest is associated with pulmonary emphysema and normal ageing. Normally the ratio of the anterior/posterior to lateral diameter of the adult chest is approximately $1 : 2$. With emphysema and normal ageing the ratio approximates $1 : 1$. The presence of thoracic kyphosis or scoliosis will affect the shape and symmetry of the chest.

---

[a]Blood pressure normally declines with inhalation and increases with exhalation. Pulsus paradoxus refers to an exaggeration of the normal blood pressure variation during the inspiration phase. It can suggest a number of conditions including cardiac tamponade, pericarditis, obstructive lung disease or chronic sleep apnoea.

Fig. 14.4 Common rib cage distortions (A funnel chest; B pigeon chest; C barrel chest)

Observe the rate and rhythm of breathing and any abnormal retraction of the supraclavicular fossae or the interspaces between the ribs during breathing (severe asthma, emphysema, tracheal obstruction) or abnormal bulging of the interspaces during expiration (asthma, emphysema). Note the use of accessory muscles including sternocleidomastoid, scalenes and upper trapezius on inspiration and abdominals on expiration during normal breathing.

FUNCTIONAL TESTS

The costovertebral joints transmit movements of the thoracic spine to the rib cage. Begin functional examination of the chest with range of motion testing of the thoracic spine (see Chapter 11).

Thoracic spine

ACTIVE RANGE OF MOTION (AROM)

Flexion

- Stand behind the client.
- Instruct the client to bend forward slowly as far as they can without pain.

Extension

- Stand at the side of the client and place hand on the spine at T12 level. Ask client to bend backwards from the contact point as far as they comfortably can.

Lateral flexion (sidebend)

- Ask the client to take their shoulder towards the hip on the same side. Stabilise the iliac crest with one hand and gently guide the client with the other hand on their shoulder as they laterally flex the trunk.
- Compare both sides and observe the coupling of the thoracic spine facet joints and posterior ribs.

Rotation

- Ask the client to turn their shoulders to the left and then the right as far as they are comfortably able.

PASSIVE RANGE OF MOTION (PROM)

Passive range of motion of the thoracic spine can be performed with the client seated. Place your forearm across the top of the client's shoulders to guide the movements. Rest your other hand on the middle thoracic spine as the client's trunk is flexed, extended, laterally flexed and rotated. Next your spinal contact is moved to the upper thoracic spine and the movements are repeated (see Chapter 11).

RESISTED RANGE OF MOTION (RROM)

The six ranges of motion of the thoracic spine tested in AROM can also be tested against resistance. Resisted range of motion tests are best performed with the client sitting on the treatment table to minimise extraneous muscle recruitment (see Chapter 11).

Resisted and length test for specific muscles[10]

Consider muscles with respect to their shortening and lengthening and also their hypoactivity and hyperactivity.[11] Mobilisers (e.g. upper trapezius) tend to tighten and shorten; stabilisers (e.g. lower trapezius and serratus anterior) tend to weaken and lengthen.[12] Length tests and resisted tests can be performed for the major muscles of the thoracic spine and chest. Resisted tests provide information about muscle strength and location of muscle strains. As with all clinical examination procedures findings from any test should be interpreted with caution and correlated with findings from other assessment procedures.

1. Pectoralis major

Resisted test: pectoralis major upper fibres (clavicular part) The client lies supine, shoulder flexed to 90°, elbow straight and palm facing towards the feet. Stand at the

Fig. 14.5 Resisted test for pectoralis major (A clavicular and B sternal divisions)

head of the table. Place one hand over the client's elevated forearm and resist as the client attempts to move their arm across their chest towards the opposite shoulder (see Figure 14.5).

Resisted test: pectoralis major lower fibres (sternal part) Use the same position as above but this time apply resistance as the client tries to move their arm towards their opposite hip (see Figure 14.5).

Length test With the client supine, shoulder level with the edge of the table, the client abducts their arm to 90° and lets their arm drop down towards the floor. Shortness of the pectoralis major (clavicular part) prevents the arm dropping to the table level. Lower fibres (sternal part) are tested as above except that the arm is abducted to 135° (see Figure 14.6).

Clinical significance Shortness is commonly observed in upper crossed and rounded shoulder postures.

2. Pectoralis minor
Resisted test The client lies supine and thrusts their shoulder forward against resistance (see Figure 14.7 on p 254).

Length test The client lies supine with their arms alongside their body, elbows extended. Normally both shoulders lie flat against the table. A short pectoralis minor holds the shoulder off the table (see Figure 14.8 on p 254).

Clinical significance Short pectoralis minor muscles are often associated with forward head carriage.[13, 14] Pectoralis minor contracture can pull the coracoid process of the scapula

Fig. 14.6 Length test for pectoralis major

Fig. 14.7 Resisted test for pectoralis minor

Fig. 14.8 Length test for pectoralis minor

downward and compress cords of the brachial plexus and axillary blood vessels causing arm pain. Weakness of pectoralis minor may reduce the strength of arm extension and could add to respiratory distress when using accessory muscles to breathe.[10]

SPECIAL TESTS

If clients experience pain while performing special tests, ask the client to indicate the exact location of the pain and continue to test only within the client's pain tolerance.

Deep breathing

Pain aggravated by deep breathing or coughing could be related to a musculoskeletal or respiratory condition. Listen for audible rhonchi (e.g. snoring sound in chronic bronchitis and emphysema), wheezing (e.g. in asthma) or rales (e.g. crackles in acute bronchitis and pneumonia).

PALPATION

Apply direct compression/pressure over the costochondral junctions, sternocostal joints, pectoral muscles and costal cartilages. Tender points and/or pain suggests musculoskeletal causes of chest pain.

With the client prone, palpate rib alignment by placing four fingertips in four consecutive intercostal spaces and sliding

them laterally from the spine. Start at the floating ribs and work up the rib cage. If the space between two consecutive ribs narrows considerably the intercostal muscles at that location may be contracted.

Respiratory excursion

To assess respiratory excursion, the client must be seated. Change in circumference of a client's chest can be measured with a tape measure at the level of the 4th intercostal space as the client inhales and exhales as far as possible. Expansion of less than 2.5 cm suggests decreased costovertebral movement, ankylosing spondylitis or respiratory pathology.[8, 15, 16]

REMEDIAL MASSAGE TREATMENT

Assessment of the chest provides essential information for development and negotiation of treatment plans, including:

- client's suitability for remedial massage therapy
- duration of the condition (i.e. acute or chronic)
- severity of the condition (i.e. grade of injury; mild, moderate or severe pain)
- type(s) of tissues involved
- priorities for treatment if more than one injury or condition is present
- whether the signs and symptoms suggest a common condition of the chest region
- special considerations for individual clients (e.g. client's preference for treatment types and styles, specific population considerations).

MUSCLE STRAIN

Muscle strains may occur as a result of sudden trauma, repetitive overuse or from coughing episodes. Chronic contractures of the pectoralis major and minor which are associated with prolonged hours of desk work, upper crossed syndrome and rounded shoulder postures may predispose the client to muscle strain.

Assessment
HISTORY

The client complains of localised chest pain associated with trauma (e.g. pectoralis major strain from performing bench

---

Assessment findings for muscle strain

- History of trauma or repetitive overuse
- Postural analysis: rounded shoulder posture or upper crossed syndrome may be associated with long-standing contractures
- Functional tests:
  Thoracic range of motion
  - AROM: positive
  - PROM: may be positive at end of range as muscle is passively stretched
  - Resisted and length tests positive for specific muscles
  - Special test usually negative
- Palpation positive for tenderness/pain and/or spasm

press exercises) or repetitive overuse. Pain is usually aggravated by movement or by inspiration, although these features may also be present with intrathoracic disease. Chronic contractures of pectoralis major and minor (as may occur in head forward postures or upper crossed syndrome) may predispose the client to chest muscle strain.

POSTURAL ANALYSIS

Contractures of pectoralis major and minor are associated with rounded shoulder posture, upper crossed syndrome and forward head carriage.

FUNCTIONAL TESTS

Thoracic spine

AROM positive.
PROM positive as the muscle is passively stretched.
RROM positive.
Resisted and length tests positive for specific muscle.
Special test: usually negative.

PALPATION

Palpation at the site of lesion elicits tenderness or pain. Muscle spasm may be palpable.

Treatment

Acute injuries are treated with ice and rest. Gentle stretching exercises are introduced as soon as pain permits.

Remedial massage techniques for chronic grade 1 or 2 muscle strains include:

- Swedish massage to the chest, upper limb, neck, upper and mid back.
- A range of specific muscle techniques including (see Table 14.3):
  - deep gliding frictions along the muscle fibres
  - cross-fibre frictions
  - soft tissue releasing techniques
  - deep transverse friction
  - trigger point therapy
  - muscle stretching.
- Myofascial release (see Chapter 8).

Address any underlying or predisposing conditions (e.g. scoliosis, post Scheuermann's disease).

CLIENT EDUCATION

Advise clients to avoid aggravating activities. Correction of weight-lifting techniques may be required. Posture advice is essential and includes avoidance of all postures and activities that cause the head to be held forward. Advise clients about lumbar supports, correct sitting posture and improving the ergonomics of the work area (see Figure 12.20). Clients often respond well to a corrective exercise program and referral for osseous manipulation may be required.

Home exercise program

Begin with gentle stretches and isometric exercises as soon as pain permits (see Table 14.3). Progressively introduce shoulder range of motion exercises and functional exercises. In clients with upper crossed syndrome, a program to strengthen

> **Key assessment findings for rib subluxation/fracture**
>
> - History of impact or blow to the chest, presence of underlying pathology or repetitive strain; sharp localised rib pain, referring laterally along the rib. Severe pain if fracture present
> - Functional tests:
>   **Thoracic spine:**
>   - AROM: limited especially rotation to the injured side
>   - PROM: limited especially rotation to injured side
>   - RROM: may be positive for associated intercostal strain
>   - Resisted and length tests: may be positive for associated intercostals strain
>   - Special tests: positive if fracture present
> - Palpation: tenderness/pain is elicited at the injury site: severe pain and muscle guarding if fracture present

weak middle and lower trapezius, rhomboids and serratus anterior should be progressively introduced for long-term biomechanical improvements.

RIB SUBLUXATION/FRACTURE

Rib subluxations or misalignments may occur at any age. Slipping rib syndrome is a rare condition associated with hypermobility of the floating ribs. Rib fractures are typically caused by impacts to the chest. However, even inconsequential traumas can fracture a rib in the presence of pre-existing weakness (e.g. osteopenia, cancer or bone infection). Onset can also be related to repetitive strain (e.g. twisting action in boxing or severe bouts of coughing).

Assessment

HISTORY

Clients with rib subluxations complain of intense sharp localised pain at the site of lesion. Subluxations can occur at the insertion of the rib into the thoracic spine posteriorly or at the sternal cartilaginous attachment anteriorly. The pain often refers laterally along the rib. Both the anterior and the posterior attachment sites may be painful simultaneously. The client will often report a recent episode of twisting, for example boxing, paddling or repetitive twisting in the workplace such as moving items through a supermarket checkout or along a production line. If fracture has occurred, the client reports severe pain in the ribs. Coughing, laughing and deep breathing are painful and make normal breathing difficult. Usually a significant traumatic event is described (e.g. a football game or car accident). If traumatic event is absent, there is usually a history of underlying pathology or symptoms suggestive of one (e.g. osteopenia, bone cancer, bone infection).

FUNCTIONAL TESTS

Thoracic spine

AROM: positive, particularly on rotation to the side of lesion. If fracture is present, range of motion on most movements is greatly limited due to pain.
PROM: positive, particularly on rotation to the side of lesion. If fracture is present, range of motion on most movements is greatly limited due to pain.
RROM: may be positive for associated muscle strains.

Table 14.3 Remedial massage techniques for muscles of the chest

Muscle	Soft tissue release	Trigger point	Stretch	Client education[17]	Home stretch
Pectoralis major	Stand at the head of the table, slightly to the involved side and place knuckles or fingers of the medial hand over the lateral aspect of pectoralis major. The client's straight arm is flexed to 90°. Hold the client's wrist with your other hand. Glide along the fibres of pectoralis major as the client's arm is passively horizontally abducted. Alternatively the client can actively perform the arm movement.			Correct standing and sitting posture, avoid mechanical overload.	In doorway stretch

Table 14.3 Remedial massage techniques for muscles of the chest—cont'd

Muscle	Soft tissue release	Trigger point	Stretch	Client education[17]	Home stretch
Pectoralis minor	Stand at the head of the table slightly to the involved side. Pressure is gently applied to the pectoralis minor with fingers, knuckles or thumbs maintained as the client protracts and retracts their shoulder. Note: clients often find this technique beyond their comfortable pain tolerance. Do not use this technique if the client reports pain of more than 7 out of 10 on a pain scale.		The client lies supine. Stand at the head of the table and gently apply downward (posterior) pressure to the shoulders with the palms of the hands.	Correct standing and sitting posture, avoid mechanical overload	The client lies supine with arms alongside body and tries to take their shoulders to the floor.
Intercostal muscles and diaphragm	Stand to one side of the client facing the client's head. Place palms on either side of the lower ribs, fingers pointing towards the floor. With elbows almost horizontal, apply pressure to the rib cage as the client exhales. Instruct the client to breathe in deeply. As the client inhales the practitioner resists the expansion of the rib cage. (Note: contraindicated in osteoporosis.)		Intercostal muscles can be stretched by raising the arms overhead, trunk lateral flexion to the opposite side and deep breathing.	Correct paradoxical breathing, correct head forward and slumped posture	Breathing exercises (e.g. Buteyko, yoga)

Resisted and length tests for specific muscles may be positive for involved muscles.

Special tests: deep breathing, coughing, sneezing and laughing are positive if fracture is present.

PALPATION

Anteriorly the rib attaches to the sternum via costocartilage. Posteriorly the tubercle of the rib articulates with the transverse process and the rib head with either two adjacent vertebral bodies (ribs 1 to 8) or one vertebral body (ribs 9 to 12). Palpation at the site of lesion (anteriorly or posteriorly) elicits acute pain. The region may be boggy and inflamed. Associated intercostal muscles are typically contracted and sore and the ribs unevenly spaced. Palpating a fracture site may invoke involuntary muscle guarding.

DIFFERENTIAL DIAGNOSIS

Rib subluxations may be difficult to distinguish from fractures. The rib cage is highly innervated to enable normal coordinated breathing. Consequently rib subluxations are initially intensely painful. The severity of the trauma or the presence of underlying pathology suggest fracture. Severe pain that does not decrease over days and the presence of involuntary muscle guarding also suggest fracture. An X-ray of the region is required in order to make a definitive diagnosis.

Costochondritis

Costochondritis refers to inflammation of one or more rib cartilages usually on one side of the sternum. It is associated with pain related to activity and localised tenderness at the costochondral joint. Tietze's syndrome is a severe form of costrochondritis characterised by swelling of the affected costal cartilages. The cause is poorly understood. It is thought to arise from minor trauma or bouts of coughing, sneezing or vomiting. The condition usually resolves within 3 months but can become chronic. It may be associated with other conditions like fibromyalgia, inflammatory bowel disease, psoriatic arthritis and ankylosing spondylitis.

Sternocostal joint sprain

Clients with sternocostal joint sprain report a history of trauma and localised sharp pain that is aggravated by movement and relieved by rest. AROM and PROM of the thoracic spine aggravate symptoms. Pain and/or tenderness elicited by palpation of the affected sternocostal joints suggests sternocostal joint sprain.

Overview of treatment and management of rib subluxation

If fracture is suspected, referral is required. Remedial massage is contraindicated until the bone has healed (a minimum of 6 weeks). Initially, Swedish massage helps to reduce muscle spasm and pain. As tolerated, deep remedial techniques may be introduced.

Rib subluxation often involves ligamentous sprain, which may take 8 weeks to heal. Acute pain and inflammation usually subside in a few days. Cryotherapy may provide pain relief. Residual intercostal protective muscle spasm will be relieved with massage therapy. The client needs to avoid excessive rotation movements in order to prevent relapse within the first 8 weeks post injury.

A typical remedial massage treatment for rib subluxation includes:

- Swedish massage to the thoracic spine and chest.
- Remedial massage techniques, which include:
  - for ligamentous sprain: cross-fibre frictions and deep transverse friction
  - for muscle strain (see Table 14.3)
    - deep gliding frictions along the muscle fibres
    - cross-fibre frictions
    - soft tissue releasing techniques
    - deep transverse friction
    - trigger point therapy
    - muscle stretching.

  Adjacent rib spaces can be treated simultaneously using fingers in the intercostal spaces to gently separate the ribs.

- Gentle thoracic and rib mobilisation help restore normal movement patterns (see Chapter 7) including:
  - thoracic longitudinal mobilisation
  - thoracic diagonal mobilisation
  - arm overhead rib mobilisation
  - rib rotation.
  (Note that mobilisations are contraindicated in clients with osteoporosis.)
- Thermotherapy may provide pain relief.
- Myofascial releasing techniques may be beneficial (see Chapter 8) (see Figure 14.9).

CLIENT EDUCATION

Advise clients to take several deep breaths each day within their pain tolerance. Heat packs may provide pain relief after the acute phase.

Home exercise program

Introduce gentle stretches as soon as they can be tolerated. For example, standing upright with hands on hips, the client raises the arm overhead on the side of rib lesion. The client slowly bends to the opposite side to open the rib cage and stretches the intercostal muscles on the side of injury.

Fig. 14.9 Myofascial release: rib subluxation

Predisposing biomechanical factors may include weak or contracted erector spinae muscles and weak core muscles. Progressively introduce a strengthening program as required.

RESPIRATORY CONDITIONS

Remedial massage therapists can assist in the management of respiratory conditions, particularly asthma and chronic obstructive pulmonary conditions. A randomised control trial of children with asthma found that symptoms of dyspnea, cough and wheeze in the massage group were reduced by 45%, 56% and 52% respectively when compared with the control group. The findings suggest that massage might reduce symptoms and anxiety in children with asthma.[18]

Encouraging findings were also reported by a recent systematic review which found that massage therapy had a significantly positive effect on children with asthma. Massage improved the function of large airway and plasma metabolism, greatly improving pulmonary function.[19] However, the included trials had high risk of bias and better quality trials are needed to confirm the results.

Symptoms of cough, shortness of breath and chest pain require referral for assessment by a medical practitioner (see red flags). Some conditions affecting the respiratory system are presented in Table 14.4.

For those clients for whom remedial massage is suitable, observe the shape of the chest and any use of accessory muscles of breathing, especially sternocleidomastoid, scalenes and upper trapezius muscles on inspiration, and abdominals on expiration. Note the breathing rate and character. Observe the client's general colour (pink colour may suggest emphysema, blue colour may suggest chronic bronchitis). Is there any clubbing of the fingers?[b]

Listen to the client's breathing. Is there any wheezing, crackles or laboured breathing? Table 14.5 contains some of the physical signs of bronchitis, bronchial asthma and emphysema.

Overview of treatment and management of respiratory conditions

Remedial massage therapists have long supported people with asthma and chronic obstructive pulmonary disease (COPD) to manage their condition. Remedial massage treatment these respiratory conditions includes the following:

- Swedish massage to the back, including T3 (nerve supply to lungs, bronchial tubes, pleura, chest), neck (the phrenic nerve, which supplies the diaphragm, originates mainly from C4) and chest (focus on intercostal muscles). Tapotement is useful in loosening mucus.
- Remedial massage techniques include:
  - specific muscle techniques, particularly for muscles of respiration (pectoralis minor, external intercostal, subclavius, scalene and sternocleidomastoid muscles). Techniques include (see Tables 14.3 and 12.4):
    - deep gliding frictions
    - cross-fibre frictions
    - soft tissue releasing techniques
    - trigger point therapy
    - muscle stretching.
- Deep gliding and cross-fibre frictions of the subclavius are useful when treating respiratory conditions. The muscle is an accessory respiratory muscle and is often overworked in asthmatics and in people with chest infections (see Figure 14.10 on p 260).

Table 14.4 Conditions of the respiratory system

Bronchial asthma	Chronic airway inflammation and narrowing of airways from smooth muscle spasm in small bronchi and bronchioles, oedema of the airway and excessive mucus. This results in dyspnoea, wheezing, chest tightness and coughing.
Chronic bronchitis	Excessive secretion of bronchial mucus and productive cough. Lasts for at least 3 months of the year for 2 consecutive years.
Coryza	Common cold caused by viruses.
Emphysema	Loss of elasticity of alveolar walls. Lungs become permanently inflated with reduced surface area for gas exchange. Inspiration is forced to obtain more oxygen. Barrel-chested.
Influenza	Chills, fever, headache, muscle aches, and cough due to infection with the influenza virus.
Pertussis (whooping cough)	Contagious disease caused by bacterium Bordetella pertussis. Dry, harassing cough developing into paroxysms followed by a long, drawn inspiration with a 'whoop' sound.
Pleurisy	Inflammation of the pleural linings of the lungs, usually accompanied by viral infection. Sharp pain on inhalation (pleuritic chest pain).
Pneumonia	Acute inflammation of the alveoli of the lungs which fill up with fluid. Decreased ventilation and gas exchange. Most commonly caused by Streptococcus pneumonia.
Pneumothorax	Lung collapse due to air in the pleural space in people with chronic lung disease or spontaneous collapse from penetrating wound.
Sinusitis	Infection and inflammation of the mucous membranes of the paranasal sinuses (maxillary, frontal, ethmoid, sphenoid). Chronic sinusitis may result in the formation of the tumour like processes called polyps (see Chapter 13).
Tuberculosis	Infection caused by Mycobacterium tuberculosis which causes inflammation of the pleura and lungs. Symptoms include fatigue, weight loss, anorexia, low-grade fever, night sweats, dyspnoea, cough and chest pain. Contagious through inhalation.

---

[b]Clubbing refers to swelling in the subcutaneous tissues over the terminal phalanges. The angle at the base of the nail is decreased (the nail turns downwards like the rounded part of an upside-down spoon). Clubbing occurs in patients with heart and lung disease, lung cancer or liver and gastrointestinal disease.

Table 14.5 Comparison of inflammatory chest conditions[20]

Condition	Asthma	Bronchitis	Emphysema
Pathogenesis	-Bronchial smooth muscle hyper-reactivity -Inflammatory bronchial wall thickening -Increased mucus production	Inflammation leads to -proliferation of glandular tissue -hypersecretion of mucus -fibrosis of smaller airways	Imbalance of inflammatory and anti-inflammatory forces that eventually leads to tissue destruction
Factors	-Genetic, associated with allergic rhinitis and eczema -Environmental, exposure to allergens, cold, exercise	Cigarette smoke exacerbates	Cigarette smoke and other irritants
Symptoms	Intermittent attacks of dyspnea, chest tightness, coughing, and wheezing during expiration	Dyspnea, productive cough, and frequent respiratory infections	Dyspnea, cough, wheezing, and a barrel chest Patients often expire against pursed lips, as a means of increasing end-expiratory pressure and keeping the airways open

Fig. 14.10 Subclavius: deep gliding and cross-fibre frictions

- Acupressure points can be incorporated into Swedish massage. Apply digital pressure to specific respiratory points along acupuncture meridians or energy lines of the body. Apply thumb or knuckle pressure on points for approximately 10 seconds. Points commonly used to treat asthma and chronic bronchitis include (see Figure 14.11 on p 261):
  - Lung 1 (L1): In the interspace between the first and second ribs, 8 fingerbreadths lateral to the midline.
  - Lung 7 (L7): Proximal to styloid process of the radius, 2 fingerbreadths above the transverse crease of the wrist.
  - Conception vessel 17 (CV17): Centre of the chest, between the nipples.
  - Pericardium 6 (P6): 2 thumb widths above the transverse crease of the wrist between the tendons of palmaris longus and flexor carpi radialis.
  - Bladder 12 (BL12): 2 fingerbreadths either side of the spinous process of T2.
  - Bladder 43 (BL43): 4 fingerbreadths either side of the spinous process of T4.
  Note that the distances refer to the client's own finger and thumb size.

Note: Lung 1 is located in the delto-pectoral groove or triangle. It is generally regarded as a forbidden point for needling although pressure and/or heat (moxibustion) may be applied. Pectoralis minor and the coracoid process also lie in this region. Circular frictions at this point may be useful for treating lung conditions.

- Gentle mobilisations of the thoracic spine including (see Chapter 7):
  - thoracic longitudinal mobilisation
  - thoracic diagonal mobilisation
  - arm overhead rib mobilisation
  - rib rotation.
  (Note: mobilisation techniques are contraindicated in clients with osteoporosis.)
- Further mobilisations include:
  - Prone
    - i) Compressions. Remove oil or cover the client with a towel and stand facing transversely across the client. Apply slow rhythmic compressions making brief contact and releasing the hand to allow the rib cage to recoil, first on one side of the rib cage and then to the other (see Figure 14.12 on p 261).
    - ii) Cat walk. Stand at the head of the table. Remove oil or cover the client with a towel. Place the heels of both hands on the upper thoracic paravertebral muscles, fingers pointing inferiorly. Apply pressure downward with one hand, release, and transfer weight to the other hand. Repeat this transfer of pressure on one side of the spine and then on the other as the hands 'walk' down the rib cage. Apply pressure slowly as the client exhales (see Figure 14.13 on p 261).
  - Sidelying
    - i) Assisted breathing: sidelying, arm overhead. The client lies on their side with their uppermost arm overhead. Face caudally and gently traction the fully abducted arm with the cephalad hand. Apply gentle pressure with your caudal palm to the lower ribs as the client exhales (see Figure 14.14 on p 262). (Note: all assisted breathing techniques are contraindicated in osteoporosis.)
  - Supine: Stand at client's head. Work in two sections: upper ribs and lower ribs above and below a towel folded

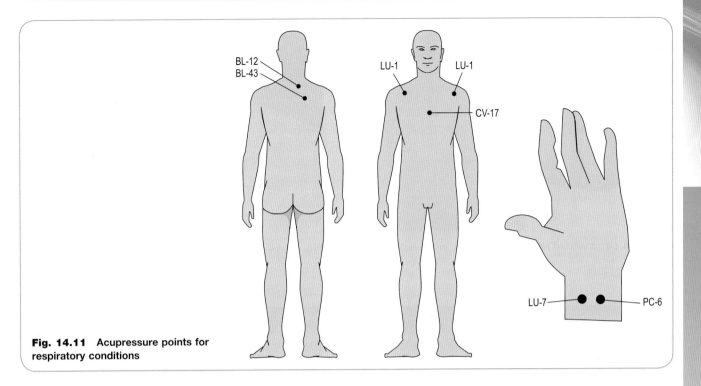

Fig. 14.11 Acupressure points for respiratory conditions

BL-12
BL-43

LU-1   LU-1

CV-17

LU-7   PC-6

Fig. 14.12 Compressions

Fig. 14.13 Cat walk

horizontally across the breasts. (It is beyond the scope of remedial massage therapy to massage breast tissue.)

i) Assisted breathing: supine, upper and lower ribs
Stand at the head of the table. Apply gentle pressure on the anterior upper chest with both palms (heels of

hands laterally and fingers pointing medially) as the client exhales, and then quickly change hand position to the posterolateral aspect of the lower ribs and lift the lower ribs as the client inhales. Repeat for several breaths (see Figures 14.15 and 14.16 on p 262).

Fig. 14.14   Assisted breathing: sidelying, arm overhead

Fig. 14.16   Assisted breathing: supine, lower ribs

Fig. 14.15   Assisted breathing: supine, upper ribs

Fig. 14.17   Diaphragm release

ii) Assisted breathing: supine, upper ribs
Stand at the head of the table. Cover the client's chest with a towel. Place the palm of one hand over the sternum. Alternatively, place palms on either side of the upper chest, fingers pointing medially. Apply downward pressure as the client exhales, then instruct the client to inhale deeply. At about half inspiration, suddenly release your palm pressure by lifting the hands rapidly off the chest. This will often cause the client to gasp. Repeat up to 3 times.

iii) Assisted breathing supine, lower ribs
Stand to one side of the client facing the client's head. Place palms on either side of the lower ribs, fingers pointing towards the floor. With elbows almost horizontal, apply pressure to the rib cage as the client exhales. Instruct the client to breathe in deeply and at about half inspiration, release the pressure.

iv) Diaphragm release
Face the client's head. Place thumb tips under the client's costal margin. Try to contract the underside of the costal margin with the thumbs. Begin lateral to the xiphoid process and, as the client exhales, slowly slide the thumbs under the costal margin from medial to lateral (see Figure 14.17).

■ Remedial massage treatments may also include aromatherapy, reflexology and Bowen therapy. Although little scientific evidence is available to support their use, these techniques are often used in clinical practice. They are part of the range of techniques available to remedial massage therapists when they negotiate treatment plans with clients.

■ Reflexology
Reflexologists use reflex points that are associated with the lungs and bronchi (see Figure 14.18). Techniques include mild pressure directly on the reflex points on the feet using fingers, thumbs or knuckles and *caterpillars* (a stroke involving repeated flexion and extension of the interphalangeal joint of the thumb).

■ Aromatherapy
An essential oil blend may be used as the lubricant in Swedish massage (5 drops in 10 mL carrier oil) or vapourised in an oil-burner during the treatment. Useful oils for asthma include aniseed, atlas cedarwood, cajeput, clary sage, Roman chamomile, cypress, fennel, frankincense, everlasting, eucalyptus radiate, hyssop var. decumbens, lavender, pinus sylvestris, spike lavender, lemon, mandarin, myrtle, peppermint, petitgrain, rosemary. (Caution: always check the client's sensitivity/allergic response before using essential oils.)

Fig. 14.18 Reflexology for lungs and bronchi

Right   Left

Sinuses   Nose   Sinuses
Throat
Thalamus
Lungs
Heart
Diaphragm
Solar plexus

CLIENT EDUCATION

Integrative medicine in the management of asthma and COPD includes evidence-based manual therapy, medications, and lifestyle and self-care strategies such as stopping smoking and avoiding allergens. As respiratory conditions are linked to distress, attention to mental and emotional health, physical activity, and nutrition are beneficial. A recent clinical trial of people with asthma found that combining inspiratory muscle training with manual therapy and an exercise program was more effective than the inspiratory muscle training on its own. Both short-term maximum inspiratory pressure and forward head posture were improved in the multimodal group.[21] Traditionally steam inhalations and humidifiers using essential oils (e.g. eucalyptus and pine) have been used. Breathing exercises, swimming, yoga, Buteyko[c] and hydrotherapy may be recommended.

The Victorian government Better Health channel recommends the following simple breathing exercises.[22]

Relaxed deep breathing

Sit down, relax your shoulders and breathe in through your nose and out through your mouth. Your abdomen should move in and out as you breathe. This shows you are using your diaphragm.

Prolonged breathing out

Breathe in for two counts and breathe out for three or four counts. This helps to expel any trapped air so there is more room for fresh air when you take your next breath.

Physical exercise to improve breathing

Discuss the possibilities of an exercise program with your doctor or healthcare professional before you start any new activities.

Examples of physical activity that can be useful include:

Walking – start with a few minutes each day and build up slowly.
Stretching – keep your muscles supple.
Weight training – use small hand-held dumbbells.
Tai chi – practise breathing techniques and slow graceful movements
Hydrotherapy – exercise in warm water.

Simons et al[17] identified paradoxical breathing (i.e. the rib cage deflating as the client inhales and inflating as they exhale) as a common perpetuating factor for trigger points in chest muscles. If there is no underlying pathology, clients can correct paradoxical breathing by placing one hand on the upper ribs and one on the abdomen and practising breathing in such a way that the hand on the rib cage rises as they inhale and falls as they exhale.

It is imperative that clients continue their usual medication. Clients can be referred to a naturopath, homoeopath, acupuncturist and/or manipulative therapist for further treatment. Allergy testing may also be required.

KEY MESSAGES

- Assessment of clients with chest conditions involves case history, outcome measures, postural observation, functional tests (including resisted tests and length tests for specific muscles) and deep breathing.
- No chest pain should ever be assumed to be musculoskeletal until other causes have been eliminated. Be vigilant for red flags for serious conditions associated with chest pain (e.g. cardiac, respiratory or gastrointestinal causes).
- Assessment findings may indicate the type of tissue involved (contractile or inert), duration of condition (acute or chronic) and severity.
- Consider Clinical Guidelines, available evidence and client preferences when planning therapy.
- Remedial massage therapy for chest conditions commonly involves treatment of chronic contractures of chest muscles (e.g. when treating clients with upper crossed syndrome or forward head carriage). Remedial massage therapists also treat chest muscle strains and rib subluxations, and provide supportive treatment for clients with chronic respiratory conditions.
- Educating clients about likely causal and predisposing factors is an essential part of remedial massage therapy. Prioritise the client self-help component of treatment wherever possible to reduce likelihood of recurrence and/or to promote health maintenance and illness prevention.

---

[c]The Buteyko breathing method is a series of exercises involving nasal breathing, relaxation and holding the breath. It is used in the treatment of asthma.

Review questions

1. A 70-year-old client presents with pain in the chest. She has recently recovered from a chest infection and cough. The pain is sharp, localised and continuing to be very painful. She is unable to take a deep breath without pain. Palpation of the injury site is very tender and there is evidence of reflex muscle guarding. This history suggests:
   a) bronchitis
   b) a fractured rib
   c) a herniated thoracic disc
   d) intercostal muscle strain

2. Describe a test for:
   i) the length of pectoralis minor
   ii) the length of pectoralis major sternal division
   iii) differentiating a musculoskeletal chest pain from a visceral one.

3. A 48-year-old man is suffering from chest pain. He has high blood pressure, is overweight and smokes about 20 cigarettes a day. He looks pale, is having difficulty breathing and appears to be in some distress. This history suggests:
   a) cardiovascular disease
   b) pectoralis major strain
   c) pericarditis
   d) shingles

4. Costochondritis may be associated with:
   a) cardiovascular disease
   b) pericarditis
   c) inflammatory bowel disease
   d) a fractured rib

5. The most common cause of chest pain in a 25-year-old athlete is:
   a) benign, e.g. referral from the thoracic spine
   b) angina
   c) rib stress fracture
   d) gastroesophageal reflux

6. A pigeon chest is associated with:
   a) normal ageing
   b) childhood asthma
   c) emphysema
   d) pertussis

7. What symptoms and signs differentiate a rib fracture and a rib subluxation?

8. List five red flags associated with chest pain.

9. Give three characteristics of musculoskeletal chest pain that differentiate it from pain of visceral or other origin.

10. What role can remedial massage play in the treatment and management of asthma?

11. List the primary and accessory muscles of respiration.

12. a) What is *paradoxical* breathing?
    b) How can it be corrected?

REFERENCES

1. Winzenberg T, Jones G, Callisaya M. Musculoskeletal chest wall pain. Aust Fam Physician 2015;44(8):540–4.
2. Burgstaller JM, Jenni BF, Steurer J, et al. Treatment efficacy for non-cardiovascular chest pain: a systematic review and meta-analysis. PLOS One 2014;9(8):e104722.
3. Chambers JB, Marks EM, Hunter MS. The head says yes but the heart says no: what is non-cardiac chest pain and how is it managed? Heart 2015;101: 1240–9.
4. Reamy BV, Williams PM, Odom MR. Pleuritic chest pain: sorting through the differential diagnosis. Am Fam Physician 2015;96(5):306–12.
5. Zitkus B. Take chest pain to heart. Nurse Pract 2010;35(9):41–7.
6. Moran B, Bryan S, Salud C, et al. Diagnostic evaluation of nontraumatic chest pain in athletes. Curr Sports Med Rep 2017;16(2):84–94.
7. Ayloo A, Cvengros T, Marella S. Evaluation and treatment of musculoskeletal chest pain. Prim Care Clin Office Pract 2013;40:863–87.
8. Bickley L. Bates' guide to physical examination and history taking. 11th edn. Philadelphia: Lippincott-Raven; 2013.
9. Kang J-I, Jeong D-K, Choi H. Correlation between pulmonary functions and respiratory muscle activity in patients with forward head posture. Journal Phys Ther Sci 2018;30:132–5.
10. Hislop H, Avers D, Brown M, et al. Daniels and Worthingham's muscle testing: techniques of manual examination and performance testing. 9th edn. St Louis, MO: Saunders; 2014.
11. Czaprowski D, Stolinski L, Tyrakowski M, et al. Non-structural misalignments of body posture in the sagittal plane. Scoliosis Spinal Disord 2018;13:6. https://doi.org/10.1186/s13013-018-0151-5
12. Chaitow L. Muscle energy techniques. 4th edn. Edinburgh: Churchill Livingstone; 2013.
13. Muscolino J. The thoracic spine: the silent saboteur. J Aust Trad Med Soc 2017;23(4):192–8.
14. Kim M-K, Lee JC, Yoo K-T. The effects of shoulder stabilization exercises and pectoralis minor stretching on balance and maximal shoulder muscle strength of healthy young adults with round shoulder posture. J Phys Ther Sci 2018;30: 373–80.
15. Vizniak N. Physical assessment. Burnaby, BC: Professional Health Systems; 2008.
16. Al-Qadi MO. Disorders of the chest wall: clinical manifestations. Clin Chest Med 2018;39:361–75.
17. Simons D, Travell J, Simons L. Myofascial pain and dysfunction: the trigger point manual. Vol 1: upper half of body. 2nd edn. Philadelphia: Williams and Wilkins; 1999.
18. Goli H, Shabestari MS. Effectiveness of massage therapy in improving symptom in children with allergic asthma: a randomized clinical trial. BMJ Open 2017;7(0):A1–A78.
19. Wu J, Yang X-W, Zhang M. Massage therapy in children with asthma: a systematic review and meta-analysis. Evid-Based Compl Alt Med. Article ID 5620568. Online. Available: https://doi.org/10.1155/2017/5620568; 2017.
20. Gunderman RB, Lydon BT. Respiratory disease: update for radiologists. Acad Radiol 2016;23: 108–11.
21. Lopez-de-Uraldo-Villanueva I, Candelas-Fernandez P, de-Diego-Cano B, et al. The effectiveness of combining inspiratory muscle training with manual therapy and a therapeutic exercise program on maximum inspiratory pressure in adults with asthma: a randomized clinical trial. Clin Rehabil 2018;32(6):752–65.
22. State Government of Victoria, Australia. Department of Health: breathing problems and exercise. Online. Available: https://www.betterhealth.vic.gov.au/health/HealthyLiving/breathing-problems-and-exercise?viewAsPdf=true; 2019.

The shoulder region

15

Learning Outcomes

- Assess clients with conditions of the shoulder region for remedial massage, including identification of red and yellow flags.
- Assess clients for signs and symptoms associated with common conditions of the shoulder region (including muscle strains, impingement syndrome, glenohumeral osteoarthritis and adhesive capulitis), and treat and/or manage these conditions with remedial massage therapy.
- Develop treatment plans for clients with conditions of the shoulder region, taking assessment findings, duration and severity of the condition, likely tissue types, clinical guidelines, the best available evidence and client preferences into account.
- Develop short- and long-term treatment plans to address presenting symptoms, underlying conditions and predisposing factors, and to progressively increase the self-help component of therapy.
- Adapt remedial massage therapy to suit individual client's needs based on duration and severity of injury, the client's age and gender, the presence of underlying conditions and other considerations for specific population groups.

INTRODUCTION

Shoulder pain impacts around 1 in 4 people in Australia. Those at higher risk are women, people over 50 years old, smokers and people living with obesity.[1] Shoulder pain may indicate intrinsic shoulder dysfunction although pain may also be referred from other structures, such as the neck, gall bladder or heart.[2] A comprehensive massage therapy assessment which includes a thorough history and physical assessment of the shoulder is key for optimal patient outcomes.

FUNCTIONAL ANATOMY

The shoulder joint comprises a relatively shallow ball and socket joint which enables the extensive mobility required for manual dexterity. Its stability relies on overlying muscles and tendons, particularly the rotator cuff muscles, the

glenohumeral ligaments, glenoid labrum, joint capsule and fascia. Normal shoulder function requires coordination of stabilising and movement forces of the glenohumeral joint, the scapula, and the acromioclavicular (AC) and sternoclavicular (SC) joints. The subacromial bursa sits on top of the supraspinatus tendon and is designed to reduce friction between the supraspinatus tendon and the acromion. This bursa extends over the superior region of the humerus and out from under the acromion process deep to the deltoid muscle (see Figure 15.1 on p 266).

Major muscles of the shoulder region are shown in Figure 15.2 on p 266 and summarised in Table 15.1. The rotator cuff muscles (see Figure 15.3 on p 268) and the coracobrachialis control the position of the head of the humerus in the glenoid fossa. The supraspinatus in particular counteracts the upward pull of the deltoid muscle on the head of the humerus when the shoulder is abducted. Smooth scapulohumeral rhythm requires strong scapular stabilisers (lower trapezius, serratus anterior, rhomboids, levator scapulae and pectoralis minor muscles) and normal length of scapulohumeral muscles (infraspinatus, teres minor and subscapularis). Most shoulder pathologies are associated with disturbances of these integrated movement and stabilising forces.

ASSESSMENT

The purpose of remedial massage assessment includes:

- determining the suitability of clients for massage (contra-indications and red flags, see Table 15.2)
- determining the duration (acute or chronic), severity and types of tissues involved in the injury/condition
- determining whether symptoms fit patterns of common conditions.

Clinical assessment alone cannot produce an accurate diagnosis of the causes of shoulder pain but positive outcomes can be achieved from treatment of many shoulder conditions without identifying the exact cause.[4]

Principles of remedial massage assessment are discussed in Chapter 2. This section presents specific considerations for assessment of the shoulder region.

CASE HISTORY

Information from case histories can alert practitioners to the presence of serious conditions requiring referral. However,

265

individual features in case histories may have low significance for diagnosis and should always be interpreted in the context of information from other assessments.[4] Use targeted questioning to collect the most useful and relevant information, including:

- Identifying red and yellow flags that require referral for further investigation.
- Identifying the exact location of the symptoms by asking clients to point to the site of pain.
- Determining if the pain is likely to have a mechanical cause. (Is the pain associated with rest or activity, certain postures or time of day?) Obtain descriptions of the specific mechanism of the injury and the forces involved. For example, falls onto the outstretched hand may be associated with acromioclavicular (AC) injuries, wrenching the arm backwards may suggest anterior dislocation, and morning pain relieved with daily activity is often associated with arthritis. Enquire about the onset of symptoms, nature of the pain, disability and functional impairment, previous injuries to the area, type of work, typical postures, sleeping posture, overuse and overhead work. Ask clients to demonstrate movements and positions that aggravate or relieve their pain and to be specific with descriptions of aggravating or relieving activities.

- Determining if pain is likely to be associated with visceral function or is neurogenic or psychosocial (yellow flags).

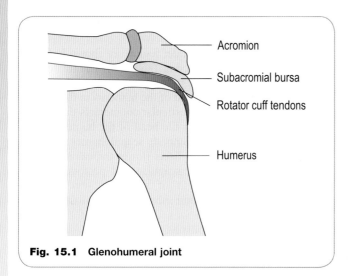

Fig. 15.1 Glenohumeral joint

- Acromion
- Subacromial bursa
- Rotator cuff tendons
- Humerus

Assessment of the shoulder region

1. Case history
2. Outcome measures, e.g. The Shoulder Pain and Disability Index (see Appendix 15.1) and The Patient Specific Functional Scale
3. Postural analysis
4. Functional tests
   Cervical spine
   Active range of motion tests
   Flexion, extension, lateral flexion, rotation
   Shoulder joint
   Active range of motion tests
   Flexion, extension, abduction, horizontal adduction, internal rotation, external rotation
   Passive range of motion tests
   Flexion, extension, abduction, horizontal adduction, internal rotation, external rotation
   Resisted range of motion tests
   Flexion, extension, abduction, horizontal adduction, internal rotation, external rotation
   Resisted and length tests for specific muscles, including supraspinatus, infraspinatus, subscapularis, teres major, teres minor, deltoid, pectoralis major
   Special tests
   Apley's scratch test
   Drop arm test
   Impingement test
   Apprehension test
   Yergason's test
   Empty can test
5. Palpation

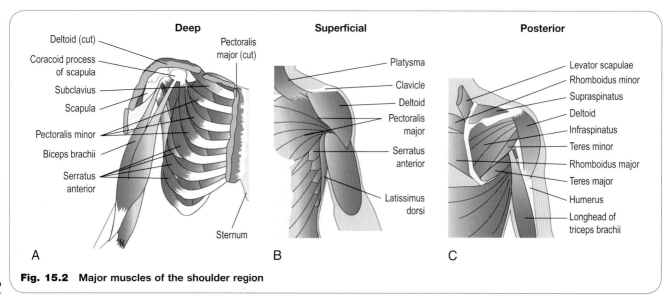

Deep — Deltoid (cut), Coracoid process of scapula, Subclavius, Scapula, Pectoralis minor, Biceps brachii, Serratus anterior, Pectoralis major (cut), Sternum

Superficial — Platysma, Clavicle, Deltoid, Pectoralis major, Serratus anterior, Latissimus dorsi

Posterior — Levator scapulae, Rhomboidus minor, Supraspinatus, Deltoid, Infraspinatus, Teres minor, Rhomboidus major, Teres major, Humerus, Longhead of triceps brachii

A   B   C

Fig. 15.2 Major muscles of the shoulder region

Table 15.1 Muscles of the shoulder region[3]

Muscles that move the humerus	Origin	Insertion	Action
Deltoid	acromial extremity of clavicle (anterior fibres), acromion of scapula (lateral fibres) and spine of scapula (posterior fibres)	deltoid tuberosity of humerus	lateral fibres abduct humerus; anterior fibres flex and medially rotate arm at shoulder joint; posterior fibres extend and laterally rotate arm at shoulder joint
Supraspinatus	supraspinatus fossa of scapula	greater tubercle of humerus	assists deltoid muscle in abducting humerus
Infraspinatus	infraspinous fossa of scapula	greater tubercle of humerus	externally rotates and adducts humerus
Teres major	inferior angle of scapula	intertubercular sulcus of humerus	extends humerus and assists in adduction and internal rotation of humerus
Teres minor	inferior lateral border of scapula	greater tubercle of humerus	externally rotates, extends and adducts the humerus
Subscapularis	subscapular fossa of scapula	lesser tubercle of humerus	internally rotates humerus
Biceps brachii	long head originates from the supraglenoid tubercle; short head originates from coracoid process of scapula	radial tuberosity and bicipital aponeurosis	flexes humerus at shoulder joint, flexes forearm at elbow joint, supinates forearm at radioulnar joints
Coracobrachialis	coracoid process of scapula	middle of medial surface of shaft of humerus	flexes and adducts humerus
Triceps brachii	long head: infraglenoid tubercle lateral head: lateral and posterior surface of humerus superior to radial groove medial head: entire posterior surface of humerus inferior to a groove for the radial nerve	olecranon of ulna	extends humerus at shoulder joint and extends forearm at elbow joint

Note: latissimus dorsi, rhomboid muscles and serratus anterior are described in Chapter 11; pectoralis major and minor are described in Chapter 14.

Table 15.2 Red flags for serious conditions associated with acute shoulder pain[4, 5]

Red flag	Condition
History of trauma Sudden onset of pain, altered sensation, pins and needles, numbness	Fracture/dislocation
Symptoms and signs of infection (e.g. fever) Risk factors for infection (e.g. underlying disease process, immunosuppression, penetrating wound)	Infections (joint, bone or possibly skin)
Past history of malignancy Age >50 years Failure to improve with treatment Unexplained weight loss Pain at multiple sites Pain at rest	Tumour
Significant limb swelling following an injury or an excessively tight bandage or cast Pain disproportionate to the injury	Acute compartment syndrome (a surgical emergency)
Bilateral shoulder pain and weakness	Polymyalgia rheumatic
Pressure, squeezing, burning, or tightness Possible feeling of indigestion	Ischaemic cardiac pain

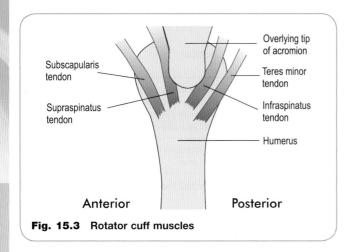

Fig. 15.3 Rotator cuff muscles

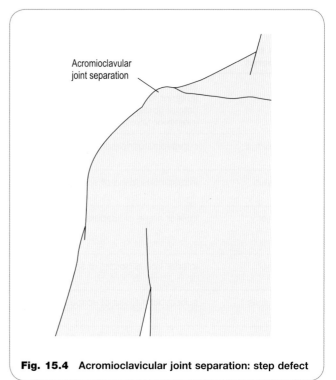

Fig. 15.4 Acromioclavicular joint separation: step defect

Referred pain occurs when the brain interprets pain generated by one structure as originating from another source. An example of this is gall bladder pain which may be perceived as shoulder pain.[6] The heart, liver, lungs and diaphragm may also refer pain to the shoulder region. Clients with numbness, pins and needles and muscle weakness associated with their shoulder condition may have brachial plexus injuries or cervical radiculopathy. Refer clients with sensory symptoms or muscle weakness for further investigation. Psychosocial factors can also contribute to the onset and development of shoulder pain. The client's social background, depression and tendency to catastrophise appear to be key considerations.[7]

OUTCOME MEASURES

Outcome measures are questionnaires that are specifically designed to assess clients' level of impairment and to define benefits of treatment. The Shoulder Pain and Disability Index can be used to assess pain and routine functional skills (see Appendix 15.1).[8] The Shoulder Pain and Disability Index has been shown to be a reliable and valid questionnaire for shoulder pain.[9] The Patient Specific Functional Scale can be used to measure progress of treatment of clients with any musculo-skeletal condition, including shoulder conditions. Activities which are difficult to perform are nominated by the client. The Patient Specific Functional Scale is considered to be a reliable, valid and responsive evaluation instrument in clients with a primary shoulder complaint.[10]

POSTURAL ANALYSIS

Postural analysis enables observation of the whole client and facilitates identification of important features through bilateral comparison. It also facilitates detection of possible predisposing or contributing factors by observing the cervical and thoracic spines, glenohumeral joints and scapula. Observe and compare the shoulders anteriorly and posteriorly noting their symmetry. The shoulder muscles normally appear full and round. Observe any bruising, colour changes, swelling, surgical incisions and scars. Differences in bony contour may be apparent in AC joint separation (the step defect, see Figure 15.4), sternoclavicular (SC) separation and clavicle fractures.

The level of the shoulders is often distorted in clients with scoliosis. Observe winging of the scapula and muscle hypertonicity or atrophy.

FUNCTIONAL TESTS

For any tests involving joint movements it is important to compare both sides and take into account any underlying pathology and the age and lifestyle of the client. Findings from physical examinations should be interpreted in the light of evidence for their diagnostic accuracy. No clinical test is both reliable and valid for any specific diagnostic entity. However, despite their limitations, functional tests help alert practitioners to the presence of potentially serious conditions and suggest types of tissues that are likely to be involved. Range of motion tests have been shown to be reliable but their diagnostic utility is unknown. Devices such as goniometers, including digital goniometers, and smartphone apps can provide accurate measurements of shoulder range of motion.[11, 12] Manual muscle strength testing also appears to be reliable.[13] Limitations of individual tests should also be taken into consideration. A recent study demonstrated reliability with shoulder manual muscle testing only when one side was at least 15–25% weaker than the other side.[14] Another study on the reliability of upper quarter physical examination for patients with shoulder pain found variable reliability. Muscle length and cervical range of motion were significantly more reliable than other tests.[15]

Active range of motion of the cervical spine (flexion, extension, lateral flexion and rotation)

Examination of the shoulder complex begins with functional tests of the cervical spine to help rule out brachial plexus and

Fig. 15.5 Dermatomes of the shoulder region

Table 15.3 Shoulder end-feel[18]

Shoulder movement	Normal end-feel
Flexion	Firm
Extension	Firm
Abduction	Usually firm
Adduction	Not typically measured
Lateral or external rotation	Firm
Medial or internal rotation	Firm

cervical radiculopathy which refer pain to the shoulder region (see Figure 15.5). If active range of motion tests of the cervical spine reproduce the shoulder symptoms, further examination of the cervical spine is indicated (see Chapter 12). Record all measurements in clinical notes as evidence of change over treatment sessions.

Active range of motion of the glenohumeral joint

The client may be standing or sitting, elbow bent or straight as convenient. Face the client and demonstrate the movements. Examine the following ranges of motion:[16]

- Flexion/extension (165°/60°)[17]
- Internal/external rotation (70°/90°)
  Instruct the client to bend their elbows and keep their elbows close to their body as they move their forearms outwards from the body and inwards across the body.
- Abduction/adduction (165°)
  Painful arc: Look for a painful arc (i.e. pain that comes on after the arm has been abducted to the middle of the arc (40°–120°) and dissipates with further abduction). The presence of a painful arc suggests rotator cuff, AC joint pathology or impingement syndrome.
- **Scapulohumeral rhythm:** Glenohumeral abduction and scapulothoracic abduction occur in the ratio 2 to 1 (beginning after the upper limb has reached 20° of abduction); that is, when the humerus is abducted 120°, the scapula abducts 60°. Disturbances to the smooth scapulohumeral rhythm may be due to weak scapula stabilisers and/or tightness of the scapulohumeral muscles (infraspinatus, teres minor, subscapularis).
- Horizontal adduction (130°).

Passive range of motion

If the client is unable to perform normal AROM in any direction, further investigation is required. PROM testing should be performed with one hand stabilising and palpating the shoulder joint while the other hand moves the upper limb. Note that PROM shoulder tests may be performed with the elbow flexed. Palpate for crepitus, capsular pattern and end-feel (see Table 15.3). The capsular pattern of restriction for the glenohumeral joint is external rotation more limited than abduction; abduction more limited than internal rotation.[16]

Resisted range of motion

RROM tests should also be performed if AROM testing indicates the likelihood of a shoulder problem. RROM tests include:

- flexion: anterior deltoid, biceps brachii, coracobrachialis, pectoralis major
- extension: posterior deltoid, latissimus dorsi, triceps brachii, teres major
- abduction: middle deltoid, supraspinatus
- adduction: latissimus dorsi, teres major, pectoralis major
- horizontal adduction: pectoralis major, coracobrachialis, anterior deltoid
- internal rotation: subscapularis, teres major, latissimus dorsi, pectoralis major
- external rotation: infraspinatus, teres minor
- scapular elevation: upper trapezius, levator scapulae, rhomboid major, rhomboid minor
- scapular retraction: rhomboid major, rhomboid minor, middle trapezius
- scapular protraction: serratus anterior

Resisted tests and length tests for specific muscles[19]

If RROM tests reproduce symptoms, then further tests may be used to help identify specific muscles involved. Always compare bilaterally. Manual muscle testing becomes reliably perceptible once the weakness becomes greater than 15–25%.[14] For increased accuracy consider the use of devices such as hand-held dynamometers.[11]

Fig. 15.6 Resisted test for middle deltoid

Fig. 15.8 Resisted test for posterior deltoid

Fig. 15.7 Resisted test for anterior deltoid

Fig. 15.9 Resisted test for supraspinatus

1. DELTOID MUSCLE

Middle deltoid

Resisted test

The client abducts their arm to 90° with their elbow flexed at 90°. Place one hand on the client's shoulder and the other on the elbow. Ask the client to hold their arm in this position against your downward pressure (see Figure 15.6).

Anterior deltoid

Resisted test

Position as above. One of your palms contacts the anterior aspect of the upper arm, the other is placed over the shoulder joint. The client tries to bring their forearm forwards against your resistance (see Figure 15.7).

Posterior deltoid

Resisted test

Position as above. One of your palms contacts the posterior aspect of the client's upper arm. The client tries to move their upper arm backwards against your resistance (see Figure 15.8).

Length test

The length of middle deltoid is tested with supraspinatus (see Figure 15.10 on p 271).

2. SUPRASPINATUS

Resisted test

Place one hand on the client's forearm or elbow, the other hand contacts the shoulder joint. The client abducts their arm to 30° against your resistance (see Figure 15.9).

Length test

Supraspinatus and middle deltoid are tested together. The client adducts their arm by reaching across their back as far as possible. The client should be able to reach the elbow if their other arm. (see Figure 15.10).

Fig. 15.10 Length test for supraspinatus

Fig. 15.12 Length test for infraspinatus/teres minor

Fig. 15.11 Resisted test for infraspinatus/teres minor

4. TERES MAJOR

Resisted test

The client places the dorsum of one hand on the posterior aspect of their iliac crest. Place one hand on the shoulder; the other hand contacts the posterior aspect of the elbow. The client tries to hold this position as you apply pressure to the elbow in the direction of abduction and flexion (see Figure 15.13 on p 272).

Length test

The length of the external rotator muscles is tested with the client supine and one hand placed behind their neck. The client's elbow should touch the table (see Figure 15.14 on p 272).

5. SUBSCAPULARIS

Resisted test

The client places their arm against their side with their elbow flexed to 90°, their forearm is semi-supinated. The practitioner places one hand on the patient's elbow to prevent abduction and the other hand on the dorsum of the wrist. The client tries to internally rotate their forearm against resistance (see Figure 15.15 on p 272). (Note: This test recruits all shoulder internal rotator muscles. Latissimus dorsi (see Chapter 11) and teres major (see above) may be distinguished from subscapularis with further resisted tests.)

3. INFRASPINATUS/TERES MINOR

Resisted test

The client places their arm against their side with their elbow flexed to 90°, their forearm is semi-supinated. Place one hand on the patient's elbow to prevent abduction and the other hand on the dorsum of the wrist. The client tries to laterally rotate their forearm against your resistance (see Figure 15.11).

Length test

The client should be able to touch the inferior tip of the opposite shoulder blade with their fingers (see Figure 15.12).

Length test

The shoulder internal rotators are tested together (see Figure 15.15 on p 272).

Fig. 15.13 Resisted test for teres major

Fig. 15.14 Length test for shoulder internal rotators

Fig. 15.15 Resisted test for subscapularis

Fig. 15.16 Resisted test for biceps brachii

Fig. 15.17 Length test for biceps brachii

6. BICEPS BRACHII

Resisted test

The client flexes their elbow to 90°. One of your hands supports the elbow, the other contacts the client's supinated wrist. Apply resistance as the client tries to flex their elbow (see Figure 15.16).

Length test

The client lies supine with their shoulder level with the edge of the table, elbow extended and forearm pronated. The client extends their shoulder, keeping their elbow fully extended (see Figure 15.17). There are no know normative data for this flexibility test.[20]

7. CORACOBRACHIALIS

Resisted test

The client is seated with elbow flexed to 90°, wrist pronated, and tries to hold this position as the practitioner applies

Fig. 15.18 Resisted test for coracobrachialis

Fig. 15.19 Resisted test for triceps brachii

Fig. 15.20 Length test for triceps brachii

pressure towards the floor (see Figure 15.18). (Note: This procedure tests all shoulder flexor muscles. Biceps brachii and anterior deltoid can be distinguished with further resisted tests described above.)

Length test

See biceps brachii length test (Figure 15.17).

8. TRICEPS BRACHII

Resisted test

Contact the client's elbow with one hand and wrist with the other and resist as the client tries to extend their elbow (see Figure 15.19).

Length test

The client tries to touch the back of the shoulder on the same side with the shoulder flexed to 180°. There are no known normative data for this flexibility test (see Figure 15.20).[20]

Special tests

Special tests are designed to reproduce the client's symptoms. If pain is reported when performing a special test, ask the client to identify the exact location of the pain and confirm

that it is the same pain as the pain described in the case history. Positive special test results should always be interpreted cautiously and in the context of other clinical findings (see Chapter 2).

APLEY'S SCRATCH TEST

The client tries to touch the opposite scapula approaching from above and from below. Pain when performing these movements or inability to perform the movements normally suggests rotator cuff pathology, labral pathology, AC arthritis or capsular/muscle contracture (see Figure 15.21 on p 274).

DROP ARM TEST

The drop arm test is designed to identify tears of the supraspinatus muscle. Stand behind the client and abduct their arms to 90° supporting their arm at the elbow. Suddenly release the elbow support and ask the client to stop their arms from dropping. Pain or weakness may indicate rotator cuff strain or tear, bursitis or impingement (see Figure 15.22 on p 274).

IMPINGEMENT TEST

The client raises their arm to 90° flexion with the palm facing up (externally rotated) and then returns their arm to the starting position. Next, the client raises their arm to 90° with the thumbs down (internally rotated). Pain during flexion with external rotation may suggest supraspinatus impingement; pain during flexion with internal rotation may suggest long head of biceps impingement (see Figure 15.23 on p 274).

APPREHENSION TEST

Stand behind the client and abduct their humerus to 90° with the elbow bent (the stop sign position). Observe the client for distress or anxiety while slow and gentle anterior pressure is

Fig. 15.21 Apley's scratch test (the client tries to touch their scapula)

Fig. 15.22 Drop arm test

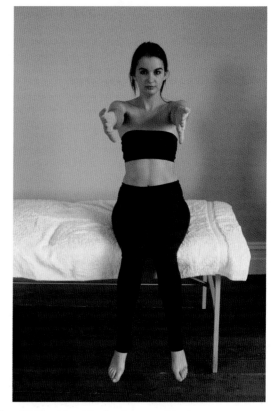

Fig. 15.23 Shoulder impingement test

applied to the shoulder joint. Apprehension on the client's part suggests anterior glenohumeral instability (see Figure 15.24 on p 275).

YERGASON'S TEST

Begin with the client's elbow flexed to 90° and wrist pronated. Demonstrate the hitchhiker movement (i.e. supinating, flexing and externally rotating their forearm). Next, palpate the long head of the biceps with one hand and hold the client's forearm with the other. The client performs the hitchhiker movement against your resistance. Pain in the region of the bicipital groove suggests biceps brachii tendinosis or strain. Pain in the shoulder suggests glenoid labrum pathology. If the transverse

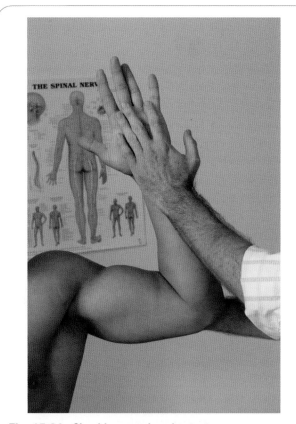

Fig. 15.24 Shoulder apprehension test

Fig. 15.25 Yergason's test

Fig. 15.26 Empty can test

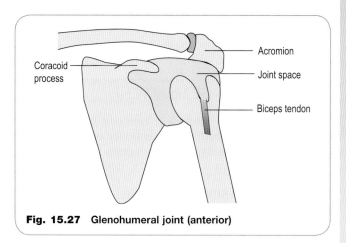

Fig. 15.27 Glenohumeral joint (anterior)

humeral ligament is torn, the tendon will snap out of the groove (bicipital tendinopathy) (see Figure 15.25).

EMPTY CAN TEST

The client abducts both arms to 120° with their palms facing upwards. Next, the client internally rotates their arm by turning their thumbs downwards towards the floor (empty can position) and, maintaining the internal rotation, slowly lowers their arms to their sides. Pain or weakness may indicate a supraspatus muscle injury (see Figure 15.26).

PALPATION

Palpatory findings, along with findings from other assessments, are used to guide treatment plans. From the suprasternal notch, palpate the sternoclavicular joints immediately laterally. Clavicular dislocations are usually easily palpated, the medial end of the clavicle displacing medially and superiorly. The tip of the coracoid process can be palpated 2.5 cm below the clavicle through the pectoralis major muscle. Palpate the AC joint and the acromion. The greater tuberosity of the humerus can be palpated lateral and inferior to the acromion. Externally rotate the client's shoulder to palpate the intertubercular groove which is anterior and medial to the greater tuberosity, and the lesser tuberosity medial to the groove. Palpate the tendon of the long head of biceps brachii in the bicipital groove (see Figure 15.27).

The deltoid attaches to the acromion and inserts into the deltoid tuberosity. It overlays the greater tuberosity of the humerus and gives the shoulder its full and rounded appearance. Three of the rotator cuff muscles (the supraspinatus, infraspinatus and the teres minor, commonly referred to by the acronym SIT muscles[21]) insert into the greater tuberosity. The fourth muscle of the rotator cuff, the subscapularis, attaches to the lesser tuberosity and is not easily palpated. When the client's arm is by their side, the supraspinatus attachment lies under the acromion, the subscapularis attachment is anterior, and the infraspinatus and teres minor attachments are posterior. Passively extending the client's shoulder moves the SIT muscles into a more easily palpable position. Tenderness elicited during palpation of the muscle attachments suggests tear or strain. Note that the supraspinatus tendon is the most commonly injured muscle in the shoulder joint.[22] The subacromial and subdeltoid bursa may be palpable immediately below the anterior and lateral aspects of the acromion when the arm is in the neutral position by the side.

Palpate the spine of the scapula posteriorly. The superior angle of the scapula and the insertion of the levator scapulae muscle are palpated through the trapezius muscle. Palpate the medial border of the scapula, inferior angle, lateral border and overlying latissimus dorsi, teres major and teres minor muscles. The latissimus dorsi muscle forms the posterior border of the axilla and the subscapularis muscle may be palpated deep to latissimus dorsi. Pectoralis major makes up the anterior border of the axilla. Ribs 2–6 and the overlying serratus anterior muscle are palpated in the medial axilla. Lymph node enlargements may be palpated at the apex of the axilla.

REMEDIAL MASSAGE TREATMENT

Shoulder pain is the third most common musculoskeletal complaint and only half of new episodes of shoulder pain show complete recovery within 6 months.[23] Shoulder pain may recur even when a full recovery appears to have been made in the short term. Strong predictors of chronicity include high scores on the SPADI questionnaire, high shoulder pain intensity, concomitant neck pain and a longer duration of complaint.[23, 24] Moderate predictors of chronicity include being male, over 55 years of age, poor general health, a gradual onset of complaints, a large amount of sick leave, the perception of high job demand, the perception of low social support, and increased visits to a healthcare professional.[23] Fear avoidance and pain catastrophising may have a negative influence on chronicity and patient outcomes. Shoulder patients with higher scores for optimism have higher shoulder function although report similar pain levels.[25]

Protective factors include an active treatment policy and avoidance of non-essential medication. Key to informing therapists' awareness of shoulder patients' treatment progress is the use of patient-reported outcome measures throughout care, not just at the start and end of treatment.[26]

Assessment of the shoulder region provides essential information for development of treatment plans, including:

- clients' suitability for remedial massage therapy
- duration of the condition (i.e. acute or chronic)
- severity of the condition (i.e. grade of injury; mild, moderate or severe pain)
- type(s) of tissues involved
- priorities for treatment if more than one injury or condition are present
- whether the signs and symptoms suggest a common condition of the shoulder region
- special considerations for individual clients (e.g. client's preference for treatment types and styles, specific population considerations).

Treatment options must always be considered in the context of the best available evidence for treatment effectiveness and clinical practice guidelines where they exist. A 2017 systematic review and meta-analysis found that the evidence for massage improving shoulder pain in the short term is large and robust. Long-term evidence exists although it is limited.[27] Deep tissue massage applied to the shoulders for 10 sessions had the greatest long-term effect. However, high-quality randomised controlled trials with a long follow-up are needed to support many remedial massage shoulder treatments. Findings of current research are summarised in Table 15.4.

NON-SPECIFIC SHOULDER AND NECK PAIN

Many people live with non-specific neck and shoulder pain which is not the result of a traumatic injury or serious disease.

Table 15.4 Summary of the evidence for the effectiveness of conservative interventions for shoulder conditions[27–30]

Shoulder condition	Intervention	Quality of evidence
Shoulder limited range of motion	Massage increased shoulder range of motion particularly in flexion and abduction	Low to moderate
Shoulder pain	Massage short-term efficacy	Large and robust
	Massage long-term efficacy	Low
Non-specific shoulder pain	Massage improving pain function and range of motion	Low
	Exercise therapy for small improvements in pain	Low
	Low level laser therapy	Moderate
Shoulder impingement syndrome	Manual therapy	Moderate
	Kinesio taping	Moderate
	Low level laser therapy	Moderate
	Pulsed electromagnetic field therapy	Moderate
	Supervised and home exercise	Moderate
Adhesive capsulitis	Manual therapy	Low to moderate
	Low level laser therapy	Low to moderate
Rotator cuff-associated disorders	Manual therapy	Low to moderate
	Physical therapy	Effective (although superior when combined with surgery)
	Extracorporeal shockwave therapy for calcific tendonitis	Moderate
	Diathermy and cortisone injections	Moderate
	Cortisone injections	Moderate

Muscles that often tender and painful include trapezius, neck extensors, levator scapulae and infraspinatus.[2]

Shoulder pathology is mostly related to either impingement or instability.[31] Common mechanisms of injury include throwing overhead, falling on the outstretched arm or shoulder tip and forcing the shoulder into external or internal rotation while the arm is abducted.

OVERVIEW

Develop a short- and a long-term plan for each client. The short-term plan directs treatment to the highest priority (usually determined by symptoms). The long-term plan can be introduced when presenting symptoms have subsided. Long-term treatment focuses on contributing or predisposing factors such as underlying structural features and lifestyle factors. A significant part of both short-term and long-term treatment involves educating clients about likely causal or aggravating factors and guiding their management of these factors.

MUSCLE STRAIN

The most common sites of pathology in the shoulder are the rotator cuff muscles (particularly supraspinatus), the sub-acromial bursa and the tendon of the long head of biceps brachii.[32, 33]

Rotator cuff tendinosis

Rotator cuff tendinosis refers to strain of the supraspinatus, infraspinatus, teres minor or subscapularis tendons. Most rotator cuff strains are partial tears. They are the result of progressive collagen breakdown and develop from prolonged repetitive strain, especially from overhead activities, throwing or lifting, shovelling, spiking in volleyball, bowling in cricket and racquet sports.[34] Strains may also arise from sudden trauma or excessive force applied to the shoulder. Full thickness tears of the tendon tend to result from serious acute injuries with high force loads.

Supraspinatus is the most commonly strained rotator cuff muscle. Repeated compression under the acromion eventually leads to tissue degeneration and fibre tearing. Decreased vascularity near the supraspinatus insertion can also lead to slower healing and calcification of the tendon.[35] The infraspinatus and teres minor muscles laterally rotate the humerus (concentric contraction) and also decelerate medial rotation of the humerus as in the eccentric contraction phase (follow through) of throwing. The subscapularis is rarely strained as other stronger accessory muscles, such as pectoralis major, latissimus dorsi and teres major provide mechanical support. Subscapularis strains are more likely in clients over 40 years and are often associated with glenohumeral dislocation.

Biceps brachii tendinosis[36]

Biceps brachii tendinosis is a result of progressive degeneration of the long head of the biceps brachii tendon as it passes from the superior aspect of the glenoid fossa through the joint capsule to the bicipital groove of the humerus. The tendon is surrounded by a synovial sheath. The tendon may be a primary or secondary source of shoulder pain and so a comprehensive evaluation is required.[36] Tendinosis is usually the result of overuse, especially with excessive weight training (e.g. excessive bench press and dips). The tendon is stabilised

in the bicipital groove by the transverse humeral ligament and may pop out of the groove if the transverse ligament is impaired. The tendon may also pull away from the glenoid labrum if excessive force is applied. Refer all severe injuries for further investigation.

Assessment

HISTORY

The client complains of shoulder pain after prolonged or repetitive overuse, especially after overhead throwing, shovelling, racquet sports or a single blow, fall onto an outstretched hand or sports injury. Pain can be experienced immediately or within the next 24–48 hours. Pain is associated with activities and generally relieved with rest.

FUNCTIONAL TESTS

AROM: limited in one or more directions.
PROM: mild to no pain except at end of range when muscle is stretched.
RROM: painful.
Resisted and length tests painful for involved muscles.
Special tests for specific muscle strains positive (e.g. Apley's scratch test, drop arm test, empty can test, Yergason's test).

PALPATION

Muscle spasm is usually evident. The client reports tenderness or pain on palpation of the affected muscle.

Overview of treatment of muscle strains

A typical remedial massage treatment for mild to moderate muscle strains of the shoulder includes:

- Swedish massage to the shoulder, upper back, neck, upper limb and chest.
- Remedial techniques including:
  - deep gliding frictions along the muscle fibres
  - cross-fibre frictions
  - soft tissue releasing techniques
  - deep transverse friction
  - trigger point therapy.

> **Key assessment findings for muscle strain**
>
> - History of trauma or repetitive overuse
> - Functional tests
>   - AROM limited in one or more directions
>   - PROM usually negative except at end of range if muscle is passively stretched
>   - RROM painful in one or more directions
>   - Resisted test and length test positive for specific muscle
>   - Special tests may be positive for specific muscles (e.g. Apley's scratch for rotator cuff pathology, empty can test for supraspinatus, Yergason's test for long head of biceps brachii)
> - Palpation positive for tenderness/pain, spasm, myofibril tears/scar tissue

Fig. 15.28 Myofascial release: Arm pull

Remedial massage techniques for muscles of the shoulder region are illustrated in Table 15.5.

- Myofascial release including cross-arm techniques and the arm pull (see Chapter 8). (Figure 15.28).
- Thermotherapy might be useful for pain relief.

Other remedial techniques for muscle strains/tightness include:

- **Horizontal fibre release (derived from Bowen)**

In its traditional form Bowen is a stand-alone therapy. A derivative form is described here which may be integrated with other remedial techniques.

The client is seated. Stand behind the client and place your foot on the table next to the client (hip and knee flexed). For hygiene purposes, place foot on paper towel. Instruct the client to raise their arm into the stop sign position (shoulder abducted to 90°, elbow flexed to 90°). The client's elbow is placed on your knee. Place both hands together over the client's shoulder joint and deltoid, with fingers anteriorly and thumbs posteriorly. Instruct the client to slowly move their hand as far forward as

they can (internal rotation) and then as far back again (external rotation). As the client moves, grip the shoulder muscles to separate the myofibrils horizontally (see Figure 15.29 on p 286).

- Shoulder passive joint articulation may be a useful supplement to the muscle-specific techniques described above (see Chapter 7):
  - shoulder rotation
  - shoulder traction
  - shoulder progressive cylindrical articulation
  - shoulder progressive external rotation
  - shoulder progressive internal rotation
  - shoulder figure-8.

Address any underlying conditions or predisposing factors (e.g scoliosis or thoracic hyperkyphosis).

CLIENT EDUCATION

Prioritise clients taking an increasingly active role in their treatment through rehabilitation and health promotion activities. Shoulders are particularly susceptible to injury from

Table 15.5 Remedial massage techniques for muscles of the shoulder region

Muscle	Soft tissue release	Trigger point	Deep transverse friction	Stretch	Corrective action[38, 39]	Home exercise
Middle deltoid	Horizontal fibre release (derived from Bowen). Practitioner: stands behind the seated client with their foot on the table (on a paper towel). Client: raises arm into stop sign position (shoulder abducted to 90°, elbow flexed to 90°) and rests flexed elbow on practitioner's knee. The practitioner places both hands together over the deltoid, with fingers anterior and thumbs posterior. The client slowly moves their hand as far forward as they can (shoulder internal rotation) and then as far back (shoulder external rotation). As the client moves, the practitioner grips the deltoid muscle to spread the fibres.			Middle deltoid: As for supraspinatus.	Eliminate perpetuating mechanical stresses (e.g. drive with two hands on steering wheel). Technique correction with overhead sports.	Stretch: Reach behind back as far as possible within pain tolerance towards opposite side of body. (Other hand can assist by pulling flexed elbow further medially.)

Continued

Table 15.5 Remedial massage techniques for muscles of the shoulder region—cont'd

Muscle	Soft tissue release	Trigger point	Deep transverse friction	Stretch	Corrective action[38, 39]	Home exercise
Supraspinatus	Client: sitting or supine with elbow bent to 90°. Practitioner: applies gentle sustained pressure to the belly of the supraspinatus using thumbs or knuckles as client slowly abducts and adducts their arm as far as possible within pain tolerance. Repeat several times. In the dynamic variation, the practitioner glides their contact along the supraspinatus belly while the client adducts the arm (i.e. lengthening supraspinatus).			CRAC stretch: Client: seated, adducts arm by reaching behind their back across their body towards their other arm as far as possible within pain tolerance. Practitioner: applies resistance at the client's flexed elbow as they try to abduct their arm for 6–8 seconds. After the resistance, the client returns their arm to their side and then adducts their arm again as far as possible within pain tolerance. Repeat the whole procedure three times.	Avoid overloading the muscle (e.g. avoid carrying heavy loads). Do not sleep with hands above head.	Stretch:

Table 15.5 Remedial massage techniques for muscles of the shoulder region—cont'd

Muscle	Soft tissue release	Trigger point	Deep transverse friction	Stretch	Corrective action[38, 39]	Home exercise
Infraspinatus/ teres minor	Client: seated, elbow flexed to 90°. Practitioner: maintains pressure on taut band/lesion of the muscle using thumbs or knuckles, as the forearm is actively or passively taken inwards across the body (shoulder internal rotation) and outwards (shoulder external rotation), keeping elbow at side of body. Dynamic variation: practitioner slowly glides along the muscle fibres as the muscle is lengthened (i.e. the humerus internally rotates) Can be performed prone, beginning with client's shoulder abducted to 90°	infraspinatus teres minor		CRAC stretch: Client: reaches behind their back towards inferior angle of opposite scapula within pain tolerance. Practitioner: holding client's wrist and elbow, resists the client's attempt to return arm to their side for 6–8 seconds. Client returns arm to their side. Next, client reaches behind their back towards inferior angle of scapula again within pain tolerance. Repeat the whole procedure three times.	Avoid overloading the muscle (e.g. reaching into back seat of car). Support arm on a pillow for pain relief when sleeping. Avoid rounded shoulder posture.	Stretch: Try to touch hands behind back with one arm overhead and the other behind the back. Can hold a small towel between hands if required. Hold for up to 30 seconds. Repeat three times. Strengthen: Resisted shoulder external rotation

Continued

281

Table 15.5 Remedial massage techniques for muscles of the shoulder region—cont'd

Muscle	Soft tissue release	Trigger point	Deep transverse friction	Stretch	Corrective action[38, 39]	Home exercise
Teres major	Client: seated, elbow flexed to 90°. Practitioner: maintains pressure on taut band/lesion of the muscle using thumbs or knuckles as the forearm is actively or passively taken inwards across the body (shoulder internal rotation) and outwards (shoulder external rotation), keeping elbow at side of body. Can be performed prone, beginning with client's shoulder abducted to 90°.			CRAC stretch: Client lies supine, elbow flexed to 90° and externally rotates forearm as far as possible within pain tolerance, keeping elbow alongside body. The practitioner applies resistance for 6–8 seconds as the client tries to bring their forearm across their body (internally rotate shoulder). When the resistance is released, the client tries to externally rotate their forearm as far as possible again. The whole procedure is repeated three times. Progress to different starting positions (e.g. humerus abducted to 30°, 60° or 90°, practitioner supporting abducted elbow), making sure the client's scapula remains flat on the treatment table throughout the stretch.	Avoid overloading the muscle (e.g. drive with two hands on the steering wheel). To sleep, lie on the affected side and place a pillow between the elbow and the front of the body. Check gym activities.	Lie supine, place both hands behind the neck and let elbows fall towards the floor as far as possible. Strengthen: Resisted internal rotation

Table 15.5 Remedial massage techniques for muscles of the shoulder region—cont'd

Muscle	Soft tissue release	Trigger point	Deep transverse friction	Stretch	Corrective action[38, 39]	Home exercise
Subscapularis	Client: supine, humerus abducted to 90° and elbow flexed to 90°. Practitioner: contacts the lateral aspect of the subscapularis using a flat finger contact and moves medially into the posterior axilla. The practitioner contacts the client's forearm at the wrist and slowly externally and internally rotates the arm while applying pressure to the subscapularis.		The distal musculotendinous junction where most tears occur is accessible. The practitioner grasps either side of the posterior axilla between thumb and index finger and applies deep friction to the fibres by dragging the contacts laterally.	CRAC stretch: Client: supine or seated, elbow flexed to 90° and externally rotates the arm as far as possible within pain tolerance. Practitioner: applies resistance for 6–8 seconds as the client tries to internally rotate their arm. After the resistance, the client tries to externally rotate their arm to their comfortable limit. Repeat the whole procedure three times.	Correct rounded shoulder posture.	Stretch: Lie supine, humerus abducted to 90° or as far as possible, elbow flexed to 90°. Let the forearm fall backwards towards the floor as far as possible within pain tolerance. Hold for 30 seconds. Make sure that the scapula remains flat on the floor throughout the stretch. Alternatively, the doorway stretch (see Chapter 14) can also be used to stretch subscapularis. Strengthen: Resisted internal rotation.

Continued

Table 15.5 Remedial massage techniques for muscles of the shoulder region—cont'd

Muscle	Soft tissue release	Trigger point	Deep transverse friction	Stretch	Corrective action[38, 39]	Home exercise
Biceps brachii	Client: supine or seated, elbow fully flexed at the beginning of this technique to shorten the biceps. Practitioner: maintains pressure with thumbs, fingers or knuckles, or performs a deep glide along the muscle fibres as the client's forearm is actively or passively extended and flexed. The client can hold a weight in their hand to recruit more fibres.		At the humeral insertion, deep friction techniques are applied in a longitudinal rather than transverse direction to prevent dislocation of the tendon from the groove.	Passive stretch: Biceps brachii is stretched by extending the shoulder, extending the elbow and then pronating the forearm.	Lift objects with forearms in pronation. Decrease load when carrying with flexed elbows. Strengthen triceps brachii. Correct sleeping posture. Check work ergonomics.	Extend the shoulder, extend the elbow and point thumb downwards. Hold for 30 seconds.

A variant of the doorway stretch can be used: stand in front of the doorway, hold the door jamb with thumbs pointing downward, elbows extended and lean forward. |

Table 15.5 Remedial massage techniques for muscles of the shoulder region—cont'd

Muscle	Soft tissue release	Trigger point	Deep transverse friction	Stretch	Corrective action[38, 39]	Home exercise
Triceps brachii	Client: prone or seated (or supine with arm extended overhead). Practitioner: maintains pressure with thumbs, fingers or knuckles or performs a deep glide along the muscle fibres as the client slowly flexes and extends their elbow.			CRAC stretch: Client: seated, elbow fully flexed, and humerus flexed to comfortable limit. Practitioner: stands behind the client, holds the elbow and resists as the client tries to extend their humerus (i.e. bring their elbow forward) for 6–8 seconds. After the resistance, the client tries to flex the humerus again to their comfortable limit. Repeat the whole procedure three times.	Avoid overload. Modify chairs with inadequate elbow support. Review arm position in repetitive manual work. Use tennis racquet with a large grip. Avoid overhead activities.	Fully flex the elbow and flex the humerus as far as possible. Use the other hand to try to pull the flexed elbow towards a vertical position within a comfortable limit. Hold the stretch for up to 30 seconds. Repeat three times.

Fig. 15.29 Horizontal fibre release (derived from Bowen)

activities and sports which place sustained demands on the arms and shoulders or where there is a risk of sudden trauma. The importance of a general and sport-specific physical conditioning program in the prevention of shoulder injuries cannot be overstated. To prevent overuse injuries technique correction (e.g. for throwing, spiking, overhead smashing, overhand serving, crawl and butterfly swimming, and tackling) may be required.

Home exercise program

A program of progressive rehabilitation should accompany remedial massage treatment. Aim for maximum strength and full length of all major muscles. Unresolved strains lead ultimately to faulty biomechanics and other conditions such as adhesive capsulitis and osteoarthritis may follow.

Introduce stretching exercises as soon as possible after injury (depending on severity and pain tolerance). Introduce non-resistive pendulum exercises gradually progressing to active resistive isometric, isotonic and isokinetic exercises after most ROM has been regained. Apply ice after exercises if pain or swelling returns (exercises should be performed initially at less than 90° flexion and abduction). Focus on glenohumeral rotation (aim for a strength ratio of 2:3 of external rotators to internal rotators).[37] Strengthening programs should progress towards functional exercises (e.g. wall push ups, overhead work, ball throwing) which should be maintained long term. Include proprioceptive exercises (e.g. gymball).

Clients may be referred for manipulation of the neck, upper back and shoulders. Refer any client who worsens or fails to improve within 2 weeks or shows only slight improvement within 4 weeks.

SHOULDER IMPINGEMENT SYNDROME

Shoulder impingement syndrome (sometimes called swimmer's shoulder) describes the compression of several soft tissue structures between the coracoacromial arch (made up of the coracoid process, the acromion and the coracoacromial ligament) and the greater tuberosity of the humerus. Soft tissues that may be compressed include the supraspinatus muscle or tendon, the tendon of the long head of biceps brachii, the upper glenohumeral joint capsule and the

subacromial bursa. When the subacromial bursa becomes inflamed it can swell to the size of a golf ball. Subacromial bursitis often occurs from repetitive compression underneath the coracoacromial arch as can occur in overhead movements (e.g. tennis serve, bowling in cricket, or freestyle swimming). Other causes of bursitis include autoimmune disease, crystal deposition, or infection.

Impingement is classified as primary or secondary. Primary impingement may be caused by reduced space under the acromion due to a flattened or tilted acromion, or osteophytes which have developed under the acromion. Secondary impingement may be caused by repeated overhead movements as occur in throwing, overhead strokes in swimming, cricket, weight lifting, water polo and tennis, decreased vascularity to the rotator cuff or biceps brachii tendons, or a raised humeral head due to a previous dislocation.

Shoulder impingement tends to initiate a cycle of degeneration. Once the shoulder muscles are impinged, they are less effective at maintaining the humeral head in the glenoid fossa, which in turn leads to further impingement. Treatment outcomes depend on how quickly treatment is commenced. Three progressive stages of impingement have been described.[40] Stage 1 is characterised by acute inflammation, oedema and haemorrhage in the rotator cuff muscles. Stage 2 progresses to fibrosis and tendinosis of the rotator cuff muscles. In Stage 3 mechanical disruption of the rotator cuff tendons and changes to the coracoacromial arch occur. As with most musculoskeletal conditions, early intervention is likely to produce the best outcomes.

Assessment

Key assessment findings for shoulder impingement syndrome

- History of repetitive overhead activity; painful abduction and flexion
- Functional tests
  - AROM positive (painful arc)
  - PROM ± painful
  - RROM positive in some directions
  - Resisted and length tests positive for affected muscles
  - Special tests: shoulder impingement test positive
- Palpation positive for pain/tenderness, spasm, myofibril tears/scar tissue

HISTORY

The client complains of pain during active flexion and abduction of the shoulder, usually between 70° and 120° (painful arc). The client may describe recurring or constant shoulder pain, often worse at night. There is often a history of several previous episodes of shoulder pain that are associated with repetitive overhead activity. Pain may refer to the lateral and posterolateral upper arm.

FUNCTIONAL TESTS

Cervical AROM negative.

Shoulder:
AROM: positive flexion and abduction (painful arc).
PROM: may be positive in flexion and abduction.

RROM: Weakness and pain depending on muscle(s) involved (e.g. if supraspinatus involved, pain ± weakness on resisted shoulder abduction; if biceps brachii tendon is involved, pain on resisted shoulder flexion).

Resisted tests and length tests are positive for affected muscles.

Special tests: Impingement test positive, empty can test and Apley's scratch test positive if supraspinatus is affected.

PALPATION

Tenderness may be elicited during palpation over the greater tuberosity and anterior acromion. (Note: tenderness may also be present in glenohumeral or AC arthrosis). Muscle atrophy may follow long-standing impingement. Crepitus/snapping may be present. (Note: crepitus/snapping is also associated with glenohumeral and AC arthrosis and labral tears.[41])

Overview of treatment and management

One of the challenges of treating impingement is that the tissues that have been compressed are often fibrotic. They are also difficult to access under the acromion. Effective techniques to accessible tissues include friction to the supraspinatus tendon, deep longitudinal stripping to the supraspinatus belly, and deep friction to the infraspinatus and teres minor muscles. Attention should be focused on tissues that can alter biomechanical function, such as tightness in the deltoid or weakness of the lateral and internal rotators which could raise the humeral head in the glenoid fossa predisposing to impingement during overhead movements.

A typical remedial massage treatment for mild or moderate impingement syndrome includes:

- Swedish massage therapy to the shoulder and upper arm, neck, upper back (and chest).
- Remedial massage techniques, including (see Table 15.5):
  - deep gliding frictions along the muscle fibres
  - cross-fibre frictions
  - soft tissue releasing techniques
  - deep transverse friction
  - trigger point therapy
  - muscle stretching.

If assessment results suggest inert structures then myofascial releasing techniques (see Chapter 8) and passive joint articulations (see Chapter 7) may be appropriate. Passive joint articulation for the shoulder includes:

- shoulder rotation
- shoulder traction
- shoulder progressive cylindrical articulation
- shoulder progressive external rotation
- shoulder progressive internal rotation
- shoulder figure-8.

CLIENT EDUCATION

Advise clients to avoid all overhead or painful activities. Posture correction especially for the cervical spine and pectoral girdle may be required. Review aggravating sporting techniques or work activities and correct if possible. A rehabilitation exercise program should be started as soon as tolerated by the client. The goal of the program is to restore normal shoulder biomechanics. This usually involves strengthening the shoulder stabilisers and rotator cuff muscles. Restoration

of normal scapular rotation about a medial to lateral axis and serratus anterior muscle function are particularly important in the rehabilitation of clients whose symptoms are related to overhead sport or work.[42, 43] For patients with rotator cuff related pain a scapula-focused approach may be more effective in reducing disability than a general approach. The benefit is particularly evident in the first 6 weeks of treatment.[42, 43] Joint mobilisation techniques may prove beneficial as part of a multimodal care plan. For example, a recent controlled trial of patients with acute shoulder and joint restriction found that patients who were prescribed internal rotation 'hand behind the back' mobilisation plus exercise and hot packs had greater benefit than those receiving exercise and hot packs alone.[44]

Care must be taken to ensure that strength-training programs do not aggravate the condition. Exercises should progress from pain-free stretches (e.g. pendulum exercises) and isometric exercises to increasingly loaded muscle strength training and functional exercises (e.g. wall push ups, overhead work, ball throwing) which should be maintained long term. Flexibility exercises should be continued through all phases of rehabilitation. Refer for spinal and shoulder manipulation. Cervicothoracic spinal manipulation and mobilisation in addition to usual care may improve self-perceived recovery in patients with non-specific shoulder pain.[45]

Note: Oral anti-inflammatory medication or subacromial corticosteroid injections are sometimes used to decrease inflammation. There are concerns about injecting corticosteroids into the connective tissue because of the long-term detrimental effects. Surgical techniques to create space under the acromion are considered when conservative approaches fail. Acromioplasty involves shaving off the underside of the acromion in order to reshape it or remove bone spurs.

OSTEOARTHRITIS

Osteoarthritis of the shoulder is uncommon unless there is a history of previous significant trauma or overuse, or osteoarthritis in other joints. Osteoarthritis is more commonly found in the AC joint than the glenohumeral joint. It has been characterised by slow loss of articular and subchondral bone with narrowing of the glenohumeral cavity (see Figure 15.30). The client is usually middle-aged or elderly or has a history of

Fig. 15.30 Radiograph of glenohumeral osteoarthritis

previous significant trauma, or work or sport that involves repetitive shoulder activity.

Assessment

Key assessment findings for osteoarthritis of the glenohumeral joint

- History of chronic shoulder pain and limitation aggravated by use; client usually over 50 years old
- Functional tests:
  - AROM limited ± painful in some directions
  - PROM limited ± painful (capsular pattern)
  - RROM usually negative
  - Special tests negative
- Palpation positive for crepitus and hard or capsular end-feel

---

HISTORY

The client complains of chronic shoulder pain and stiffness that is aggravated by use. The client is usually over 50 years old or has a history of significant previous injury or overuse. Osteoarthritis of the glenohumeral joint is not a common presenting condition although it is more common when other joints are also affected.

FUNCTIONAL TESTS

Cervical AROM does not reproduce shoulder symptoms.

Shoulder:
AROM positive (limited external rotation, abduction and medial rotation).
PROM positive (capsular pattern: limited external rotation, abduction and medial rotation), crepitus often present.
RROM negative.
Resisted and length tests for specific muscles: Osteoarthritis is often accompanied by capsule tightening and muscle contractures. In such cases, muscle length tests reveal shortening of affected muscles.
Special tests usually negative.

PALPATION

Crepitus and abnormal hard or capsular end-feel are usually palpated.

Treatment and mangement of osteoarthritis of the glenohumeral joint

Osteoarthritis is now understood as a dynamic condition where bone reparative processes are overwhelmed by destructive processes that are often related to injury and other mechanical load factors.[46] Acute episodes can occur from time to time, usually after over-activity. Reassure the client that acute episodes usually only occur 2–3 days per month and may be managed by a variety of strategies including cryotherapy for analgesia, acupressure, Reiki and reflexology.

A typical remedial massage treatment for mild or moderate subacute or chronic osteoarthritis includes:

- Swedish massage therapy to the shoulder and upper arm, neck, upper back and chest.

- Remedial massage therapy, which includes heat therapy, myofascial releasing techniques (see Chapter 8) and passive joint articulation (see Chapter 7), including:
  - shoulder rotation
  - shoulder traction
  - shoulder progressive cylindrical articulation
  - shoulder progressive external rotation
  - shoulder progressive internal rotation
  - shoulder figure-8.
- Apply remedial massage techniques to address any associated muscle contractures (see Table 15.5):
  - deep gliding frictions along the muscle fibres
  - cross-fibre frictions
  - soft tissue releasing techniques
  - deep transverse friction
  - trigger point therapy
  - muscle stretching.

CLIENT EDUCATION

The client should be advised to continue to use heat or ice therapy for pain relief and to modify or avoid aggravating activities. Home exercises should be commenced as soon as pain permits. Stretching and strengthening exercises can be introduced as indicated by assessment findings and should progress towards functional exercises (e.g. wall push-ups and overhead work) that mimic activities required for daily living. Educate clients about the importance of low impact aerobics exercises like Tai Chai, swimming, cycling and paddling.

Many clients with osteoarthritis of the shoulder joint will also have arthritis in other areas of the body including the lower cervical spine. For such clients, massage and posture advice for the neck and upper back will be beneficial.

Nutritional supplements such as glucosamine and chondroitin have been found to be ineffective or show small and possibly clinically insignificant effects.[47] Clients may be referred for other supportive therapies including specialist nutritional advice and acupuncture. Conservative medical treatment options include non-steroidal anti-inflammatory medication, and intra-articular injections of corticosteroid injection of sodium hyaluronate.[48, 49]

ADHESIVE CAPSULITIS (FROZEN SHOULDER)

Adhesive capsulitis is characterised by significantly limited movement caused when the normally loose capsule on the underside of the shoulder joint adheres to itself. Adhesive capsulitis develops over months beginning with painful early synovitis and progressing to an acute inflammatory phase with adhesion formation in the axillary fold. Stiffness and decreased range of motion ensue along with muscle atrophy and a reduction in the size of the synovial cavity and the glenohumeral space. In many cases prolonged immobility of the glenohumeral joint is related to inadequate rehabilitation of a previous shoulder injury (e.g. rotator cuff tears, bicipital tendinosis, shoulder trauma, trigger points of the subscapularis). In such cases the condition may be prevented by adequate rehabilitation of shoulder injuries, including continued shoulder movement within reasonable pain limits. The condition may also be secondary to cardiac disease or surgery, pulmonary disease, diabetes mellitus or thyroid disease. It can also be idiopathic and can subside in one shoulder only to reappear in the other. The condition tends to be self-perpetuating as clients avoid painful movements and this lack of movement further increases adhesions, immobility and pain. Without treatment incomplete improvements in range of motion will be observed after 1 to 4 years of follow-up.[50] Mobilisation therapy and therapeutic exercises have been found to reduce pain and improve range of motion and function in frozen shoulder.[51]

Assessment

HISTORY

The client is usually 40 to 60 years old and complains of significantly limited functional movement of the entire upper limb. They are often unable to lift their arms above 90° and movement is often accompanied by significant pain. They may complain of being unable to reach into their back pocket, comb their hair or hang clothes on the line. There is usually a history of previous significant trauma. There may be a history of previous adhesive capsulitis in the other shoulder.

FUNCTIONAL TESTS

Cervical AROM does not usually reproduce the shoulder symptoms.

Shoulder tests:
AROM: positive for limitation and pain (capsular pattern: motion is limited in external rotation > abduction > internal rotation). The client shrugs their shoulder when trying to abduct their arm.
PROM: limited and painful (capsular pattern). Note that muscle contractures will follow immobility, further restricting passive stretching of muscles.
RROM: Muscle contractures and atrophy are common accompaniments of adhesive capsulitis.
Resisted and length tests: Adhesive capsulitis is associated with capsule tightening and muscle contractures. Length tests reveal contractures of affected muscles.
Special tests: Apley's test positive.

Note: both adhesive capsulitis and subacromial impingement syndrome will limit abduction. However, adhesive capsulitis limits external rotation and impingement syndromes generally do not.

Treatment

A typical remedial massage treatment for adhesive capsulitis includes:

- Swedish massage therapy to the shoulder and upper arm, neck, upper back and chest.
- Remedial massage therapy, which includes heat therapy, myofascial releasing techniques (see Chapter 8) and passive joint articulation (see Chapter 7). Passive joint articulation initially focuses on restoring scapulothoracic/scapulohumeral rhythm and then progresses to restoring glenohumeral movement. Passive stretching, especially in external rotation, abduction and internal rotation, is beneficial. Joint articulations include:
  - shoulder rotation
  - shoulder traction
  - shoulder progressive cylindrical articulation
  - shoulder progressive external rotation
  - shoulder progressive internal rotation
  - shoulder figure-8.

Select appropriate remedial massage techniques to address muscle contractures, particularly subscapularis. Techniques include (see Table 15.5):
- deep gliding along the muscle fibre
- cross-fibre frictions
- soft tissue releasing techniques
- deep transverse friction
- trigger point therapy
- muscle stretching including proprioceptive neuromuscular facilitation (PNF).

A recent study of idiopathic adhesive capsulitis compared patients who received PNF and patients who received PNF and deep transverse friction of supraspinatus at the tenoperiosteal and musculotendinous junctions. Internal rotation PNF was performed supine with 90° abduction and the elbow flexed at 90°. Treatments were performed on alternate days over a 2-week period. The group receiving the addition of the deep transverse friction had a faster response in terms of pain reduction and increased range of motion.[52]

CLIENT EDUCATION

The client should be advised to use ice/heat therapy for pain relief. Home exercises (pendulum exercises, wall climbing exercise, manoeuvring with a cord to reach their hands behind their back) and a gentle strengthening program should be commenced immediately and the client advised to work within their pain tolerance. Encourage clients to find the right balance between too little activity, which leads to further capsule adhesions and muscle contractures, and too much activity which can inflame the area. Support and encourage the client (e.g. recognise even small gains in ranges of motion). Progressively introduce strengthening exercises within the client's pain-free range. Strengthening programs usually begin with isometric exercises and progress towards functional exercises (e.g. wall push-ups, overhead work, ball throwing) which should be maintained long term.

Clients may also require treatment of the upper back, neck and pectoral girdle. Some clients may benefit from referral for spinal and shoulder manipulation and acupuncture.

ACROMIOCLAVICULAR SPRAINS, CLAVICLE FRACTURES AND GLENOHUMERAL DISLOCATIONS

Clients with acute traumatic shoulder injuries such as acromioclavicular sprains, clavicle fractures and glenohumeral dislocations require assessment and treatment by medical practitioners. The rehabilitation of such injuries can be drawn out and many clients experience symptoms or dysfunction for many years after the initial injury. Remedial massage techniques, particularly those that promote optimal muscle function and address myofascial restrictions, may improve shoulder biomechanics and provide symptom relief.

AC sprains (shoulder separation)

The AC ligaments (superior and inferior acromioclavicular ligaments and coracoacromial ligament) provide anterior/posterior and medial/lateral stability of the AC joint; the coracoclavicular ligaments are designed to provide stability against vertical forces. Injury usually occurs from a direct blow on the anterolateral shoulder from falling on the shoulder or outstretched arm or severe distraction of an abducted arm.

GRADES OF AC SPRAINS

Grade 1: No visible separation, mild injury to the AC ligaments

Grade 2: Elevation of the clavicle, moderate disruption of the AC and coracoclavicular ligaments

Grade 3: Marked elevation of the clavicle, severe disruption of the AC and coracoclavicular ligaments

Presenting symptoms depend on the severity of the initial trauma and subsequent treatment. Clients with Grade 3 injuries are often left with a cosmetic deformity (see Figure 15.4 on p 268). Fibrotic tissue may be evident in affected ligaments.

Clavicle fractures

Clavicle fractures are one of the most common fractures arising from sporting activities. They are usually caused by falls onto the point of the shoulder. In rare cases a bone fragment may cause arterial or nerve damage.

Glenohumeral dislocations

Most glenohumeral dislocations are anterior. They occur from the combined movements of abduction and external rotation and damage the inferior glenohumeral ligament and the glenoid labrum. Many clients will be left with ligamentous laxity and return positive apprehension tests.

Treatment

A typical treatment for a client with a history of chronic symptoms related to previous traumatic injury includes:

- Swedish massage to the shoulder, upper back, neck, upper limb and chest.
- Remedial massage techniques to restore muscle balance including:
  - deep gliding along the muscle fibre
  - cross-fibre frictions
  - soft tissue releasing techniques
  - deep transverse friction
  - trigger point therapy
  - muscle stretching.
- Passive joint articulation may be helpful (see Chapter 7) but any technique that stretches already overstretched ligaments must be avoided.
- Provide myofascial releasing techniques for myofascial restrictions. Thermotherapy may be beneficial.

CLIENT EDUCATION

Prioritise stretching and strengthening exercises. Advise clients about good posture, especially about avoiding rounded shoulders and head forward posture when sitting. Clients may require referral for osseous manipulation. For clients with a history of glenohumeral dislocation, strengthening rotator cuff, trapezius and serratus anterior may be beneficial. Avoid strengthening pectoralis major as it pulls the humeral head anteriorly.

KEY MESSAGES

- Assessment of clients with conditions of the shoulder region involves history, outcome measures, postural analysis, functional tests and palpation.
- Assessment findings may indicate the type of tissue involved (contractile or inert, muscle, joint, fascia, ligament), duration of condition (acute or chronic) and severity (grade).
- Assessment findings may indicate common presenting conditions such as muscle strain, shoulder impingement syndrome, subacromial bursitis, osteoarthritis or adhesive capsulitis.
- Assessment findings also indicate client perception of injury and preferences for treatment.
- Consider Clinical Guidelines, available evidence and client preferences when planning therapy.
- Be conservative in treatment: if in doubt, perform pain-free Swedish massage.
- Although serious conditions of the shoulder region are rare, all clients with symptoms of neurological or vascular impairment in the upper limb should be referred for further assessment.
- The selection of remedial massage techniques depends on assessment results. Swedish massage to the shoulder, upper back, neck, upper limb and chest may be followed by muscle techniques (e.g. deep gliding, cross-fibre frictions, soft tissue releasing techniques, trigger point therapy and deep transverse friction), passive joint articulation, myofascial release and thermotherapy as indicated.
- Educating clients about likely causal and predisposing factors and exercise rehabilitation are essential parts of remedial massage therapy.
- Prioritise the client self-help component of treatment to reduce likelihood of recurrence and/or to promote health maintenance and illness prevention.

Review questions

1. Match the end-feels in Column A with the shoulder range of motion or condition in Column B

Column A	Column B
Elastic and firm	Horizontal adduction
Empty	Adhesive capsulitis
Hard and capsular	Horizontal abduction
Soft tissue	Severe instability

2. A test that would most likely be positive for a subscapularis muscle strain is:
   a) resisted shoulder adduction
   b) resisted shoulder external rotation
   c) resisted shoulder abduction
   d) resisted shoulder internal rotation

3. A client with shoulder pain has the following assessment results:
   ■ Positive active abduction (painful arc)
   ■ Positive passive abduction
   ■ Negative resisted abduction
   What is/are the most likely soft tissue structure(s) indicated by the assessment findings?
   a) muscle belly
   b) ligament
   c) tendon
   d) bursa

4. The apprehension test of the shoulder may help identify:
   a) grade 3 supraspinatus tear
   b) subacromial bursitis
   c) history of anterior glenohumeral dislocation
   d) impingement of structures between the acromion and the humerus

5. The capsular pattern for osteoarthritis describes limitations of ranges of motion that are specific to each joint. The capsular pattern for osteoarthritis of the glenohumeral joint suggests that its most restricted movement will be:
   a) abduction
   b) lateral rotation
   c) medial rotation
   d) flexion

6. A step deformity may be observed in a client with:
   a) adhesive capsulitis
   b) impingement syndrome
   c) AC joint separation
   d) a grade 3 supraspinatus tear

7. Describe a home stretch for:
   i) supraspinatus
   ii) teres major
   iii) biceps brachii

8. Home exercises for shoulder impingement syndrome usually include:
   i) stretching for _____
   ii) strengthening for _____

9. The following questions refer to the diagram below:

   i) Name the muscle that the arrows cross.
   ii) The arrows represent the direction of deep transverse friction. What are the specific indications for this technique? (For further information see Chapter 4.)

10. A 19-year-old female swimmer has recently increased her training program. She has developed pain in the left shoulder during the pull stroke. The pain seems to be getting worse. Postural analysis reveals a mild scoliosis. The results of her functional tests are as follows:
    Cervical spine:
    AROM: Negative
    Shoulder tests:
    AROM: Painful in flexion, abduction (painful arc)
    PROM: Negative
    RROM: Painful shoulder flexion
    Resisted tests: Positive for flexion
    Special tests: Impingement test positive
    What structure(s) could be involved?

11. Name five remedial massage techniques that would be suitable for a client with mild to moderate supraspinatus tendinosis.

12. Client education is an essential part of remedial massage therapy. List three recommendations for a client with chronic glenohumeral osteoarthritis.

APPENDIX 15.1

Shoulder pain and disability index[53]

The Shoulder Pain and Disability Index (SPADI) is a self-administered questionnaire that consists of two dimensions, one for pain and the other for functional activities. The pain dimension consists of five questions regarding the severity of an individual's pain. Functional activities are assessed with eight questions designed to measure the degree of difficulty an individual has with various activities of daily living that require upper-extremity use. The SPADI takes 5 to 10 minutes for a patient to complete and is the only reliable and valid region-specific measure for the shoulder.

SCORING INSTRUCTIONS

To answer the questions, patients place a mark on a 10 cm visual analogue scale for each question. Verbal anchors for the pain dimension are 'no pain at all' and 'worst pain imaginable', and those for the functional activities are 'no difficulty' and 'so difficult it required help'. The scores from both dimensions are averaged to derive a total score.

INTERPRETATION OF SCORES

Total pain score: / 50 × 100 = %
Note: If a person does not answer all questions divide by the total possible score (e.g. if 1 question missed divide by 40)
Total disability score: / 80 × 100 = %

Note: If a person does not answer all questions divide by the total possible score (e.g. if 1 question missed divide by 70)

Total Spadi score: / 130 × 100 = %

Note: If a person does not answer all questions divide by the total possible score (e.g. if 1 question missed divide by 120) The means of the two subscales are averaged to produce a total score ranging from 0 (best) to 100 (worst).

Minimum Detectable Change (90% confidence) = 13 points (change less than this may be attributable to measurement error)

SHOULDER PAIN AND DISABILITY INDEX (SPADI)

Please place a mark on the line that best represents your experience during the last week attributable to your shoulder problem.

Pain scale

How severe is your pain?	
Circle the number that best describes your pain where: 0 = no pain and 10 = the worst pain imaginable. At its worst?	0 1 2 3 4 5 6 7 8 9 10
When lying on the involved side?	0 1 2 3 4 5 6 7 8 9 10
Reaching for something on a high shelf?	0 1 2 3 4 5 6 7 8 9 10
Touching the back of your neck?	0 1 2 3 4 5 6 7 8 9 10
Pushing with the involved arm?	0 1 2 3 4 5 6 7 8 9 10

Disability scale

How much difficulty do you have?	
Circle the number that best describes your experience where: 0 = no difficulty and 10 = so difficult it requires help. Washing your hair?	0 1 2 3 4 5 6 7 8 9 10
Washing your back?	0 1 2 3 4 5 6 7 8 9 10
Putting on an undershirt or jumper?	0 1 2 3 4 5 6 7 8 9 10
Putting on a shirt that buttons down the front?	0 1 2 3 4 5 6 7 8 9 10
Putting on your pants?	0 1 2 3 4 5 6 7 8 9 10
Placing an object on a high shelf?	0 1 2 3 4 5 6 7 8 9 10
Carrying a heavy object of 10 pounds (4.5 kilograms)?	0 1 2 3 4 5 6 7 8 9 10
Removing something from your back pocket?	0 1 2 3 4 5 6 7 8 9 10

REFERENCES

1. Hill CL, Gill TK, Shanahan EM, et al. Prevalence and correlates of shoulder pain and stiffness in a population-based study: the North West Adelaide Health Study. Int J Rheum Dis 2010;13:215–22.
2. Subramanian VS, Kumar S. Prevalence and anatomical location of muscle tenderness among adults with nonspecific shoulder/neck pain but without any traumatic injuries and other chronic disease. Research J Pharm Tech 2016;9(12): 2407–14.
3. Drake R, Vogl AW, Mitchell WM. Gray's anatomy for students. 3rd edn. London: Churchill Livingstone; 2014.
4. Australian Acute Musculoskeletal Pain Guidelines Group. Evidence-based management of acute musculoskeletal pain: a guide for clinicians. Bowen Hills, Qld: Australian Academic Press; 2004.
5. Brun S. Initial assessment of the injured shoulder. Aust Fam Physician 2012;41(4):217–20.
6. Hoppenfeld JD. Fundamentals of pain medicine how to diagnose and treat your patients. Alphen aan den Rijn: Wolters Kluwer Health; 2014.
7. Wolfensberger A, Vuistiner P, Konzelmann M, et al. Clinician and patient-reported outcomes are associated with psychological factors in patients with chronic shoulder pain. Clin Orthop Relat Res 2016;474(9):2030–9.
8. Williams J, Holleman D, Simel D. Measuring shoulder function with the shoulder pain

and disability index. J Rheumatol 1995;22: 727–32.
9. Thoomes-de Graaf M, Scholten-Peeters GG, Duijin E, et al. The Dutch Shoulder Pain and Disability Index (SPADI): a reliability and validation study. Qual Life Res 2015;24:1515–19.
10. Koehorst ML, van Trijffel E, Lindeboom R. Evaluative measurement properties of the patient-specific functional scale for primary shoulder complaints in physical therapy practice. J Orthop Sports Phys Ther 2016;44(8):595–603.
11. Cools A, De Wilde L, van Tongel A, et al. Measuring shoulder external and internal rotation strength with a hand-held dynamometer, and range of motion using a goniometer and a digital inclinometer: comprehensive intra- and inter-rater reliability study of several testing protocols. Br J Sports Med 2014;48(7):560–674.
12. Correll S, Field J, Hutchinson H, et al. Reliability and validity of the halo digital goniometer for shoulder range of motion in healthy subjects. Int J Sports Physl Ther 2018;13(4):707–14.
13. Cleland J, Koppenhaver S, Su J. Netter's orthopaedic clinical examination: an evidence-based approach. 3rd edn. Philadelphia: Saunders; 2015.
14. Nagatomi T, Mae T, Nagafuchi T, et al. Shoulder manual muscle resistance test cannot fully detect muscle weakness. Knee Surg Sports Traumatol Arthrosc 2017;25:2081–8.

15. Burns SA, Cleland JA, Carpenter K, et al. Interrater reliability of the cervicothoracic and shoulder physical examination in patients with a primary complaint of shoulder pain. Phys Ther Sport 2016;19:46–55.
16. Warth RJ, Millett PJ. Physical examination of the shoulder: an evidence-based approach. New York, NY: Springer; 2015.
17. Reese N, Bandy WD, Yates C. Joint range of motion and muscle length testing. 2nd edn. St. Louis, MO: Saunders/Elsevier; 2010.
18. Norkin CD, White DJ. Measurement of joint motion: a guide to goniometry. 4th edn. Philadelphia, PA: F.A. Davis; 2009.
19. Hislop H, Avers D, Brown M, et al. Daniels and Worthingham's muscle testing: techniques of manual examination and performance testing. 9th edn. St. Louis, MO: Elsevier/Saunders; 2014.
20. Reiman M, Manske R. Functional testing in human performance. Champaign, IL: Human Kinetics; 2009.
21. Hoppenfeld S. Physical examination of the spine and extremities. Pearson New International Edition. Harlow: Pearson Education; 2013.
22. Guo L-P, Wang W-M, Wang Y-H, et al. Ultrasound in assessment of supraspinatus tendon injury: correlation with arthroscopy. Chinese M J-Peking 2016;129(3):361–3.

23. Struyf F, Geraets J, Noten S, et al. A multivariable prediction model for the chronification of non-traumatic shoulder pain: a systematic review. Pain Physician 2016;19:1–10.

24. Kooijman MK, Barten D-J, Swinkels IC, et al. Pain intensity, neck pain and longer duration of complaints predict poorer outcome in patients with shoulder pain – a systematic review. BMC Musculoskel Dis 2015;16:288. Doi: 10.1186/s12891-015-0738-4.

25. Coronado RA, Simon CB, Lentz TA, et al. Optimism moderates the influence of pain catastrophizing on shoulder pain outcome: a longitudinal analysis. J Ortho Sports Phys Ther 2017;47(1):21–30.

26. Uhl TL, Smith-Forbes EV, Nitz AJ. Factors influencing final outcomes in patients with shoulder pain: a retrospective review. J Hand Ther 2017;30:200–7.

27. Yuen Y-R. Effectiveness of massage therapy for shoulder pain: a systematic review and meta-analysis. J Phys Ther Sci 2017;29:936–40.

28. Hawk C, Minkalis AL, Khorsan R, et al. Systematic review of nondrug, nonsurgical treatment of shoulder conditions. J Manipulative Physiol Ther 2017;40(5):293–317.

29. Van den Dolder PA, Ferreira PH, Refshauge KM. Effectiveness of soft tissue massage and exercise for the treatment of non-specific shoulder pain: a systematic review with meta-analysis. Br J Sports Med 2014;28:1216–26.

30. Yuen Y-R. Effectiveness of massage therapy on the range of motion of the shoulder: a systematic review and meta-analysis. J Phys Ther Sci 2017;29:365–9.

31. Brukner P, Khan K. Clinical sports medicine. 4th edn. North Ryde, NSW: McGraw-Hill; 2012.

32. Ram H, Kuman R. Diagnostic evaluation of magnetic resonance imaging in shoulder pathologies. Int J Med Sci Public Health 2018;7(9):691–6.

33. Innes JA, Dover AR, Fairhurst K. Macleod's clinical examination. 14th edn. Edinburgh: Elsevier Health Sciences; 2018.

34. Edmonds EW, Dengerink DD. Common conditions in the overhead athlete. Ame Fam Physician 2014;89(7):537–41.

35. Karthikeyan S, Griffith DR, Parsons N, et al. Microvascular blood flow in normal and pathological rotator cuffs. J Shoulder Elbow Surg 2015;24:1954–60.

36. Wilk KE, Hooks TR. The painful long head of the biceps brachii. Nonoperative treatment approaches. Clin Sports Med 2016;35:75–92.

37. Lin H-T, Ko H-T, Chen Y-C, et al. Changes in shoulder rotation strength ratio for various shoulder positions and speeds in the scapular plane between baseball players and non-players. J Phys Ther Sci 2015;27:1559–63.

38. Simons D, Travell J, Simons L. Myofascial pain and dysfunction: the trigger point manual. Volume 1 Upper half of body. 2nd edn. Philadelphia: Williams & Wilkins; 1999.

39. Niel-Asher S. Concise book of trigger points. 3rd edn. Berkeley, CA: North Atlantic; 2014.

40. Neer CS. Impingement lesions. Clin Orthop Relat Res 1983;(173):70–7.

41. Grumet RC, Rubin BD. Injection therapies in the management of shoulder injuries. Oper Techn Sport Med 2012;20:114–23.

42. Bury J, West M, Chamorro-Moriana G, et al. Effectiveness of scapula-focused approaches in patients with rotator cuff related shoulder pain: a systematic review and meta-analysis. Manual Ther 2016;25:35–42.

43. Yoo W-G. Changes in acromion and scapular position after short-term overhead work. J Phys Ther Sci 2013;25:679–80.

44. Satpute KH, Bhandari P, Hall T. Efficacy of hand behind back mobilization with movement for acute shoulder pain and movement impairment: a randomized controlled trial. J Manipulative Physiol Ther 2015;38(5):324–34.

45. Southerst D, Yu H, Randhawa K, et al. The effectiveness of manual therapy for the management of musculoskeletal disorders of the upper and lower extremities: a systematic review by the Ontario Protocol for Traffic Injury Management (OPTIMa) collaboration. Chiropr Man Therap 2015;23:30–46.

46. Hunter DJ. Everything you ever wanted to know about osteoarthritis. The Health Report 2017. Online. Available: https://www.abc.net.au/radionational/programs/healthreport/everything-you-ever-wanted-to-know-about-osteoarthritis/8664218#transcript; 2017.

47. Liu X, Machado GC, Eylesl JP, et al. Dietary supplements for treating osteoarthritis: a systematic review and meta-analysis. Br J Sports Med 2018;52:167–75.

48. Mehl J, Imhoff AB, Beltzel K. Omarthrose: Pathogenese, Diagnostik Und Konservative Therapieoptionen. Der Orthopäde 2018;47(5):368–76.

49. Guo JJ, Wu K, Guan H, et al. Three-year follow-up of conservative treatments of shoulder osteoarthritis in older patients. Orthopedics 2016;39(4):e634–e641.

50. Wong CK, Levine WN, Deo K, et al. Natural history of frozen shoulder: fact or fiction? A systematic review. Physiotherapy 2017;103:40–7.

51. Jain TK, Sharma NK. The effectiveness of physiotherapeutic interventions in treatment of frozen shoulder/adhesive capsulitis: a systematic review. J Back Musculoskelet Rehabil 2014;27:247–73.

52. Sonkusale JT, Damke US, Bhave SM. Comparing the effectiveness of deep transverse friction massage on supraspinatus as an adjunct to PNF in idiopathic adhesive capsulitis of shoulder. Indian J Physiother Occup Thera 2016;10(2):114–20.

53. Roach K, Budiman-Mak E, Songsiridej N, et al. Development of a shoulder pain and disability index. Arthrit Care Res 1991;4(4):143–9.

16 The elbow region

INTRODUCTION

Repetitive overuse, especially of wrist extension, is the most common mechanism of elbow injury. Over 3% of the population will experience lateral epicondylitis (tennis elbow) each year.[1] Other elbow injuries arise from traumas such as falling on the outstretched arm. Conditions of the elbow often occur concurrently with conditions of the neck, shoulder and wrist. However, regardless of whether the elbow region is the primary or secondary lesion, treatment should be directed to the whole kinetic chain. Wherever possible, the practitioner should identify both the cause of the condition and aggravating factors so that treatment can be directed not only to normalising structural integrity of the region but also to underlying contributing factors.

FUNCTIONAL ANATOMY

The elbow is a combination hinge and pivot joint made up of three joints: the humeroulnar, the humeroradial and the radioulnar joints which are formed by the articulation of the distal humerus and proximal radius and ulna. The radius is on the lateral side of the joint; the ulna is on the medial side and its large olecranon process forms the posterior point of the elbow.

The humeroulnar and humeroradial joints are responsible for the hinge action. The trochlea of the humerus articulates with the semilunar notch of the ulna to form the humeroulnar joint (Figure 16.1 on p 295). The capitulum of the humerus articulates with the fovea on the head of the radius to form the humeroradial joint. The radial head also articulates with the radial notch of the ulna to form the pivot component of the joint which enable pronation and supination. The radius and ulna are connected by the interosseous membrane, a broad sheet of connective tissue which extends along their shafts and forms an attachment for tendons of some of the deep muscles of the forearm.

The medial and lateral epicondyles are prominent projections on either side of the humerus just above the elbow joint. They are the major attachment points for muscles of the forearm: the wrist flexors attach to the medial epicondyle and the wrist extensors to the lateral epicondyle. The ulna nerve (funny bone) lies on the posterior surface of the medial epicondyle.

The articular surfaces of the elbow are connected by an articular capsule which thickens either side to form the medial and lateral collateral ligaments. The radial annular ligament circles the head of the radius and attaches it to the radial notch of the ulna (Figure 16.2 on p 295).

Flexion of the forearm is largely due to the action of the brachialis muscle of the upper arm. It is assisted by biceps brachii and brachioradialis, and to a lesser extent by wrist flexors which attach to the medial epicondyle. Triceps brachii and anconeus are the main muscles responsible for elbow extension with assistance from wrist extensors attaching to the lateral epicondyle.

Supination is controlled by supinator, biceps brachii and brachioradialis (see Figure 16.3 on p 296, Figure 16.4 on p 297); pronation by pronator teres at the elbow joint and pronator quadratus at the wrist. Brachioradialis helps bring the forearm into mid-range pronation or supination depending on its starting position.

The common flexor tendon attaches to the medial epicondyle. It is shared by a number of superficial flexor muscles (flexor carpi radialis, flexor carpi ulnaris, palmaris longus, flexor digitorum superficialis) and pronator teres which is also a weak elbow flexor.

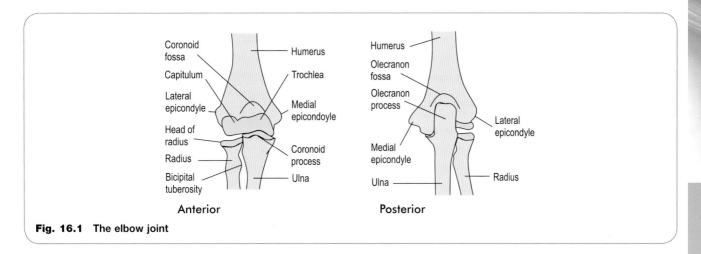

Fig. 16.1   The elbow joint

Fig. 16.2   Capsule and ligaments of the elbow joint

Assessment of the elbow region

1. Case history
2. Outcome measures, e.g. The Patient Specific Functional Scale
3. Postural analysis
4. Functional tests
   Cervical spine
   Active range of motion tests
   Flexion, extension, lateral flexion, rotation
   Shoulder joint
   Active range of motion tests
   Flexion, extension, abduction, horizontal adduction, internal rotation, external rotation
   Elbow joint
   Active range of motion tests
   Flexion, extension, supination, pronation
   Passive range of motion tests
   Flexion, extension, supination, pronation
   Resisted range of motion tests
   Flexion, extension, supination, pronation
   Resisted and length tests for specific muscles, including:
   wrist flexor muscles, wrist extensor muscles, supinator, pronator quadratus, pronator teres
   Special tests including:
   Valgus stress test
   Varus stress test
   Elbow extension test
   Resisted wrist flexion
   Resisted wrist extension
5. Palpation

At the lateral epicondyle extensor carpi radialis brevis, extensor carpi radialis longus, extensor digitorum, extensor digiti minimi and extensor carpi ulnari attach via a common extensor tendon (see Figure 16.4 on p 297).

Major muscles of the elbow region are summarised in Table 16.1 on p 299.

ASSESSING THE ELBOW AND FOREARM

The purpose of remedial massage assessment includes:

- determining the suitability of clients for massage (contra-indications and red flags)

- determining the duration (acute or chronic), severity of injury and types of tissues involved in the injury/condition
- determining whether symptoms fit patterns of common conditions.

Principles of remedial massage assessment are discussed in Chapter 2. This section presents specific considerations for assessment of the elbow and forearm.

CASE HISTORY

Information from case histories can alert practitioners to the presence of serious conditions requiring referral. Questioning should be targeted to include:

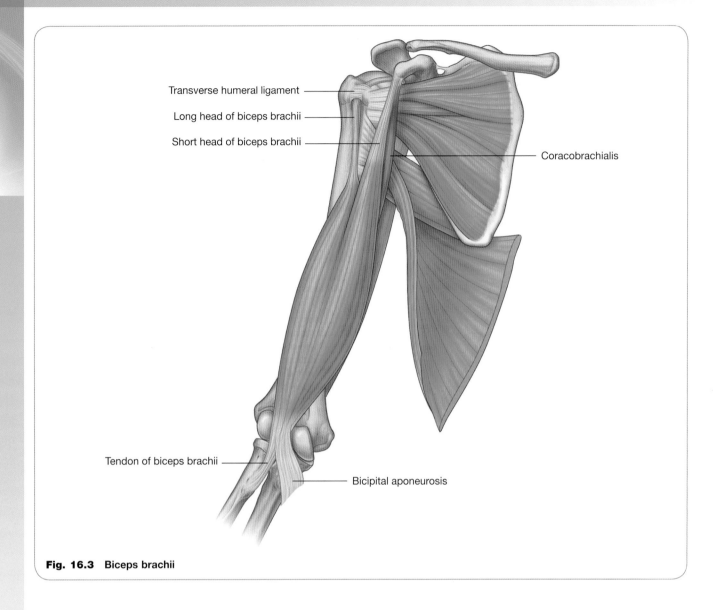

Transverse humeral ligament

Long head of biceps brachii

Short head of biceps brachii

Coracobrachialis

Tendon of biceps brachii

Bicipital aponeurosis

Fig. 16.3 Biceps brachii

- Descriptions of the specific mechanism of the injury and the forces involved. Enquire about the onset of symptoms, nature of the pain, disability and functional impairment, previous injuries to the area, type of work, typical postures, overuse and overhead work. Ask clients to demonstrate movements and positions that aggravate or relieve their pain and to be specific with descriptions of aggravating or relieving activities. Identify whether the pain is located at the lateral, medial or posterior aspect of the elbow, or the forearm.
- Identifying red and yellow flags that require referral for further investigation. Red flags for serious causes of elbow pain are summarised in Table 16.2 on p 300.
- Identifying the exact location of the symptoms by asking clients to point to the site of pain. Anatomical location of symptoms is useful in differential diagnosis.[3] For example: anterior elbow pain suggests anterior capsule strain, biceps tendinopathy, osteoarthritis; lateral elbow pain suggests lateral epicondylitis, posterolateral rotatory instability, radial tunnel syndrome; medial elbow pain suggests medial epicondylitis, cubital tunnel syndrome, ulnar collateral ligament injury; and posterior elbow pain suggests

olecranon bursitis, osteoarthritis, posterior impingement, triceps tendinopathy.
- Determining if the pain is local or referred. Local pain tends to be sharp and well-localised; referred pain tends to be dull and poorly localised. Is there any numbness, tingling or weakness? The presence of nerve impingement symptoms suggests referral from lower cervical nerves or local ulnar or radial nerve entrapment.

OUTCOME MEASURES

Outcome measures are questionnaires that are specifically designed to assess clients' level of impairment and to define benefits of treatment. There is currently no preferred outcome measure in elbow clinical trial research,[4] however the Patient Specific Functional Scale can be used to measure progress of treatment of clients with any musculoskeletal condition, including elbow conditions.

POSTURAL ANALYSIS

Postural analysis enables observation of the whole client and facilitates identification of important features through

Posterior view

Supinator
(deep head)

Supinator
(superficial head)

Anconeus

Extensor carpi
radialis longus

Interosseous
membrane

Extensor carpi
radialis brevis

Extensor
carpi ulnaris

Abductor
pollicis longus

Extensor
digiti minimi

Extensor
pollicis longus

Extensor
digitorum

Extensor indicis

Extensor
pollicis brevis

Extensor
retinaculum

Posterior view

Fig. 16.4 Muscles of the forearm

Ulnar nerve

Ulnar nerve

Humeral head of pronator teres

Brachial artery

Ulnar head of pronator teres

Ulnar artery

Median nerve

Radial artery

Flexor carpi radialis

Interroseous membrane

Pronator teres (cut)

Palmaris longus

Flexor carpi ulnaris

Flexor digitorum profundus

Flexor pollicis longus

Pronator quadratus

Flexor retinaculum

Palmar aponeurosis

Flexor digitorum superficialis tendon (cut)

Fig. 16.4, cont'd

Table 16.1 Muscles of the elbow region[2]

Muscle	Origin	Insertion	Action
Forearm Flexors			
▪ Biceps brachii	Long head: supraglenoid tubercle Short head: coracoid process of scapula	Radial tuberosity of radius and bicipital aponeurosis	Flexes forearm at elbow joint, supinates forearm at radioulnar joints, and flexes humerus at shoulder joint
▪ Brachialis	Distal anterior surface of humerus	Ulnar tuberosity and coronoid process of ulna	Flexes forearm at elbow joint
▪ Brachioradialis	Lateral border of distal end of humerus	Superior to styloid process of radius	Flexes forearm at elbow joint, supinates and pronates forearm at radioulnar joints to neutral position
Forearm Extensors			
▪ Triceps brachii	Long head: infraglenoid tubercle Lateral head: lateral and posterior surface of humerus superior to radial groove Medial head: entire posterior surface of humerus inferior to radial groove	Olecranon of ulna	Extends forearm at elbow joint and extends humerus at shoulder joint
▪ Anconeus	Lateral epicondyle of humerus	Olecranon of ulna	Extends forearm at elbow joint
Forearm Pronators			
▪ Pronator teres	Medial epicondyle of humerus and coronoid process of ulna	Middle of lateral surface of radius	Pronates forearm at radioulnar joint and weakly flexes forearm at elbow
▪ Pronator quadratus	Distal portion of shaft of ulna	Distal portion of shaft of radius	Pronates forearm at radioulnar joints
Forearm Supinator			
▪ Supinator	Lateral epicondyle of humerus and supinator crest	Lateral surface of proximal one-third of radius	Supinates forearm at radioulnar joints
Superficial flexor compartment of the forearm			
▪ Flexor carpi radialis	Medial epicondyle of humerus	Second and third metacarpals	Flexes and abducts hand (radial deviation) at wrist joint
▪ Palmaris longus	Medial epicondyle of humerus	Flexor retinaculum and palmar aponeurosis	Weakly flexes hand at wrist joint
▪ Flexor carpi ulnaris	Medial epicondyle of humerus and superior posterior border of ulna	Pisiform, hamate and base of fifth metacarpal	Flexes and adducts hand (ulnar deviation) at wrist joint
▪ Flexor digitorum superficialis	Medial epicondyle of humerus, coronoid process of ulna, anterior oblique line of radius	Middle phalanx of each finger	Flexes middle phalanx of each finger at proximal interphalangeal joint, flexes proximal phalanx of each finger at metacarpophalangeal joint, and flexes hand at wrist joint
Superficial extensor compartment of the forearm			
▪ Extensor carpi radialis longus	Lateral supracondylar ridge of humerus	Second metacarpal	Extends and abducts hand at wrist joint
▪ Extensor carpi radialis brevis	Lateral epicondyle of humerus	Third metacarpal	Extends and abducts hand at wrist joint

Continued

Table 16.1 Muscles of the elbow region—cont'd

Muscle	Origin	Insertion	Action
■ Extensor digitorum	Lateral epicondyle of humerus	Distal and middle phalanges of each finger	Extends distal and middle phalanges of each finger at interphalangeal joints, proximal phalanx of each finger at metacarpophalangeal joint, and hand at wrist joint
■ Extensor digiti minimi	Lateral epicondyle of humerus	Tendon of extensor digitorum on fifth phalanx	Extends proximal phalanx of little finger at metacarpophalangeal joint and hand at wrist joint
■ Extensor carpi ulnaris	Lateral epicondyle of humerus and posterior border of ulna	Ulnar side of fifth metacarpal	Extends and adducts hand at wrist joint

Table 16.2 Red flags for potentially serious elbow disorders[5, 6]

Disorder	Symptoms	Signs
Fracture	History of significant trauma Fall on outstretched hand Fall onto lateral elbow	Deformity consistent with fracture Reduced range(s) of motion Pain with range of motion Disturbance in the triangular relationship between the olecranon and the epicondyles Significant bruising, if subacute (unusual)
Dislocation	History of fall/trauma as above History of deformity with or without spontaneous reduction	Deformity consistent with dislocation Haemarthrosis
Infection	Pain, swelling, redness Diabetes mellitus History of immunosuppression (e.g. transplant, chemotherapy, HIV) History of systemic symptoms	Localised heat, swelling, erythema Purulence Erythematous streaks, especially from a portal of entry Systemic signs of infection
Cancer	History of cancer Unintentional weight loss Continuous pain, especially at night and not improved with rest	Palpable mass not consistent with usual diagnoses
Inflammation	History of gout or pseudogout History of rheumatoid arthritis History of other inflammatory arthritides	Effusion Localised heat, swelling, erythema, tenderness
Rapidly Progressive Neurologic Deficit	History of neurologic disease Trauma	Abnormal neurologic examination Focal or global motor weakness distal to the elbow Weakness may be limited to one nerve, such as hand intrinsic muscles
Vascular Compromise	History of diabetes mellitus Tobacco use History of fracture or dislocation History of vascular disease of any kind	Decreased or absent peripheral pulses and delayed capillary refill Oedema
Compartment Syndrome	History of trauma, surgery or extreme unaccustomed forceful activity Persistent forearm pain and 'tightness' Tingling, burning or numbness	Palpable tenderness and tension of involved compartment Pain intensified with stretch to involved muscles Paraesthesia, paresis and sensory deficits Diminished pulse and prolonged capillary refill

bilateral comparison. It also facilitates detection of possible predisposing or contributing factors that may be implicated by observing the position of the head, cervical and thoracic spines, glenohumeral joints and scapula. Observe and compare the upper limbs anteriorly and posteriorly, noting symmetry, colour, swelling, lumps, bruising and carrying angle. (When the arm is extended in anatomical position, the longitudinal axes of the upper arm and forearm form a lateral (valgus) angle at the elbow joint known as the carrying angle (see Figure 16.5 on p 301). A normal carrying angle

Fig. 16.5 Carrying angle

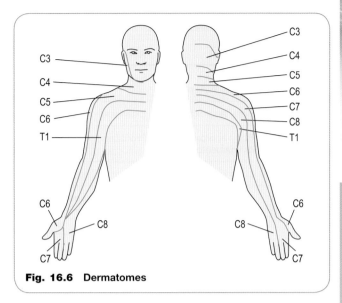

Fig. 16.6 Dermatomes

measures approximately 5° in males and 10–15° in females. The carrying angle often increases with greater elasticity of the ligaments, especially in females and is associated with extension greater than 0°. The carrying angle may increase when the lateral epicondyle is fractured or decrease as a result of trauma. A reversed carrying angle (a gunstock deformity) may result from a supracondylar fracture in a child.

Observe the elbow region for swelling. Swelling may be local (e.g. olecranon bursitis) or diffuse (e.g. fracture or crush injury). Diffuse swelling involves the entire elbow region. The client often carries their elbow flexed at 45° to accommodate the swelling with minimal pain. Look for scars (e.g. surgical scars, burns, drug addiction) and muscle hypertonicity or atrophy.

FUNCTIONAL TESTS

For any tests involving joint movements it is important to compare both sides and take into account any underlying pathology and the age and lifestyle of the client. Measuring elbow range of motion has consistently exhibited good to high reliability for assessing flexion, extension, supination and pronation.[7]

Active range of motion of the cervical spine (flexion, extension, lateral flexion and rotation)

Examination of the elbow and forearm begins with active range of motion tests of the cervical spine to help rule out cervical radiculopathy or brachial plexus neuropathy which may refer pain to the elbow region. Dermatomes which cover the elbow region are shown in Figure 16.6. If active range of motion tests of the cervical spine reproduce elbow symptoms, further examination of the cervical spine is indicated (see Chapter 12).

Active range of motion (AROM) of the glenohumeral joint (flexion, extension, abduction, horizontal adduction, external and internal rotation)

Examination of the glenohumeral joint helps identify or eliminate elbow pain referred from the glenohumeral joint or associated structures (e.g. trigger points in shoulder muscles). If AROM tests of the glenohumeral joint produce elbow or other symptoms, a full examination of the glenohumeral joint is indicated.

Active range of motion of the elbow joint

The client may stand or sit as convenient. Face the client and demonstrate the movements for the client to follow. Examine the following ranges of motion:

- Flexion/extension (140°/0°[5])
- Pronation/supination (80°/80°).

Passive range of motion (PROM)

If the client is unable to perform normal AROM in any direction, further investigation is required. PROM testing should be performed with one hand stabilising and palpating the elbow joint while the other hand moves the forearm. Palpate for crepitus, capsular pattern and end-feel (see Table 16.3 on p 302). The capsular pattern of restriction for the humeroulnar joint is flexion more limited than extension.

Table 16.3 Elbow joint: end-feel[8, 9]

	End-feel	Range of motion
Normal end-feel	Soft tissue approximation	Flexion
	Bony approximation	Extension
	Bony approximation or ligamentous	Pronation
	Ligamentous	Supination
	End-feel	**Suggested condition**
Abnormal end-feel	Boggy	Joint effusion
	Early myospasm	Acute injury
	Late myospasm	Instability
	Hard (mid range of motion)	Bony abnormality or loose body (bone fragment)
	Springy block	Loose body

Fig. 16.7 Resisted test for brachialis

Fig. 16.8 Resisted test for brachioradialis

Resisted range of motion (RROM)

RROM tests should also be performed if AROM testing indicates the likelihood of an elbow problem. RROM tests include:

- flexion: biceps brachii, brachialis, brachioradialis
- extension: triceps brachii, anconeus
- pronation: pronator teres, pronator quadratus
- supination: biceps brachii, supinator.

Resisted tests and length tests for specific muscles[10]

If RROM tests reproduce symptoms, further tests may be used to help identify specific muscles.

1. BRACHIALIS

Resisted test

This test is similar to the resisted test for biceps brachii except that it is performed with the wrist pronated. The client flexes their elbow to 90° and pronates their wrist. One of your hands supports the elbow. Your other hand applies resistance as the client tries to flex their elbow (see Figure 16.7).

Length test

The client should be able to fully extend their elbow with the wrist supinated.

2. BRACHIORADIALIS

Resisted test

This test is similar to the resisted test for biceps brachii and brachialis except that the wrist is semi-supinated (in the hand-shake position). The client flexes their elbow to 90° and semi-supinates their wrist. One of your hands supports the elbow while the other applies resistance as the client tries to flex their elbow (see Figure 16.8).

Length test

The client should be able to fully extend the elbow.

3. PRONATOR TERES

Resisted test

Stabilise the elbow to avoid shoulder movement. The client pronates the forearm with the elbow partially flexed and holds this position as you try to supinate the forearm above the wrist (see Figure 16.9 on p 303).

Length test

Shortening of the pronator muscles of the forearm is observed as limited supination which can interfere with many normal functions of the hand and forearm.

4. PRONATOR QUADRATUS

Resisted test

The test is similar to the resisted test for pronator teres except that the test is performed with the elbow fully flexed (see Figure 16.10 on p 303).

Fig. 16.9 Resisted test for pronator teres

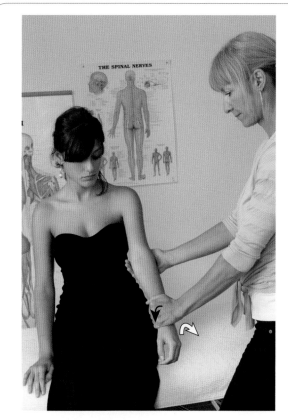

Fig. 16.11 Resisted test for supinator

Fig. 16.10 Resisted test for pronator quadratus

Length test

Shortening of the pronator muscles of the forearm is observed as limited supination, which can interfere with many normal functions of the hand and forearm.

5. SUPINATOR

Resisted test

The client sits with the forearm supinated and the elbow either fully flexed or fully extended to shorten or elongate biceps brachii. In such positions the procedure is more likely to test the action of supinator. Stabilise the elbow. The client holds the supinated position as you try to pronate the client's forearm (see Figure 16.11). (To test the biceps brachii, the test is performed with the elbow partially flexed.)

Length test

Shortening of the supinator muscles is observed as limited pronation which can interfere with many normal functions of the hand and forearm.

6. WRIST EXTENSOR MUSCLES

The wrist extensor muscles can be tested as a group. The client makes a loose fist and pronates the forearm. Apply resistance to the client's hand as the client tries to extend the wrist (see Figure 16.12 on p 304). (Tests for individual wrist extensor muscles are described in Chapter 17.)

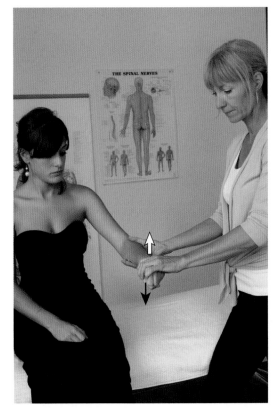

Fig. 16.12 Resisted test for wrist extensor muscles

Fig. 16.13 Resisted test for wrist flexor muscles

7. WRIST FLEXOR MUSCLES

The wrist flexor muscles can be tested as a group. The client makes a loose fist and supinates the forearm. Apply resistance to the client's palm as the client tries to flex the wrist (see Figure 16.13). (Tests for individual wrist flexor muscles are described in Chapter 17.)

Special tests

If symptoms are reported when performing a special test, ask the client to identify their exact location and confirm that they are the same as those described in the case history. Positive special test results should always be interpreted cautiously and in the context of other clinical findings (see Chapter 2).

VALGUS STRESS TEST

The client is seated with the forearm supinated. Apply valgus stress to the elbow at full extension and at 30°, 60° and 90° of elbow flexion. Pain or excessive joint movement suggests medial collateral ligament sprain or instability (see Figure 16.14).

The moving valgus stress test has been shown to exhibit superior diagnostic accuracy when compared with the valgus stress test for identifying a medial collateral tear.[7] To perform the moving valgus stress test the client is seated with the forearm supinated. Flex the elbow and then abduct the client's arm to 90° to the start position. From there apply a valgus force as you extend the elbow (see Figure 16.15).

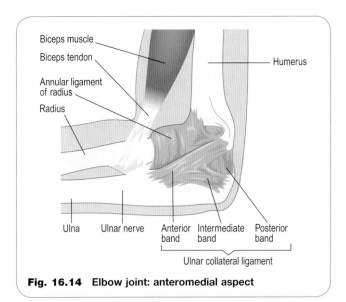

Fig. 16.14 Elbow joint: anteromedial aspect

Biceps muscle
Biceps tendon
Humerus
Annular ligament of radius
Radius
Ulna
Ulnar nerve
Anterior band
Intermediate band
Posterior band
Ulnar collateral ligament

VARUS STRESS TEST

The client is seated with the forearm supinated. Apply varus stress to the elbow at full extension and at 30°, 60° and 90° of elbow flexion. Pain or excessive joint movement suggests lateral collateral ligament sprain or instability (see Figures 16.16 and 16.17 on p 305). To date no studies have examined

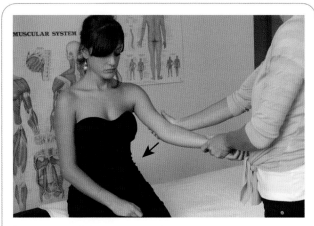

Fig. 16.15 Valgus stress test

Fig. 16.18 Elbow extension test

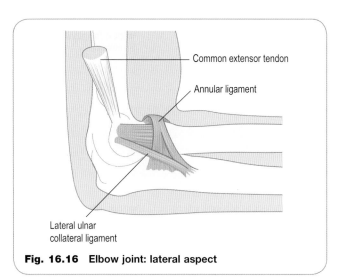

Fig. 16.16 Elbow joint: lateral aspect

Fig. 16.17 Varus stress test

the usefulness of the varus stress test for identifying the presence of lateral collateral ligament tears.[7]

ELBOW EXTENSION TEST

The client sits with arms supinated and humerus flexed to 90° at the shoulder joint. The client then extends both elbows.

Limited extension in one elbow compared with the other suggests bone or joint injury. This test has been consistently shown to be an excellent test to rule out the presence of bone or joint injury[7] (see Figure 16.18).

RESISTED WRIST FLEXION/EXTENSION

Although resisted wrist flexion and extension are not special orthopaedic tests, they are included here so that the elbow-testing procedure captures the conditions that most commonly produce elbow pain, namely flexor/extensor tendinosis. The client makes a fist and extends and flexes their wrist against the practitioner's resistance (see Figures 16.12 and 16.13 on p 304). Pain at the lateral or medial epicondyle suggests flexor/extensor tendinosis respectively.

PALPATION

Locate the olecranon process on the posterior aspect of the elbow. Move to the medial epicondyle to locate the ulnar nerve which feels soft and tubular. Avoid compressing the nerve which may cause paraesthesia in the forearm, ring and little fingers. Trace the border of the ulna to the wrist.

Palpate the epicondyles on either side of the distal humerus. On the anterior aspect of the forearm locate the medial epicondyle and just inferiorly palpate the attachment of the wrist and finger flexors and pronator quadratus. The medial collateral ligament extends from the medial epicondyle of the humerus to the coronoid process and olecranon of the ulna. Supracondylar lymph nodes may be palpable when there is an infection in the arm or hand. Palpate the wrist flexor muscles on the anteromedial medial aspect of the forearm and trace their tendons as they cross the anterior aspect of the wrist.

Palpate the cubital fossa, the brachioradialis laterally and pronator teres medially. Locate the brachial artery (a pulse medial to the biceps tendon). The median nerve is directly medial to the brachial artery.

Palpate the lateral epicondyle, the attachment site for some of the wrist and finger extensors which form the bulk of the posterolateral forearm. Brachioradialis is medial to the wrist extensor muscles. To make brachioradialis more prominent, instruct the client to make a fist with the thumb up and push

Fig. 16.19 Soft-tissue release for extensor tendinosis

Table 16.4 Evidence for some non-surgical recommendations for lateral elbow tendinopathy[13, 14]

Recommendation	Evidence
Ultrasound plus friction massage	Moderate evidence of effectiveness versus laser therapy on short-term follow-up
Laser therapy	Moderate evidence was found over plyometric exercises on short-term follow-up
Electrotherapy, extracorporeal shock wave therapy (ESWT), transcutaneous electrical nerve stimulation (TENS) and pulsed electromagnetic field therapy	Limited/conflicting evidence
Non-surgical techniques: corticosteroid injection, injection technique, iontophoresis, botulinum toxin A injection, prolotherapy, platelet-rich plasma or autologous blood injection, bracing, physical therapy, shockwave therapy, or laser therapy	No conclusive evidence for a preferred method of non-surgical treatment

the fist upwards under the table. Palpate the lateral collateral ligament of the elbow which extends from the lateral epicondyle to the annular ligament of the radius and the radial notch of the ulna. Palpate the radial head and the radial annular ligament (see Figure 16.19).

REMEDIAL MASSAGE TREATMENT

Assessment of the elbow and forearm provides essential information for development of treatment plans, including:

- client's suitability for remedial massage therapy
- duration of the condition (i.e. acute or chronic)
- severity of the condition (i.e. grade of injury; mild, moderate or severe pain)
- type(s) of tissues involved
- priorities for treatment if more than one injury or condition are present
- whether the signs and symptoms suggest a common condition of the elbow region
- special considerations for individual clients (e.g. client's preference for treatment types and styles, specific population considerations).

Clients who present to remedial massage clinics with elbow pain almost invariably have extensor tendinosis or flexor tendinosis and occasionally olecranon bursitis. Treatment options must always be considered in the context of the best available evidence for treatment effectiveness and clinical practice guidelines where they exist. A 2014 Cochrane Review of deep transverse friction massage for treating lateral elbow (or lateral knee) tendinitis found insufficient evidence to determine the effects of deep transverse friction on pain, improvement in grip strength, and functional status for patients with lateral elbow tendinitis.[11] Future trials using specific methods and adequate sample sizes were recommended. Another systematic review in 2016 by the Ontario Protocol for Traffic Injury Management (OPTIMa) Collaboration found that there may be a role for multimodal care in the management of patients with persistent lateral epicondylitis. Good outcomes were associated with education, exercise (strengthening,

stretching, occupational exercise), manual therapy (manipulation) and soft tissue therapy (massage) for five visits over a 5-week period.[12] Table 16.4 summarises some of the evidence for non-surgical treatments of lateral elbow tendinopathy. The OPTIMa Collaboration also conducted a systematic review examining the effectiveness of soft tissue therapy for the management of musculoskeletal disorders and injuries of the upper and lower extremities. The review found that myofascial release improved outcomes for lateral epicondylitis. In addition, movement re-education (contraction/passive stretching) provided better long-term benefits than a single corticosteroid injection.[15]

The most common mechanism of elbow injury is repetitive overuse, especially of wrist extension. Other causes include throwing overhead, falling on the outstretched arm, hyperextension and valgus or varus stress.

OVERVIEW

Develop a short- and a long-term plan for each client. The short-term plan directs treatment to the highest priority (usually determined by symptoms). The long-term plan can be introduced when presenting symptoms have subsided. Long-term treatment focuses on contributing or predisposing factors such as underlying structural features and lifestyle factors. A significant part of both short-term and long-term treatment involves educating clients about likely causal or aggravating factors and guiding their management of these factors. If massage therapy is being used in conjunction with other treatments, it is important to communicate with other treating practitioners.

MUSCLE STRAIN

The most common sites of pathology in the elbow are the tendinous attachments of the wrist extensors and flexors.

Lateral elbow tendinopathy (tennis elbow)

Lateral elbow tendinopathy is one of the most common repetitive strain or overuse injuries. This condition is also known as tennis elbow because it can affect tennis players, but the overall percentage of clients who develop this condition from tennis is actually small. Over 3% of the general population will experience tennis elbow each year.[1] Clients typically develop lateral elbow tendinopathy from repetitive tasks that involve wrist extension such as typing. It is thought that repeated microtrauma of the tendons from repeated stretching and contraction of the extensors of the forearm and hand causes disruption of the internal structure and degeneration of the cells and matrix.[16, 17] The condition was previously referred to lateral epicondylitis; however, lateral elbow tendinopathy is the currently preferred term as it more accurately represents the pathology. It appears that dense populations of fibroblasts, vascular hyperplasia and disorganised collagen contribute to degenerative processes.[18]

The site of injury is usually the common extensor tendon of the wrist, in particular the fibres of extensor carpi radialis brevis just inferior to its attachment at the lateral epicondyle. Populations particularly at risk are those who make repetitive movements of the forearm muscles against resistance such as manual workers and upper extremity athletes. For example carpenters, plumbers and those who play tennis, golf, cricket, baseball and squash.[1, 19] Office workers and nurses are also susceptible and the dominant arm is more frequently involved.[1] Activities that contribute to lateral elbow tendinopathy include using a racket, hammer, screwdriver, typing, using a mouse, scanning groceries or performing a massage. Clinicians and athletic trainers can advise clients to avoid extreme coupling postures of the wrist joint (such as extension with supination) with rapid contraction movements.[19] Sustained contraction of wrist muscles may lead to myofascial trigger points which will also require treatment.

ASSESSMENT

History

The client may present with intermittent lateral elbow pain. The pain usually develops gradually and may begin with morning stiffness or stiffness after rest. There is usually a history of repetitive overuse (e.g. racket sports, typing). Grasping objects may be associated with pain and weakness. Note: radial neuropathy may cause elbow pain. However, it is more commonly associated with sensory changes in the dorsum of the first web space and wrist and finger extensor weakness.

Nirschi[1] described the following pain phase scale for athletic overuse injuries:

Phase 1: stiffness or mild soreness after activity, usually gone within 24 hours
Phase 2: stiffness or mild soreness before activity that is relieved by warm-up; symptoms not present during activity but return after, lasting up to 48 hours
Phase 3: stiffness or mild soreness before specific sport or occupational activity; pain partially relieved by warm-up; pain minimally present during activity but does not cause athlete to alter activity
Phase 4: pain causes athlete to alter performance of the activity; mild pain may also be noticed with activities of daily living
Phase 5: significant (moderate or greater) pain before, during and after activity, causing alteration of activity; pain occurs with activities of daily living but does not cause a major change in them
Phase 6: pain persists even with complete rest; pain disrupts simple activities of daily living and prohibits doing household chores
Phase 7: pain also disrupts sleep consistently; pain is aching and intensifies with activity

Functional tests

Cervical AROM tests do not reproduce elbow symptoms.
Shoulder AROM tests do not reproduce elbow symptoms.

Elbow tests

AROM may be painful during wrist extension (± flexion) when the elbow is extended.
PROM may be painful at the end of wrist flexion when the elbow is extended.
RROM is usually negative for muscles that move the elbow joint but positive for muscles that extend the wrist.
Special tests: Resisted wrist extension is painful. Wrist supination may also cause pain.

Palpation

There is local tenderness around the lateral epicondyle. Fibrotic tissue is often palpable in the extensor tendon.

Key assessment findings for extensor tendinosis

- History of repetitive overuse
- Functional tests:
  - AROM painful during wrist extension and flexion with the elbow extended
  - PROM painful at end of wrist flexion with elbow extended
  - RROM may be negative for muscles that move the elbow joint, but positive for muscles that extend the wrist
  - Special tests: positive for resisted wrist extension
- Palpation: local tenderness or pain. Fibrotic tissue is usually palpable.

OVERVIEW OF TREATMENT AND MANAGEMENT

Lengthy recovery times are sometimes associated with lateral elbow tendinopathy. Acute presentations may require cryotherapy. Advise clients to avoid aggravating conditions. Tennis elbow splints which usually comprise a Velcro strap worn around the forearm below the elbow joint have traditionally been recommended although their efficacy is currently being questioned. One 2017 multicentre randomised controlled trial found that a forearm band may only have a placebo effect and did not support its use.[20] However, another study advised that the psychological benefits of the placebo effect could be beneficial.[21] A forearm spiral splint which cast the forearm in the mid-point position to limit the rotational movements of supination and rotation was also found beneficial. Tennis elbow symptoms reduced when the splint was worn for 12 hours a day, particularly when performing activities of daily living for 4 weeks.[22]

A typical remedial massage treatment for acute or chronic lateral elbow tendinopathy includes:

- Swedish massage therapy to the elbow, upper limb, neck and upper back.
- Remedial massage techniques including (see Table 16.5):
  - deep gliding frictions along the muscle fibres (including extensor carpi ulnaris, extensor digiti minimi, extensor digitorum, extensor carpi radialis brevis, anconeus, brachioradialis)
  - cross-fibre frictions
  - soft tissue releasing techniques
    The client is supine with the palm down and the hand over the edge of the table. Alternatively, a rolled towel or bolster may be placed under the client's wrist to allow full wrist flexion. Static pressure is applied to a point of hypertonicity in the wrist extensors using fingers, thumbs or knuckles. The wrist is then slowly passively or actively flexed and extended. You may also perform deep longitudinal stripping while the wrist is moving (see Figure 16.19).
  - deep transverse friction applied directly to the damaged tendon may help stimulate collagen production. A Cochrane Review of deep transverse friction massage for treating lateral elbow (or lateral knee tendinitis) found insufficient evidence to determine the effects of deep transverse friction on pain, improvement in grip strength, and functional status for patients with lateral elbow tendinitis.[11]
  - trigger point therapy for wrist extensor muscles
  - muscle stretches
- Myofascial release including cross-arm techniques (see Figure 16.20) and the arm pull (see Chapter 8).
- Cryotherapy or thermotherapy may be indicated.
- Other remedial techniques such as elbow joint articulation (see Chapter 7) may be introduced as required.

Client education

Advise the client to rest from aggravating activities to reduce the stress on the damaged tendons. Rehabilitation exercises are designed to improve overall strength, endurance and flexibility in the muscles of the entire upper limb kinetic chain. This includes the muscles of the neck, shoulder, elbow and wrist. Initially wrist extensor stretches (flexing the wrist and extending and pronating the forearm) are recommended (see Figure 16.21). Isometric exercises for muscles of the shoulder including biceps brachii, triceps brachii and rotator cuff may be introduced. Eccentric-concentric training with isometric contractions has proved to be the most effective combination.[18] When full range of wrist flexion and extension can be performed within pain tolerance, strengthening exercises for the wrist extensors, flexors, pronators and supinators are introduced. Tennis players should review their technique (e.g. a two-handed backstroke, adequate warm-up, changing racquet, avoiding high string tension). For carpenters or others regularly using a hammer, use a larger shock-absorbing handle and/or padded gloves.

Refer for osseous manipulation and for physical therapy modalities such as ultrasound, phonophoresis or electrical stimulation. Most cases of tennis elbow respond to non-surgical management. However, if conservative methods fail, surgical treatment is sometimes considered. Surgical approaches include arthroscopic debridement of the extensor carpi radialis brevis, laser and injection with botulinum toxin.

Medial elbow tendinopathy (golfer's elbow)

The common flexor tendons of the wrist that attach at the medial epicondyle are also susceptible to overuse trauma, especially flexor carpi radialis. The condition is commonly called golfer's elbow although it is also associated with repetitive overhead throwing, tennis serving and using a hammer. In golf, the problem occurs when the ball is struck at the low point of the swing. At the point of impact the wrist flexors concentrically contract to swing the club towards the ground. When the ball is hit there is a sudden eccentric load on the flexor group which is exaggerated by the length of the golf club. Medial epicondylitis rarely involves inflammation of the

Fig. 16.20 Myofascial release: cross-hand technique

Fig. 16.21 Home stretch for extensor tendinosis

Table 16.5 Remedial massage techniques for muscles of the elbow region

Muscle	Soft tissue release	Trigger point	Deep transverse friction	Stretch	Corrective action[23, 24]	Home exercise
Wrist extensors	Client: supine, wrist pronated over the edge of the table or over a bolster. Practitioner: applies static pressure or deep gliding to a taut band/lesion in the muscle using fingers, thumbs or knuckles as wrist is slowly passively or actively flexed and extended.		Common wrist extensor tendon insertion at the lateral epicondyle, distal to common extensor tendon (up to several cms) along line of tendon.	CRAC: Client: wrist flexion with elbow extension within pain tolerance. Practitioner: resists as client tries to extend wrist for 6–8 seconds. Release pressure. Client flexes wrist with elbow extension as far as possible within pain tolerance. Repeat whole procedure 3 times.	Eliminate or avoid muscle overload (e.g. avoid sustained or excessive gripping in sport). Tennis elbow splint. Check work ergonomics, especially keyboard and mouse. Change grip in tennis and golf.	Stretch: Extend elbow and flex the wrist. Use the other hand to further flex the wrist within pain tolerance. Hold 30 seconds. Repeat 3 times.
Wrist flexors	Client: supine, wrist supinated over the edge of the table or over a bolster. Practitioner: applies static pressure or deep gliding to a taut band/lesion using fingers, thumbs or knuckles as wrist is slowly passively or actively flexed and extended.		2.5 cm below medial epicondyle, common wrist flexor tendon insertion at the medial epicondyle.	CRAC: Client: wrist extension with elbow extension within pain tolerance. Practitioner: resists as client tries to flex wrist for 6–8 seconds. Release pressure. Client extends wrist with elbow extension as far as possible within pain tolerance. Repeat whole procedure 3 times.	Avoid prolonged tight gripping (e.g. power tools). Palmaris longus: avoid palmar cupping. Change golf grip.	Stretch: Extend elbow and extend the wrist. Use the other hand to further extend the wrist within pain tolerance. Hold 30 seconds. Repeat 3 times.

Continued

309

Table 16.5 Remedial massage techniques for muscles of the elbow region—cont'd

Muscle	Soft tissue release	Trigger point	Deep transverse friction	Stretch	Corrective action[23, 24]	Home exercise
Pronator teres/ pronator quadratus	For pronator teres: Client: supine, wrist supinated, elbow extended. Practitioner: applies static pressure or deep gliding using fingers, thumbs or knuckles as wrist is slowly passively or actively supinated or pronated.			Passive stretch: Practitioner stabilises the client's elbow and supinates their forearm to pain tolerance/muscle stretch end-feel and holds the stretch for up to 30 seconds.	Avoid overloading muscle (e.g. driving with two hands on the steering wheel). Change grip and technique in tennis and golf.	Stretch: Sit at a table, forearms flat on table. Keeping elbows on table, supinate wrists as far as possible, hold 30 seconds. Repeat 3 times. Strengthen: Sit or stand, arms by sides, elbows flexed to 90°. Begin holding light weight, pronate the wrist. Relax and return to starting position. Repeat to fatigue. Progress to increased weight and number of repetitions.

Table 16.5 Remedial massage techniques for muscles of the elbow region—cont'd

Muscle	Soft tissue release	Trigger point	Deep transverse friction	Stretch	Corrective action[23, 24]	Home exercise
Supinator	Palpate in space between biceps tendon, pronator teres and brachioradialis. Client: supine, forearm supinated. Practitioner: applies static pressure to supinator as the forearm is slowly actively or passively pronated and supinated.			Passive stretch: Practitioner stabilises the client's elbow and pronates their forearm to pain tolerance/muscle stretch end-feel.	Avoid overloading muscle (e.g. prolonged gripping or carrying or backpack). Correct tennis technique and grip size. Carry loads with forearms supinated.	Stretch: Sit at a table, forearms flat on table. Keeping elbows on table, pronate wrists as far as possible, hold 30 seconds. Repeat 3 times.

tendon. Rather it is a problem of collagen degeneration in the tendon fibres from chronic tensile loads. The most common site of pathology occurs 2.5 cm distal to the medial epicondyle at the interface between pronator teres and flexor carpi radialis origins.[8] Early stages of the condition, referred to as flexor tendinitis, often require cryotherapy. The wrist flexor tendons travel through the carpal tunnel and it is not uncommon to find flexor tendinosis occurring concurrently with carpal tunnel syndrome.

ASSESSMENT

History

The client complains of aching pain over the medial elbow. In the early stages the pain is brought on by activities such as overhead throwing, tennis serving or swinging a golf club and relieved by rest. Left unchecked, the condition can progress to constant pain and weakness in grip strength.

Functional tests

Cervical AROM tests do not reproduce elbow symptoms.
Shoulder AROM tests do not reproduce elbow symptoms.

Elbow tests

AROM painful during wrist flexion (± extension) when elbow is extended.
PROM painful at the end of wrist extension when elbow is extended.
RROM negative for muscles that move the elbow but positive for muscles that flex the wrist.
Special tests: Resisted wrist flexion painful. Resisted wrist pronation may also cause pain.

Palpation

There is local tenderness around the medial epicondyle. Fibrotic tissue is often palpable in the flexor tendon.

OVERVIEW OF TREATMENT AND MANAGEMENT

The approach to remedial massage treatment is similar to that for extensor tendinosis. In the acute phase, advise the client to eliminate or avoid the aggravating condition. Traditionally ice and forearm splints are prescribed.

A typical remedial massage treatment for subacute or chronic flexor tendinosis includes:

- Swedish massage therapy to the elbow, upper limb, neck and upper back.
- Remedial massage techniques for muscles including (see Table 16.5):
  - deep gliding frictions along the muscle fibres (including flexor carpi radialis, palmaris longus, flexor carpi ulnaris, flexor digitorum superficialis, pronator teres, supinator, pronator quadrates)
  - cross-fibre frictions (see Figure 16.22)
  - soft tissue releasing techniques
    The client is supine with the palm supinated and the hand over the edge of the table. Alternatively, a rolled towel or bolster can be placed under the wrist to allow for full range of wrist extension. Static pressure is applied to a point of hypertonicity/lesion in the wrist flexors using fingers, thumbs or knuckles while the wrist is slowly passively or actively flexed and extended. Alternatively, you may perform deep longitudinal stripping while the wrist is moving (see Figure 16.23).
- Deep transverse friction applied directly to the damaged tendon may help stimulate collagen production.
- Trigger point therapy, including wrist flexors and extensors and rotator cuff muscles.

Fig. 16.22 Cross-fibre frictions at the common flexor tendon

Fig. 16.23 Soft tissue release for flexor tendinosis

Key assessment findings for flexor tendinosis

- History of repetitive overuse
- Functional tests:
  - AROM painful during wrist flexion ± extension with elbow extended
  - PROM painful at end of wrist extension with elbow extended
  - RROM negative for muscles that move the elbow; positive for muscles that flex the wrist
  - Special tests: positive for resisted wrist flexion
- Palpation: local tenderness or pain. Fibrotic tissue is often palpable.

- Muscle stretching, including wrist flexors, elbow flexors, pronators and supinators.
- Myofascial release including cross-arm techniques (see Figure 16.20).
- Other remedial techniques such as elbow joint articulation (see Chapter 7) may be introduced as required.

Client education

Advise the client to reduce or eliminate aggravating activities. Ice applications may provide some pain relief. Corticosteroid injections for tendinopathy were found to reduce pain in the short term compared with other interventions but this effect reversed in the intermediate and long term.[25] Most cases respond to conservative management and exercise rehabilitation, although recovery can take time and relapse is not uncommon. Refer clients for osseous manipulation. In some instances, surgery to remove damaged tissue may be performed.

Home exercises

Stretching the wrist flexor muscles (extend the wrist and elbow and use the other hand to further extend the wrist – see Figure 16.24) and elbow flexors and forearm pronators. Progressively introduce isometric exercises and weights to strengthen the elbow and wrist flexors and extensors, forearm pronators and rotator cuff muscles. Later introduce sports-specific activities.

OLECRANON BURSITIS

Olecranon bursitis is painful inflammation of the bursa which overlies the olecranon at the back of the elbow and lubricates movement of the olecranon under the skin (see Figure 16.25). Its usual cause is either a direct blow or sustained irritation exerted by pressure, rubbing or bumping. It is commonly referred to as student's elbow. The history of its development is important since there are occasions where bleeding into the bursa may occur after direct trauma or the bursa ruptures through excessively forced flexion at the elbow. Slow onset with no apparent cause suggests infection and should be referred for medical examination.

Treatment

Apply ice and firm compression. Advise clients to eliminate the responsible activity. This may involve avoiding resting the elbow on a hard surface, modifying the work environment or wearing an elbow pad. If the aetiology is associated with a tight triceps brachii or forearm extensor muscles, include specific remedial massage techniques (including deep gliding, cross-fibre frictions, soft tissue release, trigger point therapy and muscle stretches – see Table 16.5) to restore full muscle length in the subacute or chronic phase. Myofascial release may be beneficial. Refer clients for osseous manipulation if required.

Note: Joint infection or gout can occur at the elbow. Refer any client with systemic signs such as raised temperature and inflamed lymph nodes associated with olecranon bursitis.

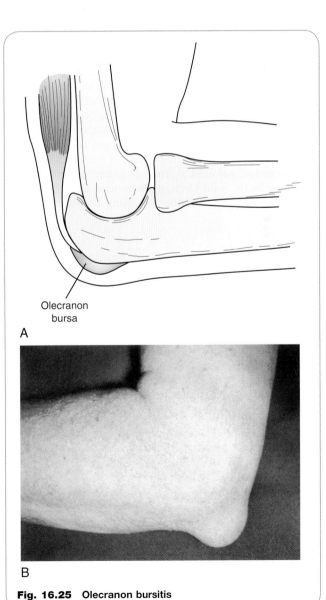

Olecranon bursa

A

B

Fig. 16.25 Olecranon bursitis

Fig. 16.24 Home stretch for flexor tendinosis

ELBOW SPRAIN

Elbow sprains are uncommon. Sprains of the medial and lateral collateral ligaments may occur as a result of trauma (e.g. falls on the outstretched arm and direct blows to the elbow) or repeated excessive varus and valgus stress (e.g. from throwing). Clients complain of pain, swelling around the elbow and limited movement. Severe sprains should be referred to a physiotherapist, osteopath or chiropractor. Remedial massage therapists may be called upon to assist in the rehabilitation of mild and moderate strains. Treatment includes ice applications for acute injuries and then deep transverse friction to the injury site within pain tolerance. Address muscle function, encourage full range of motion in the joint through gentle joint articulation in the pain-free range and eliminate myofascial adhesions using myofascial release techniques. Rehabilitation exercises should be commenced when pain tolerance allows.

FRACTURES AND DISLOCATIONS

Fractures are extremely disabling and may leave permanently restricted movement. Heavy falls on the outstretched arm can crush the head of the radius or chip the joint with similar damage to the end of the humerus. Bone chips may also break from the medial epicondyle of the humerus and the tip of the olecranon. In children the head of the radius may be dislocated through wrenching movements (pulled elbow). Dislocations are usually reduced by medical or paramedical staff by forearm rotation in flexion. Remedial massage therapists may be called upon to treat clients after fractures and dislocations have healed. At this stage the purpose of treatment is usually to promote optimal muscle function, to encourage full range of motion in the joint through gentle joint articulation, and to eliminate myofascial adhesions using myofascial release techniques.

KEY MESSAGES

- Assessment of clients with conditions of the elbow region involves case history, outcome measures, postural analysis, functional tests and palpation.
- Assessment findings may indicate the type of tissue involved (contractile or inert; muscle, joint, fascia, ligament), duration of condition (acute or chronic) and severity (grade).
- Assessment findings may indicate a common presenting condition such as wrist extensor/flexor tendinosis or olecranon bursitis.
- Assessment findings also indicate client perception of injury and preferences for treatment.
- Consider Clinical Guidelines, available evidence and client preferences when planning therapy.
- Be conservative in treatment: if in doubt, perform pain-free Swedish massage.
- Although serious conditions of the elbow region are rare, be vigilant for red flags during assessment (including history of significant trauma, constant pain, systemic signs accompanying joint pain, symptoms of neurological or vascular compromise).
- The selection of remedial massage techniques depends on assessment results. Swedish massage to the elbow, upper limb, neck and upper back may be followed by muscle techniques (e.g. deep gliding, cross-fibre frictions, soft tissue releasing techniques, trigger point therapy, deep transverse friction and muscle stretching), passive joint articulation, myofascial release and thermotherapy as indicated.
- Educating clients about likely causal and predisposing factors and exercise rehabilitation are essential parts of remedial massage therapy.
- Prioritise the client self-help component of treatment wherever possible to reduce likelihood of recurrence and/or to promote health maintenance and illness prevention.

Review questions

1. The carrying angle in an adult female is approximately:
   a) 5°
   b) 5–10°
   c) 10–15°
   d) 15–20°
2. Name four wrist flexor muscles that attach to the medial epicondyle via the common flexor tendon.
3. When performing resisted tests for forearm pronation, how can pronator teres be differentiated from pronator quadratus?
4. Which dermatomes cross the posterior aspect of the wrist?
   a) C5
   b) T1
   c) C7
   d) C8
5. Boggy end-feel during elbow range of motion testing suggests:
   a) joint effusion
   b) instability
   c) loose body
   d) capsular tightening
6. A client has pain on resisted elbow flexion. Biceps brachii, brachialis and brachioradialis all flex the elbow joint. How can resisted wrist flexion tests be modified to isolate each of the elbow flexors?
7. Massage therapists are prone to develop wrist extensor tendinosis. What recommendations would you make to a beginning therapist to help them avoid injury?
8. Extensor tendinosis most commonly involves:
   a) extensor carpi ulnaris
   b) extensor digitorim
   c) extensor carpi radialis brevis
   d) extensor carpi radialis longus
9. Name two common presentations of elbow injury to remedial massage clinics.
10. Describe your treatment for olecranon bursitis:
    i) in the acute phase
    ii) in the subacute phase
11. Name four remedial massage techniques that could be used to treat subacute extensor tendinosis.
12. A resisted test of the wrist flexors reproduces pain at the medial epicondyle. What condition does this suggest?
    a) sprained ligament
    b) tennis elbow
    c) golfer's elbow
    d) olecranon bursitis

REFERENCES

1. Nirschl R. The epidemiology and health care burden of tennis elbow: a population-based study. Ann Transl Med 2015;3(10):133. Doi: 10.3978/j.issn.2305-5839.2015.05.05.

2. Tortora GJ, Derrickson BH. Principles of anatomy and physiology. 15th edn. Stafford, Qld: Wiley; 2016.

3. Kane SF, Lynch JH, Taylor JC. Evaluation of elbow pain in adults. Am Fam Physician 2014;89(8):649–57.

4. Evans JP, Smith CD, Fine NF, et al. Clinical rating systems in elbow research—a systematic review exploring trends and distributions of use. J Shoulder Elbow Surg 2018;27(4):E98–E106.

5. American College of Occupational and Environmental Medicine (ACOEM). Elbow disorders. Elk Grove Village (IL): Reed Group; 2013.

6. ACOEM Guidelines. ACOEM Practice Guidelines: elbow disorders. J Occup Environ Med 2013;55(11):1365–74.

7. Cleland J, Koppenhaver S, Su J. Netter's orthopaedic clinical examination: an evidence-based approach. 3rd edn. Philadelphia: Saunders; 2015.

8. Carnes M, Vizniak N. Quick reference evidence-based conditions manual. 3rd edn. Burnaby, BC: Professional Health Systems; 2009.

9. Norkin CD, White DJ. Measurement of joint motion: a guide to goniometry. 5th edn. Philadephia, PA: F.A. Davis; 2016.

10. Hislop H, Avers D, Brown M, et al. Daniels and Worthingham's muscle testing: techniques of manual examination and performance testing. 9th edn. St. Louis, MO: Elsevier/Saunders; 2014.

11. Loew L, Brosseau L, Tugwell P, et al. Deep transverse friction massage for treating lateral elbow or lateral knee tendinitis. Cochrane Database Syst Rev 2014;(11):CD003528.

12. Sutton D, Gross D, Côté P, et al. Multimodal care for the management of musculoskeletal disorders of the elbow, forearm, wrist and hand: a systematic review by the Ontario Protocol for Traffic Injury Management (OPTIMa) Collaboration. Chiropr Man Therap 2016;24(8):8.

13. Dingemanse R, Randsdorp M, Koes B, et al. Evidence for the effectiveness of electrophysical modalities for treatment of medial and lateral epicondylitis: a systematic review. Br J Sports Med 2014;48(12):957–65.

14. Sims S, Miller K, Elfar J, et al. Non-surgical treatment of lateral epicondylitis: a systematic review of randomized controlled trials. Hand 2014;9(4):419–46.

15. Piper S, Shearer H, Cote P, et al. The effectiveness of soft-tissue therapy for the management of musculoskeletal disorders and injuries of the upper and lower extremities: a systematic review by the Ontario Protocol for Traffic Injury Management (OPTIMa) collaboration. Manual Ther 2016;21:18–34.

16. McMurray J, Baker R. An exploratory analysis of a novel treatment-based classification algorithm for treating tendinopathy. ProQuest Dissertations and Theses; 2016.

17. Koot W, The B, Eygendaal D. Lateral and medial non-articular elbow pain. J Orthop Trauma 2016;30(4):336–45.

18. Stasinopoulos D, Stasinopoulos I. Comparison of effects of eccentric training, eccentric-concentric training, and eccentric-concentric training combined with isometric contraction in the treatment of lateral elbow tendinopathy. J Hand Ther 2017;30(1):13–19.

19. Lee S-Y, Chieh H-F, Lin C-J, et al. The potential risk factors relevant to lateral epicondylitis by wrist coupling posture. PLOS One 2016;11(5):E0155379.

20. Nishizuka T, Iwatsuki K, Kurimoto S, et al. Efficacy of a forearm band in addition to exercises compared with exercises alone for lateral epicondylitis: a multicenter, randomized, controlled trial. J. Orthop Sci 2017;22(2):289–94.

21. Hodeaux K. The effect of floss bands on elbow range of motion in tennis. Theses and Dissertations. Online. Available: https://scholarworks.uark.edu/etd/1948; 2017.

22. Najafi M, Arazpour M, Aminian G, et al. Effect of a new hand-forearm splint on grip strength, pain, and function in patients with tennis elbow. Prosthet Orthot Int 2016;40(3):363–8.

23. Simons D, Travell J, Simons L. Myofascial pain and dysfunction: The trigger point manual. Volume 1 Upper half of body. 2nd edn. Philadelphia: Williams & Wilkins; 1999.

24. Niel-Asher S. Concise book of trigger points. 3rd edn. Berkeley, CA: North Atlantic; 2014.

25. Coombes B, Bisset L, Vicenzino B. Efficacy and safety of corticosteroid injections and other injections for management of tendinopathy: a systematic review of randomised controlled trials. Lancet (London, England). 2010;376(9754):1751–67.

17 The wrist and hand

Learning Outcomes

- Assess clients with conditions of the wrist and hand for remedial massage, including identification of red and yellow flags.
- Assess clients for signs and symptoms associated with common conditions of the wrist and hand (including muscle strains, carpal tunnel syndrome, repetitive strain injury, de Quervain's tenosynovitis, osteoarthritis and wrist sprains) and treat and/or manage these conditions with remedial massage therapy.
- Develop treatment plans for clients with conditions of the wrist and hand, taking into account assessment findings, duration and severity of the condition, likely tissue types, clinical guidelines, the best available evidence and client preferences.
- Develop short- and long-term treatment plans to address presenting symptoms, underlying conditions and predisposing factors, and to progressively increase the self-help component of therapy.
- Adapt remedial massage therapy to suit the individual client's needs based on duration and severity of injury, the client's age and gender, the presence of underlying conditions and other consideration for specific population groups.

INTRODUCTION

Injuries sustained to the hand and wrist are common, accounting for 20% of all presentations to emergency departments. Direct, indirect and intangible costs of acute hand and wrist injuries are a substantial burden to the individual and society at large.[1] Remedial massage therapists commonly encounter repetition strains of the wrist such as carpal tunnel syndrome and de Quervain's tenosynovitis, and first- and second-degree sprains. It is of concern that a number of studies have reported a high incidence of work-related musculoskeletal disorders among massage and other physical therapists. One study found that up to 90% of physical therapists experienced a work-related musculoskeletal disorder during their careers.[2] Therapists dealt with their symptoms by altering treatment techniques, improving body mechanics, and by self-treating or seeking physical therapy treatment from a colleague. Low back injuries were the most common but massage therapists also experience high rates of finger and thumb disorders.

FUNCTIONAL ANATOMY

The wrist and hand are made up of eight carpal bones in two rows (proximal row: scaphoid, lunate, triquetrum and pisiform; distal row: trapezium, trapezoid, capitate and hamate), five metacarpal bones, five proximal phalanges, four middle phalanges and five distal phalanges. The distal end of the radius articulates with the scaphoid and lunate to form the wrist or radiocarpal joint. There is no direct articulation between the distal ulna and the carpal bones. Instead, the distal ulna joins the wrist via the fibrocartilaginous disc of the distal radioulnar joint (see Figure 17.1 on p 317).

The wrist joint is enclosed by a fibrous capsule which extends from the distal radius and ulna to the proximal carpal row. The capsule is strengthened by dorsal and palmar radiocarpal ligaments and also by radial and ulnar collateral ligaments. The flexor retinaculum, a thickening of the deep fascia of the forearm, is a strong transverse band that forms the roof of the carpal tunnel. Nine flexor tendons and the median nerve pass under the flexor retinaculum as they pass through the carpal tunnel.

The metacarpals and phalanges form hinge joints for flexion and extension. The five metacarpal bones each have a base, shaft and head. The heads of the metacarpal bones articulate with proximal phalanges to form the metacarpophalangeal joints (knuckles of the hand). Each finger has three phalanges (proximal, middle and distal); the thumb only has two. The opposable thumb is formed by the rotation of the first metacarpophalangeal joint. The movements of the thumb are described as if the thumb were in line with the row of fingers (see Figure 17.2 on p 317).

Normal hand function requires complex coordination and control of muscles, many of which begin at the elbow or forearm. Muscles of the forearm often help maintain the position of the wrist and hand when the thumb and fingers perform fine motor movements or grip an object (see Figure 17.3 on p 318 and 319). Muscles of the thenar eminence (abductor pollicis brevis, opponens pollicis, flexor pollicis brevis) and the hypothenar eminence (abductor digiti minimi, flexor digiti minimi brevis, opponens digiti minimi and palmaris brevis) usually run from the carpal bones to the thumb and fingers. They enable the hand to grip and hold (see Figure 17.4 on p 320).

Nerve supply to the hand and fingers originates from the brachial plexus (C4 to T2). Three major nerves supply the hand:

1. ulnar nerve is responsible for sensation to the medial side of the hand, the medial half of the ring finger and the little finger, and motor activity of flexor carpi ulnaris, part of flexor digitorum profundus and some of the muscles of the hand
2. median nerve is responsible for sensation to the palmar surface of the thumb, index, middle and half of the ring finger, and motor activity of thenar muscles and the rest of the muscles on the front of the forearm and hand
3. radial nerve is responsible for sensation to the radial side of the forearm, dorsum of the hand, thumb, 2nd and 3rd digits, and motor activity of triceps and muscles of the back of the forearm

Table 17.1 summarises the major muscles of the wrist and hand.

ASSESSMENT

The purpose of remedial massage assessment includes:

- determining the suitability of clients for massage (contra-indications and red flags)
- determining the duration (acute or subacute), severity of injury and types of tissues involved in the injury/condition
- determining whether symptoms fit patterns of common conditions.

Principles of remedial massage assessment are discussed in Chapter 2. This section presents specific considerations for assessment of the wrist and hand.

CASE HISTORY

When assessing clients who sustain wrist injuries, case history and physical examinations are important diagnostic tools.[3] Information from case histories should always be interpreted with findings from other assessments. For example, subjective complaints do not appear to be useful in identifying carpal tunnel syndrome. Reports of dropping objects or that shaking hands improved symptoms were shown to minimally alter the probability of diagnosis (+LR = 1.7–1.9, −LR = 0.34–0.47).[4]

History questions should be targeted to include:

- describing the mechanism of the current injury, onset of symptoms, pain, disability and functional impairment and previous injuries to this area. Did the client fall on the outstretched hand? Is there any numbness, tingling, weakness?[3]
- identifying the client's type of work and habitual postures
- identifying red and yellow flags that require referral for further investigation (red flags for serious conditions of the wrist and hand are summarised in Table 17.2)
- identifying the exact location of the symptoms by asking clients to point to the site of pain/symptoms
- determining if the pain is local or referred. Local pain tends to be sharp and well-localised; referred pain tends to be dull and poorly localised. The presence of nerve impingement symptoms like numbness, tingling or weakness suggest

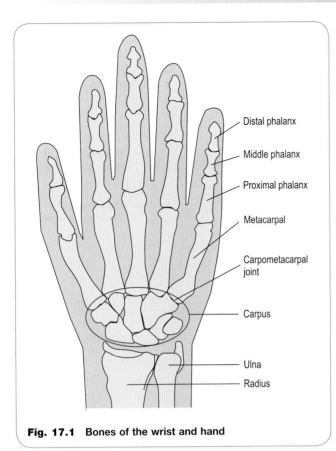

Fig. 17.1 Bones of the wrist and hand

Distal phalanx
Middle phalanx
Proximal phalanx
Metacarpal
Carpometacarpal joint
Carpus
Ulna
Radius

Flexion · Extension

Abduction · Adduction · Opposition

Fig. 17.2 Movements of the thumb

Ulnar nerve

Humeral head of
pronator teres

Brachial artery

Ulnar artery

Ulnar head of
pronator teres

Median nerve

Flexor carpi radialis

Radial artery

Pronator teres (cut)

Palmaris longus

Flexor carpi ulnaris

Palmar aponeurosis

Ulnar nerve

Humeral head of
flexor carpi ulnaris

Ulnar head of
flexor carpi ulnaris

Pisohamate ligament

Pisiform

Pisometacarpal ligament

Hook of hamate

Fig. 17.3 Major muscles of the forearm

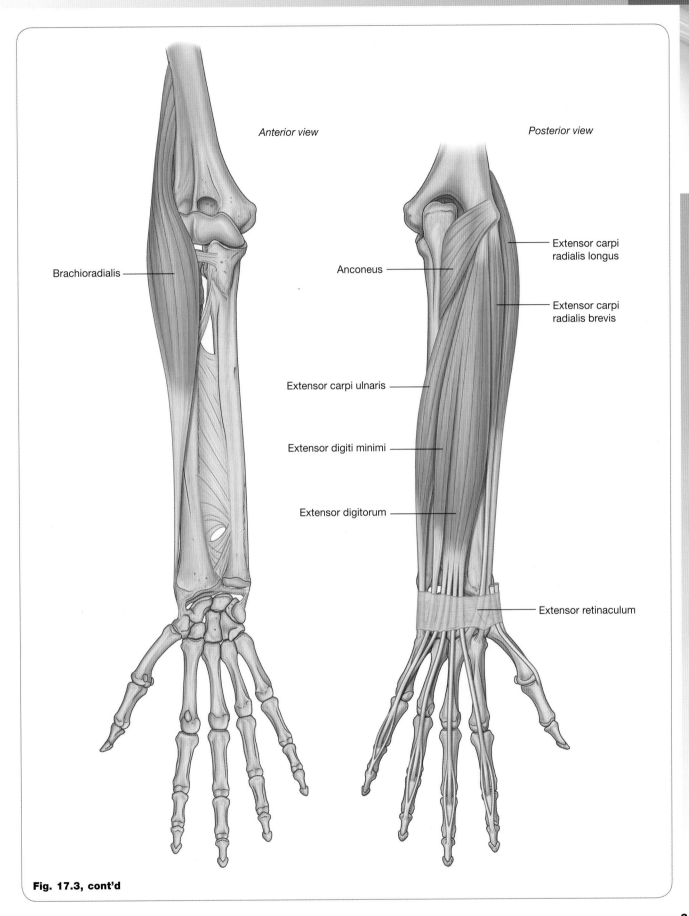

Anterior view

Posterior view

Brachioradialis

Anconeus

Extensor carpi ulnaris

Extensor digiti minimi

Extensor digitorum

Extensor carpi radialis longus

Extensor carpi radialis brevis

Extensor retinaculum

Fig. 17.3, cont'd

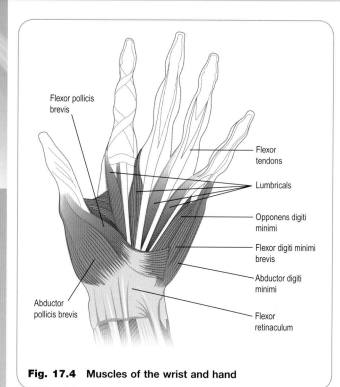

Flexor pollicis
brevis

Flexor
tendons

Lumbricals

Opponens digiti
minimi

Flexor digiti minimi
brevis

Abductor digiti
minimi

Abductor
pollicis brevis

Flexor
retinaculum

Fig. 17.4 Muscles of the wrist and hand

C6

C8

C7

Anterior

C6

C8

C7

Posterior

Fig. 17.5 Dermatomes of the wrist and hand

referral from lower cervical nerves (C6 nerve root affects the thumb, index finger, radial side of the hand and forearm, C7 affects the middle finger, and C8 affects the ring and little finger, ulnar side of the hand and forearm) (see Figure 17.5), or local nerve entrapment (median nerve affects thumb, index and middle fingers, the radial half of the ring finger and the radial half of the palm, ulnar nerve affects the little finger, the ulnar half of the ring finger and the ulnar half of the palm). Other causes of distal paraesthesia include B12 deficiency, hypothyroidism, heavy metal poisoning, diabetes, systemic lupus erythematosus, Sjögren's syndrome[a], malnutrition, HIV and HIV medications.

OUTCOME MEASURES

Outcome measures are questionnaires that are specifically designed to assess clients' level of impairment and to define benefits of treatment. The Patient Specific Functional Scale can be used to measure progress of treatment of clients with any musculoskeletal condition, including conditions of the wrist and hand (see Chapter 2).

POSTURAL ANALYSIS

Postural analysis enables observation of the whole client and facilitates identification of important features through bilateral comparison. It also facilitates detection of possible predisposing or contributing factors through observing the position of the head, cervical and thoracic spines, glenohumeral joints and scapula. Observe the alignment and symmetry of the upper limbs, carrying angle of the elbow and length of upper limbs in relation to the torso.

Observation of the wrist and hand

Observe the wrist and hand for symmetry, swelling (local or diffuse), colour, bruising, scars and muscle hypertonicity or atrophy.

Assessment of the wrist and hand

1. Case history
2. Outcome measures (e.g. The Patient Specific Functional Scale – see Chapter 2)
3. Postural analysis
4. Functional tests
   Cervical spine
   Active range of motion tests
   Flexion, extension, lateral flexion, rotation
   Glenohumeral joint
   Active range of motion tests
   Flexion, extension, abduction, horizontal adduction, internal rotation, external rotation
   Elbow joint
   Active range of motion tests
   Flexion, extension, supination, pronation
   Wrist and hand
   Active range of motion tests
   Flexion, extension, supination, pronation, adduction, abduction
   Passive range of motion tests
   Flexion, extension, supination, pronation, adduction, abduction
   Resisted range of motion tests
   Flexion, extension, supination, pronation, adduction, abduction
   Resisted and length tests for specific muscles
   Special tests including
   Phalen's test
   Tinel's test
   Finkelstein's test
5. Palpation

---

[a]Sjögren's syndrome is an autoimmune disease which causes glandular inflammation and is characterised by dry mouth and eyes. It may also be associated with connective tissue diseases like rheumatoid arthritis, systemic lupus erythematosus or scleroderma.

Table 17.1 Muscles of the wrist and hand[5]

Muscle	Origin	Insertion	Action
Forearm Pronators			
■ Pronator teres	Medial epicondyle of humerus and coronoid process of ulna	Middle of lateral surface of radius	Pronates forearm at radioulnar joint and weakly flexes forearm at elbow
■ Pronator quadratus	Distal portion of shaft of ulna	Distal portion of shaft of radius	Pronates forearm at radioulnar joints
Forearm supinator			
■ Supinator	Lateral epicondyle of humerus and supinator crest	Lateral surface of proximal one-third of radius	Supinates forearm at radioulnar joints
Wrist flexors *Superficial flexor compartment of the forearm*			
■ Flexor carpi radialis	Medial epicondyle of humerus	Second and third metacarpals	Flexes and abducts hand (radial deviation) at wrist joint
■ Palmaris longus	Medial epicondyle of humerus	Flexor retinaculum and palmar aponeurosis	Weakly flexes hand at wrist joint
■ Flexor carpi ulnaris	Medial epicondyle of humerus and superior posterior border of ulna	Pisiform, hamate and base of fifth metacarpal	Flexes and adducts hand (ulnar deviation) at wrist joint
■ Flexor digitorum superficialis	Medial epicondyle of humerus, coronoid process of ulna and anterior oblique line of radius	Middle phalanx of each finger	Flexes middle phalanx of each finger at proximal interphalangeal joint, proximal phalanx of each finger at metacarpophalangeal joint and flexes hand at wrist joint
Deep flexor compartment of the forearm			
■ Flexor pollicis longus	Anterior surface of radius and interosseous membrane (sheet of fibrous tissue that holds shafts of ulna and radius together)	Base of distal phalanx of thumb	Flexes distal phalanx of thumb at interphalangeal joint
■ Flexor digitorum profundus	Anterior medial surface of body of ulna	Base of distal phalanx of each finger	Flexes distal and middle phalanges of each finger at interphalangeal joints, proximal phalanx of each finger at metacarpophalangeal joint and hand at wrist joint
Extensors of the wrist and fingers *Superficial extensor compartment of the forearm*			
■ Extensor carpi radialis longus	Lateral supracondylar ridge of humerus	Second metacarpal	Extends and abducts hand at wrist joint
■ Extensor carpi radialis brevis	Lateral epicondyle of humerus	Third metacarpal	Extends and abducts hand at wrist joint
■ Extensor digitorum	Lateral epicondyle of humerus	Distal and middle phalanges of each finger	Extends distal and middle phalanges of each finger at interphalangeal joints, proximal phalanx of each finger at metacarpophalangeal joint and hand at wrist joint
■ Extensor digiti minimi	Lateral epicondyle of humerus	Tendon of extensor digitorum on fifth phalanx	Extends proximal phalanx of little finger at metacarpophalangeal joint and hand at wrist joint
■ Extensor carpi ulnaris	Lateral epicondyle of humerus and posterior border of ulna	Ulnar side of fifth metacarpal	Extends and adducts hand at wrist joint

Continued

Table 17.1   Muscles of the wrist and hand—cont'd

Muscle	Origin	Insertion	Action
Deep extensor compartment of the forearm			
▪ Abductor pollicis longus	Posterior surface of middle of radius and ulna and interosseous membrane	First metacarpal	Abducts and extends thumb at carpometacarpal joint and abducts hand at wrist joint
▪ Extensor pollicis brevis	Posterior surface of middle of radius and interosseous membrane	Base of proximal phalanx of thumb	Extends thumb at carpometacarpal and metacarpophalangeal joints; assists in abduction of the wrist
▪ Extensor pollicis longus	Middle third of posterior aspect of ulna and interosseous membrane	Base of distal phalanx of thumb	Extends distal phalanx of thumb at interphalangeal joint, assists in extension of metacarpophalangeal and carpometacarpal joints of the thumb and assists in abduction and extenson of the wrist
▪ Extensor indicis	Posterior surface of ulna	Tendon of extensor digitorum of index finger	Extends distal and middle phalanges of index finger at interphalangeal joints, proximal phalanx of index finger at metacarpophalangeal joint and hand at wrist joint
Intrinsic muscles of the hand			
▪ Adductor pollicis	Oblique head: capitate and second and third metacarpals Transverse head: third metacarpal	Medial side of proximal phalanx of thumb by a tendon containing a sesamoid bone	Adducts thumb at carpometacarpal and metacarpophalangeal joints
Thenar eminence			
▪ Abductor pollicis brevis	Flexor retinaculum, scaphoid and trapezium	Lateral side of proximal phalanx of thumb	Abducts thumb at carpometacarpal joint
▪ Opponens pollicis	Flexor retinaculum and trapezium	Lateral side of first metacarpal (thumb)	Moves thumb across palm to meet little finger (opposition) at the carpometacarpal joint
▪ Flexor pollicis brevis	Flexor retinaculum, trapezium, capitate and trapezoid	Lateral side of proximal phalanx of thumb	Flexes thumb at carpometacarpal and metacarpophalangeal joints
Hypothenar eminence			
▪ Abductor digiti minimi	Pisiform and tendon of flexor carpi ulnaris	Medial side of proximal phalanx of little finger	Abducts and flexes the little finger at metacarpophalangeal joint
▪ Flexor digiti minimi brevis	Flexor retinaculum and hamate	Medial side of proximal phalanx of little finger	Flexes little finger at carpometacarpal and metacarpophalangeal joints
▪ Opponens digiti minimi	Flexor retinaculum and hamate	Medial side of fifth metacarpal	Moves little finger across palm to meet thumb (opposition) at the carpometacarpal joint
Intermediate midpalmar			
▪ Lumbricals	Lateral side of tendons and flexor digitorum profundus of each finger	Lateral sides of tendons of extensor digitorum on proximal phalanges of each finger	Flex each finger at metacarpophalangeal joints and extends each finger at interphalangeal joints
▪ Palmar interossei	Sides of shafts of metacarpals of all digits (except the middle one)	Sides of bases of all proximal phalanges (except the middle one)	Adduct each finger at metacarpophalangeal joints; flex each finger at metacarpophalangeal joints
Dorsal interossei	Adjacent sides of metacarpals	Proximal phalanx of each finger	Abducts fingers at metacarpophalangeal joints; flex fingers at metacarpophalangeal joints; extend each finger at interphalangeal joints

Note: Biceps brachii supinates the forearm. It is described in Chapter 15.

Table 17.2 Red flags for potentially serious conditions of the wrist and hand

Condition	Red flag – history	Red flag – physical examination
Fracture/dislocation	History of significant trauma (e.g. fall on outstretched hand) Focal, severe non-radiating pain combined with history of trauma Inability to use the joint	Significant swelling Deformity with displaced, rotated or spiral fractures Point tenderness Pain with motion
Infection	History of systemic symptoms (e.g. fever, chills/rigor) Recent cut or puncture wound such as a human or animal bite History of immunosuppression (e.g. chemotherapy) Diabetes mellitus	Localised heat, swelling, erythema, erythematous streaks, especially from a portal of entry Systemic signs of infection Tenderness with motion
Tumour (melanoma)	History of cancer History of rapidly growing, painful firm or hard mass of hand or wrist History of immunosuppression (e.g. chemotherapy) Melanoma: Female <40 years, male >40 years Fair skin, history of sunburns Unintentional weight loss Continuous pain, especially at night and not improved with rest	Asymmetrical or irregular-shaped lesion, not consistent with ganglion or other benign lesion Melanoma: Borders are notched, scalloped or vaguely defined Colour unevenly distributed or defined Diameter >6 mm
Joint inflammation	History of gout or pseudogout History of rheumatoid arthritis History of other inflammatory arthritides	Swelling and deformity Mostly symmetrical joint involvement for more common inflammatory arthropathies (e.g. rheumatoid arthritis) Localised heat, swelling, erythema, usually solitary joint for crystal arthropathies (e.g. gout) Pain, usually without systemic symptoms
Rapidly progressive neurologic compromise	Rapidly progressive numbness, paresthesia or weakness in radial, ulnar or median nerve distribution Trauma History of stroke, cervical spine disorders or other CNS compromise	Sensory deficit in radial, ulnar or median distribution Loss of finger or grip strength when picking up objects Atrophy
Vascular compromise	History of diabetes mellitus History of fracture or dislocation History of vascular disease Compartment syndrome Inflammatory arthropathies with vasculitis	Decreased peripheral pulses Delayed capillary refill Cold, cool or pale hand
Raynaud's phenomenon	Positive family history Women on oestrogen therapy Cold exposure/frostbite injury Underlying collagen vascular disease	Skin pallor, cyanosis, and/or hyperaemic erythema of the fingers Taking medication promoting vasoconstriction such as β-blockers, amphetamines, decongestants and caffeine
Compartment syndrome	History of trauma, surgery or extreme unaccustomed activity Persistent forearm pain and tightness Tingling, burning or numbness	Palpable tenderness and tension of involved compartment Pain intensified with stretch to involved muscles Paraesthesia, paresis and sensory deficits Diminished pulse and prolonged capillary refill
Complex regional pain syndrome (Reflex sympathetic dystrophy)	History of trauma or surgery Severe burning/boring/aching pain out of proportion to the inciting event Pain not responsive to typical analgesics Secondary hyperalgesia/hypersensitivity	Area swollen (pitting oedema), warm and erythematous Temperature difference between involved and uninvolved extremity, hot or cold

(Adapted from Occupational Medicine Guidelines[6])

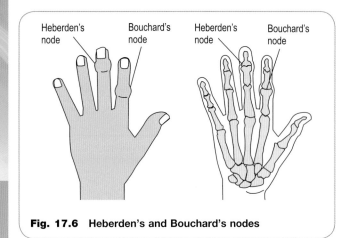

Fig. 17.6 Heberden's and Bouchard's nodes

Fig. 17.8 Dupuytren's contracture

Fig. 17.7 Mallet finger

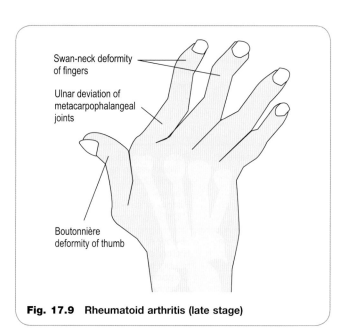

Fig. 17.9 Rheumatoid arthritis (late stage)

Common conditions of the hand include:

- Heberden's nodes at distal interphalangeal joints (associated with osteoarthritis) (see Figure 17.6)
- Bouchard's nodes at the proximal interphalangeal joint (usually associated with rheumatoid arthritis) (see Figure 17.6)
- Boutonnière deformity at the proximal interphalangeal joint (rupture of the extensor tendon at the middle phalanx, associated with rheumatoid arthritis and severe sprains) (see Figure 17.9)
- Mallet finger (rupture of the extensor tendon attachment at the distal phalanx) (see Figure 17.7)
- Dupuytren's contracture (hypertrophic nodular fibroplasia of the palmar aponeurosis producing flexion contracture usually of the ring and little fingers) (see Figure 17.8)
- Claw hand (flexion contracture of all digits from ulnar and median nerve palsy)
- Ulnar deviation of fingers and wrist (associated with rheumatoid arthritis) (see Figure 17.9)
- Swan neck deformity (proximal interphalangeal joint hyperextension and distal interphalangeal joint flexion associated with severe rheumatoid arthritis) (see Figure 17.9)
- Trigger finger (snapping during flexion and extension of the metacarpophalangeal joint which progresses to locking the digit in flexion due to fusiform swelling in flexor digitorum superficialis or flexor pollicis longus just proximal to the metacarpophalangeal joint, associated with osteoarthritis, rheumatoid arithritis or tendon trauma)
- Ganglia (swellings overlying tendon sheaths or joint capsules occurring commonly in the wrist and hand). Generally no treatment is required.

Table 17.3 Fingernail signs

Fingernail signs	Associated condition
Clubbing (thickening of end of digits, loss of normal angle between the nailbed and the skin of the distal phalanx)	Chronic decreased oxygen supply to ends of digits; associated with severe respiratory disease, cardiac condition
Spoon nails (thin, concave nails)	Anaemia, local injury, fungal infection, chronic diabetes
Thick, hard, brittle nails	Silica deficiency
Thin, soft, pliable nails	Calcium phosphate deficiency
Lateral ridges (Beau's lines)	Nutritional deficiencies, uncontrolled diabetes, peripheral artery disease, systemic disease, repetitive trauma to nails
White spots	Silica, calcium phosphate, zinc deficiency
White bands under nails	(Muehrcke lines) albumin deficiency (liver and kidney disease) (Mee's lines) arsenic poisoning
Pink-brown bands	Cirrhosis, heart disease, diabetes, cancer
Opaque nails, tip has dark band (Terry's nails)	Congestive heart failure, diabetes, liver disease, malnutrition
Distal half brown	Chronic renal failure
Splinter haemorrhages	Bacterial endocarditis, trauma, glomerulonephritis, vasculitis, cirrhosis, scurvy, psoriasis, trichinosis
No moons	Poor circulation
Blue moons	Naevus (birth mark), argyria (silver poisoning), Wilson's disease
Growths	Fungal infections
Longitudinal ridges	Small or large intestine disease
Pitting (small depressions in nails)	Psoriasis, nail injuries, chronic dermatitis
Yellow nails	Respiratory condition (e.g. chronic bronchitis), lymphoedema

Observe the fingernails of both hands for signs of certain conditions. Table 17.3 lists some fingernail signs and possible associated conditions.

FUNCTIONAL TESTS

For any tests involving joint movements it is important to compare both sides and take into account any underlying pathology and the age and lifestyle of the client. Measuring wrist range of motion appears to be highly reliable but of unknown diagnostic utility. Measuring finger and thumb range of motion is less reliable, even when performed by the same examiner.[4]

Active range of motion of the cervical spine (flexion, extension, lateral flexion and rotation)

Examination of the wrist and hand begins with active range of motion tests of the cervical spine to help rule out brachial plexus injury which may refer pain and other symptoms to the wrist and hand (see Figure 17.5 on p 320). If active range of motion tests of the cervical spine reproduce wrist and hand symptoms, further examination of the cervical spine is indicated (see Chapter 12). Patients with neck pain frequently report functional limitation in the upper limb.[7]

Active range of motion of the glenohumeral joint (flexion, extension, abduction, horizontal adduction, external and internal rotation)

If active range of motion tests of the glenohumeral joint produce symptoms, a full examination of the glenohumeral joint is indicated (see Chapter 15).

Active range of motion of the elbow joint (flexion, extension, pronation and supination)

If the client experiences pain or other symptoms during elbow movement, a full examination of the elbow joint is indicated (see Chapter 16).

Active range of motion of the wrist and fingers[8]
Wrist

Flexion/extension 80°/70°
Supination/pronation 80°/80°
Abduction (radial deviation)/adduction (ulnar deviation) 20°/30°
1st carpometacarpal joint
Flexion/extension 15°/20°
Abduction 70°

Fingers and thumb

Metacarpophalangeal joints
Fingers: Flexion/extension 90°/20°
Thumb: Flexion/extension 50°/0°
Interphalangeal joints
Fingers: PIP flexion/extension 100°/0°
DIP flexion/extension 70°/0°
Thumb: IP flexion/extension 65°/10–20°

Passive range of motion of the wrist and hand

If the client is unable to perform normal AROM in any direction, further investigation is required. PROM testing for the wrist should be performed by stabilising and palpating the wrist with one hand and moving the client's wrist through its ranges of motion with the other. To isolate finger joints, place one contact either side of the joint (e.g. to isolate the PIP, one hand contacts the proximal phalanx, the other contacts the distal phalanx). Palpate for crepitus, capsular pattern and end-feel as the joints are being moved.

CAPSULAR PATTERNS

Wrist joint   flexion more limited than extension
1st carpometacarpal joint   abduction more limited than extension
Fingers: metacarpophalangeal joints   flexion more limited than extension
Fingers: interphalangeal joints   flexion more limited than extension.

Resisted range of motion

RROM tests should also be performed if AROM testing indicates the likelihood of a wrist or hand problem. RROM tests include:

Wrist

Flexion: flexor carpi radialis, flexor carpi ulnaris, palmaris longus, flexor digitorum superficialis and profundus
Extension: extensor carpi radialis longus and brevis, extensor carpi ulnaris, extensor digitorum
Pronation: pronator teres, pronator quadratus
Supination: supinator
Abduction: extensor carpi radialis longus and brevis, flexor carpi radialis
Adduction: flexor carpi ulnaris, extensor carpi ulnaris

Fingers

Flexion: flexor digitorum profundus and superficialis, lumbricals
Extension: extensor digitorum
Abduction: dorsal interossei
Adduction: palmar interossei

Thumb

Flexion: flexor pollicis longus and brevis
Extension: extensor pollicis longus and brevis
Abduction: abductor pollicis longus and brevis
Adduction: adductor pollicis

Resisted tests and length tests for specific muscles[9]

If RROM tests reproduce symptoms, then further tests may be used to help identify specific muscles involved. Refer to Chapter 16 for resisted and length tests of biceps brachii, supinator, pronator teres and pronator quadratus.

1. FLEXOR CARPI RADIALIS

Resisted test

The client holds their wrist flexed towards the radial side, fingers relaxed. Apply pressure to extend their wrist towards the ulnar side. Note that palmaris longus may also be activated during this test (see Figure 17.10).

Length test

Contracture of flexor carpi radialis prevents the wrist from fully extending and deviating towards the ulnar side.

2. FLEXOR CARPI ULNARIS

Resisted test

The client holds their wrist flexed towards the ulnar side, fingers relaxed. Apply pressure against the hypothenar eminence in the direction of extension towards the radial side (see Figure 17.11).

Fig. 17.10   Resisted test for flexor carpi radialis

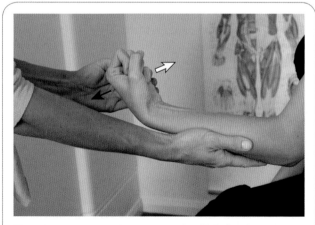

Fig. 17.11   Resisted test for flexor carpi ulnaris

Fig. 17.12 Palmaris longus and brevis resisted test

Fig. 17.14 Resisted test for flexor digitorum superficialis

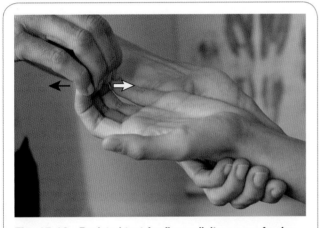

Fig. 17.13 Resisted test for flexor digitorum profundus

Fig. 17.15 Resisted test for flexor pollicis longus

Length test

Contracture of flexor carpi ulnaris prevents the wrist from fully extending and deviating towards the radial side.

3. PALMARIS LONGUS AND BREVIS

Resisted test

The client strongly cups their palm and flexes their wrist. Apply pressure to both thenar and hypothenar eminences to flatten the hand and extend the wrist as the client tries to hold the position (see Figure 17.12).

Length test

Contracture of palmaris longus and brevis muscles limits the client's ability to open their palm and extend their wrist.

4. FLEXOR DIGITORUM PROFUNDUS

Resisted test

The client flexes the distal interphalangeal joints of the 2nd to 5th digits. Contact the palmar surface of the distal phalanges and try to extend their fingers (see Figure 17.13).

Length test

Contracture of flexor digitorum profundus prevents full extension of the distal phalanges of 2nd to 5th fingers. It

can cause a flexion deformity of the distal phalanges of the fingers.

5. FLEXOR DIGITORUM SUPERFICIALIS

Resisted test

This test is similar to the test for flexor digitorum profundus except that pressure is applied at the middle phalanges (see Figure 17.14).

Length test

Contraction of flexor digitorum superficialis limits extension of the middle phalanges of digits 2 to 5. It can cause flexion of the middle phalanges of the fingers if the wrist is extended or flexion of the wrist if the fingers are extended.

6. FLEXOR POLLICIS LONGUS

Resisted test

The client flexes the distal phalanx of the thumb and holds this position. Contact the palmar surface of the distal phalanx and apply pressure in the direction of extension (see Figure 17.15).

Length test

Contracture of flexor pollicis longus limits extension of the distal phalanx of the thumb. It can cause a flexion deformity of the distal interphalangeal joint of the thumb.

327

Fig. 17.16 Resisted test for flexor pollicis brevis

Fig. 17.18 Resisted test for abductor pollicis brevis

Fig. 17.17 Resisted test for abductor pollicis longus

Fig. 17.19 Resisted test for adductor pollicis

7. FLEXOR POLLICIS BREVIS

This test is similar to the test for flexor pollicis longus except that the client flexes the proximal phalanx of the thumb and the practitioner applies pressure to its palmar surface in the direction of extension (see Figure 17.16).

Length test

Contracture of flexor pollicis brevis limits extension of the proximal phalanx of the thumb. It can cause a flexion deformity of the proximal interphalangeal joint of the thumb.

8. ABDUCTOR POLLICIS LONGUS

The client abducts the thumb. Apply pressure to the lateral surface of the first metacarpal bone in the direction of adduction (see Figure 17.17).

Length test

If abductor pollicis longus is contracted, adduction of the carpometacarpal joint of the thumb is limited. Contracture can cause the first metacarpal to be abducted and slightly extended with slight radial deviation of the hand.

9. ABDUCTOR POLLICIS BREVIS

Resisted test

The test is similar to the test for abductor pollicis longus except that you apply pressure against the proximal phalanx in the direction of adduction towards the palm (see Figure 17.18).

Length test

If abductor pollicis brevis is contracted, adduction of the carpometacarpal and metacarpophalangeal joints of the thumb is limited.

10. ADDUCTOR POLLICIS

Resisted test

Contact the medial surface of the thumb and resist as the client tries to adduct the thumb towards the palm (see Figure 17.19).

Length test

Contracture of adductor pollicis limits abduction of the thumb and can create an adduction deformity of the thumb.

Fig. 17.20 Resisted test for opponens pollicis and opponens digiti minimi

Fig. 17.22 Resisted test for extensor carpi ulnaris

Fig. 17.21 Resisted test for extensor carpi radialis longus and brevis

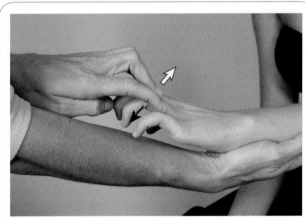

Fig. 17.23 Resisted test for extensor digitorum

11. OPPONENS POLLICIS/OPPONENS DIGITI MINIMI

Resisted test

Opponens pollicis and opponens digiti minimi can be tested at the same time. The client touches the tip of their little finger with the tip of their thumb and holds this position as you try to separate finger and thumb (see Figure 17.20).

Length test

Contracture of opponens pollicis limits extension of the carpometacarpal joint of the thumb and contracture of opponens digiti minimi limits extension of the fifth metacarpal.

12. EXTENSOR CARPI RADIALIS LONGUS AND BREVIS

The client extends their wrist towards the radial side and holds the position as you apply pressure against the dorsum of the hand in the direction of flexion towards the ulnar side (see Figure 17.21).

Length test

Contracture of extensor carpi radialis longus and brevis muscles limits flexion and ulnar deviation of the wrist. It can cause the wrist to be held in extension with radial deviation.

13. EXTENSOR CARPI ULNARIS

The client extends their wrist towards the ulnar side and holds the position as you apply pressure against the dorsum of the hand in the direction of flexion towards the radial side (see Figure 17.22).

Length test

Contracture of extensor carpi ulnaris limits radial deviation and flexion of the wrist. It can cause the wrist to be held in ulnar deviation with slight extension.

14. EXTENSOR DIGITORUM

Resisted test

The client extends the proximal phalanges of the 2nd to 5th digits. The interphalangeal joints are relaxed. Apply pressure against the dorsal surface of the proximal phalanges in the direction of flexion (see Figure 17.23).

Length test

Contracture of extensor digitorum limits flexion of the 2nd to 5th metacarpophalangeal joints. It may create a hyperextension deformity of the metacarpophalangeal joints if the wrist

329

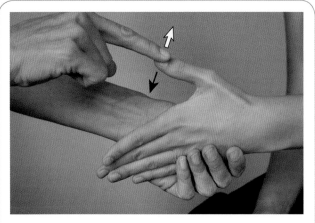

Fig. 17.24 Resisted test for extensor pollicis longus

Fig. 17.26 Phalen's test

Fig. 17.25 Resisted test for extensor pollicis brevis

Fig. 17.27 Tinel's sign at the wrist

is flexed, or extension of the wrist when the metacarpophalangeal joints are flexed.

15. EXTENSOR POLLICIS LONGUS

Resisted test

The client extends the distal phalanx of the thumb. Apply pressure against the dorsal surface of the distal phalanx of the thumb in the direction of flexion (see Figure 17.24).

Length test

Contracture of extensor pollicis longus limits flexion of the interphalangeal joint of the thumb.

16. EXTENSOR POLLICIS BREVIS

This test is similar to the test for extensor pollicis longus except that you apply pressure against the dorsum of the proximal phalanx of the thumb in the direction of flexion (see Figure 17.25).

Length test

Contracture of extensor pollicis brevis limits flexion and adduction of the carpometacarpal joint and flexion of the metacarpophalangeal joint of the thumb.

Special tests

If the client reports symptoms when performing a special test, ask the client to identify the exact location of the symptoms and confirm that they are the same as the symptoms described in the case history. Positive special test results should always be interpreted cautiously and in the context of other clinical findings (see Chapter 2).

PHALEN'S TEST

The client presses the backs of both hands together for up to one minute to maximally flex the wrists. Carpal tunnel is suggested if this position causes numbness and tingling in the thumb, index and middle finger (the median nerve distribution), wrist pain or weakness (see Figure 17.26).

TINEL'S SIGN

Tap over the median nerve in the carpal tunnel with the fingertips. Numbness, tingling or shooting pain into the thumb, index and middle finger (median nerve distribution) suggests median nerve neuropathy (see Figure 17.27).

FINKELSTEIN'S TEST

Instruct the client to make a fist with the thumb tucked inside the other fingers and then to move the wrist to the ulnar side.

Fig. 17.28 Finkelstein's test

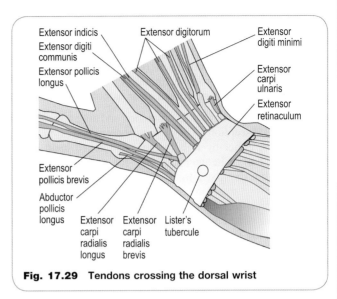

Fig. 17.29 Tendons crossing the dorsal wrist

Pain in the area of the abductor pollicus longus and extensor pollicus brevis tendons indicate stenosing tenosynovitis of these tendons of the thumb (de Quervain's tenosynovitis) (see Figure 17.28).

PALPATION

Palpate the radial styloid process on the lateral aspect of the wrist. The depression distal to the radial styloid process is the anatomical snuff box which is bordered posteriorly by the extensor pollicis longus tendon and anteriorly by the extensor pollicis brevis and abductor pollicis longus tendons. Scaphoid and trapezius form the floor. The scaphoid is the most commonly injured carpal bone. Tenderness in the snuffbox could indicate fractured scaphoid or de Quervain's tendinitis.

Medial to the styloid process of the radius on the anterior aspect of the wrist, palpate the radial artery and flexor carpi radialis tendon.

The tubercle on the dorsum of the radius (Lister's tubercle), the lunate, capitate and third metacarpal are in a straight line (see Figure 17.29). This is a useful guide when palpating. The lunate is the most frequently dislocated bone in the wrist and the second most frequently fractured.

Locate the ulnar styloid process, the most prominent structure on the dorsum of the wrist, and the triquetrum in the proximal carpal row. The triquetrum is more easily palpated when the wrist is radially deviated. The pisiform within the flexor carpi ulnaris tendon and the hook of the hamate can be palpated through the hypothenar muscles distal to the ulna. The hook of the hamate forms the lateral border of the tunnel of Guyton which transports the ulnar nerve and artery to the hand. The pulse of the ulnar artery may be felt just proximal to the hook of the hamate.

Palpate the flexor tendons as they cross the palm and any nodules in the palmar fascia. From Lister's tubercle on the dorsum of the distal radius, palpate the tendons of the extensor carpi radialis longus and brevis, abductor pollicis longus and extensor pollicis brevis on the radial side. On the ulnar side of Lister's tubercle, palpate tendons of the extensor pollicis longus, extensor indicis, extensor digitorum communis, extendor digitorum, extensor digiti minimi and extensor carpi ulnaris.

Palpate the thenar and the hypothenar eminences. The thenar muscles are the abductor pollicis brevis, opponens pollicis and flexor pollicis brevis; the hypothenar muscles are the abductor digiti minimi, opponens digiti minimi and flexor digiti minimi brevis.

REMEDIAL MASSAGE TREATMENT

Assessment of the wrist and hand provides essential information for development of treatment plans, including:

- client's suitability for remedial massage therapy. Wrist and hand conditions can lead to significant disability. Referral to a specialist medical or physiotherapist may be required.
- duration of the condition (i.e. acute or chronic)
- severity of the condition (i.e. grade of injury; mild, moderate or severe pain)
- type(s) of tissues involved
- priorities for treatment if more than one injury or condition are present
- whether the signs and symptoms suggest a common condition of the wrist and hand
- special considerations for individual clients (e.g. client's preference for treatment types and styles, specific population considerations).

Conditions of the wrist, hand and forearm have been classified into four broad groups:[6]

- mechanical disruption (e.g. fractures, dislocations from trauma)
- degenerative disorders (e.g. osteoarthritis, tendinosis)
- potentially serious conditions (e.g. fractures, infections, neurovascular compromise, tumours)
- non-specific disorders without clear pathological cause

The wrist and hand have little protection and are easily injured (mechanical disruption). They are most commonly injured by direct blows, either by falls to the outstretched hand or by catching a ball. Clients presenting for remedial massage therapy within the first 2 to 3 days after an injury should be checked for fracture. However, most clients wait until they are in the chronic phase before consulting remedial massage therapists for wrist and hand conditions and are often concurrently receiving treatment from other healthcare providers.

Many clients have occupational or sporting overuse syndromes caused by repetitive movements or awkward postures, including lateral elbow tendinopathy (see Chapter 16), carpal tunnel syndrome, de Quervain's disease and tenosynovitis of the wrist or hand.

OVERVIEW

Develop a short- and a long-term plan for each client. The short-term plan directs treatment to the highest priority (usually determined by symptoms). The long-term plan can be introduced when presenting symptoms have subsided. Long-term treatment focuses on contributing or predisposing factors such as underlying structural features and lifestyle factors. A significant part of both short-term and long-term treatment involves educating clients about likely causal or aggravating factors and guiding the management of these factors. If massage therapy is being used in conjunction with other treatments it is important to communicate with other treating practitioners.

TENDINOPATHY AND TENOSYNOVITIS

Any of the flexor and extensor tendons around the wrist may become injured with excessive activity, particularly with typing or using a computer mouse. Tendons commonly affected include abductor pollicis longus, extensor pollicis brevis, flexor digitorum superficialis and flexor pollicis longus. It is thought that repeated microtears may occur in the tendon or tendon sheath that initially cause inflammation but with continued overuse eventually lead to degeneration of the collagen fibre structure. However, the pathophysiology remains unclear and some authors have suggested that repetitive strain injuries may be diffuse neuromuscular illnesses involving peripheral tissues and affecting the regulatory structures of the central nervous system. Other authors suggest that both degeneration and inflammation work together in the pathogenesis of tendinopathies.[10]

Assessment

HISTORY

The client presents with pain usually on the dorsum of the hand aggravated by movement. The pain develops gradually and may begin with stiffness after rest. There is usually a history of repetitive overuse (e.g. typing, writing, using a computer mouse).

> **Key assessment findings for tendinopathy tenosynovitis**
>
> - History of repetitive overuse
> - Functional tests:
>   - AROM painful when the involved muscle contracts
>   - PROM painful when involved tendons are passively stretched
>   - RROM positive for involved muscles
>   - Resisted and length tests positive for involved muscles
>   - Special tests: Finkelstein's test positive for de Quervain's tenosynovitis
> - Palpation: linear tenderness along the tendon. Fibrotic tissue is usually palpable. Crepitus is often present in tenosynovitis.

FUNCTIONAL TESTS

Cervical AROM tests do not reproduce wrist or hand symptoms.

Shoulder AROM tests do not reproduce wrist or hand symptoms.

Elbow AROM tests do not usually reproduce wrist or hand symptoms.

Wrist tests

AROM is painful when the involved muscles are contracted.

PROM may be painful as the involved muscles are passively stretched.

RROM is painful for involved muscles.

Resisted and length tests are positive for involved muscles.

Special tests: Tinel's sign and Phalen's test are negative.

PALPATION

Tenderness is elicited along the line of the tendon as it crosses the wrist and extends above the wrist. Fibrotic tissue is often palpable in the tendon or tendon sheath. Fine crepitus may be palpated (and heard) when the involved tendon moves.

Overview of treatment and management

Resting the affected tendon by avoiding the responsible activity helps manage symptoms. Acute presentations may require cryotherapy for pain relief.

A typical remedial massage treatment for subacute or chronic tendinopathy or tenosynovitis of the wrist includes:

- Swedish massage therapy to the wrist and hand, upper limb, neck and upper back.
- Remedial massage techniques including (see Table 17.4 on p 333):
  - deep gliding frictions along the muscle fibres
  - cross-fibre frictions
  - soft tissue releasing techniques
  - deep transverse friction applied directly to the damaged tendon, which may help stimulate collagen production.
  - trigger point therapy
  - muscle stretching.
- Myofascial release including cross-arm techniques and the arm pull (see Chapter 8).
- Thermotherapy may be beneficial for pain relief.

Table 17.4 Remedial massage techniques for muscles of the wrist and hand

Muscle	Soft tissue release	Trigger point	Deep transverse friction	Stretch	Corrective action	Home exercise
Abductor pollicis longus and brevis	Practitioner: applies static pressure to the taut band/lesion using fingers or thumbs as the client's thumb is slowly passively or actively abducted and adducted. In the dynamic variant, the practitioner performs a deep glide as the muscle is slowly lengthened (i.e. adducted). The technique can also be performed with passive or active abduction and adduction of the wrist.	 Abductor pollicis longus and extensor pollicis brevis Extensor pollicis longus Not yet described		Passive stretch: Flex the client's thumb and adduct the client's wrist to their comfortable limit. Stretch all associated shortened muscles of the wrist and hand, upper limb, upper back and neck. 	Avoid aggravating activity.	Flex the thumb and adduct the wrist as far as possible within pain tolerance. Hold for up to 30 seconds. Repeat 3 times. General mobilisation and strengthening exercises as indicated: ■ Gently make a fist and then spread the fingers as far as possible ■ Gentle mobilisations of the wrist (flexion, extension, rotation, abduction and adduction) ■ Strengthening exercises including squeeze ball and elastic band exercises

Continued

Table 17.4 Remedial massage techniques for muscles of the wrist and hand—cont'd

Muscle	Soft tissue release	Trigger point	Deep transverse friction	Stretch	Corrective action	Home exercise
Extensor pollicis longus and brevis	Practitioner: applies static pressure to the taut band/lesion using fingers or thumbs as the thumb is slowly passively or actively flexed and extended. In the dynamic variant, the practitioner performs a deep glide along the muscle as it lengthens (i.e. flexes). The technique can also be performed with passive or active abduction and adduction of the wrist.	Abductor pollicis longus and extensor pollicis brevis / Extensor pollicis longus	Not yet described	Passive stretch: The thumb is flexed from the carpometacarpal joint and the wrist adducted and flexed. Stretch all associated shortened muscles of the wrist and hand, upper limb, upper back and neck.	Avoid aggravating activities. Correct workplace ergonomics.	Make a fist with the thumb inside and slowly flex and adduct the wrist. Stretch within pain tolerance. Hold for up to 30 seconds. Repeat 3 times. Include general mobilisation and strengthening exercises as indicated.
Flexor pollicis longus	Practitioner: applies static pressure to the taut band/lesion using fingers or thumbs as the thumb is slowly passively or actively flexed and/or extended. In the dynamic variant, the practitioner performs a deep glide along the muscle as it lengthens (i.e. extends).			Passive stretch: The practitioner extends the thumb from the distal phalanx. Stretch all associated shortened muscles of the wrist and hand, upper limb, upper back and neck.	Avoid prolonged tight gripping.	Hold the end of the thumb and stretch it slowly to the side as far as you can comfortably. Hold for up to 30 seconds. Repeat 3 times. Include general mobilisation and strengthening exercises as indicated.

Wrist flexors and wrist extensors are described in Chapter 16.

- Other remedial techniques such as wrist joint articulation may also be introduced as required (see Chapter 7):
  - Wrist pronated longitudinal thenar kneading
  - Wrist pronated traction and circumduction
  - Wrist semi-supinated traction and circumduction
  - Wrist overhead traction and supination
  - Metacarpophalangeal and interphalangeal mobilisation
  - Metacarpal shearing
  - Rotation and traction of phalanges.

Correct underlying biomechanical and predisposing factors if possible (e.g. upper crossed syndrome, rounded shoulder posture, forearm muscles tightness and weakness).

CLIENT EDUCATION

Advise the client to eliminate or avoid all aggravating activities to reduce the stress on the damaged tendons. A wrist splint or brace is sometimes worn to limit wrist movement and rest the affected tendons. Rehabilitative exercises are designed to improve overall strength, endurance and flexibility in the muscles of the entire upper limb kinetic chain. This includes muscles of the neck, shoulder, elbow, wrist and hand. Initially a stretching program is introduced to restore pain-free range of motion. As soon as possible, strengthening exercises are introduced (e.g. using a squeeze ball or stretching an elastic band with the fingers). The emphasis is usually on restoring function in the muscles that cross the wrist. Ergonomic and posture correction is usually required. Refer for osseous manipulation if required.

DE QUERVAIN'S TENOSYNOVITIS

Tenosynovitis of the abductor pollicis longus and/or extensor pollicis brevis is known as de Quervain's tenosynovitis. It is commonly associated with repetitive overuse among people who perform repetitive hand movements, including typists, cashiers, massage therapists and mechanics. It also occurs in sports which involve gripping or throwing. It is sometimes associated with osteoarthritis or rheumatoid arthritis of the thumb (see Figure 17.30).

Assessment

HISTORY

The onset of pain at the posterolateral aspect of the wrist and thumb is usually insidious. The client reports a history of repetitive overuse such as excessive typing, use of a computer mouse, palm-held computer or mobile phone, playing a keyboard or playing a racquet sport. The pain is described as aggravated by movement of the thumb and relieved by rest and may radiate several centimetres up the forearm.

FUNCTIONAL TESTS

Cervical AROM tests do not reproduce wrist and thumb symptoms.
Shoulder AROM tests do not reproduce wrist and thumb symptoms.
Elbow AROM tests do not reproduce wrist and thumb symptoms.

Wrist and hand tests:

AROM painful for thumb extension and/or abduction. Crepitus may be present.
PROM may be painful for thumb flexion and/or adduction when the tendon is passively stretched.
RROM painful for thumb extension and/or abduction.
Resisted and length tests positive for involved muscles.
Special tests: Finkelstein's test positive.

PALPATION

There is local tenderness on palpation of the involved tendons. Fibrotic tissue is often palpable in extensor pollicis brevis and/or abductor pollicis longus tendons.

Overview of treatment and management

Remedial massage treatment is similar for all cases of tendinopathy or tenosynovitis. Advise the client to eliminate or avoid all aggravating activities. Traditionally ice and splints have been prescribed for acute inflammation.

A typical remedial massage treatment for subacute or chronic de Quervain's tenosynovitis includes:

- Swedish massage therapy to the wrist and hand, upper limb, neck and upper back.

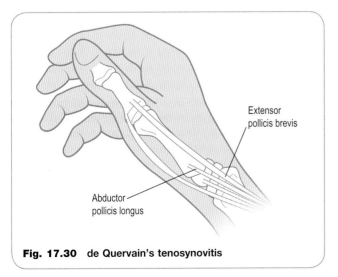

Fig. 17.30 de Quervain's tenosynovitis

Extensor pollicis brevis

Abductor pollicis longus

Key assessment findings for de Quervain's tenosynovitis

- History: insidious onset of pain on the posterolateral aspect of the wrist; pain aggravated by movement of the thumb, relieved by rest; history of repetitive overuse
- Functional tests:
  - AROM painful thumb extension and/or abduction
  - PROM painful thumb flexion and adduction (passive stretch of involved tendon)
  - RROM positive for resisted thumb extension and/or abduction
  - Resisted and length tests positive for involved muscles
  - Special tests: Finkelstein's test positive
- Palpation: local tenderness or pain. Fibrotic tissue (± crepitus) is often palpable.

335

- Remedial massage techniques for muscles (see Table 17.4) including:
  - deep gliding frictions along the muscle fibres
  - cross-fibre frictions
  - soft tissue releasing techniques
  - deep transverse friction applied directly to the damaged tendon, which may help stimulate collagen production
  - trigger point therapy
  - muscle stretching.
- Myofascial release including cross-arm techniques and the arm pull (see Chapter 8).
- Thermotherapy may assist with pain relief. Episodes of acute inflammation may require cryotherapy.
- Other remedial techniques such as wrist and thumb joint mobilisation may be introduced as required including (see Chapter 7):
  - wrist pronated longitudinal thenar kneading
  - wrist pronated traction and circumduction
  - wrist semi-supinated traction and circumduction
  - wrist overhead traction and supination
  - metacarpophalangeal and interphalangeal mobilisation
  - metacarpal shearing
  - rotation and traction of phalanges.

Correct any underlying or predisposing factors where possible.

CLIENT EDUCATION

The evidence supporting corticosteroid injections and splints for wrist and hand conditions is mixed. Moderate evidence exists for corticosteroid injections for very short-term benefits for trigger finger and de Quervain disease but not for Dupuytren's contracture. A thumb splint in addition to corticosteroid injection seems to be effective (moderate evidence) for de Quervain's contracture (short term and mid-term). Moderate evidence also exists for splinting after Dupuytren surgery in the short term.[11, 12]

Home exercises

Advise the client to avoid aggravating activties and to begin stretching and strengthening the wrist muscles as soon as pain permits: stretch the wrist in all directions, stretch the thumb in flexion and opposition and progress to include wrist, thumb and grip-strengthening exercises.[13] Progressively introduce stretching and stretching of muscles of the entire upper limb as required.

Refer for osseous manipulation and splinting. Kinesio tape or a thumb spica cast may provide short-term benefit for de Quervain's contracture.[14] Occasionally surgical decompression is required if conservative treatment fails to resolve the symptoms.

CARPAL TUNNEL SYNDROME

The carpal tunnel is the space between the carpal bones and the flexor retinaculum which runs across the anterior aspect of the wrist between the pisiform and the hamate medially and the trapezium and scaphoid laterally. The tunnel transports nine flexor tendons (flexor pollicis longus, four flexor digitorum superficialis tendons and four flexor digitorum profundus tendons) and the median nerve which is the most superficial and consequently most likely to be compressed against the flexor retinaculum[17] (see Figure 17.31).

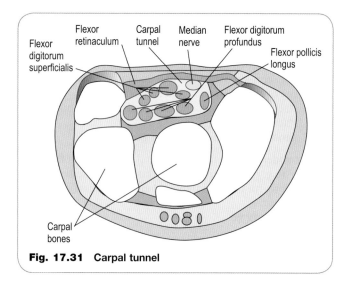

Fig. 17.31   Carpal tunnel

Carpal tunnel syndrome is the most common peripheral neuropathy and is a disabling condition from the early stages.[15] It is an entrapment neuropathy of the median nerve as it passes through the carpal tunnel. It may be accompanied by wrist flexor tendinopathy. The prevalence of carpal tunnel syndrome in the general population ranges from 1% and 5% with women at 2–3 times greater risk.[16] The age distribution peaks in the 50s. Work tasks demanding hand grip with high forces or vibrating tools are associated with the condition particularly if the tasks are repetitive.

A number of causes have been identified including:

- Mechanical compression: The flexor tendons are enclosed within a synovial sheath to reduce friction as they bend when the wrist is fully flexed or extended. When overused inflammation or adhesions may develop between the tendons and their synovial sheaths causing tenosynovitis. The increasing size of the tendon sheaths reduces space in the tunnel causing compression of the median nerve. Other causes of mechanical compression include osteoarthritis, neuroma and ganglia that develop in the tunnel, subluxation of the lunate bone, constant vibration (e.g. using a jack hammer) and trauma.
- Fluid retention/metabolic disease (e.g. diabetes, obesity, fluid retention during pregnancy).

Assessment

HISTORY

The most common symptoms of carpal tunnel syndrome include intermittent numbness, paraesthesia and pain in the median nerve distribution of the hand (i.e. the radial half of the palm including the thumb, index and middle fingers). Symptoms are often worse at night because people have a tendency to sleep with their wrists flexed, which increases compression within the tunnel. A wrist splint worn at night often alleviates the symptoms.

As the condition progresses there is likely to be a decrease in tactile sensitivity in the fingertips. Motor symptoms usually develop and are indicated by clumsiness, loss of dexterity and eventually a weakening of hand grip strength. If the condition progresses, it is also common to see a decrease in two-point

Fig. 17.32 Myofascial release for the flexor retinaculum

discrimination ability, further sensory loss, and wasting of the thenar muscles. Sensory symptoms (paraesthesia, numbness and pain) are usually the first to appear because the median nerve at the wrist is composed of over 90% sensory fibres. If motor symptoms are present it is usually an indication of the severity of nerve compression.

FUNCTIONAL TESTS

Cervical AROM tests do not reproduce symptoms.
Shoulder AROM tests do not reproduce symptoms.
Elbow AROM tests do not reproduce symptoms.

Wrist and hand tests

AROM positive for wrist flexion ± pronation. Crepitus may be present.
PROM positive for wrist flexion. Crepitus may be present.
RROM negative unless there is accompanying flexor tendinopathy.
Special tests: Phalen's test, Tinel's sign positive. Note that evidence on the utility of these tests is highly variable.[4]

PALPATION

Swelling may be palpable in the carpal tunnel. In long-standing cases thenar and hypothenar muscles may atrophy.

Overview of treatment and management

Advise the client to eliminate or avoid the aggravating condition. Traditionally, ice and splints are prescribed in the acute presentations. Night splints may be recommended.

A typical remedial massage treatment for subacute or chronic carpal tunnel syndrome includes:

- Swedish massage therapy to the wrist and hand, upper limb, neck and upper back.
- Remedial massage techniques (see Tables 17.4 and 16.5) including:
  - deep gliding frictions along the muscle fibres (e.g. wrist flexors and pronators)
  - cross-fibre friction to the flexor retinaculum and bellies of muscles that pass through the carpal tunnel
  - soft tissue releasing techniques
  - deep transverse friction applied directly to the damaged tendon, which may help stimulate collagen production
  - trigger point therapy
  - muscle stretching, including stretching of the wrist flexor muscles.

- Myofascial release to the flexor retinaculum:
  An example of a stretching technique for the flexor retinaculum is illustrated in Figure 17.32: The client's hand is supinated. The practitioner approaches distally and contacts either side of the flexor retinaculum with the pads of the thumbs, fingers resting on the dorsum of the hand. Gentle pressure is maintained for 3–5 minutes. The cross-arm technique and the arm pull (see Chapter 8) may also be beneficial.
- Joint articulation techniques may be useful including (see Chapter 7):
  - wrist pronated longitudinal thenar kneading
  - wrist pronated traction and circumduction
  - wrist semi-supinated traction and circumduction
  - wrist overhead traction and supination
  - metacarpophalangeal and interphalangeal mobilisation
  - metacarpal shearing.

Carpal bone mobilisation and median nerve mobilisation have both been shown to improving pain.[17]

- Neural stretching for median nerve entrapment may be helpful. This procedure is designed to enhance mobility of the median nerve. A systematic review found that median nerve excursion was reduced in people with carpal tunnel syndrome when compared with healthy controls.[18]
  The client is supine with their arms by their side. The wrist is in a neutral position. Take the client's upper limb through the following steps as long as the client remains symptom-free. As soon as symptoms are felt, return to the starting position. Note that this series of procedures can be done actively or passively (see Figure 17.33).
  Begin with upper limb supinated, elbow extended.
  Flex elbow.
  Hyperextend wrist.
  Externally rotate shoulder.
  Repeat the cycle several times.

Caution: The aim of treatment for carpal tunnel syndrome is to reduce nerve compression and to restore normal pain-free function. Avoid any techniques that place further pressure on this region. It is also important to evaluate other regions of median nerve entrapment as they may aggravate carpal tunnel

Fig. 17.33 Median nerve stretch

Key assessment findings for wrist sprain

- History of trauma, especially hyperextension of the wrist; immediate pain followed by swelling.
- Functional tests:
  - AROM decreased on all wrist movements
  - PROM decreased on all wrist movements
  - RROM negative unless associated muscle strain
  - Special tests: negative
- Palpation: local tenderness or pain. There may be excessive joint movement.

syndrome symptoms. These include the lower cervical spine, between the anterior and middle scalene muscles, under the clavicle, under the pectoralis minor muscle, near the anterior aspect of the elbow and between the two heads of the pronator teres muscle (a third of the way along the forearm from the cubital fossa; pronator teres attaches to the medial epicondyle). The absence of night pain usually indicates entrapment in a location proximal to the carpal tunnel.

Correct any underlying or predisposing factors. It is important to address the muscles of the entire upper limb kinetic chain.

CLIENT EDUCATION

If repetitive overuse is a likely causative factor, clients should eliminate or reduce aggravating activities. Many of the carpal tunnel syndrome rehabilitation strategies have focused on work equipment and ergonomics. Interventions include ergonomic re-education, keyboard supports and computer mouse and tool redesign. Diuretics may be used if compression is due to fluid retention. Night wrist splints may be helpful in the long term.[14] Surgery may be required for severe cases, most commonly an incision release of the flexor retinaculum. Multimodal care has been shown to relieve symptoms and improve function in patients with mild to moderate carpal tunnel syndrome. These treatments included splinting, oral drugs, injections, electrotherapy, electroacupuncture, specific manual techniques, and neural gliding exercises.[14, 15] Other soft tissue techniques have also shown good results although additional evidence is required for confirmation.[15] Oral steroids and corticosteroid injections appear to be beneficial in the short term but the benefits are not maintained in the long term.[19] A poor prognosis may be predicted by a positive Phalen's test, thenar wasting and long duration of symptoms.[20]

Home exercises

Stretching and strengthening the wrist muscles, including stretching the wrist in all directions, stretching the neck, shoulder, elbow, hand and fingers. One study found that supervised progressive strength training added to advice to continue normal physical activity provided no additional benefit for patients with hand pain.[21] Exercises to improve muscle

function of the entire upper limb, upper back and neck can be introduced as required.

SPRAINS

Ligament sprains are common in contact sports and falls onto the outstretched hand and most are hyperextension injuries. Because of the pain and swelling it may be difficult to distinguish from a fracture initially.

Assessment

HISTORY

The client describes a traumatic injury to the wrist, often during a contact sport or from a fall onto the outstretched hand. The client may describe popping or tearing at the time of the trauma. Pain is felt immediately and swelling follows approximately one hour later.

FUNCTIONAL TESTS

Cervical AROM tests do not reproduce wrist symptoms.
Shoulder tests do not reproduce wrist symptoms.
Elbow AROM tests do not reproduce wrist symptoms.

Wrist tests

AROM decreased in all ranges.
PROM decreased in all ranges.
RROM may be positive if there is associated muscle strain. Resisted and length tests may be positive for affected muscles if there is associated muscle strain.
Special tests negative.

PALPATION

Palpation at the site of injury elicits tenderness or pain. If ligaments have been stretched or completely torn, the affected joints have excessive movement.

Overview of treatment and management

In the acute phase, the recommended treatment is to apply ice, compression and elevation as required to the sprained ligament. The area is usually strapped for 3 to 4 weeks if severe. Commence isometric strengthening exercises as soon as pain permits.

A typical remedial massage treatment for subacute or chronic sprains of the wrist and hand includes:

- Swedish massage therapy to the wrist and hand, upper limb, neck and upper back.

- Remedial massage techniques (caution: make sure that injured ligaments are not stretched during treatment).
- Deep transverse friction to the site of injury.
- Myofascial release techniques (see Chapter 8).
- Joint mobilisation of the wrist and hand as required including (see Chapter 7):
  - wrist pronated traction and circumduction
  - wrist semi-supinated traction and circumduction
  - wrist overhead traction and supination
  - metacarpophalangeal and interphalangeal mobilisation
  - metacarpal shearing
  - rotation and traction of phalanges.
- Thermotherapy may provide pain relief.
- Muscle-specific techniques for associated muscle spasm, including (see Table 16.5 and Table 17.4):
  - deep gliding frictions along the muscle fibres
  - cross-fibre frictions
  - soft tissue releasing techniques
  - trigger point therapy
  - muscle stretching.

Correct any underlying or predisposing factors where possible.

CLIENT EDUCATION

Advise the client to rest and reduce or eliminate any aggravating activity. Treatment options may include a splint or orthotic brace and consider non-steroidal anti-inflammatory medication or corticosteroid injection.[22] Discuss injury prevention strategies such as sturdy footwear, improving lighting, installing handrails and exercise such as Tai Chi to improve strength and balance.[23] Also advise about safe landing strategies which include flexing the elbow to reduce the impact to the wrist.

Home exercises

Encourage the client to return to normal activities as soon as possible. There may be no additional benefit to grip strength exercises for the hand such as squeeze ball.[21] For wrist rehabilitation begin strengthening exercises of the wrist flexors, extensors, pronators and supinators.

SPRAINED THUMB

The thumb is commonly sprained in sports. For example, the thumb may be forced back during a fend in rugby or a mistimed basketball catch. Firm strapping is required to support the thumb base but it may be modified on return to play to allow some degree of movement and protection without necessarily permitting full abduction. A severe sprain may rupture the ulnar collateral ligament leaving the joint liable to further damage. Surgical repair may be required.

SPRAINED FINGER

A sprained finger may be extremely painful and persist for up to a year. Participation in sporting activities is still permitted, although in contact sports protective strapping may be required as much for confidence as for healing. In cricket, for example, extra padding inside the glove may be required. As a general rule, hand and finger movements are encouraged as soon as possible after injury and there have to be strong medical reasons for immobilising any part of the hand for long periods.

In any case, only the affected finger should be immobilised. Stiffness of the fingers may persist after sprains or fractures and can cause considerable disability.

Treatment

The client should make every effort to move the hand. Passive movements and stretches during convalescence are essential and massage is useful.

MALLET FINGER

A blow to the finger, such as can occur in cricket, basketball or goal keeping, may sprain the interphalangeal joints or rupture the extensor tendon insertion into the terminal phalanx. This causes the end of the finger to develop a mallet deformity (see Figure 17.7 on p 324).

Treatment

A straight finger splint worn for about 4 to 6 weeks and followed by persistent exercise ensures recovery with minimal loss of movement. Massage therapy may be beneficial in the rehabilitation phase.

FRACTURES AND DISLOCATIONS

Fractures are usually obvious because of the pain and deformity following injury. Fracture of the distal radius (Colles' fracture) is the most common of all fractures. It usually occurs as a result of a fall onto the outstretched arm, forcing the hand backwards and upwards. The lower part of the radius is displaced dorsally (dinner fork deformity of the wrist contour). Fracture of the scaphoid, the most common carpal fracture, can also occur from falls onto the outstretched hand. It is a common injury in roller-blading, skating and skiing. Initially fractures may be difficult to distinguish from wrist sprains. Swelling occurs for about 24 hours and then may subside. The most useful diagnostic sign for scaphoid fracture is pain on direct pressure to the floor of the anatomical snuffbox. The blood flow to the scaphoid is easily compromised and fractures tend to heal poorly.

Minor fractures of the fingers are treated simply by taping two adjacent fingers together. Contact sports are excluded but considerable activity and general training can be continued.

The lunate is the most commonly dislocated carpal bone. It usually occurs as a result of a fall onto the thenar eminence which forces the lunate anteriorly as the wrist is forcefully extended. In some cases anterior lunate dislocation is associated with median nerve compression which can cause paraesthesia in the thumb, index and middle fingers. Refer all suspected dislocations for further investigation.

Injury prevention strategies currently include improving lighting, installing handrails, not hurrying when walking, using a mobility device and exercise training such as muscle strengthening and Tai Chi to improve balance.[23] Advice about safe landing strategies have a significant effect on reducing impact load: advise clients to flex their elbow in a forward fall to significantly reduce the impact force applied to the wrist.

OSTEOARTHRITIS AND RHEUMATOID ARTHRITIS

Both osteoarthritis and rheumatoid arthritis can affect the wrist and hand. Osteoarthritis is a common presenting condition

Table 17.5 Comparison of osteoarthritis and rheumatoid arthritis of the wrist and hand

	Osteoarthritis	Rheumatoid arthritis
Pathology	Breakdown of articular cartilage, subchondral bone sclerosis, osteophyte formation	Autoimmune disease, synovial membrane thickens and produces pannus that corrodes cartilage, joints may fuse
Age of onset	Middle aged and elderly	20 to 40 years
Gender	Males = females	Females > males
Joints affected	Weight-bearing joints asymmetrically In hands, distal interphalangeal joints most affected, Heberden's nodes may be present	Small joints of hands, wrists, elbows symmetrically Metacarpophalangeal and proximal interphalangeal joints most affected. In late stage, Bouchard's nodes, ulnar deviation of fingers and swan neck deformity may be present
Systemic signs	No	Yes
Treatment	Prioritise exercise and self-management of acute episodes. Swedish massage, thermotherapy, myofascial release, remedial massage techniques muscles, weight loss, shock-absorbing footwear is recommended for osteoarthritis of the low back and joints of the lower limb), supplementation (e.g. curcumin celery seed extract)	In the chronic phase, Swedish massage, thermotherapy, myofascial release, remedial massage techniques muscles, refer for dietary modification, supplementation, acupuncture

in older clients or those with previous significant trauma or history of overuse. The distal interphalangeal joints are most affected and Heberden's nodes may develop in affected joints (see Figure 17.6 on p 324). Treatment involves educating clients about the nature of osteoarthritis (that it is a dynamic condition that can be managed), appropriate exercises and how to manage acute episodes.[24] Remedial massage therapy usually consists of Swedish massage to the entire upper limb and lower cervical and upper thoracic spines, local heat applications (e.g. hot wax treatments), gentle joint articulation, myofascial release techniques and muscle-focused techniques, including muscle stretches. For patients with base of thumb (trapeziometacarpal) osteoarthritis high-quality evidence showed that unimodal and multimodal physical therapy treatments can result in clinically beneficial improvements in pain and function.[25] Worthwhile unimodal treatments included orthosis and splinting. Multimodal treatments included a combination of frequent therapeutic exercise, heat, orthoses, joint mobilisations, and neurodynamic techniques. Recommendations for arthritis of the wrist and hand also include avoiding aggravating conditions, heat applications at home and stretching exercises. The most widely used supplements (e.g. glucosamine, chondroitin and vitamin D) may not provide a clinically important effect on knee, hip or hand osteoarthritis.[26] Some less well-known supplements (e.g. Boswellia serrata extract, pycnogenol and curcumin) appear to have effects in the short term, although the quality of the current evidence is low.

Rheumatoid arthritis affects women more than men and usually begins when the client is between 20 and 40 years of age. The first symptoms are usually in the hands and wrists. Typically the client reports waking with swelling and pain, especially in the proximal remed interphalangeal joints. Symptoms occur in both hands and several joints are involved.

Swelling and pain are not related to activity. In severe cases, ulnar deviation of the metacarpophalangeal joints and swan-neck deformity may develop (see Figure 17.9 on p 324). Systemic signs such as fatigue and night sweats also accompany joint symptoms. In the subacute and chronic phases, remedial massage therapy is directed to symptomatic relief. Treatments can include Swedish massage, heat applications, gentle joint articulation and myofascial releasing techniques. Clients may be referred to a general medical practitioner, naturopath, herbalist or acupuncturist for further treatment.

A comparison of clinical presentation and treatments of osteoarthritis and rheumatoid arthritis of the wrist and hand is presented in Table 17.5.

KEY MESSAGES

- Assessment of clients with conditions of the wrist and hand involves case history, outcome measures, postural analysis, functional tests and palpation.
- Assessment findings may indicate the type of tissue involved (contractile or inert: muscle, joint, fascia, ligament), duration of condition (acute or chronic) and severity (grade).
- Assessment findings may indicate a common presenting condition such as tendinopathy tenosynovitis, de Quervain's tendinitis and carpal tunnel syndrome.
- Assessment findings also indicate client perception of injury and preferences for treatment.
- Consider Clinical Guidelines, available evidence and client preferences when planning therapy.
- Although serious conditions of the wrist and hand are rare, be vigilant for red flags (e.g. indications of fractures, dislocations, infections and vascular compromise) during assessment.

- The selection of remedial massage techniques depends on assessment results. Swedish massage to the wrist and hand, upper limb, neck and upper back may be followed by muscle techniques (e.g. deep gliding, cross-fibre frictions, soft tissue releasing techniques, trigger point therapy, deep transverse friction and muscle stretching), joint mobilisation, myofascial release and thermotherapy as indicated.

- Educating clients about likely causal and predisposing factors and exercise rehabilitation are essential parts of remedial massage therapy.
- Prioritise the client self-help component of treatment wherever possible to reduce likelihood of recurrence and/or to promote health maintenance and illness prevention.

Review questions

1. Name the nine tendons that pass through the carpal tunnel.
2. What is the most commonly fractured bone in the wrist? What is the most useful diagnostic indicator for a fracture of this bone?
3. De Quervain's tendinitis commonly involves strains of:
   a) abductor pollicis longus and brevis
   b) extensor carpi radialis
   c) flexor pollicis longus
   d) extensor pollicis longus and brevis
4. List three conditions that could be classified as repetitive strain injuries.
5. The lunate is the most commonly dislocated bone of the wrist. What is the usual mechanism of injury for its dislocation?
6. A resisted test of the wrist extensor muscles produces pain at the dorsum of the wrist. This result suggests
   a) ligament strain
   b) lateral epicondylitis
   c) wrist extensor tendinopathy tenosynovitis
   d) osteoarthritis of the wrist
7. Special tests that may reproduce the symptoms of carpal tunnel include:

   a) Apley's test
   b) Tinel's sign
   c) Phalen's test
   d) Finkelstein's test
8. Carpal tunnel syndrome is often caused by mechanical compression of the median nerve. By what other mechanisms can carpal tunnel syndrome occur?
9. The median nerve at the wrist is composed of sensory and motor fibres. Compression of the median nerve in the carpal tunnel can alter:
   i) sensation in _____
   ii) motor activity in _____
10. List three different signs or symptoms that can be useful in distinguishing osteoarthritis from rheumatoid arthritis of the wrist and hand.
11. List five muscle-specific remedial massage techniques that are commonly used in the treatment of de Quervain's tenosynovitis.
12. What remedial massage techniques are likely to be beneficial for a client with osteoarthritis of the wrist or finger joints?

REFERENCES

1. Robinson LS, Sarkies M, Brown T, et al. Direct, indirect and intangible costs of acute hand and wrist injuries: a systematic review. Injury 2016;47(12):2614–26.
2. Vieira E, Schneider P, Guidera C, et al. Work-related musculoskeletal disorders among physical therapists: a systematic review. J Back Musculoskelet Rehabil 2016;29(3):417–28.
3. Padegimas E, Ilyas A. Distal radius fractures: emergency department evaluation and management. Orthop Clin N Am 2015;46(2):259–70.
4. Cleland J, Koppenhaver S, Su J. Netter's orthopaedic clinical examination: an evidence-based approach. 3rd edn. Philadelphia: Saunders; 2015.
5. Tortora GJ, Derrickson BH. Principles of anatomy and physiology. 15th edn. Stafford, Qld: Wiley; 2016.
6. Occupational medicine practice guidelines: evaluation and management of common health problems and functional recovery in workers. Beverly Farms, MA: OEM Press; 2016.
7. Alreni AS, Harrop D, Mclean SM. Measures of upper limb function for people with neck pain: a systematic review of measurement and practical properties. Manual Ther 2016;25:E75.

8. Reese N, Bandy WD, Yates C. Joint range of motion and muscle length testing. 2nd edn. St. Louis, MO: Saunders/Elsevier; 2010.
9. Hislop H, Avers D, Brown M, et al. Daniels and Worthingham's muscle testing: techniques of manual examination and performance testing. 9th edn. St. Louis, MO: Elsevier/Saunders; 2014.
10. Abate M, Gravare-Silbernagel K, Siljeholm C, et al. Pathogenesis of tendinopathies: inflammation or degeneration? Arthritis Res Ther 2009;11(3):235. Doi: 10.1186/ar2723.
11. Huisstede BM, Gladdines S, Randsdorp MS, et al. Effectiveness of conservative, surgical, and postsurgical interventions for trigger finger, Dupuytren disease, and de Quervain disease: a systematic review. Arch Phys Med Rehabil 2018;99:1635–49.
12. Neiduski R. Clinical relevance commentary on: hand therapy versus corticosteroid injections in the treatment of de Quervain's disease: a systematic review and meta-analysis. J Hand Ther 2016;29(1):12–13.
13. Carnes M, Vizniak N. Quick reference evidence-based conditions manual. 3rd edn. Burnaby, BC: Professional Health Systems; 2009.

14. D'angelo K, Sutton D, Côté P, et al. The effectiveness of passive physical modalities for the management of soft tissue injuries and neuropathies of the wrist and hand: a systematic review by the Ontario Protocol for Traffic Injury Management (OPTIMa) collaboration. J Manipulative Physiol Ther 2015;38(7):493–506.
15. Jimenez del Barrio SJ, Bueno Gracia E, Garcia H, et al. Conservative treatment in patients with mild to moderate carpal tunnel syndrome: a systematic review. Neurologia 2016:33(9):590–601.
16. Shiri R, Miranda H, Heliövaara M, et al. Physical work load factors and carpal tunnel syndrome: a population-based study. Occup Environ Med 2009;66(6):368–73.
17. Vikranth GR, Vinod Kumar KC, Mathias L. Comparative effect of carpal bone mobilization versus neural mobilisation in improving pain, functional status and symptoms severity in patient with carpal tunnel syndrome. Int J Physiother 2015;2(3):524–30.
18. Ellis R, Blyth R, Arnold N, et al. Is there a relationship between impaired median nerve excursion and carpal tunnel syndrome? A systematic review. J Hand Ther 2017;30(1):3–12.
19. Huisstede BM, Randsdorp MS, Van Den Brink J, et al. Effectiveness of oral pain medication and

corticosteroid injections for carpal tunnel syndrome: a systematic review. Arch Phys Med Rehabil 2018;99(8):1609–22.e10.

20. Burton CL, Chesterton LS, Chen Y, et al. Clinical course and prognostic factors in conservatively managed carpal tunnel syndrome: a systematic review. Arch Phys Med Rehabil 2016;97(5): 836–52.e1.

21. Menta R, Randhawa K, Côté P, et al. The effectiveness of exercise for the management of musculoskeletal disorders and injuries of the elbow, forearm, wrist, and hand: a systematic review by the Ontario Protocol for Traffic Injury Management (OPTIMa) collaboration. J Manipulative Physiol Ther 2015;38(7):507–20.

22. Woo S-H, Lee Y-K, Kim J-M, et al. Hand and wrist injuries in golfers and their treatment. Hand Clin 2017;33(1):81–96.

23. Moon Y, Sosnoff JJ. Safe landing strategies during a fall: systematic review and meta-analysis. Arch Phys Med Rehabil 2017;98(4):783–94.

24. Hunter DJ. Everything you ever wanted to know about osteoarthritis. The Health Report 2017. Online. Available: https://www.abc.net.au/radionational/programs/healthreport/everything-you-ever-wanted-to-know-about-osteoarthritis/8664218#transcript; 2017.

25. Ahern M, Skyllas J, Wajon A, et al. The effectiveness of physical therapies for patients with base of thumb osteoarthritis: systematic review and meta-analysis. Musculoskelet Sci Pract 2018;35: 46–54.

26. Liu X, Machado G, Eyles J, et al. Dietary supplements for treating osteoarthritis: a systematic review and meta-analysis. Br J Sports Med 2017;52(3):167–75.

The hip region

INTRODUCTION

True hip pathologies are a less common presenting condition to remedial massage clinics than pain referring to the lower limbs from the low back and for this reason assessment protocols should routinely include a scan of the low back. The age of the client is a particularly useful consideration in assessing hip complaints. Generally, older clients with hip pain are likely to have osteoarthritis of the hip. (The hip is more susceptible to degeneration than to trauma.)[1] Young adults present with muscle strains and femoroacetabular impingement. All children presenting with hip or knee pain must be carefully assessed to rule out hip pathologies that require referral (see Table 18.1 on p 344).

Childhood conditions of the hip are discussed in Chapter 21.

FUNCTIONAL ANATOMY

The hip or acetabulofemoral joint is a synovial ball and socket joint composed of the head of the femur and the acetabulum of the ilium. In normal activities the hip joint carries the greatest load of any joint in the body. In standing, the weight of the upper body is transmitted to the sacrum and then to the iliofemoral ligaments so that the body can remain in equilibrium with minimal muscle activity. The stability of the hip joint is enhanced by the depth of the acetabulum and the presence of the acetabular labrum (cartilaginous ring) and ligamentum teres, which keeps the head of the femur in the socket. Other ligaments of the hip joint include the pubofemoral ligament, ischiofemoral ligament, zona orbicularis and the transverse ligament of the acetabulum.

The pelvis contains five joints: two sacroiliac joints, the symphysis pubis and two acetabulofemoral joints (see Figure 18.1 on p 344). The acetabulofemoral joints are the most mobile joints of the pelvis and osteoarthritis of the hip or weak gluteus medius, gluteus maximus, quadriceps or hamstrings disturb the biomechanics of the pelvis and the rate and rhythm of normal gait. The major muscles that move the hip joint include (see Figure 18.2 on p 344):

- Flexion
    Iliopsoas
    Rectus femoris
- Extension
    Gluteus maximus
    Hamstrings
- Abduction
    Gluteus medius
    Gluteus minimus
    Tensor fasciae latae
- Adduction
    Adductor magnus
    Adductor longus
    Adductor brevis
    Gracilis
- Lateral rotation
    Piriformis
- Medial rotation
    Gluteus minimus
    Tensor fasciae latae

Major muscles of the hip are described in detail in Table 18.2 on p 345.

Blood supply to the femoral head comes from three sources: medial circumflex femoral artery (the most important source),

Table 18.1   Hip conditions according to age group

Age of onset	Hip pathology
0–5 years	Congenital hip displacement (unilateral or bilateral dislocation, more common in female infants and breech babies)
5–10 years	Perthes' disease (idiopathic aseptic necrosis of the femoral capital epiphysis)
10–15 years	Slipped femoral capital epiphysis (affects tall and thin or obese boys)
20–40 years	Muscle strains; femoroacetabular impingement
>40 years	Osteoarthritis
>60 years	Osteoarthritis, fracture of the neck of femur, Paget's disease (chronic disorder of the adult skeleton which affects normal bone remodelling. Localised areas of bone become soft, enlarged, brittle and prone to fracture)

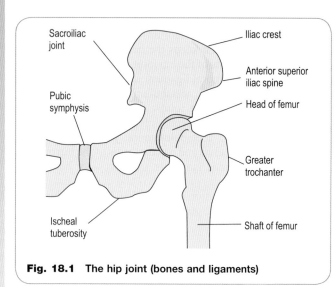

Fig. 18.1   The hip joint (bones and ligaments)

Fig. 18.2   Major muscles that move the hip

lateral circumflex artery, and artery of the ligamentum teres (a minor blood source in adults). The region is supplied by the femoral nerve (which supplies rectus femoris), the obturator nerve (anterior division of lumbar plexus) and the superior gluteal nerve (which supplies quadratus femoris). Dermatomes covering the region are illustrated in Figure 18.3 on p 346.

ASSESSMENT

The purpose of remedial massage assessment includes:

- determining the suitability of clients for massage (contra-indications and red flags)
- determining the duration (acute or chronic), severity and types of tissues involved in the injury/condition
- determining whether symptoms fit patterns of common conditions.

Always refer clients for further assessment and treatment if there is any doubt about their suitability for remedial massage therapy.

Serious conditions of the hip in children and adolescents should not be missed.

- Hip pain in the presence of more than a low-grade fever or in children who appear ill should be assessed for a septic joint.
- Polyarticular pain suggests juvenile rheumatoid arthritis.
- Perthes' disease (avascular necrosis of the femoral head) causes hip pain in children 3 to 12 years old.
- Slipped capital femoral epiphysis occurs most commonly in 10- to 17-year-old boys who are either tall and slim or obese.

Principles of remedial massage assessment are discussed in Chapter 2. This section presents specific considerations for assessment of the hip region.

CASE HISTORY

Subjective history, physical examination, and radiographic examination each have their own limitations and an integrative approach is needed. Studies suggest that a history provides key information in 56–90% of all cases whereas the physical exam provides 30%.[3]

Information from case histories can alert practitioners to the presence of serious conditions requiring referral. Several complaints have also been found to be useful in identifying specific hip pathologies. For example, a complaint of clicking in the hip is strongly associated with acetabular labral tear.[4] Reports of constant low back/buttock pain and ipsilateral groin pain are moderately helpful in diagnosing osteoarthritis

Table 18.2 Muscles that move the hip[2]

Muscles that move the hip	Origin	Insertion	Action
Hip flexors • Psoas major	Transverse processes and bodies of lumbar vertebrae	With iliacus into lesser trochanter of femur	Psoas major and iliacus muscles acting together flex thigh at hip joint, rotate thigh laterally and flex trunk on the hip
• Iliacus	Iliac fossa and sacrum	With psoas major into lesser trochanter of femur	
• Psoas minor	Bodies of T12 and L1 and intervening intervertebral disc	Fascia over psoas major and iliacus	Present in about half the population; when present sits on top of psoas major
• Rectus femoris (this is the only muscle of the quadriceps group that crosses the hip joint)	Anterior inferior iliac spine	Patella via quadriceps tendon and then tibial tuberosity via patellar ligament	Extends leg at knee joint; flexes thigh at hip joint
• Sartorius	Anterior inferior iliac spine	Medial surface of body of tibia	Flexes leg at knee joint; flexes, abducts and laterally rotates thigh at hip joint
Hip extensors • Gluteus maximus	Iliac crest, sacrum, coccyx and aponeurosis of sacrospinalis	Iliotibial band of fascia lata and lateral part of linea aspera under greater trochanter (gluteal tuberosity) of femur	Extends thigh at hip joint and laterally rotates thigh
Hamstrings • Biceps femoris	Long head arises from ischial tuberosity; short head arises from linea aspera of femur	Head of fibula and lateral condyle of tibia	Flexes leg at knee joint and extends thigh at hip joint
• Semitendinosus	Ischial tuberosity	Proximal part of medial surface of shaft of tibia	Flexes leg at knee joint and extends thigh at hip joint
• Semimembranosus	Ischial tuberosity	Medial condyle of tibia	Flexes leg at knee joint and extends thigh at hip joint
Hip abductors • Gluteus medius	Ilium	Greater trochanter of femur	Abducts thigh at hip joint and medially rotates thigh
• Gluteus minimus	Ilium	Greater trochanter of femur	Abducts thigh at hip joint and medially rotates thigh
• Tensor fasciae latae	Iliac crest	Tibia by way of the iliotibial tract	Flexes and abducts thigh at hip joint
Hip lateral rotators • Piriformis	Anterior sacrum	Superior border of greater trochanter of femur	Laterally rotates and abducts thigh at hip joint
• Obturator internus	Inner surface of obturator foramen, pubis and ischium	Greater trochanter of femur	Laterally rotates and abducts thigh at hip joint
• Obturator externus	Outer surface of obturator membrane	Deep depression inferior to greater trochanter (trochanteric fossa)	Laterally rotates and abducts thigh at hip joint
• Superior gemellus	Ischial spine	Greater trochanter of femur	Laterally rotates and abducts thigh at hip joint
• Inferior gemellus	Ischial tuberosity	Greater trochanter of femur	Laterally rotates and abducts thigh at hip joint
• Quadratus femoris	Ischial tuberosity	Elevation superior to mid-portion of intertrochanteric crest (quadrate tubercle) on posterior femur	Laterally rotates and stabilises hip joint

Continued

Table 18.2 Muscles that move the hip—cont'd

Muscles that move the hip	Origin	Insertion	Action
Hip adductors			
• Adductor longus	Pubic crest and pubic symphysis	Linea aspera of femur	Adducts and flexes thigh at hip joint and medially rotates thigh
• Adductor brevis	Inferior ramus of pubis	Superior half of linea aspera of femur	Adducts and flexes thigh at hip joint and medially rotates thigh
• Adductor magnus	Inferior ramus of pubis and ischium to ischial tuberosity	Linea aspera of femur	Adducts thigh at hip joint and medially rotates thigh; anterior part flexes thigh at hip joint, and posterior part extends thigh at hip joint
• Pectineus	Superior ramus of pubis	Pectineal line of femur, between lesser trochanter and linea aspera	Flexes and adducts thigh at hip joint

Fig. 18.3 Dermatomes of the hip region

Assessment of the hip region

1. Case history
2. Outcome measures, e.g. The Patient Specific Functional Scale
3. Postural analysis
4. Gait analysis
5. Functional tests
   Lumbar spine
   Active range of motion tests
   Flexion, extension, lateral flexion, rotation
   Hip joint
   Active range of motion tests
   Flexion, extension, abduction, adduction, internal rotation, external rotation
   Passive range of motion tests
   Flexion, extension, abduction, adduction, internal rotation, external rotation
   Resisted range of motion tests
   Flexion, extension, abduction, adduction, internal rotation, external rotation
   Resisted and length tests for specific muscles, including iliopsoas, rectus femoris, sartorius, gluteus maximus, hamstrings, gluteus medius, gluteus minimus, tensor fasciae latae, adductor muscles, piriformis and lateral hip rotators
   Special tests
   Patrick's/Fabere test
   Thomas test
   Trendelenburg test
   Ober's test
   Modified Ober's test
   Impingement/FADIR test
6. Palpation

of the hip. Use targeted questioning to collect the most useful and relevant information, including:

- Identifying red and yellow flags that require referral for further investigation (see Table 18.3 for red flags for acute hip pain in adults).
- Identifying the exact location of the symptoms by asking clients to point to the site of pain.
- Determining if the pain is likely to have a mechanical cause. (Is the pain associated with rest or activity, certain postures or time of day?) Obtain descriptions of the specific mechanism of the injury and the forces involved. For example, morning pain relieved with daily activity is often associated with arthritis. Enquire about the onset of symptoms, nature of the pain, disability and functional impairment, previous injuries to the area, type of work, typical postures and overuse. Ask clients to demonstrate movements and positions that aggravate or relieve the pain and to be specific with descriptions of aggravating or relieving activities.

- Determining if pain is likely to be associated with visceral function or is neurogenic, or psychosocial (yellow flags). Pain can be referred to the hip from conditions like appendicitis, urinary tract infections, gynaecological conditions and rheumatic conditions like ankylosing spondylitis.

Table 18.3 Red flags for acute hip pain in adults[5, 6]

Feature or risk factor	Condition
Symptoms and signs of infection (e.g. fever, malaise, night sweats) Risk factors for infection (e.g. underlying disease process, immunosuppression, penetrating wound)	Infection (e.g. septic arthritis, osteomyelitis)
History of trauma, fall, motor vehicle accident Sudden onset of pain	Fracture/dislocation
Past history of malignancy Age >50 years Failure to improve with treatment Unexplained weight loss Night pain Pain at multiple sites Pain at rest Pain that is out of proportion to the reported diagnosis or injury	Cancer

Clients with numbness, pins and needles and muscle weakness associated with their hip condition may have referred pain from the lumbar spine or sciatica. Refer all clients with sensory symptoms or muscle weakness for further investigation.

OUTCOME MEASURES

Outcome measures are questionnaires that are specifically designed to assess clients' level of impairment and to define benefits of treatment. The Patient Specific Functional Scale can be used to measure progress of treatment of clients with any musculoskeletal condition, including conditions of the hip.

POSTURAL ANALYSIS

Postural analysis enables observation of the whole client and facilitates identification of important features through bilateral comparison. It also facilitates detection of possible predisposing or contributing factors that may be implicated by observing the position of the thoracic and lumbar spines and pelvis. Observe and compare the lower limbs posteriorly, laterally and anteriorly, noting their symmetry. Observe any bruising, colour changes, swelling, scars and varicose veins. Observe Q-angle,[a] tibial torsion,[b] everted/inverted feet, leg length and muscle hypertonicity or atrophy.

GAIT ANALYSIS

Observe the client walking and note any disturbances in the rate and rhythm of gait. Identify the phase of gait that is altered. Gait disturbances are more evident in stance phase than swing phase, when the hip joint takes the load of the

upper body. For example, painful osteoarthritis can cause clients to reduce the duration of the weight-bearing phase. Weakness of gluteus minimus, gluteus maximus and quadriceps may be manifested as Trendelenburg gait, hip extensor gait and back knee gait respectively.

FUNCTIONAL TESTS

For any tests involving joint movements it is important to compare both sides and to take into account any underlying pathology and the age and lifestyle of the client. Findings from physical examinations should be interpreted in the light of evidence for their diagnostic accuracy. Measuring hip range of motion has consistently been shown to be highly reliable and when limited in three planes can be fairly useful in identifying hip osteoarthritis (+LR = 4.5–4.7).[4] Assessing pain during range of motion measurements can be helpful in identifying both osteoarthritis and lateral tendon pathologic conditions. Lateral hip pain during passive abduction is strongly suggestive of lateral tendon pathologic disorders (+LR = 8.3), whereas groin pain during active hip abduction or adduction is moderately suggestive of osteoarthritis (+LR = 5.7). Limited hip abduction in infants can also be very helpful in identifying hip dysplasia or instability.

Active range of motion (AROM) of the lumbar spine (flexion, extension, lateral flexion and rotation)

Examination of the hip begins with functional tests of the lumbar spine and pelvis to help rule out lumbar radiculopathy which refers pain to the hip region (see Figure 18.3 on p 346). If active range of motion tests of the lumbar spine and pelvis reproduce hip symptoms, further examination of the lumbar spine and pelvis is indicated (see Chapter 10).

Active range of motion (AROM) of the hip joint

The client stands and faces you. The client holds on to the back of a chair, the table or other support if needed. Demonstrate the movements for the client to follow and instruct the client to perform the movements as far as they can comfortably. Note that the knee should be flexed during hip flexion to minimise the influence of hamstring tightness on the range of motion. Examine the following ranges of motion:

- Flexion/extension (120°/20°)[7]
- Internal/external rotation (35–40°/35–40°)
  Instruct the client to turn their whole leg outwards and inwards.
- Abduction/adduction (40–45°/25–30°)

An alternative routine that is commonly used for assessing hip AROM involves asking clients to:

- sit down without using their arms (hip flexion)
- stand up without using their arms (hip extension)
- stand with both feet pointed inwards (hip internal rotation)
- stand with both feet pointed outwards (hip external rotation)
- stand with feet apart as far as they are comfortably able (hip abduction)
- cross one leg over the other to place the lateral border of one foot alongside the medial border of the other (hip adduction).

---

[a]The Q-angle is the angle between a line from the ASIS to the middle of the patella and a line from the middle of the patella to the tibial tubercle. In males, the Q-angle is approximately 14° and in females 17°.
[b]Tibial torsion refers to the anatomical twist of the proximal articular axis of the tibia compared to the distal articular axis.

Table 18.4 Hip joint: end-feel[8]

Normal end-feel	Flexion and adduction	Elastic or tissue approximation
	Extension and abduction	Elastic tissue stretch
	Internal/external rotation	Elastic tissue stretch
Abnormal end-feel	Bony (hard)	Osteoarthrosis
	Late myospasm	Instability
	Empty	Instability or subluxation
	Firm	Contracture or capsular tightness

This quick hip screen enables bilateral comparisons of functional movements.

Passive range of motion (PROM)

If the client is unable to perform normal active range of motion in any direction, further investigation is required. PROM testing should be performed with the client supine and prone, with one hand stabilising and palpating the hip joint while the other hand moves the lower limb. Note that PROM hip tests may be performed with the knee flexed or extended. (Note that hip flexion is usually performed with knee flexion to avoid the complication of hamstring shortness.) Palpate for crepitus, capsular pattern and end-feel (see Table 18.4). The capsular pattern of restriction for the acetabulofemoral joint is internal rotation more limited than extension; extension more limited than abduction.[8]

Resisted range of motion (RROM)

RROM tests should also be performed if AROM testing indicates the likelihood of a hip problem. RROM tests include:

- **flexion**
  iliopsoas, rectus femoris, sartorius
- **extension**
  gluteus maximus, hamstrings
- **abduction**
  gluteus medius and minimus, tensor fasciae latae
- **adduction**
  adductor magnus, gracilis, adductor longus and brevis
- **internal rotation**
  tensor fasciae latae, gluteus medius and minimus
- **external rotation**
  piriformis, quadratus lumborum, superior and inferior gemellus, obturator internus and externus

Resisted tests and length tests for specific muscles[9, 10]

If RROM tests reproduce symptoms, then further tests may be used to help identify specific muscles.

Assessment of hip muscle strength has been shown to be fairly reliable, but it appears to be less helpful in identifying lateral tendon pathologic conditions than reports of pain during resisted tests, especially of the gluteus minimus and medius muscles (+LR = 3.27).[4]

Fig. 18.4 Resisted quadriceps test

1. RECTUS FEMORIS
Resisted test

As a group the quadriceps can be tested with the client seated. Place one hand over the knee and the other over the ankle. Apply resistance at the ankle as the client tries to straighten their leg (see Figure 18.4).

As rectus femoris is the only muscle of the quadriceps group to cross the hip joint, it can be identified from the other muscles in the group by resisting hip flexion. If hip flexion were performed first and found to be painful or weak, resisting knee extension isolates rectus femoris from iliopsoas. Alternatively, if resisted knee extension were found to be painful or weak, resisting hip flexion would differentiate rectus femoris from the other quadriceps muscles.

Length test

Shortening of the quadriceps restricts knee flexion. Shortened rectus femoris can be observed as restricted knee flexion when the hip is extended or restricted hip extension when the knee is flexed (see Figure 18.5 on p 349).

2. SARTORIUS
Resisted test

The client lies supine with one foot across the knee of the other leg (figure 4 position). Place one hand on the knee and the other on the ankle. Instruct the client to hold this position while you try to straighten the leg (i.e. push knee

Fig. 18.5 Length test for quadriceps

Fig. 18.7 Resisted test for gluteus medius

Fig. 18.6 Resisted test for sartorius

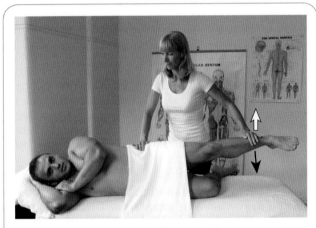

Fig. 18.8 Resisted test for gluteus minimus

into extension and adduction and the hip into extension) (see Figure 18.6).

Alternatively, the client may be seated. Kneel at the side of the client and hold the lateral aspect of their knee with one hand and the ankle with the other. Instruct the client to try to place their foot on the opposite knee as you resist the movement.

Length test

The length of sartorius is tested with other hip flexors, abductors and lateral rotators. A short sartorius muscle would limit the client's ability to sit cross-legged. A contracture of sartorius can produce flexion, abduction and lateral rotation deformity of the hip, along with flexion of the knee.

3. GLUTEUS MEDIUS

Resisted test

The client lies on their side with their lower leg flexed at the hip and knee for stability. The client's upper hip is abducted, slightly extended and externally rotated and the knee is extended. Place one hand over the client's upper hip and the other contacts the lateral side of the upper leg proximal to the ankle. The client tries to hold the position as the practitioner

applies pressure in the direction of adduction and slight flexion (see Figure 18.7).

Note that the Trendelenburg test (see Figure 18.14 on p 351) also tests gluteus medius strength.

Length test

Shortness of the hip abductors limits hip adduction. Contracture of the hip abductors may be observed as a pelvic drop on the side of tightness and abduction of the lower limb.

4. GLUTEUS MINIMUS

Resisted test

The resisted test for gluteus minimus is similar to the resisted test for gluteus medius except that the client's upper leg is abducted in the neutral position (no flexion, extension or internal or external rotation of the hip). Your pressure is applied in the direction of adduction and very slight extension (see Figure 18.8).

Length test

Shortness of gluteus minimus limits hip abduction and lateral rotation. Contracture may be observed as a pelvic drop towards the side of tightness and medial rotation of the hip joint.

Fig. 18.9　Resisted test for tensor fasciae latae

Fig. 18.10　Resisted test for hip adductors

5. TENSOR FASCIAE LATAE

Resisted test

The client lies supine and flexes and abducts their straight leg to about 45° and medially rotates the hip. Place one hand on the lateral pelvis to stabilise the hip, and place the other hand on the lateral aspect of the leg proximal to the ankle. Ask the client to move the leg outwards diagonally in the direction of abduction and flexion as you resist the movement by pushing in the direction of adduction and extension (see Figure 18.9).

Length test

Bilateral contraction of tensor fasciae latae may cause anterior pelvic tilt and occasionally genu valgus. Unilateral tightness of tensor fasciae latae and other hip abductors is associated with pelvic drop to the side of tightness. The knee on the side of tensor fasciae latae tightness tends to genu valgus.

6. HIP ADDUCTORS

Resisted test

The hip adductors (adductor magnus, gracilis, adductor longus, adductor brevis and pectineus) are tested as a group. The client lies supine, knees flexed and feet on the table. Contact the medial aspects of both knees and ask the client to bring their knees together against your resistance (see Figure 18.10).

Length test

Short hip adductors limit hip abduction (e.g. sitting cross-legged). Hip adduction contracture is associated with lateral pelvis tilt with the pelvis high on the contracted side. (The knee and hip on the opposite side may be flexed or abducted to compensate.)

7. HIP LATERAL ROTATORS

Resisted test

The lateral rotators of the hip (piriformis, quadratus femoris, obturator internus, obturator externus, gemellus superior and gemellus inferior) are tested as a group. The client sits and flexes their knees over the side of the treatment table. Place one hand on the lateral aspect of the knee; the other on the

Fig. 18.11　Resisted test for hip lateral rotators

medial aspect of the leg proximal to the ankle. The client tries to bring their foot towards the midline (i.e. externally rotate their hip) against your resistance (see Figure 18.11).

This test can also be performed with the client prone, knee flexed to 90°. The client tries to move their foot medially against your resistance.

Length test

Short lateral rotators of the hip limit internal rotation. Out-toeing gait may be observed.

Note that the medial rotators of the hip can be tested either as individual muscles (see gluteus medius, gluteus minimus, tensor fasciae latae) or as a group. As a group the medial rotators are tested similarly to the lateral rotators except that the client tries to move their foot laterally against your resistance.

Special tests

Generally, special tests of the hip have not been demonstrated to be especially helpful in identifying specific hip pathologic conditions.[4, 11] The Patrick (FABER) test (see below) is widely used but it may have little diagnostic utility. Although less reliable than strength tests, the Trendelenburg test (see below) is also moderately useful in identifying both lateral tendon pathologic conditions and gluteus medius tears (+LR = 3.2 to 3.6). As with all assessments, findings should be interpreted cautiously and in the context of other clinical findings (see Chapter 2).

PATRICK'S/FABERE TEST

The client is supine and crosses one foot over the other knee in a figure-4 position so that the hip is flexed, abducted and externally rotated. The examiner stabilises the hip on the straight leg side and applies gentle downward pressure to the knee on the opposite side. Inguinal pain has been used as an indication of hip joint pathology or strains in surrounding muscles. (FABERE refers to the testing procedure: flexion, abduction, external rotation and then passive extension.) (See Figure 18.12.)

THOMAS TEST

The client lies supine and brings one knee to their chest keeping the other leg straight. Elevation of the straight leg indicates hip contracture, tight iliopsoas or rectus femoris (see Figure 18.13).

TRENDELENBURG TEST

The patient stands on one leg and the practitioner observes the level of the pelvis. A client with normal hip abductor strength on one side will be able to maintain a level pelvis when they raise the opposite leg off the ground (see Figure 18.14).

Fig. 18.13 Thomas test

Fig. 18.12 Patrick's test

Fig. 18.14 Trendelenburg test

Fig. 18.15   Ober's test

Fig. 18.16   Modified Ober's test

OBER'S TEST

The client lies on their side with their involved leg uppermost. Hold the client's ankle and flex the knee to 90°, abduct and extend the hip; then internally rotate the hip (see Figure 18.15). Hip pain on this manoeuvre suggests hip joint pathology; trochanteric pain suggests trochanteric bursitis.

(Caution with clients with knee joint pathology.)

MODIFIED OBER'S TEST

The client lies on their side with the involved leg uppermost. Stabilise the client's pelvis with one hand on the upper ilium and adduct the involved leg behind the lower leg. Iliotibial band tightness is suggested if the client is unable to lower the leg to the table (see Figure 18.16).

IMPINGEMENT/FADIR TEST

The client lies supine with the affected hip and knee flexed to 90°. The hip is then adducted and internally rotated in this flexed position. A positive test is indicated if the client experiences a sudden, often sharp, pain in the hip.

PALPATION

Palpatory findings are interpreted with findings from other assessments and used to guide treatment plans.

In the sidelying position the greater trochanter is palpated at the widest part of the pelvis. Gluteus medius is palpable from its origin just below the iliac crest to its insertion into the upper part of the greater trochanter. Gluteus minimus is not usually palpable under the gluteus maximus. The trochanteric bursa separates the greater trochanter from the insertions of gluteus medius and minimus. It is palpable only when it becomes inflamed. From the anterior aspect of the iliac crest palpate tensor fasciae latae to its insertion into the iliotibial tract. Palpate the ischial tuberosity posteriorly. The sciatic nerve is palpable in the sidelying position with the knee flexed. It is located halfway between the greater trochanter and the ischial tuberosity.

With the client prone, trace the arc of the iliac crests to the posterior superior iliac spines (PSISs) slightly inferolateral to the back dimples (dimples of Venus). The PSISs are level with the second sacral segment. The sacroiliac joints are not palpable under the ilia. The gluteus maximus is the largest and most superficial muscle of the pelvis. It runs from the inner upper ilium, sacrum and coccyx to the iliotibial tract and gluteal tuberosity of the femur. Its upper border runs from the PSIS to slightly above the greater trochanter. Its lower border runs from the coccyx to the iliotibial tract. The piriformis is deep to gluteus maximus. It runs from the sacrum to the superior border of the greater trochanter. It can be identified when the client's knee is flexed to 90° and hip lateral rotation is resisted (i.e. the client tries to move their foot towards the midline against your resistance). The sciatic nerve exits below the pirifomis and occasionally through it. The ischial tuberosity is located midway along the gluteal fold. A bursa separates the ischial tuberosity and the overlying gluteal muscle. Palpate the insertion of the hamstrings at the ischial tuberosity. Tenderness over the ischial tuberosity could indicate bursitis or hamstring strain. Palpate the biceps femoris laterally and the semitendinosus and semimembranosus medially.

In the supine position, palpate the iliac crest, greater trochanter and the anterior superior iliac spine (ASIS). The pubic tubercle is located in the midline level with the greater trochanter. The inguinal ligament runs between the ASIS and the pubic tubercle and is not usually palpable. With the client's lower limb in the figure-4 position (i.e. hip abducted and externally rotated, knee flexed and foot placed across the other knee) and appropriately draped, palpate structures in the femoral triangle, which is bounded by the sartorius, adductor longus and inguinal crease (see Figure 18.17 on p 353). The pulse of the femoral artery is palpated halfway along and slightly below the inguinal ligament. The femoral nerve, which runs lateral to the femoral artery, and the femoral vein, which runs medial to the femoral artery, are not palpable. Inguinal lymph nodes are often palpable below and parallel to the inguinal ligament. The iliopsoas may be palpable in the floor of the femoral triangle. Adductor longus is the most superficial muscle of the adductor group. It runs from the symphysis pubis to the middle third of the linea aspera. It forms a prominent cord in the medial upper thigh. The attachment of sartorius is palpable from the ASIS. Rectus femoris arises from the anterior inferior iliac spine and lies lateral to sartorius.

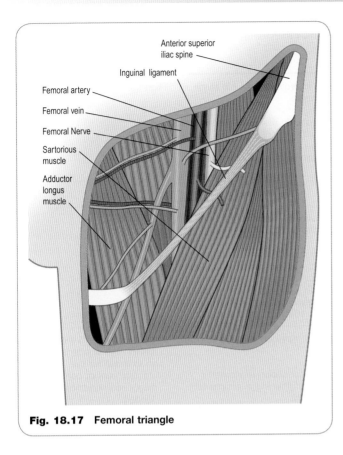

Fig. 18.17 Femoral triangle

OVERVIEW

Develop a short- and a long-term plan for each client. The short-term plan directs treatment to the highest priority (usually determined by symptoms). The long-term plan can be introduced when presenting symptoms have subsided. Long-term treatment focuses on contributing or predisposing factors such as underlying structural features and lifestyle factors. A significant part of both short-term and long-term treatment involves educating clients about likely causal or aggravating factors and an exercise program to improve or restore normal muscle function. If massage therapy is used in conjunction with other treatments, it is important to communicate with other treating practitioners and to integrate treatments where possible for the best outcomes.

MUSCLE STRAIN

Muscle strains are usually collagen tears in the connective tissue in and around a muscle.[14] Acute injuries commonly result from an eccentric contraction where external load exceeds muscle force.[15] The most common injury site is the musculotendinous junction.[16] Muscle strains frequently occur in muscles that cross two joints (e.g. hamstrings, rectus femoris and gastrocnemius).[17] The tendon in muscles like rectus femoris and biceps femoris extends for a significant distance within the muscle belly. Difficult quadriceps and hamstring injuries that require lengthy rehabilitation or that reoccur may have an injury at the musculotendinous junction and also in the intramuscular tendon itself.[18]

Repair of damaged muscle tissue leads to cross-linkages and adhesions in collagen and the muscle typically shortens and becomes less flexible. Muscle strains occur as a result of an acute traumatic injury or from overuse. They are common injuries in sport. Athletes who sprint, jump, leap or kick are most susceptible to muscle strains. Hamstring strains, the most frequently strained muscle in the lower extremity, can lead to significant disability.[17] The 2017 AFL Injury Survey reported that hamstring strains occurred at a rate of 4.9 new injuries per club per season and were the most common cause of matches missed (16.6 matches missed per club per season). Comparatively the incidence for other lower limb new muscle strains were calf 2.1, groin 1.2 (adductors 0.8 and iliopsoas 0.4) and quadriceps 1.0.[19] Although research evidence is scarce, anecdotal evidence suggests that massage therapy may assist in restoring normal function to muscle tissue.

REMEDIAL MASSAGE TREATMENT

Assessment of the hip region provides essential information for development of treatment plans, including:

- client's suitability for remedial massage therapy
- duration of the condition (i.e. acute or chronic)
- severity of the condition (i.e. grade of injury; mild, moderate or severe pain)
- type(s) of tissues involved
- priorities for treatment if more than one injury or condition are present
- whether the signs and symptoms suggest a common condition of the hip region
- special considerations for individual clients (e.g. client's preference for treatment types and styles, specific population considerations).

Treatment options must always be considered in the context of the best available evidence for treatment effectiveness and clinical practice guidelines where they exist. Little research has been conducted into the effectiveness of massage treatments for conditions of the hip. Some relevant studies are summarised in Table 18.5. Results should be interpreted in light of the variable quality of the trials.

The predominant conditions of the hip treated in remedial massage clinics are mild to moderate thigh muscle strains and osteoarthritis of the hip and occasionally impingement syndrome and trochanteric bursitis. Remedial massage treatments for these conditions are described below.

Groin (adductor and iliopsoas) strains

Groin strains are relatively common in such activities as soccer, football, water skiing, gymnastics and dancing. Strains may occur when athletes have a low adductor to abductor ratio or decreased hip range of motion.[20] Athletes who are involved in repetitive kicking, quick starts, or changes in direction have a high incidence of adductor injury. Groin injuries are frequent in soccer and a 25-player squad can expect two to four acute groin injuries each season with the adductor longus tendon being affected most frequently.[21] Acute adductor longus injuries in soccer occur in a variety of situations. Player actions can be categorised into closed-chain (change of direction and reaching) and open-chain (kicking and jumping) movements involving hip motion in three planes. A rapid muscle activation during a rapid muscle lengthening appears

Table 18.5 Evidence of the efficacy of non-pharmalogical conservative management of hip conditions[12, 13]

Condition	Conservative treatment	Quality of evidence
Hip joint (acetabularfemoral) osteoarthritis	Manual therapy is effective in improving pain, hip range of motion and physical function Specifically: • Manual therapy can relieve pain in the short term • Manual therapy combined with patient education can relieve pain in the long term • Manual therapy increases hip range of motion in the short term • Manual therapy improves physical function immediately after treatment	High quality
	Exercise therapy (ET) is effective in improving pain, hip range of motion and physical function Specifically: • Nordic walking relieves pain more than strength training (supervised or unsupervised) at 4 months of follow-up • ET was more effective combined with hot packs and ultrasound at 1- and 3-month follow-up • ET plus patient education shows better benefit than patient education at 10- and 16-month follow-up	High quality
Chronic adductor related groin pain	Clinic-based exercise programs may benefit patients with persistent groin pain Specifically: • clinic-based group exercises consisting of isometric and concentric resistance strengthening exercises for the adductors, trunk, and pelvis • balance and agility exercises for the lower extremity • stretching for the abdominals, back, and lower extremity (with the exception of the adductor muscles)	Limited high-quality evidence, further high-quality studies on exercise for the management of commonly diagnosed conditions needed
Commonly diagnosed conditions such as • hamstring sprain • strain injuries, • hamstring tendinopathy • trochanteric bursitis • capsular injuries of the hip	Clinic-based exercise programs	High-quality studies are lacking

to be the fundamental injury mechanism for acute adductor longus injuries.

Groin strains are also associated with overuse activities such as running with increased foot flare, breast stroke and gymnastics. As with any other muscle, groin strains can be graded as either mild (Grade 1), moderate (Grade 2) or severe (Grade 3). A Grade 3 strain indicates a complete rupture of the muscle tendon or an avulsion of the tendon from its attachment site on the bone and requires referral.

Hamstring strain

Hamstring strains, the most frequently strained muscle in the lower extremity, can lead to significant disability.[17] Hamstring tightness in athletes and non-athletes is associated with various musculoskeletal injuries such as lower back, hip, and knee strain and impairment. A tear can occur in any of the three hamstring muscles (biceps femoris, semitendinosus and semimembranosus), however, they occur most frequently in biceps femoris at the proximal musculotendinous junction. Strain can result from trauma or from overuse (e.g. in sprinters due to high eccentric forces[22]). Injury is common during eccentric contraction and particularly when the muscle is required to stop the leg at the end of its forward swing. Previous hamstring injury also appears to be a significant risk

factor for hamstring strain. Predictors of hamstring re-injury include the number of previous hamstring injuries, active knee extension deficit, isometric knee flexion force deficit at 15° and presence of localised discomfort on palpation just after return to play. MRI imaging findings have not been found to be a useful predictor of re-injury.[23]

There are several possible risk factors that contribute to the high incidence of hamstring strain:

- strength imbalances between the quadriceps and hamstrings
- the hamstrings cross two joints (with the exception of the short head of the biceps femoris) making it more susceptible to injury
- sciatic nerve tension may have a role in hamstring hypertonicity
- muscle fatigue
- insufficient warm-up
- age, ethnicity, flexibility.[22]

Stretching techniques

Hamstring tightness in athletes and non-athletes is associated with various musculoskeletal injuries such as lower back, hip, and knee strain and impairment.

Hold-Relax or Contract Relax with Agonist Contraction (CRAC) stretching is based on proprioceptive neuromuscular facilitation (PNF) (see Chapter 5). These techniques stimulate sensory receptors that provide information about body position and movement.[24]

A 2019 systematic review found low to moderate evidence that CRAC stretching is safe and effective in increasing hamstrings flexibility short term. Conflicting or limited evidence from low to moderate quality trials demonstrates that CRAC stretching has long-term effects and is superior to other stretching techniques.[24]

Quadriceps strain

The quadriceps are the most powerful and bulky muscles in the body and injury may result in marked functional disability. Injury often results from sudden contraction of the muscle, especially when it is stretched (e.g. sprinting, jumping or kicking). The injury may be felt as a sudden sharp pain or muscle pull in the anterior thigh during an activity requiring explosive muscle contraction.

Assessment

HISTORY

The client often complains of sudden onset of acute pain at the site of lesion (e.g. near the pubic bone in adductor strain, in the anterior thigh in quadriceps strain) and large areas of bruising may develop. Pain is often aggravated by exercise and relieved by rest. In some cases, the client reports hearing a loud pop or snap when the injury occurs. Symptoms may persist for long periods and re-injury is common.

For suspected groin strains it is important to consider a wide range of differential diagnoses before focusing solely on musculoskeletal causes of pain. Pain in the groin can be referred from such conditions as appendicitis, urinary tract infection, gynaecological pathology or rheumatoid conditions like ankylosing spondylitis, or structures may refer pain to the groin (e.g. appendix, urinary tract).[25] The upper sacroiliac joint may also refer pain to the groin.[26]

FUNCTIONAL TESTS

Lumbar AROM tests do not reproduce symptoms.

Hip tests

AROM: positive in one or more directions.
PROM: may be positive when the affected muscle is passively stretched (e.g. in quadriceps strain the client may have difficulty bringing their heel to their buttock).

Key assessment findings for muscle strain

- History of trauma or repetitive overuse
- Functional tests of the hip
  - AROM positive in one or more directions
  - PROM may be positive at the end of the range when affected muscle is stretched
  - RROM positive for affected muscle
  - Resisted and length test positive for affected muscle
  - Special tests: positive for specific muscle test (e.g. Thomas test positive, Ober's test)
- Palpation positive for tenderness/pain; ± spasm, myofibril tears/scar tissue

---

RROM: pain and/or weakness in the affected muscles.
Resisted tests and length tests: positive for affected muscles.
Special tests: may be positive (e.g. Thomas test positive for rectus femoris shortening).

PALPATION

Tenderness or pain may be elicited during palpation at the injury site. Spasm and myofibril tears may be evident. In chronic strains, fibrotic tissue may be palpable.

Key indicators of muscle strain:
- Resisted test is painful.
- Muscle stretch is painful.
- Palpation at the site of lesion is painful.

Overview of treatment and management of muscle strains

Rest, ice, compression and elevation is often recommended for acute injuries. Advise the client to avoid or reduce the responsible activity.

In the chronic phase, remedial massage techniques for muscle strains including Swedish massage to the lumbar spine and hip is followed by:

- muscle specific techniques (see Tables 10.4 on p 154 and 18.6 on p 356).
  - deep gliding frictions along the muscle fibres
  - cross-fibre frictions
  - soft tissue releasing techniques
  - deep transverse friction at the site of the lesion. Deep transverse friction is thought to stimulate collagen production and create mobile scar tissue. Apply the technique for several minutes within the client's pain threshold, alternating with other forms of tissue mobilisation including effleurage, sweeping cross-fibre frictions and stretching.
  - Trigger point therapy
  - Muscle stretching
- Myofascial release including cross-arm techniques and the leg pull (see Figure 18.18 on p 359).
- Thermotherapy may be beneficial for pain relief.

Note:

i) Treating adductor strains requires appropriate draping. Instruct the client to hold the draping in place to protect modesty.
ii) The femoral artery, vein and nerve travel through the femoral triangle. Care should be taken to avoid compressing these structures when massaging the area.

Other remedial techniques for muscle strains/tightness include:

- hip passive joint articulation (see Chapter 7)
  - hip rotation
  - hip figure-8
  - hip traction
  - hip rotation sidelying.

Address any underlying conditions or predisposing factors (e.g scoliosis, ankle pronation, pes planus).

Table 18.6 Remedial massage techniques for muscles of the hip

Muscle	Soft tissue release	Trigger point	DTF	Stretch	Corrective action[27, 28]	Home stretch
Gluteus medius and minimus	Client: Sidelying, towel draped around the upper leg, knee bent or straight as preferred. A pillow may be placed between the client's knees. Practitioner: stands behind the client, contacts the lesion/taut band in the muscle with fingers, thumbs or elbows as the client slowly abducts and adducts the upper leg.	Gluteus medius Gluteus minimus		Client supine: flex one knee and place the foot on the table near the outside of the knee of the other leg. Practitioner: stands at side facing towards the client's head. The practitioner stabilises the lateral pelvis with one hand. The other hand contacts the client's flexed knee and slowly moves the knee across the client's body keeping their foot on the table.	Sleep on the uninvolved side with a pillow between the knees. Avoid prolonged immobility.	As for the assisted stretch Alternatively, stand side on to a wall with hand on the wall for support. Place the leg closer to the wall behind the other and slowly lean the pelvis towards the wall. Hold up to 30 seconds. Repeat 3 times.

Table 18.6 Remedial massage techniques for muscles of the hip—cont'd

Muscle	Soft tissue release	Trigger point	DTF	Stretch	Corrective action[27, 28]	Home stretch
Tensor fasciae latae	Client: sidelying, towel draped around the upper leg, knee bent or straight as preferred. A pillow may be placed between the client's knees. Practitioner: stands behind the client, contacts the lesion/taut band in the muscle with fingers, thumbs or pincer grip as the client slowly abducts and adducts the upper leg. **For iliotibial band** Client: as above. Practitioner: faces cephalad. Using a double thumb contact, interphalangeal joints or knuckles, perform a slow deep glide as the muscle lengthens. In another variation the practitioner performs cross-fibre frictions as the thigh is abducted and adducted. 			Client: sidelying, back close to the edge of the table, holding the side of the table in front. Practitioner: stands behind the client and gently lowers the top leg over the side of the table. (This stretch can also be performed supine, adducting one leg over the other.) The client tries to abduct their leg against the practitioner's resistance for 6–8 seconds, then relaxes and allows the leg to drop into adduction again. This whole procedure is repeated three times.	Avoid sitting cross-legged or prolonged hip flexion. Place a pillow between the thighs when sleeping. Adequate warm-up before running. Running technique assessment.	Stand side on to a wall with hand on the wall for support. Place the leg closer to the wall behind the other and slowly lean the pelvis towards the wall. Hold up to 30 seconds. Repeat 3 times.

Continued

Table 18.6 Remedial massage techniques for muscles of the hip—cont'd

Muscle	Soft tissue release	Trigger point	DTF	Stretch	Corrective action[27, 28]	Home stretch
Adductor group	Client: supine, knee flexed, hip slightly abducted (appropriate draping). Practitioner: stands ipsilaterally, facing towards the client's head. The practitioner performs a deep glide over a short range from the proximal knee as the client slowly abducts the thigh to their comfortable limit.			Client: supine. Practitioner: stands to the side of the table, stabilises the pelvis with one hand and abducts the leg as far as possible within the client's comfort. The client tries to adduct the leg against the practitioner's resistance for 6–8 seconds. Next the client relaxes and the practitioner tries to adduct the leg again to its comfortable limit. Repeat the process three times. Alternatively, the same procedure can be performed with the client's hip and knee flexed and the client's foot placed on the table level with the knee of the other leg.	Avoid immobility that places the adductor muscles in a shortened position for long periods. Avoid overuse at the gym. Review skiing, cycling technique.	Sit on the floor with the soles of the feet together. Gently push the knees towards the floor. Hold for 30 seconds and repeat three times.

(Resisted and length tests for iliopsoas, piriformis, gluteus maximus and the hamstring muscles are described in Chapter 10.)

Fig. 18.18 Leg pull

CLIENT EDUCATION

Advise clients of the importance of a rehabilitation program which should be commenced as soon as possible and continued until optimal function has been restored. There are no agreed criteria for return to play. Some commonly used criteria include pain resolution, normal strength, subjective feeling of full recovery reported by the player and normal flexibility, although these are not a safeguard and do not maximise performance. There is little consensus on how to assess return to play.[29] Clients may also be referred for manipulation of the low back and pelvis, hip, knee, ankle and foot. Refer any client whose condition worsens or fails to improve within 2 weeks, or shows only slight improvement within 4 weeks.

Home exercise program

A program of progressive rehabilitation should accompany remedial massage treatment. Aim for maximum strength and full length of all major muscles while maintaining general fitness levels. Unresolved strains lead to faulty biomechanics and ultimately to other conditions such as shin splints and plantar fasciitis.

Introduce stretching exercises within 1–2 weeks after injury (depending on severity and pain tolerance). Introduce low-resistance high-repetition exercises as soon as pain permits, including both concentric and eccentric exercises. Progress to functional training and sports-specific skills before returning to sport.

Quadriceps contusion

A quadriceps contusion (charley horse or cork thigh) is a common injury resulting from a direct blow to the anterior thigh. The area becomes swollen and tender. Pain worsens when the muscle is actively contracted or passively stretched.

TREATMENT

The first 24 hours is most important in controlling the haemorrhage. Ice, compression and elevation are usually recommended. As with all acute injuries, massage therapy is contraindicated in the first 24 hours but may be useful in restoring range of motion and functional rehabilitation in the subacute phase.

OSTEOARTHRITIS

Osteoarthritis is a common condition affecting the acetabulofemoral (hip) hip joint. It is a condition affecting the whole joint with a complex pathomechanism involving interaction between multiple joint tissues including articular cartilage, subchondral bone, synovial membrane and menisci. It has genetic, biological and biomechanical components. Chronic, low-grade inflammation contributes to symptoms and disease progression and a number of mediators that regulate the process have been identified.[30, 31] According to the ACR American College of Rheumatology criteria, diagnosis of osteoarthritis is confirmed if imaging findings (i.e. osteophytes and detectable joint space narrowing) are concurrently present together with one of the following: age over 50 years, joint stiffness, or crepitus.[31] The maximum BMI over one's lifespan is also a factor in hip osteoarthritis and the knee joint appears to be even more sensitive to obesity as both current and maximal lifetime BMI are a predictor of knee osteoarthritis.[32] Faster progression of the condition may be more likely in patients with a co-morbidity, a family history of osteoarthritis, a high level of baseline pain, a low self-reported global assessment, and imaging findings indicating atypical shape and advancing osteoarthritis.[33] The chief complaint in hip osteoarthritis is chronic pain which is worse after weight-bearing and better with rest. The pain can be felt in the groin, thigh or knee. The pain may be variable with different ranges of motion. Passive internal rotation is usually the most limited movement (capsular pattern of the hip).

Assessment

HISTORY

The client complains of chronic pain in the groin, thigh and knee and stiffness that is aggravated by use and relieved by rest. The client is usually over 50 years or has a history of significant previous injury or overuse. Pain, stiffness and limited range of motion are common complaints and the client may walk with a limp. A report of posterior pain with a squat is fairly useful in identifying hip osteoarthritis (+LR = 6.1).[4]

FUNCTIONAL TESTS

Lumbar AROM tests do not reproduce hip symptoms.

Hip tests

AROM positive (limited internal rotation, extension and abduction).
PROM positive (limited internal rotation, extension and abduction), crepitus often present, hard (bony) end-feel.
RROM negative (unless osteoarthritis is accompanied by muscle contractures and weaknesses).
Special tests: Patrick's FABERE test positive.

Key assessment findings for osteoarthritis of the acetabulofemoral joint

- History of chronic hip pain and limitation aggravated by use; deep gnawing pain; stiffness after rest; usually over 50 years old
- Functional tests of the hip:
  - AROM limited ± painful in some directions
  - PROM limited ± painful (capsular pattern); crepitus; hard end-feel
  - RROM usually negative unless associated muscle strain
  - Special tests: Patrick's FABERE test positive
- Palpation may elicit deep pain in the groin, anterior or posterior thigh or referred to the medial thigh and knee

---

PALPATION

Palpation may elicit deep pain in the groin, posterior or anterior thigh, or pain referred to the thigh and knee.

Treatment of osteoarthritis of the acetabulofemoral joint

Although osteoarthritis is a chronic condition, acute episodes can occur from time to time, usually after overuse. If acute inflammation is present, treatment could include cryotherapy for analgesia, acupressure, Reiki, reflexology or anti-inflammatory medication. The client should be advised to modify activities to avoid aggravating the condition.

A typical remedial massage treatment for mild or moderate subacute or chronic osteoarthritis includes:

- Swedish massage therapy to the low back, pelvis and lower limb.
- Remedial massage therapy, which includes heat therapy, myofascial releasing techniques and joint articulation (see Chapter 7) including:
  - hip rotation
  - hip figure-8
  - hip traction
  - hip rotation sidelying.
- Remedial massage techniques (e.g. deep gliding, cross-fibre frictions, soft tissue release and muscle stretching) for associated muscle contractures.

CLIENT EDUCATION

The client should be advised to continue to use heat or ice therapy for pain relief and to modify or avoid all aggravating activities priorities for ongoing management of osteoarthritis are weight loss (if required), physical exercise and self-management of acute episodes.[34] Range of motion exercises should be commenced as soon as possible within the client's pain tolerance. Stretching and strengthening exercises can be introduced as indicated by assessment findings. Non-weight-bearing activities such as water aerobics are often beneficial. Use of shock-absorbing soles and weight loss are recommended. Nordic walking has proven to be effective in reducing pain in the short and medium term.[13] The Royal Australian College of General Practitioners strongly recommend land-based exercise for all people with hip osteoarthritis, although the type of exercise that is most beneficial has not been determined. An individualised program that suits the client's preference, capability and the availability of local facilities is recommended.[35]

Injury prevention strategies currently include improving lighting, installing handrails, not hurrying while walking, using a mobility device and exercise training such as muscle strengthening and Tai Chi to improve balance.[36] In addition advice regarding safe landing strategies have a significant effect on reducing the impact of falls. For example, martial arts fall techniques, characterised by rolling movements of the trunk, have been observed to efficiently protect the hips in sideways falls. The most widely used supplements (e.g. glucosamine, chondroitin and vitamin D) do not appear to provide a clinically important effect on knee, hip or hand osteoarthritis.[37] However, less well-known supplements like Boswellia serrata extract, pycnogenol and curcumin appear to have beneficial effects in the short term, although the quality of the current evidence is low. Clients may be referred for other supportive therapies including specialist nutritional advice, acupuncture and osseous mobilisation and manipulation of the pelvis and spine. Medical treatment may include medication such as non-steroidal anti-inflammatory drugs although these are linked to significant morbidity and mortality in this population. Other pain medications cause nausea, constipation and drowsiness.[38] Hip intra-articular steroid injections may help to reduce osteoarthritis hip pain in the short term although the quality of the evidence is currently poor. For the population of elderly high risk fallers, hip protectors may help reduce hip fractures. Hip protectors are soft or hard shell pads embedded in specialised outer or under garments. They reduce peak impact force to the hip by up to 40% during simulated sideways falls from standing.[39]

FEMOROACETABULAR IMPINGEMENT/ HIP IMPINGEMENT

In recent years, femoroacetabular impingement has been increasingly recognised as an important contributor to hip pain in the adult population and a precursor to labral tears and hip osteoarthritis later in life.[40] Femoroacetabular impingement is a collection of bony morphologic abnormalities of the hip joint that result in abnormal contact during motion. Cam-type femoroacetabular impingement relates to a non-spherical osseous prominence of the proximal femoral neck or head–neck junction. Pincer-type femoroacetabular impingement relates to excessive acetabular coverage over the femoral head, which can occur as a result of several morphologic variants.[40]

Clients with femoroacetabular impingement present with chronic, deep, or aching anterior groin pain most commonly in the sitting position, or during or after activity. Clients might also experience occasional sharp pains during activity.[41] A thorough history should be taken that includes incidence of trauma and exercise frequency. A physical examination should be performed that includes a full hip, low back and abdominal examination to assess for other causes of anterior groin pain. Diagnosis of femoroacetabular impingement should be confirmed with radiography.

Femoroacetabular impingement can be managed conservatively with rest, modification of activities, medications, and physical therapy. Some cases require surgical correction. Osteoarthritis and total hip arthroplasty might be avoided with early recognition and intervention.

Assessment

HISTORY

The client is usually a physically active young adult who complains of deep aching pain in the anterior groin area that is aggravated by sitting and during or after activity. Symptoms can follow an injury or can emerge insidiously after prolonged exercise. History taking should include incidence of trauma and exercise frequency. Occasionally pain is also felt on the side of the hip or in the buttock. When asked to point to the site of pain, clients often use their thumb and index finger to grip either side of the affected hip just above the greater trochanter (the C sign).

FUNCTIONAL TESTS

Lumbar AROM negative.

Key assessment findings for femoroacetabular impingement

- Pain and tenderness anterior groin; pain worse on sitting or during or after exercise; often a young physically active adult
- Functional tests:
  - AROM positive (flexion, adduction, internal rotation)
  - PROM positive (flexion, adduction, internal rotation)
  - RROM may be positive for associated muscles
  - Tests for specific muscles: positive for affected muscles
  - Special tests: Impingement/FADIR test positive
- Palpation positive for pain and tenderness over anterior and lateral hip.

Hip tests

AROM: positive (flexion, adduction and internal rotation).
PROM: positive (flexion, adduction and internal rotation).
RROM: may be positive for associated muscle strains.
Resisted tests and length tests may be positive for affected muscles.
Special tests: Hip impingement test/FADIR test (flexion, adduction, internal rotation) positive.

PALPATION

Tenderness may be elicited during palpation of the hip joint and associated muscles (e.g. iliopsoas, adductors, lateral hip muscles, gluteals).

Overview of treatment and management

The goals of treatment include relieving pain, improving the range of motion of the hip and advising the client of self-management strategies (e.g. avoiding aggravating activities). An individualised program of stretching tight hip muscles and ligaments and passive joint articulation within pain tolerance may be beneficial. An appropriately modified exercise program is required to prevent progression to osteoarthritis later in life.

A typical remedial massage treatment for chronic femoroacetabular impingement includes:

- Swedish massage therapy to the low back, pelvis and lower limb.
- Remedial massage techniques, including heat therapy, myofascial releasing techniques and joint articulation (see Chapter 7):
  - hip rotation
  - hip figure-8
  - hip traction
  - hip rotation sidelying.
- Remedial massage techniques (e.g. deep gliding, cross fibre frictions, soft tissue release, trigger point therapy and muscle stretching) for associated muscle and ligament contractures. Sidelying position with the affected side uppermost may provide good access.

Correct any underlying or predisposing conditions (e.g. leg length discrepancy) where possible.

CLIENT EDUCATION

Advise the client to avoid all aggravating activities. A rehabilitation exercise program should be started as soon as tolerated by the client. The goal of the program is to restore optimal hip function. This usually involves both stretching and strengthening as indicated. Refer for spinal and hip manipulation.

TROCHANTERIC BURSITIS

The trochanteric bursa lies directly over the greater trochanter and has the role of reducing friction between overlying structures (e.g. iliotibial band, gluteus medius and minimus attachments). The bursa may become inflamed from a direct blow or, more commonly, from chronic compression and friction from the ilitotibial band as it rubs over the greater trochanter during flexion and extension of the hip. Consequently trochanteric bursitis is aggravated by climbing stairs and getting into and out of a car. The condition is often secondary to biomechanical imbalance such as muscle hypertonicity (e.g. tight gluteus maximus or hip abductor muscles) or from overuse injury (e.g. running on a sloped surface). It is more common in the middle to older age groups and more common in women than men.

Assessment

HISTORY

The client complains of aching pain in the region of the greater trochanter, aggravated by direct pressure and by lying on that side in bed or performing activities such as running or climbing stairs. Pain may also refer to the groin or lateral thigh. Note that tendinopathy and myofascial trigger points of the gluteus medius and minimus are often mistaken for trochanteric bursitis. (Caution: rule out other sources of lateral hip pain such as femoral neck stress fracture or hip arthritis.)

FUNCTIONAL TESTS

Lumbar AROM negative.

Hip tests

AROM: positive (flexion and extension).
PROM: positive (flexion and extension).
RROM: may be positive for associated muscle strains (e.g. gluteal and abductor muscles).
Resisted tests and length tests may be positive for affected muscles.
Special tests: negative.

Key assessment findings for trochanteric bursitis syndrome

- Pain and tenderness posterolateral to the greater trochanter: history of repetitive overuse (e.g. running on sloped surfaces), tight iliotibial band, or trauma: the client is usually a middle-aged female
- Functional tests:
  - AROM positive (flexion and extension)
  - PROM positive (flexion and extension)
  - RROM may be positive for associated muscles (e.g. gluteal and hip abductor muscles)
  - Tests for specific muscles: positive for affected muscles
  - Special tests: negative
- Palpation positive for pain and tenderness posterolateral to greater trochanter. Inflamed bursa may palpate as boggy.

PALPATION

Tenderness may be elicited during palpation posterolateral to the greater trochanter. Inflamed bursa may palpate as boggy.

Overview of treatment and management

The aim of treatment is to reduce inflammation in the bursa with rest and ice. Avoid all aggravating activities such as climbing stairs and running on hills, slopes or uneven surfaces. Stretching the gluteal muscles and iliotibial band may be recommended, provided they do not aggravate symptoms.

An indirect approach is required as direct massage will aggravate an inflamed bursa. A typical remedial massage treatment for subacute or chronic trochanteric bursitis includes:

- Swedish massage therapy to the low back, pelvis and lower limb.
- Remedial massage techniques, which are directed to tensor fasciae latae, iliotibial band, gluteus maximus, gluteus minimus and gluteus medius. Sidelying position with the affected side uppermost may provide better access. Muscle-specific techniques include (see Tables 10.4 and 18.6):
  - deep gliding frictions along the muscle fibres
  - cross-fibre frictions
  - soft tissue releasing techniques
    For example: **Soft tissue release for tensor fasciae latae** The client lies on their side close to the edge of the table so that the top leg can be lowered below the level of the table. The client's lower leg is slightly flexed and the client holds on to the side of the table in front of them. Instruct the client to actively abduct the top leg. Apply static pressure to the tensor fasciae latae with thumbs, fingers, knuckles or elbows and instruct the client to actively and slowly lower and raise the leg a number of times while your pressure is maintained (Figure 18.19).
  - trigger point therapy
  - muscle stretching.
- Myofascial release of the iliotibial band may be beneficial.
- Other remedial techniques including joint articulation may be beneficial (see Chapter 7):
  - hip rotation
  - hip figure-8
  - hip traction
  - hip rotation sidelying.

Fig. 18.19 Soft tissue release for tensor fasciae latae

Correct any underlying or predisposing conditions (e.g. leg length discrepancy) where possible.

CLIENT EDUCATION

Advise the client to avoid all aggravating activities such as climbing stairs or running on uneven surfaces. A rehabilitation exercise program should be started as soon as tolerated by the client. The goal of the program is to restore normal muscle balance to the muscles around the hip joint. This usually involves stretching the tensor fasciae latae/iliotibial band and gluteal muscles. Demonstrate the use of a Pilates-style foam roller to self-massage the lateral upper leg and lateral hip. This may be initially painful although it may help to relieve tension in the ITB and TFL, areas which may be challenging to stretch. Refer for spinal and hip manipulation.

KEY MESSAGES

- Assessment of clients with conditions of the hip region involves case history, outcome measures, postural analysis, gait analysis, functional tests and palpation.
- Assessment findings may indicate the type of tissue involved (contractile or inert, muscle, joint, fascia, ligament), duration of condition (acute or chronic) and severity (grade).
- Assessment findings may indicate a common presenting condition such as muscle strain, osteoarthritis, impingement syndrome or trochanteric bursitis.
- Assessment findings also indicate client perception of injury and preferences for treatment.
- Consider Clinical Guidelines, available evidence and client preferences when planning therapy.
- Although serious conditions of the hip region are rare, all clients with symptoms of neurological or vascular impairment in the lower limb should be referred for further assessment.
- The selection of remedial massage techniques depends on assessment results. Swedish massage to the hip, lower back, pelvis and lower limb may be followed by muscle techniques (e.g. deep gliding, cross-fibre frictions, soft tissue releasing techniques, trigger point therapy and deep transverse friction), passive joint articulation, myofascial release and thermotherapy as indicated.
- Educating clients about likely causal and predisposing factors and exercise rehabilitation are essential parts of remedial massage therapy.
- Prioritise the client self-help component of treatment wherever possible to reduce likelihood of recurrence and/or to promote health maintenance and injury prevention.

Review questions

1. An overweight 14-year-old boy limps into your clinic complaining of vague knee pain. He must be examined to eliminate the possibility of:
   a) Osteoarthritis of the knee
   b) Perthes disease
   c) Femoral capital slipped epiphysis
   d) Paget's disease

2. A client's pain is reproduced on resisted hip flexion. A likely assessment is:
   a) Quadriceps muscle strain
   b) Osteoarthritis of the hip joint
   c) Perthes disease
   d) Hamstring muscle strain

3. The following diagram represents a stretch for:
   a) biceps femoris
   b) vastus lateralis
   c) rectus femoris
   d) vastus intermedialis

4. The age group usually affected by Perthes disease of the hip joint is:
   a) 0 – 5 years
   b) 5 – 10 years
   c) 10 – 15 years
   d) 15 – 20 years

5. The most limited movement (i.e. the capsular pattern) of an osteoarthritic hip is usually:
   a) Extension
   b) Abduction
   c) Internal rotation
   d) External rotation

6. i) Name all the muscles that attach to the greater trochanter.
   ii) What is trochanteric bursitis?
   iii) Describe the mechanism(s) which contribute to the development of trochanteric bursitis

7. What anatomic features of the hip joint contribute to its stability?

8. Resisted hip extension produces pain. What resisted test(s) would help determine the specific muscle or muscles which are causing the pain?

9. A client presents with pain in the lateral hip region. How will you determine if the client's pain is likely to be related to a lumbar problem or an acetabulofemoral joint problem?

10. Name a muscle that could be implicated if the following special tests are painful:
    i. Trendelenburg test
    ii. Ober's test
    iii. Patrick's test

11. Briefly outline the main features of a remedial massage treatment for osteoarthritis of the hip.

12. A client has a mild strain of the rectus femoris. List five remedial massage techniques that would be suitable for their treatment.

REFERENCES

1. Hendrickson T. Massage for orthopedic conditions. 2nd edn. Philadelphia, PA: Lippincott Williams and Wilkins; 2010.

2. Tortora G, Derrickson B. Principles of anatomy and physiology. 15th edn. Milton, Qld: John Wiley; 2016.

3. Reiman MP, Thorborg K. Clinical examination and physical assessment of hip joint-related pain in athletes. Int J Sports Phys Ther 2014;9(6): 737–55.

4. Cleland J, Koppenhaver S, Su J. Netter's orthopaedic clinical examination: an evidence-based approach. 3rd edn. Philadelphia: Saunders; 2015.

5. Margo K, Drezner J, Motzkin D. Evaluation and management of hip pain: an algorithmic approach. J Fam Pract 2003;52(8):607–17.

6. Van Wye W. Patient screening by a physical therapist for non-musculoskeletal hip pain. Phys Ther 2009; 89(3):248–56.

7. Reese N, Bandy W. Joint range of motion and muscle length testing. 3rd edn. St Louis, MO: Saunders; 2016.

8. Vizniak N. Evidence informed orthopedic conditions. 3rd edn. Burnaby, BC: Professional Health Systems; 2019. https://prohealthsys.com/.

9. Kendall McCreary E, Provance P, McIntyre Rodgers M, et al. Muscles, testing and function, with posture and pain. 5th edn. Philadelphia: Lippincott Williams and Wilkins; 2005.

10. Avers D, Brown M. Daniels and Worthingham's muscle testing: techniques of manual examination and performance testing. 10th edn. Oxford: Saunders; 2018.

11. Rahman LA, Adie S, Naylor JM, et al. A systematic review of the diagnostic performance of orthopedic physical examination tests of the hip. BMC Musculoskel Dis 2013;14(1):257.

12. Brown CK, Southerst D, Côté O, et al. The effectiveness of exercise on recovery and clinical outcomes in patients with soft tissue injuries of the hip, thigh, or knee: a systematic review by the Ontario Protocol for Traffic Injury Management (OPTIMa) Collaboration. J Manipulative Physiol Ther 2016;39(2):110–20.e1.

13. Ceballos-Laita L, Estébanez-de-Miguel E, Martín-Nieto G, et al. Effects of non-pharmacological conservative treatment on pain, range of motion and physical function in patients with mild to moderate hip osteoarthritis. a systematic review. Complement Ther Med 2019; 42:214–22.

14. Takaza M, Cooney GM, McManus G, et al. Assessing the microstructural response to applied deformation in porcine passive skeletal muscle. J Mech Behav of Biomed 2014;40(C): 115–26.

15. Kelly B, Maak T, M Larson C, et al. Sports hip injuries: assessment and management. AAOS Instr Cours Lec 2013;62:515–31.

16. Resnick P, Jurch S, Ribeiro C. Sports massage: Injury recovery: Get in-depth knowledge on common sports injuries, the healing process and the role massage therapy can play in keeping athletes healthy. Massage Ther J 2017;56(3):46.

17. Sarwark J, LaBella C. Pediatric orthopaedics and sport injuries: a quick reference guide. American Academy of Pediatrics. Online. Available: http://ebookcentral.proquest.com/lib/uwsau/detail.action?docID=1988088; 2014.

18. Brukner P, Connell D. Serious thigh muscle strains: beware the intramuscular tendon which plays an important role in difficult hamstring and quadriceps muscle strains. Br J Sports Med 2015;50(4):205–8.

19. AFL Doctors Association, AFL Physiotherapists Association and AFL Football Operations Department. 2017 AFL Injury Survey. Online. Available: http://www.afl.com.au/staticfile/AFL%20Tenant/2017AFLInjuryReport.pdf; 2017.

20. Kelly B, Bedi A. Sports hip injuries: diagnosis and management. Thorofare, NJ: Slack Inc; 2015.

21. Serner A, Mosler A, Tol J, et al. Mechanisms of acute adductor longus injuries in male football players: a systematic visual video analysis. Br J Sports Med 2019;53:158–64.

22. Opar DA, Williams MD, Shield AJ. Hamstring strain injuries: factors that lead to injury and re-injury. Sports Med (NZ) 2012;42(3):209–26. Doi: http://dx.doi.org.ezproxy.uws.edu.au/10.2165/11594800-000000000-00000.

23. De Vos R, Reurink G, Goudswaard G, et al. Clinical findings just after return to play predict hamstring re-injury, but baseline MRI findings do not. Br J Sports Med 2014;48(18):1377–84. Doi: http://dx.doi.org.ezproxy.uws.edu.au/10.1136/bjsports-2014-093737.

24. Cayco CS, Labro AV, Gorgon EJ. Hold-relax and contract relax stretching for hamstrings flexibility: a systematic review with meta-analysis. Phys Ther Sports 2019;35:42–55.

25. Cohn RM, Lerebours F, Strauss EJ. Sports hernia and extra-articular causes of groin pain in the athlete. Bulletin NYU Hospital Joint Diseases 2015;73(2):90–9. Retrieved from https://search-proquest-com.ezproxy.uws.edu.au/docview/1690743022?accountid=36155.

26. Kurosawa D, Murakami E, Aizawa T. Referred pain location depends on the affected section of the sacroiliac joint. Eur Spine J 2015;24(3):521–7.

27. Simons D, Travell J, Simons L. Myofascial pain and dysfunction: the trigger point manual. Volume 1 Upper half of body. 2nd edn. Philadelphia: Williams & Wilkins; 1999.

28. Niel-Asher S. Concise book of trigger points. 3rd edn. Berkeley, CA: North Atlantic; 2014.

29. Valle X, Tol JT, Hamilton B, et al. Hamstring muscle injuries, a rehabilitation protocol purpose. Asian J Sports Med 2015;6(4):e2541. Doi: 10.5812/asjsm.25411.

30. Iolascon G, Gimigliano F, Moretti A, et al. Early osteoarthritis: how to define, diagnose, and manage: a systematic review. Eur Geriatr Med 2017;8(5-6): 383–96.

31. Mobasheri A, Batt M. An update on the pathophysiology of osteoarthritis. Ann Phys Rehabil Med 2016;59:333–9.

32. Singer S, Dammerer P, Krismer D, et al. Maximum lifetime body mass index is the appropriate predictor of knee and hip osteoarthritis. Arch Orthop Trauma Surg 2018;139:99–103.

33. Teirlinck C, Dorleijn D, Bos K, et al. Factors predicting progression of hip osteoarthritis: a systematic review. Osteoarthr Cartilage 2017;25: S203–204.

34. Hunter DJ. Everything you ever wanted to know about osteoarthritis. The Health Report 2017. Online. Available: https://www.abc.net.au/radionational/programs/healthreport/everything-you-ever-wanted-to-know-about-osteoarthritis/8664218#transcript; 2017.

35. Royal Australian College of General Practitioners. Guideline for the management of knee and hip osteoarthritis. 2nd edn. Online. Available: http://www.acsep.org.au/content/Document/guideline-for-the-management-of-knee-and-hip-oa-2nd-edition.pdf; 2018.

36. Moon Y, Sosnoff JJ. Safe landing strategies during a fall: a systematic review and meta-analysis. Arch Phys Med Rehabil 2017;98:783–94.

37. Liu X, Machado GC, Eylesl JP, et al. Dietary supplements for treating osteoarthritis: a systematic review and meta-analysis. Br J Sports Med 2018;52: 167–75.

38. McCabe PS, Maricar N, Parkes MJ, et al. The efficacy of intra-articular steroids in hip osteoarthritis: a systematic review. Osteoarthr Cartilage 2016;24(9):1509–17.

39. Korall AM, Feldman F, Scott VJ, et al. Facilitators of and barriers to hip protector acceptance and adherence in long-term care facilities: a systematic review. J Am Med Dir Assoc 2015;16(3):85–93.

40. Wright AA, Naze GS, Kavchak AE, et al. Radiological variables associated with progression of femoroacetabular impingement of the hip: a systematic review. J Sci Med Sport 2015;18: 122–7.

41. Zhang C, Li L, Forster BB, et al. Femoroacetabular impingement and osteoarthritis of the hip. Can Fam Physician 2015;61(12):1055–60.

The knee

19

Learning Outcomes

- Assess clients with conditions of the knee for remedial massage, including identification of red and yellow flags.
- Assess clients for signs and symptoms associated with common conditions of the knee (including muscle strains, iliotibial band syndrome, patellofemoral pain syndrome, ligament sprains, osteoarthritis and Osgood-Schlatter's disease), and treat and/or manage these conditions with remedial massage therapy.
- Develop treatment plans for clients with conditions of the knee, taking into account assessment findings, duration and severity of the condition, likely tissue types, clinical guidelines, the best available evidence and client preferences.
- Develop short- and long-term treatment plans to address presenting symptoms, underlying conditions and predisposing factors, and to progressively increase the self-help component of therapy.
- Adapt remedial massage therapy to suit individual client's needs based on duration and severity of injury, the client's age and gender, the presence of underlying condition and co-morbidities and other consideration for specific population groups.

INTRODUCTION

Knee pain is commonly reported by older clients. A survey in Malaysia found that approximately 1 in 5 people had experienced knee pain during the previous 6 months.[1] Three main mechanisms are responsible for knee injury: (1) overuse injuries, often associated with co-existing predisposing factors like genu valgus, or varus; (2) twisting or explosive movements as occur in sports like basketball and soccer; and (3) direct blows to the knee joint. The knee joint is also subject to arthritic changes associated with overuse, sporting injuries, obesity and ageing.

Fifteen per cent of middle-aged or elderly individuals have knee symptoms associated with osteoarthritis.[2] The knee joint is particularly sensitive to obesity. Current BMI and maximal lifetime BMI are predictors of knee osteoarthritis.[3] Knee surgery has been increasing at a concerning rate in Australia for some time. There has also been a 36% rise in the rate of

total knee replacements for osteoarthritis for the decade from 2005–06 to 2015–16.[4] The incidence of anterior cruciate ligament reconstructions in Australia is the highest in the world, and is increasing. Reconstructions have increased on average over 5% annually in Australia for a decade and a half, equating to a 43% rise from 2000–2015.[5]

FUNCTIONAL ANATOMY

The knee complex consists of:

- knee joint between the lateral and medial condyles of the distal femur and the lateral and medial condyles of the proximal end of the tibia
- patella, a sesamoid bone within the quadriceps tendon, which protects the tendon as it moves across the knee joint and acts as a pully to increase mechanical leverage
- tibial tuberosity, the insertion of the patella ligament
- fibula head which articulates with the lateral tibial condyle.

The knee joint is a modified hinge joint. Its main function is to maintain upright stance with as little energy expenditure as possible. This is achieved by the locking mechanism of the knee and its supporting ligaments. When the femur medially rotates on the tibia during the final stages of extension, the articulating surfaces are in the position of greatest contact and the supporting ligaments are taut. This is also referred to as the close-packed position of the knee. The knee is tight and stable and minimal muscle contraction is required to maintain upright stance (see Figure 19.1 on p 366).

The knee joint capsule (capsular ligament) encloses the patella, ligaments, menisci and bursae. It consists of a synovial and fibrous membrane separated by fat pads. The joint capsule is strengthened by a number of ligaments:

Extra-capsular ligaments

- Patella tendon (ligament), separated from the synovial membrane by an infrapatella fat pad and patella retinaculum (extensions of the aponeuroses of vastus medialis and lateralis).
- Oblique popliteal ligament (under the tendon of semimembranosus), from the medial condyle of tibia to the lateral condyle of femur.
- Arcuate popliteal ligament from the lateral condyle of the femur to the head of the fibula.

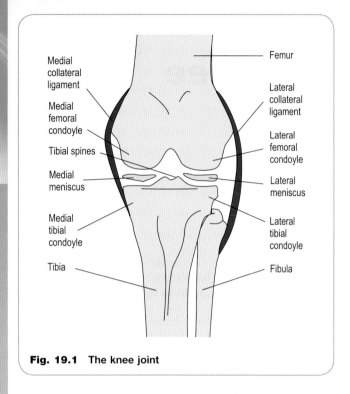

Fig. 19.1 The knee joint

Labels:
- Medial collateral ligament
- Medial femoral condoyle
- Tibial spines
- Medial meniscus
- Medial tibial condoyle
- Tibia
- Femur
- Lateral collateral ligament
- Lateral femoral condoyle
- Lateral meniscus
- Lateral tibial condoyle
- Fibula

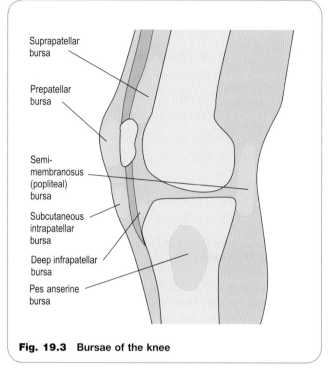

Fig. 19.3 Bursae of the knee

Labels:
- Suprapatellar bursa
- Prepatellar bursa
- Semi-membranosus (popliteal) bursa
- Subcutaneous intrapatellar bursa
- Deep infrapatellar bursa
- Pes anserine bursa

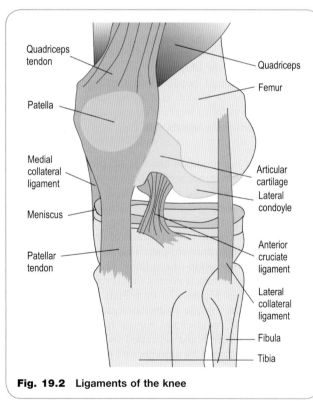

Fig. 19.2 Ligaments of the knee

Labels:
- Quadriceps tendon
- Patella
- Medial collateral ligament
- Meniscus
- Patellar tendon
- Quadriceps
- Femur
- Articular cartilage
- Lateral condyle
- Anterior cruciate ligament
- Lateral collateral ligament
- Fibula
- Tibia

Intra-capsular ligaments

- Anterior cruciate which runs from the anterior intercondylar area of the tibia to the medial surface of the lateral femoral condyle. It prevents anterior movement of the tibia on the femur or posterior movement of the femur on the tibia.
- Posterior cruciate which runs from the posterior intercondylar area of the tibia to the lateral surface of the medial femoral condyle. It prevents anterior movement of the femur on the tibia and posterior movement of the tibia on the femur. (Note: the anterior and posterior ligaments are named by their tibial attachments.)
- Coronary ligaments are extensions of fibrous capsule that attach the menisci to the tibia.
- Transverse ligament which runs between the anterior horns of the two menisci.

Two fibrocartilaginous discs cover the surface of tibial condyles. They improve the conformity of the articulating surfaces and cushion the joint.

- Lateral meniscus is oval-shaped and thicker and shorter than the medial meniscus. It is more mobile.
- Medial meniscus is C-shaped, thinner and larger. It is less mobile because of its attachment to the medial collateral ligament.

Bursa of the knee include (see Figure 19.3):

- Prepatellar bursa which overlies the patella below the skin.
- Deep infrapatellar bursa between superior part of tibia and patellar ligament.
- Suprapatellar bursa between inferior part of femur and the quadriceps femoris muscle (communicates directly with the knee joint cavity).
- Popliteal bursa behind the knee joint, a communicating bursa.

- Medial collateral ligament which runs from the medial femoral condyle to the medial tibial condyle. It also attaches to the medial meniscus.
- Lateral collateral ligament which runs from the lateral femoral condyle to the head of the fibula. It is not part of the joint capsule and does not attach to the lateral meniscus (see Figure 19.2).

Muscles

The prime movers of the knee joint are the quadriceps muscles (knee extension) and the hamstrings (knee flexion). The main function of the popliteus muscle is to unlock the extended (weight-bearing) knee. Popliteus laterally rotates the femur on the tibia and moves the lateral meniscus posteriorly at the beginning of knee flexion. External rotation when the knee is semi-flexed is a function of biceps femoris. Popliteus medially rotates the tibia when the knee is flexed along with sartorius, gracilis and semitendinosus (see Figure 19.4). The major muscles of the knee are described in Table 19.1.

The following nerves supply the muscles that move the knee:

- Femoral nerve innervates the quadriceps and sartorius muscle.
- Sciatic nerve innervates the hamstrings and popliteus.
- Obturator nerve innervates gracilis.

Normally the knee joint has a slight valgus. The Q angle measures the angle between a line from the anterior superior iliac spine and the centre of the patella and a line through the centre of the patella and the tibial tuberosity. If the Q angle

Fig. 19.4 Muscles that move the knee

Table 19.1 Muscles that move the knee[6]

Muscles that move the knee	Origin	Insertion	Action
Anterior compartment of the thigh **Quadriceps femoris**			
• Rectus femoris	Anterior inferior iliac spine	Patella via quadriceps tendon and then tibial tuberosity via patellar ligament	Extends leg at knee joint; acting alone also flexes thigh at hip joint
• Vastus lateralis	Greater trochanter and linea aspera of femur	Patella via quadriceps tendon and then tibial tuberosity via patellar ligament	Extends leg at knee joint
• Vastus medialis	Linea aspera of femur	Patella via quadriceps tendon and then tibial tuberosity via patellar ligament	
• Vastus intermedialis	Anterior and lateral surfaces of body of femur	Patella via quadriceps tendon and then tibial tuberosity via patellar ligament	
• Sartorius	Anterior superior iliac spine	Proximal part of medial surface of tibia near anterior border	Flexes leg at knee joint; flexes, abducts and laterally rotates thigh at hip joint; medial rotates tibia when knee is semi-flexed
Posterior compartment of the thigh **Hamstrings**			
• Biceps femoris	Long head arises from ischial tuberosity; short head arises from linea aspera and proximal ⅔ of supracondylar line of femur	Lateral side of head of fibula and lateral condyle of tibia	Flexes leg at knee joint and extends thigh at hip joint; externally rotates the knee when it is semi-flexed
• Semitendinosus	Ischial tuberosity	Proximal part of medial surface of shaft of tibia	Flexes leg at knee joint and extends thigh at hip joint; internally rotates tibia on femur when knee is semi-flexed
• Semimembranosus	Ischial tuberosity	Posteromedial aspect of medial condyle of tibia	
• Popliteus	Posterior aspect of lateral femoral condyle and lateral meniscus	Proximal part of posterior surface of tibia	Laterally rotates femur on tibia when the knee is extended: medially rotates tibia on the femur when the knee is flexed

Note: Gastrocnemius assists in flexion of the knee joint. It is described in Chapter 20.

exceeds 15° to 20° (slightly more in females), the patella is likely to track laterally causing it to rub against the lateral femoral condyle. Conditions affecting normal alignment, such as genu valgus, genu varum, genu recurvatum and tibial torsion, can predispose the knee to injury (see Figure 19.5 on p 369).

ASSESSMENT

The purpose of remedial massage assessment includes:

- determining the suitability of clients for massage (contraindications and red flags)
- determining the duration (acute or chronic), severity and types of tissues involved in the injury/condition
- determining whether symptoms fit patterns of common conditions.

Principles of remedial massage assessment are discussed in Chapter 2. This section presents specific considerations for assessment of the knee.

CASE HISTORY

Information from case histories can alert practitioners to the presence of serious conditions requiring referral. Little is known about the utility of subjective complaints with knee pain. The lack of self-noticed swelling seems moderately helpful in ruling out knee joint effusion. Similarly, the absence of weight bearing during trauma may help rule out a meniscal tear (both LRs = .40).[7]

Use targeted questioning to collect the most useful and relevant information, including:

- Identifying red flags requiring immediate referral (e.g. significant trauma, evidence of severe local inflammation, sepsis)[6] (see Table 19.2).

Fig. 19.5 Conditions affecting normal alignment of the knee

Genu varum | Genu valgus | Genu recurvatum | Increased Q-angle | Tibial torsion

Rotation of the leg

Q°

Assessment of the knee

1. Case history
2. Outcome measures (e.g. The Patient Specific Functional Scale)
3. Postural analysis
4. Gait analysis
5. Functional tests
   Lumbar spine
   Active range of motion tests
   Flexion, extension, lateral flexion, rotation
   Hip joint
   Active range of motion tests
   Flexion, extension, abduction, adduction, internal rotation, external rotation
   Knee joint
   Active range of motion tests
   Flexion, extension, internal rotation, external rotation
   Passive range of motion tests
   Flexion, extension, internal rotation, external rotation
   Resisted range of motion tests
   Flexion, extension, internal rotation, external rotation
   Resisted and length tests for specific muscles, including:
   Hamstrings, quadriceps, sartorius, popliteus
   Special tests
   Patellofemoral grind test
   Patella apprehension test
   Moving patella apprehension test
   Valgus/varus stress tests
   Anterior/posterior draw tests
   Lachman test
   Apley's compression test
   Thessaly test
6. Palpation

- Identifying yellow flags that require referral for further investigation.
- Identifying the exact location of the symptoms by asking clients to point to the site of pain.
- Determining if the pain is likely to have a mechanical cause. (Is the pain associated with rest or activity, certain postures or time of day?) Obtain descriptions of the specific mechanism of the injury and the forces involved, including:[9]
  - Was the limb weight bearing at the time of injury?
  - Was there any valgus or varus stress or rotational force at the time of injury?
  - Did the knee contact the ground or an opponent?
  - Was there a sound or pop/shift in the knee? (A pop is often associated with a torn anterior cruciate ligament; a shift can occur with anterior cruciate ligament rupture or patella dislocation.)
  - What happened after the injury? (Collapse, inability to continue playing, inability to weight bear suggest fracture or serious ligament injury.)
  - Did the knee swell and, if so, how quickly did it occur? (Swelling in the first hour suggests haemarthrosis from ruptured cruciate ligament or fracture: swelling developing more slowly suggests traumatic synovitis associated with meniscal tears and chondral pathology.)
  - Did the knee click, lock or is it unstable? (Painful clicking suggests meniscal tear or chondral pathology.)
- Determining if the client has a history of gout, pseudogout, rheumatoid arthritis or osteoarthritis.
- Refer any client with evidence of neurological compromise (e.g. change in cutaneous sensation, weakness of foot/toe muscles) or vascular compromise.

OUTCOME MEASURES

Outcome measures are questionnaires that are specifically designed to assess clients' level of impairment and

Table 19.2 Red flags for serious conditions associated with anterior knee pain[7, 9, 10]

Feature or risk factor	Condition
Symptoms and signs of infection (e.g. unexplained fever, night sweats, large warm red effusion) Risk factors for infection (e.g. underlying disease process, immunosuppression, penetrating wound, prosthetic joint)	Infection
History of trauma Sudden onset of pain Minor trauma if >50 years, history of osteoporosis and taking corticosteroids The Ottawa Knee Rule for Radiography is highly sensitive for knee fractures in both adults and children. When patients are younger than 55 years, can bear weight and flex the knee to 90°, and have no tenderness on the patella or fibular head, knee fracture can be confidently ruled out (–LR = .05 to .07).	Fracture/dislocation
Pallor, fever, malaise, recurrent infections, weight loss, night sweats, pain that is unchanged with rest or change in position, night pain, and pain that does not diminish with non-steroidal anti-inflammatory medications (NSAIDs) Past history of malignancy Age >50 years Pain at multiple sites (e.g. hip, groin, knee) Swelling unrelated to trauma in knee and other sites Note paediatric osteosarcoma red flags: limp or refusal to walk and bone pain, which are associated with the following clinical characteristics: - pain that wakes the child at night, lasts more than 2 weeks, is localised, is associated with swelling or deformity, and does not improve with NSAIDs - any palpable mass of recent origin that is located deep in the fascia, is non-tender, firm, and more than 2 cm in diameter or is associated with regional lymphadenopathy or neurological signs.	Cancer

to define benefits of treatment. The Patient Specific Functional Scale can be used to measure progress of treatment of clients with any musculoskeletal condition, including knee conditions.

POSTURAL ANALYSIS

Postural analysis enables observation of the whole client and facilitates identification of important features through bilateral comparison. It also facilitates detection of possible predisposing or contributing factors that may be implicated, observing the position of the cervical, thoracic and lumbar spines, pelvic balance and alignment of the lower limb (e.g. increased Q-angle, genu valgus, genu varum, genu recurvatum and tibial torsion – see Figure 19.5 on p 369). Observe and compare the knees posteriorly, laterally and anteriorly, noting their symmetry. Observe any bruising, colour changes, swelling or bumps. The level of the popliteal creases can indicate leg length. Observe the contour of

the thigh and lower leg muscles, noting muscle hypertonicity or atrophy.

GAIT ANALYSIS

During the gait cycles the knee flexes and extends: it flexes to absorb the impact of heel strike (quadriceps eccentrically contracts), extends during mid-stance (quadriceps concentrically contracts) and flexes again for toe-off and swing (gastrocnemius concentrically contracts) (see Chapter 2).

Observe any disturbance to the rate and rhythm of normal gait and the phase of the gait cycle in which it occurs. Impaired knee flexion can result in the trunk being thrust forward at heel strike or manually extending the knee by pressing on their thigh. Impaired knee flexion could prevent the leg from clearing the ground. In this case the pelvis may be hiked up in swing phase. Note any toe-in gait which may be associated with tibial torsion.

FUNCTIONAL TESTS

For any tests involving joint movements it is important to compare both sides and take into account any underlying pathology, previous surgical procedures and the age and lifestyle of the client. Findings from physical examinations should be interpreted in the light of evidence for their diagnostic accuracy. Measuring knee range of motion has consistently been shown to be highly reliable but is of unknown diagnostic utility. The assessment of end-feel during range of motion measurements, however, has been shown to be unreliable, especially between different examiners.[7] Generally, combining tests seems to be useful for identifying and ruling out various knee conditions. The Thessaly test has been shown to be excellent at both detecting and ruling out meniscal tears (+LR = 1.79 to 39.3, –LR = .08 to .73). Although the anterior draw test and pivot shift test are good at identifying anterior cruciate ligament tears (+LR = 1.5 to 36.5), the Lachman test is best at ruling them out (–LR = .10 to .24).

Varus and valgus testing, while not particularly reliable, is fairly good at ruling out medial collateral ligament tears (–LR = .20 to .30). The moving patella apprehension test seems to show very good diagnostic utility in both identifying and ruling out patella instability (+LR = 8.3, –LR = .00).[7]

Active range of motion (AROM) of the lumbar spine (flexion, extension, lateral flexion and rotation)

Examination of the knee begins with functional tests of the lumbar spine to help rule out conditions which refer pain to the knee. Look for dermatomal distribution of symptoms (see Figure 19.6). If active range of motion tests of the lumbar spine reproduce the lower limb symptoms, further examination of the lumbar spine is indicated (see Chapter 10).

AROM of the hip joint

Examine the hip joint to help rule out hip joint pathology that refers pain to the knee and/or lower leg. If active range of motion tests of the hip joint reproduce the lower limb symptoms, further examination of the hip is indicated (see Chapter 18).

Fig. 19.6 Dermatomes that cross the knee and the lower leg

AROM of the knee

The client may be seated on the treatment table. Face the client and demonstrate the movements. Examine the following ranges of motion:

- Flexion/extension (130–150°/0–5°[11])
- Internal/external rotation (5°/5°). Stabilise the thigh proximal to the knee and instruct the client to turn their lower leg outwards and inwards.

Passive range of motion (PROM)

If the client is unable to perform normal AROM in any direction, further investigation is required. The client may be seated or supine. Passive flexion and extension should be tested with one hand contacting the front of the knee and the other hand above the ankle. For passive internal and external rotation, stabilise the thigh above the knee and with the other hand holding the leg above the ankle, externally and internally rotate the lower leg. In the supine position, the client's hip and knee are flexed to 90° to perform passive internal and external rotation. Normal end-feel for knee flexion is described as soft tissue compression and for extension elastic/firm capsular.[12]

Resisted range of motion (RROM)

RROM tests should also be performed if AROM testing indicates the likelihood of a knee or lower leg strain. RROM tests include:

- flexion: hamstrings (semitendinosus, semimembranosus, biceps femoris), sartorius
- extension: quadriceps (vastus medialis, vastus lateralis, vastus intermedius, rectus femoris)
- internal rotation: popliteus with pes anserine muscles (knee flexed)
- external rotation: popliteus (knee extended); biceps femoris (knee flexed).

Fig. 19.7 Resisted hamstring test

Resisted tests and length tests for specific muscles[13, 14]

If RROM tests reproduce symptoms, then further tests may be used to help identify specific muscles.

1. HAMSTRINGS

Resisted tests

To test the hamstrings as a group, the client lies prone with their knee flexed to 90°. The client tries to bring their heel towards the buttock against your resistance (see Figure 19.7).

The lateral and medial hamstring muscles may also be tested separately.

Lateral hamstrings (biceps femoris)

The client's knee is flexed to 50° to 70° with the thigh in slight lateral rotation. Apply resistance as the client tries to flex their knee (see Figure 19.8).

Fig. 19.8   Resisted biceps femoris test

Fig. 19.10   Length test for the hamstring muscles

Fig. 19.9   Resisted semimembranosus and semitendinosus test

Fig. 19.11   Resisted quadriceps test

Medial hamstrings
(semimembranosus, semitendinosus)

This test is similar to the test for biceps femoris except that the client's thigh is placed in slight medial rotation. In this position the client tries to flex their knee against your resistance (see Figure 19.9).

Length test

Shortened hamstring muscles restrict knee extension when the hip is flexed or restrict hip flexion when the knee is extended (see Figure 19.10).

2. QUADRICEPS

Resisted test

As a group, the quadriceps can be tested with the client seated. Place one hand over the knee and the other over the ankle. Apply resistance as the client tries to straighten their knee.

Quadriceps can also be tested with the client in the prone position. Apply resistance as the client tries to take their heel to their buttock (see Figure 19.11).

Quadriceps activation differs in open chain (non-weight-bearing) and closed chain (weight-bearing) positions. In open chain positions, vastus medialis obliquus is activated last and

Fig. 19.12 Length test for rectus femoris

Fig. 19.13 Resisted test for sartorius

Fig. 19.14 Resisted test for popliteus

with smaller amplitude (30% of maximal voluntary contraction) and may be distinguished from other quadriceps muscles by resisting near end range extension. In closed chain positions, there is more activation of vastus medialis obliquus than vastus lateralis at 40° of semisquat with the hip medially rotated 30° degrees.[15] Double leg squat with simultaneous isometric hip adduction may be useful in selectively strengthening vastus medialis obliquus.[16]

Length test

Shortening of the quadriceps restricts knee flexion. Shortened rectus femoris can be observed as restricted knee flexion when the hip is extended or restricted hip extension when the knee is flexed (see Figure 19.12).

3. SARTORIUS

Resisted test

The client lies supine with one foot across the knee of the other leg (figure 4 position). Place one hand on the knee and the other on the ankle. The client is instructed to hold this position while you try to straighten the leg (i.e. move the hip into extension, medial rotation and adduction, and the knee into extension) (see Figure 19.13).

Alternatively, the client may be seated and instructed to try to place one foot on the opposite knee against your resistance.

Length test

A shortened sartorius muscle limits hip flexion, abduction and external rotation and knee flexion. For example, a client with shortened sartorius muscles has difficulty sitting cross-legged. A contracture of sartorius can produce a flexion, abduction and lateral rotation deformity of the hip, along with flexion of the knee.

4. POPLITEUS

Resisted test

The client sits with their knee flexed at 90° and is instructed to rotate their leg medially against resistance (see Figure 19.14). Note that weakness in popliteus can lead to hyperextension of the knee and lateral rotation of the tibia against the femur.

Popliteus weakness is commonly associated with hamstring imbalance where lateral hamstrings are relatively strong and medial hamstrings weak.[13]

Test for contracture

Contracture of popliteus results in slight flexion of the knee and medial rotation of the tibia against the femur.

Special tests

Special tests are designed to reproduce the client's symptoms. If symptoms are reported when performing a special test, ask the client to identify their exact location and confirm that they are the same as those described in the case history. Positive special test results should always be interpreted cautiously and in the context of other clinical findings (see Chapter 2).

PATELLA

Patellofemoral grind test

The client is supine, legs extended. Gently compress the patella onto the femur using one palm on top of the other. Maintaining the pressure, gently move the patella inferiorly. Pain and/or crepitus suggests patellofemoral syndrome, osteo-arthritis or osteochondritis of the patella (see Figure 19.15).

Patella apprehension test

This test is designed to determine if the patella is prone to lateral dislocation. The client lies supine. Gently move the patella laterally while observing the client for signs of apprehension. A positive test suggests patella instability (see Figure 19.16).

Moving patella apprehension test

The client lies supine with their ankle off the massage table and their knee fully extended. The therapist flexes the knee to 90° and back to extension while holding the patella in lateral translation. The procedure is then repeated with medial translation. Client apprehension or quadriceps contraction during lateral glide and not during medial glide suggests lateral dislocation of the patella.

LIGAMENTS

Valgus/varus stress tests

The client lies supine, legs extended. Stand at the side of the table just below the knee and stabilise the medial ankle with one hand. With the other hand apply lateral to medial (valgus) pressure at the knee. This tests the integrity of the medial collateral ligament. To test the lateral collateral ligament, the lateral ankle is stabilised and medial to lateral (varus) stress is applied to the knee (see Figure 19.17 on p 375).

Anterior/posterior draw test

The client lies supine with the knee flexed to 90° and the foot flat on the table. Place a folded towel across the client's foot and sit on the end of the table to stabilise the client's foot. Place both your hands around their leg just distal to the knee joint and gently draw the proximal tibia forward. Pain during

Fig. 19.15 Patellofemoral grind test

Fig. 19.16 Patella apprehension test

the test suggests anterior cruciate ligament sprain; excessive movement suggests rupture.[17]

The client maintains the same position for the anterior and posterior draw tests. In the posterior draw test the proximal tibia is pushed posteriorly to test the integrity of the posterior cruciate ligament. Pain during the procedure suggests ligament sprain; excessive movement suggests rupture (see Figure 19.18).

Lachman test

The client lies supine with the hip in slight external rotation and the knee in 15° flexion. Stand facing the client and stablise the femur with your lateral hand just proximal to the knee joint. The other hand is placed just distal to the knee joint on the medial side with the thumb on the anteromedial joint line. Apply pressure with the medial hand to the posterior upper tibia to lift it anteriorly. Anterior translation of the tibia associated with a soft 'mushy' end-feel indicates a positive test for anterior cruciate ligament injury.

MENISCUS

Apley's compression test

The client lies prone with knee flexed to 90°. Place both hands on the plantar surface of the foot and apply sufficient pressure to compress the medial and lateral menisci between the tibia and femur. The pressure is maintained while the tibia is internally and externally rotated on the femur. Pain on this manoeuvre suggests meniscal damage (see Figure 19.19 on p 376).

Note: Apley's distraction test can help distinguish between meniscal and ligamentous or capsular lesions. The client's

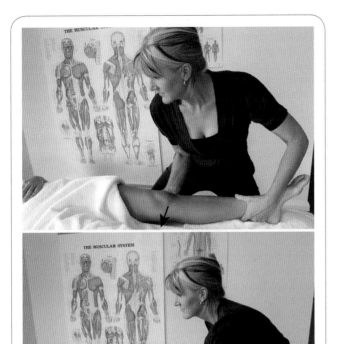

Fig. 19.17 Valgus/varus stress tests

A   B

Fig. 19.18 Anterior/posterior draw tests

Fig. 19.19 Apley's compression

position is the same as for Apley's compression test. Stabilise the knee by placing one knee on the client's mid thigh. Using both hands, hold the ankle and apply traction to the leg while rotating the tibia internally and externally. This manoeuvre reduces pressure on the meniscus and puts strain on the coronary ligaments and joint capsule.

Thessaly test

The client stands on the symptomatic leg and holds the therapist's hands for balance. The client bends their knee to 5° and rotates the body and leg internally and externally. This procedure is repeated with the knee bent to 20°. If the client feels pain and/or a click in the joint line a meniscal tear is indicated.

PALPATION

Palpatory findings along with findings from other assessments are used to guide treatment plans.

With the client supine, palpate the patella which lies entirely above the level of the knee joint. To palpate its underside move the patella gently from side to side. Palpate the quadriceps muscle just proximal to the patella and compare the lateral and medial muscles. (In patellofemoral syndrome, vastus lateralis is hypertonic and vastus medialis palpates as hypotonic or atrophied.)

Palpate the patella tendon inferior to the patella and its attachment to the tibial tuberosity. Tenderness at the tibial tuberosity suggests quadriceps tendinitis or, in an athletic

child, Osgood-Schlatter's disease. The superficial infrapatellar bursa and prepatellar bursa are normally not palpable although they may palpate as boggy when inflamed.

Bend the client's knee and place their foot on the table. From the depression at the side of the infrapatellar tendon, palpate medially to the upper edge of the medial tibial plateau and the attachment point of the medial meniscus. Move superiorly to palpate the medial femoral condyle immediately medial to the patella. Palpate the medial femoral epicondyle and the attachment of the medial collateral ligament. Trace the medial collateral ligament to the medial surface of the tibia.

The adductor tubercle is a useful landmark. Grasp the medial side of the proximal lower leg and press laterally and inferiorly with the thumb. Resisting hip adduction makes the tendon of adductor magnus become prominent. Sartorius, gracilis and semitendinosus muscles attach to the tibia at the pes anserine insertion. Palpate the posterior medial knee and resist knee flexion to detect the prominent semitendinosus.

From the depression at the side of the infrapatellar tendon, palpate the lateral tibial plateau and the lateral tubercle just below it. Palpate the lateral femoral condyle and epicondyle. The lateral collateral ligament runs between the lateral femoral condyle and the fibular head. It may be more easily palpated by placing the client's foot on the knee of the other leg. In this position it is palpated as a cord in front of the biceps tendon under the client's flexed knee.

The head of the fibula is inferior and posterior and approximately level with the tibial tuberosity. The common peroneal nerve crosses the neck of the fibula. Avoid heavy pressure on the nerve which can cause pain and/or paraesthesia. With the knee extended the anterior border of the iliotibial tract becomes prominent. When the client flexes their knee against resistance the iliotibial tract is palpable lateral to the patella.

With the client's knee bent, resist knee flexion. Feel the biceps tendon laterally and trace it to the head of the fibula. Palpate the prominent semitendinosus tendon medially. Biceps femoris forms the superior lateral border of the popliteal fossa and semimembranosus and semitendinosus form its superior medial border. The two heads of gastrocnemius form its inferior borders. The posterior tibial nerve bisects the fossa vertically. The popliteal vein and artery are medial to the tibial nerve.

REMEDIAL MASSAGE TREATMENT

Assessment of the knee provides essential information for development of treatment plans, including:

- client's suitability for remedial massage therapy
- duration of the condition (i.e. acute or chronic)
- severity of the condition (i.e. grade of injury; mild, moderate or severe pain)
- type(s) of tissues involved
- priorities for treatment if more than one injury or condition are present
- whether the signs and symptoms suggest a common condition of the knee region
- special considerations for individual clients (e.g. client's preference for treatment types and styles, specific population considerations).

Table 19.3 Interventions for the management of knee osteoarthritis (adapted from the Royal Australian College of General Practitioners' Guideline for the Management of Knee and Hip Osteoarthritis[21])

Intervention	Strength of recommendation	Quality of evidence
Exercise: Land-based exercise such as muscle strengthening exercises, walking and Tai Chi	Strong	Low (all land-based, Tai Chi) Very low (walking, muscle-strengthening exercise)
Weight management	Strong	Very low
Exercise: Stationary cycling, hatha yoga and aquatic exercise, hydrotherapy	Conditional	Low
Behavioural therapy (CBT)	Conditional	Low
Heat packs or hot water bottles	Conditional	Very low
Using a cane or other devices	Conditional	Low
A short course of manual therapy or massage	Conditional	Very low and low respectively
Transcutaneous electrical nerve stimulation (TENS)	Conditional	Very low
Ultrasound	Conditional	Moderate
Shockwave therapy	Conditional	Very low
Laser therapy	Conditional	Low
Interferential therapy	Conditional	Very low
Footwear marketed for knee OA	Conditional	Low – very low
Cold therapy	Conditional	Very low
Valgus braces and lateral wedge insoles for medial knee osteoarthritis	Conditional	Very low
Patellofemoral braces	Conditional	Very low
Kinesio taping	Conditional	Very low
Medication: Non-steroidal anti-inflammatory drugs taken orally at low doses for short periods recommended for some people (monitor for possible adverse effects, especially gastrointestinal, renal and cardiovascular)	Conditional	Moderate
Paracetamol: short trial	Conditional	Very low
Corticosteroid injections for short-term symptom relief	Conditional	Very low

Treatment options must always be considered in the context of the best available evidence for treatment effectiveness and clinical practice guidelines where they exist. Remedial massage treatments for osteoarthritis of the knee have been the subjects of a number of systematic reviews. A 2018 systematic review on the effect of manual therapy on knee osteoarthritis evaluated 11 randomised controlled trials. The authors concluded that manual therapy provides short-term benefits in reducing pain, improving function, and physical performance in patients with knee osteoarthritis.[18] These results were supported by another systematic review in the same year.[19]

A number of studies have examined the effectiveness of massage on muscles. For example, a 2014 study of the effects of massage and cryotherapy on knee extensor muscles in soccer players found that both interventions could increase isokinetic parameters and decrease perceived fatigue. Both massage and cryotherapy are likely more effective than rest as a strategy to return to normal state.[20]

Current research on interventions for knee osteoarthritis are summarised in Table 19.3.

OVERVIEW

Develop a short- and a long-term plan for each client. The short-term plan directs treatment to the highest priority (usually determined by symptoms). The long-term plan can be introduced when presenting symptoms have subsided. Treatment of all knee problems should include attention to contributing or predisposing factors such as underlying structural features, especially of the lower back, pelvis, hip, ankle and foot, and lifestyle factors. A significant part of both short-term and long-term treatment is educating clients about likely causal or aggravating factors and guiding their management of these factors. If massage therapy is used in conjunction with other treatments it is important to communicate with other treating practitioners. Health conditions can be complex and do not always conform to assessment protocols. Working with other practitioners provides an opportunity to develop integrative treatment practices for the best outcomes for clients.

MUSCLE STRAIN

Biomechanical imbalances arise when muscles develop shortness and tightness or become inhibited and weak. These imbalances cause dysfunctional movement patterns.[22] Muscles of the low back, pelvis and lower limb can affect knee function:

Muscles that tend to be tight and short:

- Iliopsoas, tensor fasciae latae, rectus femoris, quadratus lumborum, pectineus, gracilis, hip adductors, hamstrings (lateral hamstrings more than medial), soleus, gastrocnemius, piriformis and other external rotators of the hip.

Muscles that tend to be weak:

- Gluteus maximus, hip abductors, hip internal rotators (gluteus minimus and medius), vastus lateralis, intermedius and especially vastus medius obliquus, dorsiflexors of the ankle, especially tibialis anterior.

Quadriceps tendinopathy at the knee

Quadriceps muscle strains tend to occur at three common sites: (1) tenoperiosteal junction at the superior aspect of the patella, (2) infrapatella tendon (jumper's knee) and (3) the quadriceps expansion.[23] The client presents with pain at the front of the knee after excessive or sudden contraction of the quadriceps (e.g. running, hiking, dancing, squats or repetitive deep knee bends in weight lifting).

Hamstring tendinopathy at the knee

Hamstring strain is a common muscle strain in activities and sports that involve excessive eccentric contractions of the hamstrings such as running, kicking and dancing. The muscle is vulnerable to strain when it is eccentrically contracting to fully extend the knee at heel strike, particularly when a fuller or more intense stretch than usual is required (e.g. running on slippery or hilly surfaces). Ankle pronation and hip anteversion may predispose to hamstring tendinopathy. Pain is felt at the medial or lateral tenoperiosteal insertions of the hamstring muscles either side of the knee.

Muscle imbalance occurs in the hamstrings (or the quadriceps) when bilateral asymmetry (strength of one side compared to the other) exists. Depending on the sport, hamstring asymmetry greater than 8–15% will be detrimental to performance and athletes will be at increased risk of muscle strains and ligament (anterior cruciate) injury. For example, Australian football players with 8% asymmetries have been found to be at an increased risk. The hamstring to quadriceps strength balance or H:Q ratio is typically 2/3 and frequently used as part of the return-to-play criteria.[23]

Key assessment findings for muscle strain

- History of repetitive overuse or episode of intense use
- Functional tests of the knee:
  - AROM: positive in one or more directions
  - PROM: may be positive at end of range (passive muscle stretch)
  - RROM: positive for affected muscle(s)
  - Resisted and length tests: positive for affected muscle(s)
- Palpation positive for tenderness/pain. Muscle spasm and myofibril tears/scar tissue may also be evident.

Assessment

HISTORY

The client complains of localised knee pain that is aggravated by activity and relieved by rest. There is a history of repetitive overuse (e.g. excessive running, kicking, dancing) or an episode that required more than usual intensity of muscle contraction (e.g. running on slippery or hilly surfaces).

FUNCTIONAL TESTS

Lumbar AROM tests do not reproduce knee symptoms. Hip AROM tests do not reproduce knee symptoms (except for resisted hip flexion for rectus femoris strains and resisted hip extension for hamstring strains).

Knee tests

AROM: positive in one or more directions.
PROM: positive at the end of the range of motion when the affected muscle is passively stretched.
RROM: positive for affected muscles.
Resisted tests and length tests positive for affected muscles.
Special tests: negative.

PALPATION

Tenderness or pain may be elicited during palpation at the site of lesion. Muscle spasm, myofibril tears or scar tissue may be evident.

Overview of treatment for muscle strains

For acute muscle strains ice, compression and elevation are recommended. Advise the client to avoid the responsible activity. An elastic knee brace with cutout and horseshoe pad may be useful, especially if patellar tracking correction is required. Pain-free stretches and isometric exercises of the affected muscle should be introduced as soon as possible.

A typical treatment for grades 1 or 2 muscle strains includes:

- Swedish massage to the lower limb including ankle and foot, low back and pelvis.
- Remedial massage techniques for muscle strains include (see Table 19.4 on p 379):
  - deep gliding frictions along the muscle fibres
  - cross-fibre frictions
  - soft tissue releasing techniques
  - deep transverse friction
  - trigger point therapy
  - muscle stretching.

Table 19.4 Remedial massage techniques for muscles that move the knee

Muscle	Soft tissue release	Trigger point	Deep transverse friction	Stretch	Corrective action	Home exercise
Hamstring	Client: prone, knee flexed to 90°. Practitioner: Using knuckles of one hand glide along the muscle fibres or apply pressure at the site of the muscle lesion while the other hand holds the ankle and slowly flexes and extends the client's leg. Active: as above but the client flexes and extends their leg unassisted			Client: supine and raises their leg until they feel the muscle stretch. Practitioner: Using hands or shoulder, the practitioner resists the client as they attempt to return their leg to the table. Hold the resistance for 6–8 seconds. The client tries to raise their leg further within the pain-free range. Repeat the whole procedure three times.	Use chairs that match the client's leg length and a seat with a well-rounded and padded edge. Use a foot stool when seated. Take frequent breaks during long-distance driving.	There are a number of ways to stretch the hamstrings including: i) The client sits with their legs straight out in front of them or with one leg bent. The foot of the bent leg is placed on the floor alongside the thigh of the other leg and the knee rests on the floor. The client reaches forward towards their toes. ii) The client stands or kneels with one leg straight out in front. The client leans forward from their hips towards their toes. Hold stretches for up to 30 seconds and repeat three times.

Continued

Table 19.4 Remedial massage techniques for muscles that move the knee—cont'd

Muscle	Soft tissue release	Trigger point	Deep transverse friction	Stretch	Corrective action	Home exercise
Quadriceps	Client: supine, towards the side of the table, with knee flexed and leg over the side of the table. Practitioner: applies pressure to the muscle lesion with fingers, thumbs, knuckles or elbows and glides along the muscle fibres. Ask the client to slowly straighten and bend their leg as the technique is applied.			Client prone. Knee flexed to their comfortable limit Practitioner: Faces cephalad, holding the client's ankle. The practitioner applies resistance as the client tries to straighten their leg for 6–8 seconds. After the contraction the client tries to take their heel to their buttocks again. Repeat the procedures three times. Alternatively the practitioner can sit on the side of the table and apply resistance with their medial shoulder.	Avoid shortening and/or prolonged immobilisation of the quadriceps muscles. Avoid deep knee bends and complete squats. Avoid prolonged sitting with hips at 90°. Avoid full flexion of the hip when sleeping on the side.	Lying prone or standing, take the heel towards the buttocks. Hold the stretch for up to 30 seconds and repeat three times.

- Myofascial release including cross-arm techniques and the leg pull (see Chapter 8).

Other remedial techniques for muscle strains/tightness include:

- The popliteus release.
  The client lies prone and flexes the affected knee to 80–90°. Palpate the popliteus in the popliteal fossa just inferior to the knee joint under the heads of the gastrocnemius. Slowly glide the fingers across the muscle, keeping the depth within the client's pain tolerance. The knee can also be passively or actively flexed and extended during the technique (see Figure 19.20).
- Knee passive joint articulation may be introduced after the acute phase including (see Chapter 7):
  - Knee articulation inferior approach
  - Knee articulation lateral approach.

Address any underlying conditions or predisposing factors (e.g. ankle pronation, hip anteversion, scoliosis).

CLIENT EDUCATION

Advise clients about stretching, warm-up and graduated return to activity. Runners may need to replace worn-out footwear. Rehabilitation exercises usually involve pain-free isometric and later isotonic contractions of the affected muscles and stretching of quadriceps, hamstrings, iliotibial band, gastrocnemius, soleus and iliopsoas as required.

Fig. 19.20 Popliteus release

Clients may be referred for manipulation of the low back, pelvis, knee, ankle and foot.

ILIOTIBIAL BAND SYNDROME

Iliotibial band syndrome is an overuse impingement syndrome of the distal iliotibial band near the lateral femoral condyle. Iliotibial band syndrome may have multiple etiologic subtypes including in some cases the bursa between the iliotibial band and the condyle or the vascularised fat pad in the sub-iliotibial band space.[24] At full knee extension the iliotibial band is anterior to the lateral condyle but when the knee is flexed to 30° or more, the iliotibial band moves posterior to the condyle. Iliotiibial band syndrome is the most common running injury of the lateral knee and often affects cyclists, soccer and basketball players. Postural variances such as limb length discrepancy, genu varum, foot over-pronation, hip adductor weakness and myofascial restriction have a robust association with iliotibial band syndrome.[24] A 2014 Cochrane Review examining deep transverse friction massage for iliotibital band syndrome concluded that there was insufficient evidence to determine the effects of deep transverse friction on pain, improvement in grip strength, and functional status for patients with iliotibial band syndrome (or lateral elbow tendinitis).[25]

Assessment

HISTORY

The client complains of diffuse knee pain during activity and there is often a history of repetitive overuse (e.g. excessive running, cycling). Pain may be aggravated by downhill running. Occasionally the client reports crepitus or snapping during walking and running.

FUNCTIONAL TESTS

Lumbar AROM tests do not reproduce symptoms.
Hip AROM tests do not reproduce symptoms (may be positive for passive stretch).

Knee tests

AROM: may be positive as iliotibial band rubs across the condyle during flexion/extension.
PROM: may be positive as iliotibial band rubs across the condyle during flexion/extension.

Key assessment findings for iliotibial band syndrome

- History of repetitive overuse (e.g. excessive downhill running, cycling)
- Functional tests of the knee:
  - AROM: may be positive during flexion/extension
  - PROM: may be positive during flexion/extension
  - RROM: positive for associated muscles
  - Resisted and length tests positive for associated muscles (e.g. hamstring, quadriceps, gluteal muscle)
  - Special test: Modified Ober's test positive
- Palpation positive for pain in iliotibial band approximately 3 cm above the knee joint line; possible crepitus or snapping with knee flexion and extension; myospasm may be present in gluteal muscles or tensor fasciae latae.

RROM: may be positive in abduction due to associated myospasm.

Resisted tests and length tests for specific muscles may be positive for affected muscles (e.g. gluteal muscles, tensor fasciae latae, hamstrings, quadriceps).

Special tests: Modified Ober's test positive (see Chapter 18).

PALPATION

Tenderness may be elicited during palpation of the iliotibial band approximately 3 cm above the knee joint line.

Overview of treatment for iliotibial band syndrome

In the acute phase, ice, compression and elevation are recommended. Advise the client to decrease the intensity of exercise and avoid aggravating activities like downhill running.

A typical treatment for chronic iliotibial band syndrome includes:

- Swedish massage to the lower limb including ankle and foot, low back and pelvis.
- A range of remedial massage techniques including the following:
  - Deep transverse friction and cross-fibre frictions to the iliotibial band. Sidelying position provides easy access to the iliotibial band and tensor fasciae latae.
  - Myofascial release including cross-arm techniques and the leg pull (see Chapter 8).
  - For associated myospasm, deep gliding frictions along the muscle fibres, cross-fibre frictions, soft tissue releasing techniques, trigger point therapy (see Table 19.4).
  - Knee and hip passive joint articulation (see Chapter 7).

Address any underlying conditions or predisposing factors (e.g. ankle over-pronation and under-pronation).

CLIENT EDUCATION

Advise clients about stretching, warm-up and graduated return to activity. Poor shock-absorbing shoes should be replaced. Hard surfaces, hills and uneven surfaces should be avoided. Cyclist may need to lower the bicycle seat and adjust the pedals. Rehabilitation exercises include stretching and strengthening of tensor fasciae latae, gluteal muscles, hamstrings and quadriceps as required.

Clients may be referred for manipulation of the low back, pelvis, knee, ankle and foot.

PATELLOFEMORAL PAIN SYNDROME

The incidence of patellofemoral pain syndrome is estimated to be as high as 25–43% in sports injury clinics. The condition often becomes chronic with approximately 9 out of 10 patients still experiencing symptoms 4 years after onset.[26] The term is used to describe anterior knee pain that may originate from a variety of causes. (Chondromalacia patellae is sometimes used as a synonym for patellofemoral pain syndrome, although patellofemoral pain syndrome is really a precursor for it.) Patellofemoral pain syndrome is characterised by anterior knee pain that is worse with knee extension in activities like ascending or descending stairs. The primary cause of the problem appears to be related to the tracking of the patella during knee extension movements.

The patella is embedded in the quadriceps tendon. Its primary function is to improve the angle of pull of the quadriceps on the proximal tibia. The patella is pulled superiorly during quadriceps contraction along the line of the pull of the quadriceps. The degree to which this pull deviates from a vertical line is indicated by the Q angle, that is the angle between a line that connects the tibial tuberosity and the midpoint of the patella, and a line that connects the midpoint of the patella and the anterior superior iliac spine (see Figure 19.5 in p 361). An excessive Q angle is considered to be >15° for women and >10° for men.

A number of factors play a role in the development of patellofemoral pain syndrome with increasing evidence that proximal factors may be associated with its pathogenesis:

- Excessive femoral internal rotation in weight bearing leads to increased lateral patella tracking and reduction in patellofemoral contact area.[27]
- A large Q angle can lead to patella tracking disorders.
- Vastus medialis obliquus, the distal portion of the vastus medialis muscle, is important in counteracting the tendency of the other quadriceps to pull the patella in a lateral direction. Imbalances between the strength of the vastus medialis obliquus, vastus lateralis and iliotibial band, with its lateral patella expansion, can contribute to tracking disorders.
- Intrinsic factors such as patella alta (a hypermobile and unstable patella that is displaced proximally) and patella baja (a patella that is displaced distally so that the articular surfaces are incongruent) may also be involved.

Current evidence shows that there are hip strength deficits, delayed onset and shorter activation of gluteus medius in people with patellofemoral pain syndrome.[27]

Assessment

HISTORY

The client complains of anterior knee pain that is aggravated by activities like ascending or descending stairs or squatting. Clients also complain of knee pain on standing after a prolonged period of sitting. Prolonged sitting with knee flexion maintains the quadriceps in a stretched position and a sudden change in position may elicit knee pain (the movie sign). Clients sometimes report the knee giving way which may be due to reflex muscular inhibition in response to strong pain sensation in the knee extensors.[28]

Key assessment findings for patellofemoral pain syndrome

- History of repetitive activity (e.g. running)
- Functional tests of the knee:
  - AROM positive knee extension
  - PROM may be positive in knee flexion
  - RROM positive knee extension
  - Resisted and length tests positive for affected muscles.
  - Special test: Patellofemoral compression test positive.
- Palpation of the patella positive for pain; atrophy of vastus medialis obliquus may be present.

FUNCTIONAL TESTS

Lumbar AROM tests do not reproduce symptoms.
Hip AROM tests do not reproduce symptoms.

Knee tests

AROM: positive extension.
PROM: may be positive in flexion.
RROM: pain on resisted knee extension.
Resisted tests and length tests for specific muscles positive for affected muscles.
Special tests: Patellofemoral compression test positive.

PALPATION

Tenderness may be elicited during palpation on the undersurface of the patella (palpate by pushing the patella medially and laterally). Differences in muscle tone may also be palpated in the vastus lateralis and vastus medialis obliquus: vastus lateralis may be hypertonic and vastus medialis obliquus may be hypotonic or atrophied.

Overview of treatment and management

Conservative treatment includes eliminating or avoiding responsible activities, bracing and quadriceps strengthening exercises. Since a significant part of the problem with patellofemoral pain syndrome appears be associated with soft tissues around the pelvis, hip and knee, massage is helpful in treating this problem. Changes may not be immediate as altered biomechanical patterns have usually been established for some time. However, the client should feel some improvement in 3 to 4 treatments. A typical remedial massage treatment for mild or moderate patellofemoral pain syndrome includes:

- Swedish massage therapy to the knee, anterior and posterior thigh, hip, lower back and pelvis.
- Remedial massage techniques, which are aimed at promoting optimal function in the quadriceps and iliotibial band. Techniques (especially to vastus lateralis) include the following:
  - Deep gliding frictions along the muscle fibres.
    Short stripping strokes can be performed in several directions on the quadriceps retinaculum
  - Cross-fibre frictions.
  - Active and passive soft-tissue releasing techniques.
    In later stages of treatment, resistance to the eccentric contraction of the quadriceps during their elongation can enhance the active techniques further. Additional eccentric load can be added with resistance bands, weights or with your hand.
  - Deep transverse friction.
    The patella may be displaced to the medial and lateral sides for better access to the tissues just adjacent to it. Although the retinacular fibres are mostly oriented in a superior/inferior direction, stripping in several directions will help improve the overall mobility in the retinaculum.
  - Trigger point therapy (include all quadriceps muscles).
  - Muscle stretches.

Passive joint articulation (see Chapter 7) and thermotherapy may be helpful. Address causative and predisposing factors where possible, including muscle tightness in the lower back, pelvis and hip.

CLIENT EDUCATION

Advise clients to avoid all aggravating activities and on progressive and gradual return to activities. Evidence suggests that clinic-based exercise programs may benefit patients with patellofemoral pain syndrome.[29] A 2016 systematic review on hip exercise for patellofemoral pain syndrome found that both hip and knee strengthening programs were equally effective. Hip strengthening exercise addressing abductor and external rotator muscles and neuromuscular exercise had a beneficial effect on pain and function in people with patellofemoral syndrome.[27] Strengthening vastus medialis obliquus may offset the tendency of the other quadriceps to pull the patella laterally. Vastus medialis obliquus may be most active in the last 20–30° of knee extension. Recommend repeated short arc quadriceps extension exercises over the last 20–30° of knee extension against some resistance (see Figure 19.21). Begin by repeating the exercise to fatigue twice a day and progressively increase the number of repetitions and the resistance. Stretching lateral quadriceps muscles may also help restore quadriceps muscle balance.

Patella taping has been found to have benefit as an adjunct to exercise therapy.[30] Factors that predict a favourable response to off-the-shelf foot orthoses for individuals with patellofemoral pain syndrome who:

- demonstrate increased foot pronation during gait
- typically wear less supportive footwear
- report lower levels of patellofemoral pain
- exhibit less ankle dorsiflexion range of motion and report immediate reduction in pain with foot orthoses when performing a single leg squat.[31]

Refer for osseous manipulation where indicated. Surgical intervention may be called for if conservative methods are unsuccessful. Surgical options include articular cartilage procedures and lateral retinacula release which involves cutting the retinacula to reduce the lateral pull on the patella. There is little research to support the use of many current treatments for patellofemoral pain syndrome and further high-quality studies are needed.

Fig. 19.21 Strengthening vastus medialis obliquus

CHONDROMALACIA PATELLA

Patellofemoral pain syndrome is a likely precursor for chondromalacia patella. In chondromalacia clients describe pain under the patella whereas in patellofemoral pain syndrome pain the pain is described more superficially in the front of the knee. In chondromalacia patella the hyaline cartilage on the underside of the patella becomes eroded as a result of friction that occurs when the patella fails to track properly in the groove between the two femoral condyles. The client is likely to report crepitus (grating or grinding sensations) during flexion and extension of the knee. Pain may be experienced anteriorly and deep to the patella. The actual pain source is not the cartilage but subchondral bone just below the surface of the cartilage.

TREATMENT

Assessment and treatment approaches for patellofemoral pain syndrome and chondromalacia are similar. Treatment focuses on avoiding all aggravating activities, bracing and an exercise program to promote optimal muscle function, especially strengthening vastus medialis obliquus by resisting the last 20–30° of knee extension. Compressive knee braces may encourage activation of specific muscles. Surgical remodelling of the cartilage on the undersurface of the patella may be considered in persistent cases.

Remedial massage techniques are similar to those for patellofemoral syndrome. Caution should be taken to avoid undue pressure directly on the patella.

PATELLA DISLOCATION

Patella dislocation occurs when the patella moves laterally onto the lateral femoral condyle. It is usually the result of a twisting injury, such as sudden turning in football sports. It often reduces spontaneously. Predisposing factors include femoral anteversion, shallow femoral groove, genu valgus, loose medial retinaculum, tight lateral retinaculum, congenital absence of vastus medialis, increased Q angle and excessive subtalar pronation. The client often reports severe pain and an episode of instability. Clinically, clients have swelling, bruising and pain over the medial aspect of the patella and knee joint.[8] The patella apprehension test and moving patella apprehension tests are positive.

Treatment

Arthroscopy may be required to inspect the articular surfaces and remove any osteochondral fragments. The most important aim of rehabilitation is to minimise recurrence. Strengthening vastus medialis and stretching the lateral structures is required. Prolonged taping may also be required.

LIGAMENT SPRAIN

The medial collateral ligament is the most commonly injured ligament of the knee. The terrible triad (or unhappy triad) which consists of the anterior cruciate ligament, the medial collateral ligament and the medial meniscus was so named because of the frequency with which these structures were injured together from a single injury, usually involving a strong valgus or rotary force to the knee. The new unhappy triad (anterior cruciate and medial collateral ligaments and the lateral meniscus) has been found to occur more frequently in athletes than the originally described triad.[32]

Medial collateral ligament sprain

The medial collateral ligament is the larger of the two collateral ligaments. Its function is to enhance medial stability of the knee. It runs from the medial epicondyle to the medial side of the tibia about 2.5 cm below the condyle, just posterior to the pes anserine insertion (the common insertion of sartorius, gracilis and semitendinosus). Its deep part is firmly attached to the medial meniscus. Consequently injury to the medial collateral ligament may cause damage to the joint capsule and damage to the medial meniscus, however, most medial collateral ligament injuries can be treated conservatively. (The lateral collateral ligament is not connected to the joint capsule or the lateral meniscus and injuries to this ligament are rarely as severe as injuries to the medial collateral ligament.) The pes anserine muscles cross over the lower part of the medial collateral ligament and are separated from it by the pes anserine bursa.

Anterior cruciate ligament sprain

The anterior cruciate ligament runs from the anterior part of the intercondylar area of the tibial plateau to the medial side of the lateral femoral condyle. It is a primary knee stabiliser preventing forward displacement of the tibia on the femur (or preventing the femur slipping backwards on the tibia). Anterior cruciate ligament sprains are relatively common, especially in strenuous physical activities. Excessive loads on the anterior cruciate ligament may be incurred during sharp deceleration, deceleration before a change in direction or from landing from a jump or other activity. Predisposing factors may include the role of oestrogen, a large Q angle, narrowness of the intercondylar notch, weak hamstrings relative to quadriceps and pes planus. Female athletes experience non-contact anterior cruciate ligament injuries at 5 times the rate of male athletes possibly due to altered muscle activation.[33, 34]

Posterior cruciate ligament sprain

The posterior cruciate ligament runs from the back of the intercondylar area of the tibia to the lateral surface of the medial femoral condyle. Sprains of the posterior cruciate are much less common than anterior cruciate ligament or medial collateral ligament. It is usually injured by a direct blow to the tibia, often when the knee is bent (e.g. dashboard injury) or by falls that hyperflex the knee. Clients report a sense of popping or giving way. The posterior cruciate ligament is mostly extracapsular, has a good blood supply and good healing capacity.

Assessment

HISTORY

- Collateral ligament sprains: History of valgus or varus stress through the flexed knee. Pain ± instability in the medial or lateral knee, especially with change of direction.
- Anterior cruciate ligament sprains: History of heavy landing on an extended or slightly flexed knee with internal tibial rotation. Sensation of popping or shifting. Immediate severe pain. Swelling develops rapidly.

- Posterior cruciate ligament sprains: History of fall onto the knee with impact to the anterior tibia. May have instability descending stairs and walking downhill.

FUNCTIONAL TESTS

Lumbar AROM tests do not reproduce knee symptoms.
Hip AROM tests do not reproduce knee symptoms.

Knee tests

AROM: positive for limitation and pain.
PROM: limited and painful.
RROM: Protective muscle spasm may accompany sprains. Resisted and length tests may be positive for associated muscle strain or protective muscle spasm (e.g. hip adductors in medial collateral ligament sprain, quadriceps and hamstrings in cruciate ligament sprains).
Special tests: Ligament stress tests positive (e.g. valgus stress positive for medial collateral ligament sprain; anterior draw test and Lachman test positive for anterior cruciate ligament sprain and posterior draw test for posterior cruciate).

Overview of treatment and management

Medial collateral ligament sprains are often treated non-operatively with good success. Treatment immediately after injury includes cryotherapy, anti-inflammatory medication, splints or hinged knee braces and elastic wrap. Range of motion and resistance exercises for muscles that stabilise the joint (e.g. quadriceps and pes anserine muscles) should be commenced as soon as possible.

The anterior cruciate ligament is inaccessible to manual treatment. In the acute phase protective weight-bearing (e.g. using crutches, knee brace or splints), reducing weight-bearing, ice, elastic wrap and electrotherapy are used. More severe injuries may require surgical intervention including total reconstruction of the ligament using part of the patella tendon. The length of rehabilitation to full levels of activity is usually 9 to 12 months.[35] The hamstring muscles act as synergists to the anterior cruciate ligament and strengthening exercises for the hamstring muscles provide important support for the damaged ligament.

Appropriate rehabilitation can return good results for posterior cruciate ligament sprains. Acute sprains are treated with ice, elastic wrap and, if severe, a knee splint may be required. Range of motion exercises should be introduced as soon as possible.

A typical remedial massage treatment for mild or moderate ligament sprain includes:

- Swedish massage therapy to the knee, lower limb, back and pelvis.
- Remedial massage therapy including the following:
  - Deep transverse friction. The most tender part of the ligament is usually the primary site of tissue damage. Deep transverse friction is applied to promote collagen production and to prevent the formation of adhesions to surrounding tissue. Deep transverse friction could be applied for 2–3 minutes working at a pain level of 4 or 5 out of 10. (Note that the cruciate ligaments are not accessible for direct massage techniques.)
  - Techniques that focus on muscles that cross the joint (e.g. hypertonic hip adductors associated with medial collateral ligament sprain, hypertonic hamstring muscles associated with anterior cruciate ligament sprain). Techniques include:
    - deep gliding along the muscle fibres
    - cross-fibre frictions
    - muscle stretches provided they do not stress the ligament
    - soft tissue releasing techniques
    - trigger point therapy.
  Note that in some cases increased muscle tone may stabilise the joint while the ligament heals.
- Other remedial techniques include heat therapy, myofascial release and passive joint articulation (e.g. knee articulation inferior approach and knee articulation lateral approach). Clients may also require treatment of the lower back, pelvis, lower leg, ankle and foot. Some clients may benefit from referral for osseous manipulation and/or acupuncture.

CLIENT EDUCATION

The client should be advised to use ice/heat therapy for pain relief. A typical rehabilitation program for grade 1 or 2 medial collateral ligament sprain would be:

First weeks post injury

The aim is to decrease pain and swelling. Initially, depending on severity, weight bearing should be avoided or minimsed. The joint is protected with a hinged knee brace. Commence active range of motion as soon as possible within the client's pain tolerance. Progress to isometric exercises for quadriceps, hamstrings and hip abductors. Recommend swimming to maintain fitness. After the first few days introduce a stationary bicycle.

Second week post injury

Improve mobility and flexibility. Full weight bearing with brace is encouraged. Increase stationary bicycle work. Introduce light leg press, squats and jogging. Commence isotonic quadriceps and hamstring exercises.

Third week post injury

Re-establish co-ordination and proprioception. Increase strengthening exercises. Commence agility skill (skipping, hopping, running longer distances and at a higher speed). Use brace only for jogging and agility work.

Four weeks post injury

Functional training. Increase proprioceptive tasks (e.g. wobble board). Begin sport-specific skills. Use brace only for agility work and return to sport drills.

MENISCAL INJURY

The two fibrocartilaginous menisci help shock absorption and provide a larger contact surface between the femur and the tibia. They also help counteract the tendency of the femur to roll off the top of the tibial plateau. When a meniscus is removed or severely damaged, osteoarthritis often follows.

The meniscus may be damaged by trauma or degeneration. Compressive forces can break, chip or tear the meniscus; tensile forces such as acute valgus injury can tear the meniscus. Meniscal extrusion (where the meniscal margin extends beyond the tibial margin) is a common finding in patients with a medial meniscus root tear (a tear in the periphery of the meniscus where the meniscus attaches to the central tibial plateau). However, it is rare in patients with a lateral meniscus root tear, which is more commonly associated with a history of trauma and an anterior cruciate ligament tear.[36] The medial meniscus is attached to the deep fibres of the medial collateral ligament which restricts its movement and makes it more readily injured than the more mobile lateral collateral ligament. In fact, the medial meniscus is involved in 75% of meniscal injuries, particularly to the posterior horn.[37] In some instances, pieces of meniscus become separated and cause the knee to lock from time to time as they move around the joint. Table 19.5 compares signs and symptoms of meniscal injury, anterior cruciate ligament sprain and patella dislocation.

Assessment

HISTORY

Traumatic meniscal damage is characterised by a twinge or sudden pain over the medial or lateral joint line with clicking, catching or locking. Swelling occurs in about 50% of cases. Meniscal damage can also be the result of degenerative changes which may be without symptoms and progress to recurring pain, crepitus, catching ± swelling.

Key assessment findings for meniscal injuries

- History of trauma, often characterised by a sudden twinge over medial or lateral joint line with clicking, catching or locking.
- Functional tests of the knee:
  - AROM limited and painful, especially extension
  - PROM limited and painful, especially extension
  - RROM may be positive if associated muscle strain
  - Resisted and length tests may be positive for affected muscles
  - Special tests: positive Apley's compression and Thessaly test.
- Palpation positive for joint line tenderness.

FUNCTIONAL TESTS

Lumbar AROM tests do not reproduce the knee symptoms. Hip AROM tests do not reproduce the knee symptoms.

Knee tests

AROM: limited and painful, especially extension.
PROM: limited and painful, especially extension.
RROM: positive if associated muscle strains.
Resisted and length tests: positive for affected muscles.
Special tests: Apley's compression test and Thessaly test positive.
Palpation: positive for joint line tenderness.

Overview of treatment and management

If the meniscal damage is not severe, physical therapy will often be successful. Tears that occur on the outer third of the meniscus, which has a good vascular supply, have a better chance of healing; tears on the inner two-thirds and deep regions of the posterior horn are poorly vascularised and may require surgery (see Table 19.6).

In the subacute phase, remedial massage treatment focuses on restoring muscle balance around the joint. Muscle techniques include cross-fibre friction on the joint line followed by cryotherapy. Heat packs may be beneficial after the first post-injury week.

CLIENT EDUCATION

Avoid sudden changes of speed and direction, rotation of the knee and prolonged standing on hard surfaces. Refer to an osteopath, chiropractor or physiotherapist for manipulation. Refer for correction of ankle pronation if necessary. Advise clients that extensive rehabilitation is required.

Table 19.5 Differential diagnosis of anterior knee pain and swelling

	History	Special test
Anterior cruciate ligament	Painful pop in the knee after sudden change in direction with foot as pivot; immediate swelling	Anterior draw test and Lachman test positive
Meniscal injury	Locking knee, unable to extend knee after twisting with knee flexed; swelling within hours to one day	Apley's and Thessaly test positive
Patella dislocation	Patella dislocated after sudden change in direction of knee, twisting, or direct trauma	Patella apprehension test and moving patella apprehension test positive

Home exercises

Continue pain-free activities including stretching and strengthening hamstrings, quadriceps, gastrocnemius, tibialis anterior, hip abductors and rotators. Discontinue exercise if pain or swelling occurs during or after exercises. Gradually resume ballistic movements, high impact, direction changes and twisting. Progressively increase strengthening and stretching program.

OSTEOARTHRITIS

Osteoarthritis of the knee is very common in older clients, those with a history of a significant previous trauma to the knee or those whose work or sport involves repetitive loads to the knee. It is a condition where reparative processes are overwhelmed by destructive processes as a result of injury or mechanical load factors like being overweight. Familial predisposition is also a factor (see Figure 19.22).[38, 39]

Assessment

HISTORY

The client complains of chronic knee pain and stiffness that is aggravated by use and relieved by rest. Symptoms are usually better in the morning and worsen as the day progresses but do not usually occur at night. The client is usually over 50 years or has a history of significant previous injury or overuse. The client may report occasional swelling.

FUNCTIONAL TESTS

Lumbar AROM tests do not reproduce knee symptoms.
Hip AROM tests do not reproduce knee symptoms.

Table 19.6 Management of meniscal injury

Minor injury	Major injury
Conservative treatment	Surgery required
Symptoms develop 24–48 hours post injury	Unable to continue playing
Able to bear weight (no locking)	Joint locking
Minimal swelling	Swelling
Pain at end of range of motion	Little improvement with conservative treatment after 3 weeks or worsening over time

Key assessment findings for osteoarthritis of the knee joint

- History of chronic pain and limitation worse after weight bearing and relieved by rest. Occasional swelling. Usually over 50 years old.
- Functional tests of the knee:
  - AROM limited ± painful, especially in flexion
  - PROM limited ± painful in flexion (capsular pattern), hard end-feel
  - RROM usually negative.
- Palpation positive for crepitus and hard or capsular end-feel.

Fig. 19.22 Radiographs of osteoarthritis of the knee *(Source: Goldman: Cecil Medicine, 23rd edn. Copyright © 2007 Saunders).*

Knee tests

AROM positive (limited flexion).

PROM positive (capsular pattern: limited flexion), hard end-feel, crepitus often present.

RROM negative (Note that osteoarthritis is often accompanied by capsule tightening and muscle contractures. In such cases, passive muscle stretching is often painful and limited.)

Special tests usually negative.

PALPATION

Crepitus and abnormal hard or capsular end-feel are usually palpated. Client reports tenderness at several sites around the joint.

Treatment of osteoarthritis of the knee joint

Current evidence recommends behavioural management, including exercise, weight loss and self-management.[38] Acute episodes occur from time to time, usually after over-activity. If acute inflammation is present, treatment could include cryotherapy for analgesia, acupressure, Reiki, reflexology or anti-inflammatory medication. The client should be advised to modify activities to avoid aggravating the condition.

A typical remedial massage treatment for mild or moderate subacute or chronic osteoarthritis includes:

- Swedish massage therapy to the knee, lower limb, ankle and foot, lower back and pelvis.
- Remedial massage therapy includes:
  - heat therapy
  - passive joint articulation (see Chapter 7):
    - knee articulation inferior approach
    - knee articulation lateral approach
  - myofascial releasing techniques (see Chapter 8)
  - remedial massage techniques (e.g. deep gliding, cross-fibre frictions, soft tissue releasing techniques, trigger point therapy and muscle stretching) to address any associated muscle contractures.

CLIENT EDUCATION

The client should be advised to continue to use heat therapy for pain relief and to modify or avoid all aggravating activities. Weight loss and the use of shock-absorbing soles in shoes may reduce the load on the joint and provide symptom relief. Home exercises should be commenced as soon as pain permits. Stretching and strengthening exercises can be introduced as indicated by assessment findings. A 2014 systematic review and meta-analysis on the efficacy of rehabilitation programs for improving muscle strength in people with knee (or hip) osteoarthritis found moderate evidence supporting high intensity resistance exercise for large and sustained improvements for knee muscle strength in knee osteoarthritis patients.[40] Non-weight-bearing activities such as swimming, Tai Chi and paddling are often beneficial.

Supplements may provide moderate and clinically meaningful treatment effects on pain and function in patients with hand, hip or knee osteoarthritis in the short term, although the quality of evidence is very low. The most widely used supplements (e.g. glucosamine and chondroitin) have not been found to provide a clinically important effect on osteoarthritis. However, Boswellia serrata extract, pycnogenol and curcumin appear to have larger effects.[41] Clients may be referred for other supportive therapies including specialist nutritional advice and acupuncture.

The Royal Australian College of General Practitioners have made a number of recommendations for knee (and hip) osteoarthritis patients based on current evidence. They strongly recommend exercise and weight management. They also recommend short courses of manual and massage therapy. They strongly oppose the use of opioid medication and some other specific medical treatments in the management of knee OA.[21]

BURSITIS

Bursae are fluid-filled sacs located at sites where tissues move across one another. Their function is to minimise friction between the tissues as they move. Bursitis (inflammation of a bursa) can arise from friction with repetitive motion or direct trauma. Five common sites where bursitis occurs in the knee are the prepatellar bursa, pes anserine bursa, gastrocnemius bursa, popliteal bursa and iliotibial band bursa (see Figure 19.3 on p 366).

Prepatellar bursitis

Prepatellar bursitis (housemaid's knee) is common. A painless or slightly painful swelling is localised over the anterior aspect of the patella and the patellar tendon. (If there is redness, significant tenderness or a nearby break in the skin, the swelling must be tapped to rule out infection.) It is usually the result of prolonged kneeling, kneeling on a hard surface or from direct trauma from a fall.

TREATMENT

In the acute phase, bursitis is often managed with cryotherapy. The client should avoid kneeling or use a knee pad. The bursitis usually resolves when the aggravating activity is removed. In the subacute phase, heat, massage to the surrounding area and electrophysical therapy may be useful. Note that friction massage applied directly to the bursa is contraindicated.

OSGOOD-SCHLATTER'S DISEASE

Osgood-Schlatter's disease is a traction apophysitis of the tibial tuberosity in active children and young adolescents which causes pain at the tibial tuberosity. It is three times more common in males than females. It is caused by excessive traction on the soft apophysis of the tibial tuberosity by the powerful patellar tendon. It is associated with high levels of activity during a period of rapid growth.

Assessment

HISTORY

The client is an active young male (10–15 years old) or female (8–13 years old) who complains of pain at the tibial tuberosity. Pain may be felt during walking up or down hills and stairs or kneeling.

FUNCTIONAL TESTS

Lumbar AROM tests do not reproduce knee symptoms.

Hip AROM tests do not reproduce knee symptoms.

(Note: knee pain can be the main presenting complaint of a child with a serious disease of the hip.)

Key assessment findings for Osgood-Schlatter's disease

- Pain at the tibial tuberosity in an active child or young adolescent.
- Functional tests of the knee:
  - AROM painful in extension
  - PROM painful in flexion (passive quadriceps stretching)
  - RROM painful extension
  - Resisted and length tests positive for quadriceps femoris.
- Palpation: pain and tenderness on palpation at the tibial tuberosity.

Knee tests

AROM positive, especially on extension.

PROM positive with passive knee flexion (stretching quadriceps).

RROM positive on extension.

Resisted and length tests positive for quadriceps.

Special tests negative.

PALPATION

Clients report pain and tenderness at the tibial tuberosity. There may be local swelling.

Treatment

In the acute phase, recommend rest, or at least reduced participation in the responsible activity for at least two weeks. Ice and taping to reduce the pull of the quadriceps on the tibial tuberosity may be beneficial. In the chronic phase, heat and massage therapy may help reduce pain but the most important factor is reduction of activity until the end of the rapid growth phase. Avoid vigorous quadriceps stretching until the tibial tuberosity fuses to the tibia at about 16 years of age. After fusion, stretching and strengthening quadriceps and hamstrings as required to restore normal knee biomechanics.

KEY MESSAGES

- Assessment of clients with conditions of the knee involves history, outcome measures, postural analysis, gait analysis, functional tests and palpation.
- Assessment findings may indicate the type of tissue involved (contractile or inert, muscle, joint, fascia, ligament), duration of condition (acute or subacute) and severity (grade).
- Assessment findings may indicate a common presenting condition such as muscle strain, patellofemoral syndrome, ligament sprains, meniscal injury, osteoarthritis bursitis and Osgood-Schlatter's disease.
- Assessment findings also indicate client perception of injury and preferences for treatment.
- Consider Clinical Guidelines, available evidence and client preferences when planning therapy.
- Conditions requiring referral are common (e.g. acute knee injuries such as ligament sprains and meniscal tears). Refer all clients with symptoms of neurological or vascular impairment in the lower limb for further assessment (e.g. decreased sensation, muscle atrophy, unexplained swelling, discolouration of the lower limb, diminished dorsalis pedis pulse, delayed capillary refilling after compression).
- The selection of remedial massage techniques depends on assessment results. Swedish massage to the lower limb, lower back and pelvis may be followed by muscle techniques (e.g. deep gliding, cross-fibre frictions, soft tissue releasing techniques, trigger point therapy and deep transverse friction), passive joint articulation, myofascial release and thermotherapy as indicated.
- Educating clients about likely causal and predisposing factors and exercise rehabilitation are essential parts of remedial massage therapy.
- Prioritise the client self-help component of treatment wherever possible to reduce likelihood of recurrence and/or to promote health maintenance and illness prevention.

Review questions

1. Match the ligaments in Column A with the characteristics in Column B.

Column A	Column B
Medial collateral ligament	Prevents anterior movement of the tibia on the femur
Lateral collateral ligament	Resists valgus stress
Anterior cruciate ligament	Attaches to the tibial tuberosity
Posterior cruciate ligament	Attaches to the head of the fibula
Patellar ligament	Runs between the posterior intercondylar area of the tibia to the lateral surface of the medial femoral condyle

2. The popliteus can act as both a medial rotator and a lateral rotator of the knee. Explain how this can occur.
3. Describe resisted tests for the following muscles:
   i) Quadriceps as a group
   ii) Rectus femoris
   iii) Vastus medialis obliquus
4. Name a special test which could suggest the following conditions:
   i) Damage to the medial collateral ligament of the knee
   ii) Rupture to the anterior cruciate ligament of the knee
   iii) Torn cartilage (meniscus)
5. What is the movie sign? What condition does it suggest?
6. The prognosis of a meniscal tear depends on the location of its damage. What is the prognosis of a meniscal tear affecting its outer third?

Continued

Review questions—cont'd

7. Name the three structures of the knee that are referred to in the 'unhappy triad'.
8. Which statement does NOT accurately describe the lateral meniscus:
   a) Oval shaped
   b) Larger than the medial meniscus
   c) More mobile than the medial meniscus
   d) Not attached to the lateral collateral ligament
9. The effect of weak knee flexor muscles on gait can include:
   a) trunk thrown forwards over the centre of gravity
   b) lifting the hip during swing phase
   c) in-toeing gait
   d) manually pushing the knee into extension

10. The pes anserine muscles include all of the following except:
    a) sartorius
    b) semimembranosus
    c) semitendinosus
    d) gracilis
11. A runner is diagnosed with patellofemoral pain syndrome.
    i) Briefly describe the pathogenesis of the condition.
    ii) List three factors which can predispose to patellofemoral pain syndrome.
    ii) What is the usual focus of remedial massage treatment for patellofemoral pain syndrome?
12. Briefly describe the home advice that would be beneficial for a client with osteoarthritis of the knee.

REFERENCES

1. Chia YC, Beh HC, Ng CJ, et al. Ethnic differences in the prevalence of knee pain among adults of a community in a cross-sectional study. BMJ Open 2016;6(12):E011925.
2. Turkiewicz A, Gerhardsson De Verdier M, Engström G, et al. Prevalence of knee pain and knee osteoarthritis in Southern Sweden and the proportion that seeks medical care. Rheumatology 2015:54(5):827–35.
3. Singer S, Dammerer P, Krismer D, et al. Maximum lifetime Body Mass Index is the appropriate predictor of knee and hip osteoarthritis. Arch Orthop Trauma Surgery 2018;138(1):99–103.
4. Australian Institute of Health and Welfare. What is osteoarthritis? Online. Available: https://www.aihw.gov.au/reports/chronic-musculoskeletal-conditions/osteoarthritis/contents/what-is-osteoarthritis; 2019.
5. Zbrojkiewicz D, Vertullo C, Grayson JE. Increasing rates of anterior cruiciate ligament reconstruction in young Australians, 2000–2015. MJA 2018;208(8):354–8.
6. Tortora G, Derrickson B. Principles of anatomy and physiology. 15th edn. Milton, Qld: John Wiley; 2016.
7. Cleland J, Koppenhaver S, Su J. Netter's orthopaedic clinical examination: an evidence-based approach. 3rd edn. Philadelphia: Saunders; 2015.
8. Lee LH, Khan MN, Anand S. Acute soft tissue knee injuries. InnovAiT 2014;7(7):428–36.
9. Peter WF, Jansen MJ, Hurkmans EJ, et al. Physiotherapy in hip and knee osteoarthritis: development of a Practice Guideline concerning initial assessment, treatment and evaluation. Acta Reumatologica Portuguesa 2011;36(3):268–81.
10. Rankin A. An evidence-based case study of unilateral shin splints: do red flags function in paediatric osteosarcoma? Physiotherapy Canada 2015;67(4):365–8.
11. Reese N, Bandy W. Joint range of motion and muscle length testing. Philadelphia, PA: Saunders; 2016.
12. Carnes M, Vizniak N. Quick reference evidence-based conditions manual. 3rd edn. Burnaby, BC: Professional Health Systems; 2009.
13. Kendall McCreary E, Provance P, McIntyre Rodgers M, et al. Muscles, testing and function, with posture and pain. 5th edn. Philadelphia: Lippincott Williams and Wilkins; 2005.

14. Avers D, Brown M. Daniels and Worthingham's muscle testing: techniques of manual examination and performance testing. 10th edn. Oxford: Saunders; 2018.
15. Irish S, Millward A, Wride J, et al. The effect of closed-kinetic chain exercises and open-kinetic chain exercise on the muscle activity of vastus medialis oblique and vastus lateralis. J Strength Condit Res 2010;25(5):1256–62.
16. Miao P, Xu Y, Pan C, et al. Vastus medialis oblique and vastus lateralis activity during a double-leg semisquat with or without hip adduction in patients with patellofemoral pain syndrome. BMC Musculoskel Dis 2015;16:289. Doi 10.1186/s12891-015-0736-6.
17. Ellanti P, Mulhall KJ. Patient self-demonstration of the anterior drawer test in an ACL deficient knee. BMJ Case Reports 2015. Doi:10.1136/bcr-2014-207516.
18. Anwer S, Alghadir A, Zafar H, et al. Effects of orthopaedic manual therapy in knee osteoarthritis: a systematic review and meta-analysis. Physiotherapy 2018;104(3):264–76.
19. Chen B, Zhan H, Marszalek J, et al. Manual therapy for knee osteoarthritis pain: a systematic review and meta-analysis. Osteoarthr Cartilage 2018;26:S318–S319.
20. Razeghi M, Nouri H. Comparison of the effects of massage and cryotherapy on the knee extensor muscles fatigue and isokinetic parameters in soccer players. J Rehabil Sci Res 2015;2(1):1–7.
21. Royal Australian Collelge of General Practitioners. Guideline for the management of knee and hip osteoarthritis. Second edition. Online. Available: http://www.acsep.org.au/content/Document/guideline-for-the-management-of-knee-and-hip-oa-2nd-edition.pdf; 2018.
22. Rinke M. The relationship between muscle imbalance and associated injuries and re-injuries in collegiate athletes. Parkway: ProQuest Dissertations and Theses; 2015. UMI Number: 1587825.
23. Kox L, Wiegerinck E, Maas M. I-test: A gymnast with anterior knee pain: not a typical case of jumpers knee. Quadriceps femoris tendinopathy. Brit J Sports Med 2014;48(6):476. Doi:10.1136/bjsports-2012-091773.
24. Flato R, Passanante G, Skalski M, et al. The iliotibial tract: imaging, anatomy, injuries, and other pathology. Skeletal Radiology 2017;46(5):605–22.

25. Loew L, Brosseau L, Tugwell P, et al. Deep transverse friction massage for treating lateral elbow or lateral knee tendinitis. Cochrane Database System Rev 2014;(11):CD003528.
26. Leibbrandt D, Louw Q. Kinematic factors associated with anterior knee pain during common aggravating activities: a systematic review. Phys Ther Rev 2017;22(1-2):34–47.
27. Thomson C, Krouwel O, Kuisma R, et al. The outcome of hip exercise in patellofemoral pain: a systematic review. Manual Ther 2016;26:1–30.
28. Lefevre C, Thomas A, Gribble P, et al. Determining clinical impairments that lead to changes in dynamic knee valgus following a 4-week feedback intervention. Parkway: ProQuest Dissertations and Theses; 2014.
29. Brown CK, Southerst D, Côté P, et al. The effectiveness of exercise on recovery and clinical outcomes in patients with soft tissue injuries of the hip, thigh, or knee: a systematic review by the Ontario Protocol for Traffic Injury Management (OPTIMa) Collaboration. J Manipulative Physiol Ther 2016;39(2):110–20.e1.
30. Logan C, Bhashyam A, Tisosky A, et al. Systematic review of the effect of taping techniques on patellofemoral pain syndrome. Sports Health 2017;9(5):456–61.
31. Barton C, Levinger P, Crossley K, et al. Clinical and kinematic predictors of foot orthoses efficacy in individuals with patellofemoral pain syndrome. J Foot Ankle Res 2011;4(Suppl 1):O5.
32. Ravikanth R, Singh JK, Pavithran A, et al. A review of sports-related injuries: head to toe spectrum. Apollo Med 2018;15(2):79–87.
33. Collins G, Thompson RW, Mensch J, et al. The effects of a game simulation on muscle activation and knee kinematics in females. Parkway: ProQuest Dissertations and Theses; 2017.
34. Kinsey M, Wenner M, Breedlove K, et al. Estrogen effects on ACL laxity and neurocognitive function in young women. Parkway: ProQuest Dissertations and Theses; 2017.
35. Data on anterior cruciate ligament reported by researchers at Duke University. Med Devices Surg Technology Week 2017; 68.
36. Koo J, Choi S. Comparison of medial and lateral meniscus root tears. PLoS One 2015;10(10):E0141021.

37. Carnes M, Vizniak N. Quick reference evidence-based conditions manual. 3rd edn. Burnaby, BC: Professional Health Systems; 2009.

38. Hunter DJ. Everything you ever wanted to know about osteoarthritis. The Health Report 2017. Online. Available: https://www.abc.net.au/radionational/programs/healthreport/everything-you-ever-wanted-to-know-about-osteoarthritis/8664218#transcript; 2017.

39. Jiang Y, Tuan R. Origin and function of cartilage stem/progenitor cells in osteoarthritis. Nature Reviews Rheumatology 2015;11(4):206–12.

40. Zacharias A, Green RA, Semciw AI, et al. Efficacy of rehabilitation programs for improving muscle strength in people with hip or knee osteoarthritis: a systematic review with meta-analysis. Osteoarthr Cartilage 2014;22(11):1752–73.

41. Liu X, Machado G, Eyles J, et al. Dietary supplements for treating osteoarthritis: a systematic review and meta-analysis. Brit J Sports Med 2017;52(3):167–75.

20

The leg, ankle and foot

INTRODUCTION

Ankle and foot pain has a significant detrimental effect on health-related quality of life. Foot pain alone was found to affect nearly 1 in 5 people in the community.[1] It was associated with increased age, female sex, obesity and pain in other body regions.[2] Ankle ligaments are perhaps the most commonly injured ligaments in the body and gastrocnemius strains and Achilles tendinopathy are the most common athletic injuries of the ankle and foot. For example, male orienteering runners have a 10 times greater age-adjusted risk of developing Achilles tendinopathy than their non-running counterparts.[3] The foot is prone to osteoarthritis and is also subject to systemic diseases like diabetes mellitus. Although a rare presentation to remedial massage therapy clinics, one particular condition to be watchful for is deep venous thrombosis of the leg. Clients with suspected deep venous thrombosis should be referred for medical investigation.

DEEP VENOUS THROMBOSIS

In many cases the most significant indicator is history of recent surgery or a long plane or bus trip. Suspect deep venous thrombosis when the client has constant pain, tenderness, increased temperature and swelling in the calf. Homan's sign (passive dorsiflexion of the ankle) may reproduce pain (but would also be painful for calf muscle strains). The presence of deep venous thrombosis may be confirmed by Doppler scan and venography. Serious complications include pulmonary embolism and postphlebitic syndrome. Treatment consists of anticoagulant therapy, elevation of the limb, fibrinolytic therapy and sometimes thrombectomy.

FUNCTIONAL ANATOMY

The ankle (talocrural) joint is made up of the lateral malleolus of the fibula, the medial malleolus of the tibia and the talus. The distal ends of the tibia and fibula form a mortise into which the dome of the talus fits to form a hinge for plantarflexion and dorsiflexion of the foot. There are seven tarsal bones: talus, calcaneus, cuboid, navicular and the three cuneiform bones. The medial aspect of the ankle joint is supported by the deltoid ligament: three lateral ligaments (anterior talofibular, posterior talofibular and calcaneofibular ligament) support the lateral side (see Figure 20.1 on p 393).

The foot can be divided into three regions: the hindfoot, midfoot and forefoot. The hindfoot contains the calcaneus, the largest of the tarsal bones, and the talus which rests on top. About half the body weight is transmitted to the calcaneus, the other half to the other tarsal bones. The subtalar joint between the calcaneus and the talus is bound by several talocalcaneal ligaments and supported by part of the medial and lateral ligaments of the ankle. There are no muscle attachments to the talus. The sinus tarsi is a channel between the two bones just anterior to the lateral malleous. On the posteromedial aspect of the calcaneus is the sustentaculum tali, a shelf-like projection for the attachment of flexor hallucis longus. The Achilles tendon attaches to the calcaneal tuberosity. A fibroelastic fat pad cushions the heel when weight bearing. Anteriorly the calcaneus articulates with the cuboid bone.

The midfoot is made up of five of the seven tarsal bones which are arranged in two rows, the cuboid occupying both rows. The proximal row contains the navicular medially and the cuboid laterally. The distal row contains the three cuneiforms medially and the cuboid laterally. The

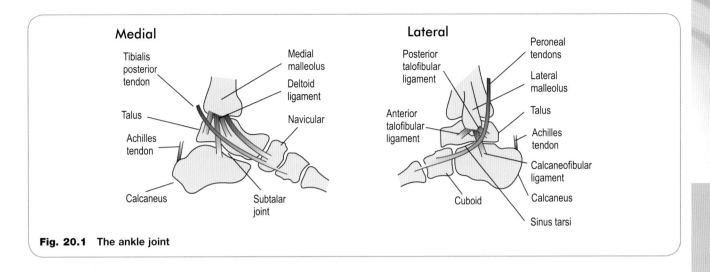

Fig. 20.1   The ankle joint

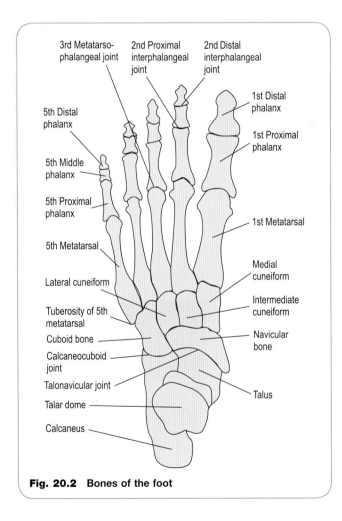

Fig. 20.2   Bones of the foot

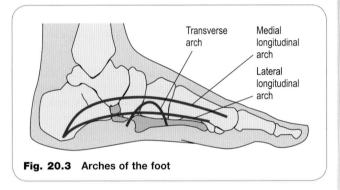

Fig. 20.3   Arches of the foot

although the peroneus tendon crosses the cuboid tuberosity. The cuboid also provides attachment for the long plantar ligament and the calcaneocuboid ligament.

The five metatarsals and phalanges make up the forefoot. The first metatarsal bone is thicker than the other metatarsals because it bears more weight and is important in the push-off phase of gait. The first metatarsal also provides attachments for tibialis anterior and peroneus longus. Two sesamoid bones are located in the flexor hallucis brevis tendon on its plantar surface. Peroneus brevis tendon attaches to the lateral side of the fifth metatarsal. Several ligaments connect the metatarsophalangeal joints and the interphalangeal joints. The interphalangeal and metatarsophalangeal joints can plantarflex and dorsiflex. Abduction and adduction of the toes are functions of metatarsophalangeal joints.

All the joints in the hindfoot and midfoot from the subtalar joint to the tarsometatarsal joints contribute to inversion and eversion of the foot. These are complex movements: inversion involves both medial rotation and supination; eversion involves lateral rotation and pronation.

The arches of the foot are important for weight bearing and propulsion. They are usually developed by 12 or 13 years of age. Pliability to adapt to uneven surfaces is provided by the multiple bones and joints of the foot. The arches are maintained by the irregular and interlocking shape of the bones, supporting ligaments and muscles and tendons of the foot. The three arches are (see Figure 20.3):

tarsometatarsophalangeal joints form the boundary between the midfoot and the forefoot. The cuneiform bones articulate with the first, second and third metatarsals; the cuboid articulates with the fourth and fifth metatarsals (see Figure 20.2). Tibialis posterior attaches to the tuberosity on the medial surface of the navicular bone. No muscles attach to the cuboid

- medial longitudinal arch: calcaneus, talus, navicular, cuneiform bones and first three metatarsals
- lateral longitudinal arch: calcaneus, cuboid, fourth and fifth metatarsals
- transverse arch: wedge-shaped cuneiforms, cuboid and bases of the five metatarsal bones.

The deep fascia of the foot forms the plantar fascia that extends from the tuberosity of the calcaneus to the heads of the metatarsal bones. The plantar aponeurosis which encloses the flexor tendons of the foot forms the central part of the plantar fascia. It supports the longitudinal arch of the foot.

The muscles of the foot are classified as intrinsic or extrinsic. Intrinsic muscles are located within the foot itself. They are responsible for movements of the toes and provide support for the arches of the foot. The extrinsic muscles arise in the lower leg. Their long tendons cross the ankle and insert into bones of the foot. They are responsible for movements of the ankle and toes and provide some support for the foot arches. Muscles of the leg and foot are described in Table 20.1 (see Figure 20.4).

NERVE SUPPLY TO MUSCLES OF THE LEG, ANKLE AND FOOT

- Deep peroneal nerve: tibialis anterior (L4, L5), extensor hallucis longus (L5) and extensor digitorum longus (L5)
- Superficial peroneal nerve: peroneus longus and brevis (L5, S1)

- Tibial nerve: gastrocnemius (S1, S2), soleus (S1, S2), flexor hallucis longus (L5), flexor digitorum longus (L5) and tibialis posterior (L5)

ASSESSMENT

The purpose of remedial massage assessment includes:

- determining the suitability of clients for massage (contraindications and red flags)
- determining the duration (acute or chronic), severity of injury and types of tissues involved in the injury/condition
- determining whether symptoms fit patterns of common conditions.

Principles of remedial massage assessment are discussed in Chapter 2. This section presents specific considerations for assessment of the leg, ankle and foot.

CASE HISTORY

Information from case histories can alert practitioners to the presence of serious conditions requiring referral. To date no studies of acceptable quality have assessed either the reliability or diagnostic utility of items from the subjective history in patients with foot and ankle problems.[4] Information from case histories needs to be integrated with findings from other

Fig. 20.4 Muscles of the ankle and foot

Table 20.1 Muscles of the leg and foot

Muscles that move the foot and toes	Origin	Insertion	Action
Anterior Compartment of the Leg			
• Tibialis anterior	Lateral condyle and body of tibia and interosseous membrane	First metatarsal and first (medial) cuneiform	Dorsiflexes foot at ankle joint and inverts foot at intertarsal joints
• Extensor hallucis longus	Anterior surface of fibula and interosseous membrane	Base of distal phalanx of great toe	Dorsiflexes foot at ankle joint and extends proximal phalanx of great toe at metatarsophalangeal joint
• Extensor digitorum longus	Lateral condyle of tibia, proximal ⅔ of anterior surface of fibula and interosseous membrane	Middle and distal phalanges of toes 2–5	Dorsiflexes foot at ankle joint and extends distal and middle phalanges of each toe at interphalangeal joints and proximal phalanx of each toe at metatarsophalangeal joint
• Fibularis (Peroneus) tertius	Distal third of fibula and interosseous membrane	Base of fifth metatarsal	Dorsiflexes foot at ankle joint and everts foot at intertarsal joints
Lateral (Fibular) Compartment of the Leg			
• Fibularis (Peroneus) longus	Head and body of fibula and lateral condyle of tibia	Base of first metatarsal and first cuneiform	Plantar flexes foot at ankle joint and everts foot at intertarsal joints
• Fibularis (Peroneus) brevis	Lateral distal ⅔ of body of fibula	Lateral aide of base of fifth metatarsal	Plantar flexes foot at ankle joint and everts foot at intertarsal joints
Superficial Posterior Compartment of the Leg			
• Gastrocnemius	Lateral and medial condyles of femur and capsule of knee	Calcaneus via calcaneal (Achilles) tendon	Plantar flexes foot at ankle joint and flexes leg at knee joint
• Soleus	Posterior surface of head of fibula and medial ⅓ of its body, and middle ⅓ of medial border of tibia	Calcaneus via calcaneal (Achilles) tendon	Plantar flexes foot at ankle joint
• Plantaris	Distal part of lateral supracondylar ridge, adjacent popliteal surface and oblique popliteal ligament	Calcaneus via calcaneal (Achilles) tendon	Plantar flexes foot at ankle joint and flexes leg at knee joint
Deep Posterior Compartment of the Leg			
• Popliteus	Lateral condyle of femur	Proximal to soleal line on posterior tibia	Flexes leg at knee joint and medially rotates tibia to unlock the extended knee
• Tibialis posterior	Lateral part of posterior tibia, proximal ⅔ medial fibula and interosseous membrane	Metatarsals 2–4, navicular, all three cuneiforms and cuboid	Plantar flexes foot at ankle joint and inverts foot at intertarsal joints
• Flexor digitorum longus	Posterior surface of tibia	Bases of distal phalanges of toes 2–4	Plantar flexes foot at ankle joint; flexes middle and distal phalanges of each toe at interphalangeal joints and proximal phalanx of each toe at metatarsophalangeal joint
• Flexor hallucis longus	Posterior surface of distal ⅔ of fibula, interosseous membrane and intermuscular septum	Base of distal phalanx of great toe	Plantar flexes foot at ankle joint; flexes distal phalanx of great toe at interphalangeal joint and proximal phalanx of great toe at metatarsophalangeal joint

Continued

Table 20.1   Muscles of the leg and foot—cont'd

Muscles that move the foot and toes	Origin	Insertion	Action
Intrinsic muscles of the foot **Dorsal**			
• Extensor digitorum brevis	Anterior and lateral surfaces of calcaneus and inferior extensor retinaculum	Tendons of extensor digitorum longus on toes 2–4 and proximal phalanx of great toe Note: The tendon that inserts into the proximal phalanx of the great toe is also described as extensor hallucis brevis.	Extends toes 2–4 at interphalangeal joints Extensor hallucis brevis extends great toe at metatarsophalangeal joint
Plantar First Layer (most superficial)			
• Abductor hallucis	Medial process of tuberosity of calcaneus, plantar fascia and flexor retinaculum	Medial side of proximal phalanx of great toe with the tendon of the flexor hallucis brevis	Abducts and flexes great toe at metatarsophalangeal joint
• Flexor digitorum brevis	Medial process of tuberosity of calcaneus and plantar fascia	Sides of middle phalanges of toes 2–5	Flexes toes 2–5 at proximal interphalangeal and metatarsophalangeal joint
• Abductor digiti minimi	Medial process of tuberosity of calcaneus and plantar fascia	Lateral side of proximal phalanx of little toe with the tendon of the flexor digiti minimi brevis	Abducts and flexes little toe at metatarsophalangeal joint
Second Layer • Quadratus plantae	Medial head: medial surface of calcaneus Lateral head: lateral border of plantar surface of calcaneus	Tendon of flexor digitorum longus	Assists flexor digitorum longus to flex toes 2–5 at metatarsophalangeal joints
• Lumbricals	Tendons of flexor digitorum longus	Tendons of extensor digitorum longus on proximal phalanges of toes 2–5	Extends toes 2–5 at interphalangeal joints and flexes toes 2–5 at metatarsophalangeal joints
Third Layer • Flexor hallucis brevis	Medial plantar surface of cuboid and 3rd (lateral) cuneiform	Medial and lateral sides of base of proximal phalanx of great toe	Flexes great toe at metatarsophalangeal joint
• Adductor hallucis	Metatarsals 2–4, ligaments of 3–5 metatarsophalangeal joints, and tendon of peroneus longus	Lateral side of proximal phalanx of great toe	Adducts and flexes great toe at metatarsophalangeal joint
• Flexor digiti minimi brevis	Base of 5th metatarsal and tendon of peroneus longus	Lateral side base of proximal phalanx of little toe	Flexes little toe at metatarsophalangeal joint
Fourth layer (deepest) • Dorsal interossei	Adjacent side of metatarsals	Proximal phalanges: both sides of 2nd toe and lateral side of toes 3 and 4	Abduct and flex toes 2–4 at metatarsophalangeal joints and extend toes at interphalangeal joints
• Plantar interossei	Bases and medial sides of metatarsals 3–5	Medial side of bases of proximal phalanges of toes 3–5	Adduct and flex proximal metatarsophalangeal joints and extend toes at interphalangeal joints

assessments and interpreted with caution. In the case of an injury, understanding the mechanism of action responsible is paramount for identifying the correct diagnosis.[5] Questioning should be targeted to include:

- description and mechanism of current injury, onset of symptoms, pain, disability and functional impairment,

previous injuries to this area. Was there a popping sound? Is there bruising and swelling, or numbness, tingling or weakness?[6]

- type of work, footwear, wear patterns on shoes
- identifying red and yellow flags that require referral for further investigation (red flags for serious causes of ankle and foot pain are summarised in Table 20.2)

Table 20.2 Red flags for potentially serious conditions of the leg, ankle and foot[6,7]

Condition	Red flag – history	Red flag – physical examination
Fracture and/or dislocation	History of recent trauma, crush injury, motor vehicle accident, falls from heights, sports injuries, osteoporosis in the elderly	Joint effusion, haemarthrosis, bruising, swelling, throbbing pain, point tenderness, unwilling to bear weight on involved leg
Infection (septic arthritis)	History of recent infection, surgery, injection, immunosuppressive disorder	Constant ache and/or throbbing pain, joint swelling, tenderness, warmth Systemic signs of infection (e.g. fever, tachycardia)
Peripheral arterial occlusive disease	Age >55 years, history of type II diabetes, ischaemic heart disease, smoking, sedentary lifestyle, intermittent claudication	Unilateral cool extremity, prolonged capillary refill time (>2 sec), decreased pulses in arteries below level of occlusion
Cancer	Unexplained weight loss, fatigue, masses, decreased or absent sensation	Palpable mass, decreased sensation in feet and ankles, motor loss in specific distribution, painless swelling
Deep venous thrombosis	Recent surgery, malignancy, pregnancy, trauma or leg immobilisation (e.g. long plane or bus trip), smoking	Unilateral calf pain, oedema, tenderness, warmth. Pain increases with standing or walking, relieved by rest and elevation. Possible pallor and loss of dorsalis pedis pulse
Cellulitis	History of recent skin ulceration or abrasion, venous insufficiency, congestive heart failure or cirrhosis	Pain, skin swelling, warmth, advancing irregular margin of erythema/reddish streaks Fever, chills, malaise, weakness
Compartment syndrome	History of blunt trauma, crush injury, or recent participation in rigorous unaccustomed exercise	Severe persistent leg pain that is aggravated by stretching the involved muscles Swelling, exquisite tenderness and palpable tension/hardness of involved compartment Paraesthesia, paresis, absence of pulse

---

Assessment of the leg, ankle and foot

1. Case history
2. Outcome measures (e.g. The Patient Specific Functional Scale)
3. Postural analysis
4. Gait analysis
5. Functional tests
   Lumbar spine and pelvis
   Active range of motion tests
   Flexion, extension, lateral flexion, rotation
   Hip joint
   Active range of motion tests
   Flexion, extension, abduction, adduction, internal rotation, external rotation
   Knee joint
   Active range of motion tests
   Flexion, extension, internal rotation, external rotation
   Ankle joint and foot

Active range of motion tests
Flexion, extension, inversion, eversion
Passive range of motion tests
Flexion, extension, inversion, eversion
Resisted range of motion tests
Flexion, extension, inversion, eversion
Resisted and length tests for specific muscles, including:
gastrocnemius, soleus, tibialis anterior, tibialis posterior, peroneus longus and brevis, extensor digitorum longus and brevis, flexor digitorum longus and brevis
Special tests
Thompson test
Anterior/posterior draw
Lateral ligament stability
Ankle impingement sign
Windlass test
Morton's foot test
6. Palpation

- eliminating other conditions that can cause symptoms in the ankle and foot (e.g. diabetes, Raynaud's phenomenon[a])
- identifying the exact location of the symptoms by asking clients to point to the site of symptoms

- determining if pain is local or referred. Local pain tends to be sharp and well localised; referred pain tends to be dull and poorly localised. Is there any numbness, tingling or weakness? The presence of nerve impingement symptoms suggests local nerve entrapment or referral from the lumbosacral radiculopathy. Dermatomes of the foot indicate the level of impingement (see Figure 20.5 on p 398). Other causes of distal paraesthesia include B12 deficiency, hypothyroidism, heavy metal poisoning, diabetes, systemic lupus erythematosus, malnutrition, HIV, HIV medications.

---

[a]Raynaud's phenomenon is characterised by impaired blood flow to the fingers, toes, ears and nose. Cold temperatures or strong emotions cause sudden constriction of blood vessels.

Fig. 20.5 Dermatomes of the leg and foot

OUTCOME MEASURES

Outcome measures are questionnaires that are specifically designed to assess clients' level of impairment and to define benefits of treatment. The Patient Specific Functional Scale is a generic assessment tool that can be used to measure progress of treatment of clients with any musculoskeletal condition, including leg, ankle and foot conditions.

POSTURAL ANALYSIS

Postural analysis enables observation of the whole client and facilitates identification of important features through bilateral comparison. It also facilitates detection of possible predisposing or contributing factors that may be implicated by observing the position of the thoracic and lumbar spines, pelvis and lower limbs. Note in particular the presence of scoliosis, femoral anteversion or retroversion, excessive Q angle, tibial torsion, genu valgus, varum or recurvatum (see Chapter 19), ankle pronation, pes cavus or planus and any abnormalities of the toes.

Observing the ankles and feet

Observe the ankles and feet for symmetry, swelling (local or diffuse), colour, bruising, scars and muscle hypertonicity or atrophy.

Common conditions of the ankles and feet include:

- Ankle pronation: Observe the Achilles tendons. Medial deviation suggests ankle pronation (see Figure 20.6). Pronation syndrome accounts for approximately 90% of all soft tissue injuries treated by podiatrists. Management is directed to correction of the underlying causes which include forefoot varus, rearfoot varus, tibia varum, genu varum and valgus, gastrocnemius and soleus contracture, hallux valgus, leg length asymmetry and spinal or pelvic asymmetry.[8]
- Pes planus (flat foot): absent or reduced medial longitudinal arch of the foot. The talus displaces medially and towards

Fig. 20.6 (A) Ankle pronation. (B) Normal alignment

the plantar surface of the foot. Pes planus deformity can be asymptomatic; or can also cause mechanic back pain through a chain reaction of kinetic and kinematic changes on the lower extremity.[9] A 2017 study found the prevalence of pes planus in a random population sample to be approximately 27%. Patients with flat foot were significantly older, showed a higher co-morbidity index, had a greater BMI and greater foot size. The presence of flat foot measurably diminished quality of life.[10] Management includes wearing shoes with shock-absorbing soles, strengthening intrinsic muscles of the foot (e.g. picking up objects with toes), strengthening quadriceps and hamstrings, stretching gastrocnemius and soleus and referral for orthotics (see Figure 20.7 on p 399).

Fig. 20.7 Pes planus

Fig. 20.8 Pes cavus

Fig. 20.9 Hallux valgus

Fig. 20.10 Claw toes

- Pes cavus: Abnormally high arches, often associated with claw toes. Pes cavus occurs in approximately 20% of adults.[8] The foot is rigid and absorbs shock poorly. Management includes mobilisation and manipulation of the foot, shock-absorbing shoes and stretches to gastrocnemius, plantar fascia and toe flexors (see Figure 20.8).
- Hallux valgus: an anatomical variant involving abduction of the 1st metatarsal and adduction of the proximal phalanx of the hallux, often associated with bunion formation. Management includes padding, wide shoes with a low heel, mobilisation and manipulation, stretches to abduct the big toe.
- Hallux rigidus: decreased dorsiflexion of the matatarsophalangeal joint of the hallux, usually from osteoarthritis. Management includes mobilisation, massage and referral for orthotics (see Figure 20.9).
- Claw toes: hyperextension of the metatarsophalangeal joint and hyperflexion of the proximal and distal interphalangeal joints, often accompanies pes cavus. Management includes padding, appropriate shoes, manipulation and mobilisation of the foot and ankle (see Figure 20.10).
- Hammer toes: hyperflexion of the proximal interphalangeal joint, some extension of the metatarsophalangeal joint,

often at the 2nd toe. The best prognosis occurs when hammer toe is treated in childhood. Later treatment includes padding, appropriate shoes, splinting and surgery (see Figure 20.11 on p 400).
- Morton's foot: the 2nd metatarsal is longer than the first (approximately 20% of the population). Clients should be advised to wear proper-fitting shoes. Morton's foot is associated with pronation-related injuries.

Fig. 20.11 Hammer toes

GAIT ANALYSIS

During the gait cycle the ankle dorsiflexes and plantarflexes. The ankle dorsiflexors, particularly tibialis anterior, concentrically contract during the swing phase so that the foot clears the ground. Tibialis anterior eccentrically contracts to control the lowering of the foot to the ground. The ankle plantarflexors are responsible for push-off along with eccentrically contracting toe extensors (see Chapter 2).

Observe any ankle over-pronation and over-supination as the foot takes the weight of the body. Compare the duration of stance phase for both lower limbs. A shortened time in stance phase (antalgic gait) can occur in any condition causing pain on weight bearing. Avoiding heel strike suggests retrocalcaneal bursitis or heel spurs. Weak tibialis anterior may cause drop foot gait. Walking on the balls of the toes suggests gastrocnemius or soleus shortening or strain, or heel or foot pain. A flat foot gait which avoids forceful push-off suggests weak gastrocnemius, soleus or hallux rigidis. Steppage gait in swing phase suggests weak dorsiflexors. Limited ankle movement is observed in clients with osteoarthritis of the ankle.

FUNCTIONAL TESTS

For any tests involving joint movements it is important to compare both sides and take into account any underlying pathology and the age and lifestyle of the client. Measuring ankle range of motion has consistently been shown to be highly reliable when one person does the measuring, but it is much less reliable when different people do the measuring.[4]

Active range of motion of the lumbar spine and pelvis (flexion, extension, lateral flexion and rotation)

Examination of the leg, ankle and foot begins with active range of motion tests of the lumbar spine and pelvis to help rule out lumbosacral radiculopathy which may refer pain and other symptoms to the lower limb. If active range of motion tests of the lumbar spine and pelvis reproduce leg, ankle or foot symptoms, further examination of the lumbar spine and pelvis is indicated (see Chapter 10).

Active range of motion of the hip joint (flexion, extension, abduction, adduction, external and internal rotation)

If active range of motion tests of the hip joint reproduce leg, ankle or foot symptoms, a full examination of the hip joint is indicated (see Chapter 18). Note that hip disease often manifests as knee pain.

Active range of motion of the knee joint (flexion, extension, internal and external rotation)

If the client experiences pain or other symptoms during knee movement, a full examination of the knee joint is indicated (see Chapter 19).

Active range of motion of the ankle and foot[11]

Talotibial joint
Dorsiflexion/plantarflexion 15–20°/40–50°
Subtalar and midtarsal joints
Inversion/eversion 30–35°/20°
1st metatarsophalangeal joint
Flexion/extension 20°/80°
2nd–5th toes metatarsophalangeal joints
Flexion/extension 75°/35°
2nd–5th toes interphalangeal joints
Flexion/extension ~60°/20°

Ankle and foot active range of motion is often tested using functional movements. Ask the client to:

- Walk on toes.
- Walk on heels.
- Walk on the outsides of their feet.
- Walk on the insides of their feet (see Figure 20.12 on p 401).

Passive range of motion of the ankle and foot

If the client is unable to perform normal AROM in any direction, further investigation is required. PROM testing for the ankle and foot may be performed with the client supine. For the toes, isolate the joint by placing one contact proximal and the other distal to the joint (e.g. to isolate the proximal interphalangeal joint, one hand contacts the proximal phalanx, the other contacts the distal phalanx). Palpate for crepitus, capsular pattern and end-feel. Capsular patterns of restriction of the ankle and foot are described as:[8]

- talotibial joint: plantar flexion more limited than dorsiflexion
- subtalar joint: varus and valgus equally limited
- midtarsal joints: dorsiflexion more limited than plantarflexion
- 1st metatarsophalangeal joint: flexion more limited than extension
- 2nd–5th metatarsophalangeal joints: variable
- interphalangeal joints: flexion more limited than extension.

Fig. 20.12 Functional active range of motion test of the ankle joint

Resisted range of motion

RROM tests should also be performed if AROM testing indicates the likelihood of a leg, ankle or foot problem. RROM tests include:

ANKLE

Dorsiflexion: tibialis anterior, extensor digitorum longus, extensor hallucis longus
Plantarflexion: Soleus, gastrocnemius, tibialis posterior, flexor digitorum longus, flexor hallucis longus
Inversion: tibialis anterior, tibialis posterior
Eversion: fibularis longus, brevis and tertius

HALLUX

Flexion: flexor hallucis longus and brevis
Extension: extensor hallucis longus and brevis
Abduction: abductor hallucis
Adduction: adductor hallucis

2ND TO 5TH TOES

Flexion: flexor digitorum longus and brevis, lumbricals
Extension: extensor digitorum longus and brevis
Abduction: dorsal interossei, abductor digiti minimi
Adduction: plantar interossei

Resisted tests and length tests for specific muscles

If RROM tests reproduce symptoms, further tests may be used to help identify specific muscles.

1. GASTROCNEMIUS

Resisted test

The client lies supine, knees straight, and tries to point their toes against your resistance (see Figure 20.13). Alternatively, ask the client to stand on their toes while resistance is applied by pushing down on their shoulders.

2. SOLEUS

Resisted test

The client lies prone with their knee flexed to 90°. Apply resistance as the client tries to plantarflex their ankle (see Figure 20.14).

Length test for ankle plantarflexors

Shortened gastrocnemius and soleus limit ankle dorsiflexion. When walking, it can interfere with heel strike and the client may tend to walk on their toes (see Figure 20.15).

3. TIBIALIS ANTERIOR

Resisted test

The client's foot is placed in inversion and dorsiflexion. Instruct the client to hold this position while resistance is applied in the direction of flexion and eversion (see Figure 20.16).

Fig. 20.14 Resisted test for soleus

Fig. 20.13 Resisted test for gastrocnemius

Fig. 20.15 Length test for ankle plantarflexors

Fig. 20.16 Resisted test for tibialis anterior

Fig. 20.18 Resisted test for tibialis posterior

Fig. 20.17 Length test for tibialis anterior

Fig. 20.19 Resisted test for fibularis longus and brevis

Length test

Contracted tibialis anterior limits plantarflexion and eversion (see Figure 20.17). In some cases contracture may cause inversion of the foot (calcaneovarus).

4. TIBIALIS POSTERIOR

Resisted test

Plantarflex and invert the client's foot and instruct the client to hold this position. Apply resistance against the medial and plantar surface of the foot in the direction of dorsiflexion and eversion (see Figure 20.18).

Length test

Contraction of tibialis posterior limits dorsiflexion and eversion.

5. FIBULARIS (PERONEUS) LONGUS AND BREVIS

Resisted test

Plantarflex and evert the client's foot and instruct them to hold the position while pressure is applied to the lateral border and sole of the foot in the direction of inversion and dorsiflexion (see Figure 20.19).

Length test

Contraction of fibularis longus and brevis limits inversion. In some cases contraction causes an everted or valgus position of the foot.

6. FLEXOR DIGITORUM LONGUS

Resisted test

The client flexes the distal phalanges of toes 2 to 5. Pressure is applied against the plantar surface of the distal phalanges of toes 2 to 5 in the direction of extension (see Figure 20.20 on p 404).

Length test

Contracture of flexor digitorum longus can cause flexion deformity of the distal phalanges of toes 2 to 5.

7. FLEXOR DIGITORUM BREVIS

Resisted test

This test is similar to the test for flexor digitorum longus except that the client flexes the proximal phalanx of toes 2 to 5 and you apply pressure to their plantar surface in the direction of extension (see Figure 20.21 on p 404).

403

Fig. 20.20 Resisted test for flexor digitorum longus

Fig. 20.22 Resisted test for extensor digitorum longus and brevis

Fig. 20.21 Resisted test for flexor digitorum brevis

Length test

Shortened flexor digitorum brevis limits extension of the proximal interphalangeal and metatarsophalangeal joints of toes 2 to 5.

8. EXTENSOR DIGITORUM LONGUS AND BREVIS

Resisted test

Extensor digitorum longus and brevis are tested together, as their tendons fuse, extending all joints of toes 2 to 5. To perform a resisted test on the muscles, pressure is applied against the dorsal surface of toes 2 to 5 in the direction of flexion (see Figure 20.22).

Length test

Shortened extensor digitorum longus and brevis muscles limit flexion of all joints of toes 2 to 5. Contracture of extensor digitorum longus and brevis leads to hyperextension of the metatarsophalangeal joints.

9. FLEXOR HALLUCIS LONGUS

Resisted test

Pressure is applied against the plantar surface of the distal phalanx of the big toe in the direction of extension (see Figure 20.23).

Fig. 20.23 Resisted test for flexor hallucis longus

Length test

Contracture of flexor hallucis longus can cause a hammer toe deformity of the big toe.

10. FLEXOR HALLUCIS BREVIS

Resisted test

This test is similar to the test for flexor hallucis longus except that you contact the plantar surface of the proximal phalanx of the big toe and apply pressure in the direction of flexion (see Figure 20.24 on p 405).

Fig. 20.24 Resisted test for flexor hallucis brevis

Fig. 20.25 Resisted test for extensor hallucis longus and brevis

Length test

Contracture holds the proximal phalanx of the big toe in flexion.

11. EXTENSOR HALLUCIS LONGUS AND BREVIS

Resisted test

Extensor hallucis brevis extends the proximal phalanx of the big toe; extensor hallucis longus extends both distal and proximal phalanges. Both muscles are tested simultaneously. The client tries to extend the metatarsophalangeal joints and interphalangeal joints of the big toe against your resistance (see Figure 20.25).

Length test

Contraction of extensor hallucis longus and brevis causes extension of the big toe.

Fig. 20.26 Resisted test for abductor hallucis

12. ABDUCTOR HALLUCIS

Resisted test

The client is asked to resist pressure applied against the medial side of the proximal phalanx of the big toe (see Figure 20.26).

Length test

If abductor hallucis is contracted, the big toe is abducted and the forefoot is pulled into varus.

13. ADDUCTOR HALLUCIS

Resisted test

The client is asked to resist pressure applied against the lateral side of the proximal phalanx of the big toe (see Figure 20.27 on p 406).

Test for contracture

Contracture of adductor hallucis can cause hallux valgus.

405

Fig. 20.27 Resisted test for adductor hallucis

Fig. 20.28 (a) Ankle anterior and (b) posterior draw

Special tests

If symptoms are reported when performing a special test, ask the client to identify their exact location and confirm that they are the same symptoms described in the case history. Functional tests have varying level of reliability and diagnostic utility and test results should always be interpreted cautiously and in the context of other clinical findings (see Chapter 2).

THOMPSON TEST

The client lies prone with their foot over the end of the table. Squeeze the calf muscle and observe plantar flexion of the foot. If the Achilles tendon is ruptured no plantar flexion will be observed. The Thompson test has very good diagnostic utility in both identifying and ruling out subcutaneous tears of the Achilles tendon ($+LR = 13.47$, $-LR = .04$).[4]

ANKLE DRAW TESTS

- Anterior draw: The client is supine with the knee on the involved side flexed and foot flat on the table. Stabilise the foot with one hand and hold the leg just proximal to the ankle with the other. Push the leg posteriorly (i.e. the foot becomes relatively anterior). Pain or excessive movement suggests anterior talofibular sprain or laxity ($LR+ = 3.1$, $LR- = 0.29$) (see Figure 20.28).
- Posterior draw: This test is similar to the anterior draw except that the leg is pulled anteriorly (i.e. the foot becomes relatively posterior). Pain or excessive movement suggests posterior talofibular ligament sprain or laxity (see Figure 20.28).

LATERAL LIGAMENT STABILITY TEST (TALAR TILT TEST)

The client is supine with knee and hip flexed. Invert the calcaneus by applying lateral pressure on the medial malleolus. Pain or excessive movement could suggest sprain or laxity of the calcaneofibular ligament and anterior talofibular ligament (see Figure 20.29).

IMPINGEMENT SIGN

The client is seated or lying supine. The therapist's lateral hand grasps the calanques, finger around the back of the head and thumb over the anterolateral aspect of the ankle. The

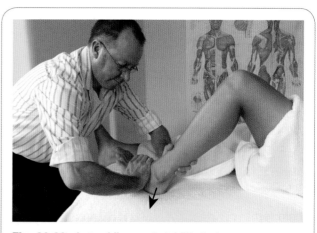

Fig. 20.29 Lateral ligament stability test

therapist's medial hand holds the forefoot and moves the foot into full plantar flexion. Apply pressure to the ankle joint with the examining thumb and maintain the pressure while the foot is fully dorsiflexed. The test is positive if the pain is greater in dorsiflexion than plantar flexion during this technique. The impingement sign has very good diagnostic utility in both identifying and ruling out anterolateral ankle impingement ($+LR = 7.9$, $-LR = .06$).[4]

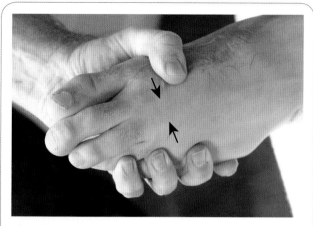

Fig. 20.30 Morton's test

WINDLASS TEST

The windlass test is designed to stretch the plantar aponeurosis and appears highly reliable but is of unknown diagnostic utility in identifying plantar fasciitis.[4]

- non-weight bearing. The client is seated on the massage table with their feet over the side. The therapist stabilises the ankle with one hand and extends the metatarsophalangeal joint of the hallux while allowing the proximal interphalangeal joint of the hallux to flex.
- weight bearing. With the client standing, extend the metatarsophalangeal joint of the hallus while allowing the proximal interphalangeal joint to flex. Heel pain reproduced during the test suggests plantar fasciitis.

MORTON'S TEST

With the client supine, squeeze the client's foot medially and laterally across the metatarsal heads. Pain on this manoeuvre suggests Morton's neuroma, metatarsal joint arthritis or fracture of the metatarsal heads (see Figure 20.30).

PALPATION

The client lies supine. Palpate the anterior border of the tibia from above the tibial tuberosity to below the medial malleolus. Palpate the muscles of the anterior compartment (tibialis anterior, extensor digitorum longus, extensor hallucis longus and peroneus tertius) lateral to the tibial border. Further lateral, palpate the lateral compartment (peroneus longus and brevis). Palpate the head of the fibula posterolateral to the knee. The common peroneal nerve runs along the lateral aspect of the head of the fibula. Palpate the circumference of the lateral malleolus at the distal end of the fibula. Compare the blunt end of the medial malleolus at the distal end of the tibia to the sharp end of the lateral malleolus. The level of the lateral malleolus is just below and slightly posterior to the level of the medial malleolus.

Medial aspect of the ankle and foot

- The first metatarsophalangeal joint is easily located. This is a common site of bunion formation, often as a result of lateral deviation of the proximal phalanx of the big toe, and of gouty arthritis, which is usually associated with redness, heat and pain. Palpate the sesamoids under the head of the first metatarsal as they slide when the big toe is passively articulated.
- Palpate the navicular tubercle, the large bony prominence on the medial side of the midfoot.
- The talar head is found approximately halfway between the medial malleolus and the navicular tubercle. Everting the foot makes the talar head more prominent.
- The sustentaculum tali of the calcaneus is palpated more than a finger's breadth below the medial malleolus posteriorly. Approach from below and press upwards. Tibialis posterior tendon and the spring ligament run from the sustentaculum tali to the navicular bone.
- The medial collateral ligament (deltoid ligament) lies under tibialis posterior and flexor digitorum longus. It can be mapped as a triangle with its apex at the medial malleolus and its base extending from the navicular to the sustentaculum tali.
- From the medial malleolus to the Achilles tendon palpate, in order, tendons of tibialis posterior and flexor digitorum longus, the posterior tibial artery and nerve and flexor hallucis longus.
- Abductor hallucis occupies the concavity of the instep (see Figure 20.31).

Lateral aspect of the ankle and foot

- Palpate the styloid process of the fifth metatarsal bone. This is the attachment site for peroneus brevis.
- Move posteriorly to the cuboid. Peroneus longus tendon winds around the lateral malleolus and runs in a groove under the cuboid towards its insertion at the medial cuneiform and first metatarsal.
- Palpate the tendons of peroneus longus and brevis (brevis is more anterior).
- Palpate the calcaneus and the peroneal tubercle (where peroneus longus and brevis tendons separate) distal to the lateral malleolus.
- Palpate the sinus tarsi area, a depression just anterior to the lateral malleolus. The talar dome is palpable here when the client's foot is plantarflexed.
- Abductor digiti minimi forms the lateral border of the foot (see Figure 20.31 on p 408).
- The lateral collateral ligament is made up of three ligaments:
  - Anterior talofibular ligament runs from the anterior aspect of the lateral malleolus to the lateral talus. Tenderness and swelling in the sinus tarsi usually indicate a sprain of the anterior talofibular ligament.
  - Calcaneofibular ligament runs from the inferior lateral malleolus to the lateral calcaneus.
  - Posterior talofibular ligament runs from the posterior lateral malleolus to the posterior talus (see Figure 20.1 on p 393).

Posterior aspect of the ankle

- Palpate the Achilles tendon from the lower third of the calf to the calcaneus. Trace the belly of the gastrocnemius up the calf and palpate the two heads to their insertions into the medial and lateral condyles of the femur. When the client stands on their toes the gastrocnemius muscle becomes prominent with the soleus bulging on either side of it.

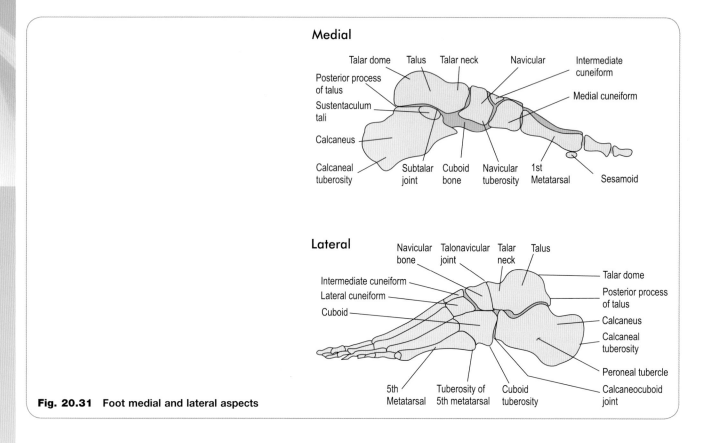

Medial

Talar dome | Talus | Talar neck | Navicular | Intermediate cuneiform

Posterior process of talus

Sustentaculum tali

Medial cuneiform

Calcaneus

Calcaneal tuberosity | Subtalar joint | Cuboid bone | Navicular tuberosity | 1st Metatarsal | Sesamoid

Lateral

Navicular bone | Talonavicular joint | Talar neck | Talus

Intermediate cuneiform

Lateral cuneiform

Cuboid

Talar dome

Posterior process of talus

Calcaneus

Calcaneal tuberosity

Peroneal tubercle

Calcaneocuboid joint

5th Metatarsal | Tuberosity of 5th metatarsal | Cuboid tuberosity

Fig. 20.31   Foot medial and lateral aspects

- The subcutaneous calcaneal bursa (between the Achilles insertion and the skin) and retrocalcaneal bursa (between the Achilles tendon and the superior angle of the calcaneus) are normally not palpable. When inflamed they often feel warm and palpate as boggy.

Dorsal aspect of the ankle and foot

- Ask the client to invert the foot and dorsiflex the ankle to bring tibialis anterior into prominence. Trace its insertion to the first metatarsal base and first cuneiform.
- Extensor hallucis longus is made prominent when the client extends their big toe.
- The anterior tibial artery runs from the neck of the fibula to midway between the malleoli. It lies lateral to the tibialis anterior and extensor hallucis longus and medial to extensor digitorum longus and peroneus tertius. Identify these tendons when the client dorsiflexes the ankle. The dorsalis pedis artery (the continuation of the anterior tibial artery) continues to the proximal end of the first intermetatarsal space.
- The superior extensor retinaculum is a broad band connecting the anterior border of the tibia to the anterior border of the fibula just above the malleoli. It forms the upper part of the anterior annular ligament.
- Palpate extensor digitorum brevis in front of the lateral malleolus when the foot is at 90° to the ankle (see Figure 20.32).

Plantar surface of the foot

- Palpate the metatarsal heads and note the integrity of the transverse arch.

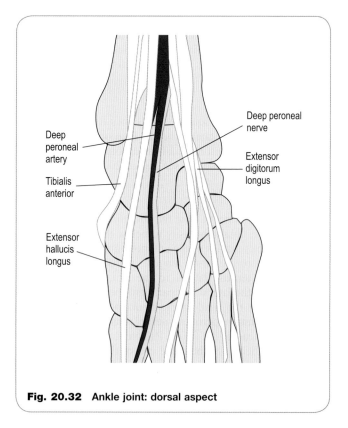

Deep peroneal artery

Tibialis anterior

Extensor hallucis longus

Deep peroneal nerve

Extensor digitorum longus

Fig. 20.32   Ankle joint: dorsal aspect

- The plantar fascia consists of bands of fascia that run from the medial tuberosity of the calcaneus to the metatarsal heads. In plantar fasciitis tenderness is often elicited when the anteromedial aspect of the calcaneus is palpated.
- Most of the muscles of the plantar surface of the foot originate from the calcaneus.

Phalanges

- Palpate each tarsometatarsal and interphalangeal joint. Note any swelling, tenderness and abnormal alignment.

REMEDIAL MASSAGE TREATMENT

Assessment of the leg, ankle and foot provides essential information for development of treatment plans, including:

- client's suitability for remedial massage therapy
- duration of the condition (i.e. acute or chronic)
- severity of the condition (i.e. grade of injury; mild, moderate or severe pain)
- type(s) of tissues involved
- priorities for treatment if more than one injury or condition are present
- whether the signs and symptoms suggest a common condition of the leg, ankle or foot
- special considerations for individual clients (e.g. client's preference for treatment types and styles, specific population considerations).

OVERVIEW

Develop a short- and a long-term plan for each client. The short-term plan directs treatment to the highest priority (usually determined by symptoms). The long-term plan can be introduced when presenting symptoms have subsided. Long-term treatment focuses on contributing or predisposing factors such as underlying structural features and lifestyle factors. Treatment should also include associated functional impairments in other parts of the kinetic chain (foot/ankle/knee/hip/low back). A significant part of both short-term and long-term treatment involves educating clients about likely causal or aggravating factors and guiding their management of these factors. If massage therapy is used in conjunction with other treatments it is important to communicate with other treating practitioners and to integrate treatment for the best outcome for the client.

LEG

MUSCLE STRAINS OF THE LEG

Muscle strains in the leg include gastrocnemius strain (tennis leg), tibialis anterior and posterior strain and strains of the peroneal muscles. Assessment and treatment of all muscle strains follow similar procedures. Tennis leg is presented here and can be used as a guide for treatment of other muscle strains of the leg.

GASTROCNEMIUS STRAIN (TENNIS LEG)

This injury tends to occur in older athletes (30 to 50 years) following a sudden explosive push off from a stationary

> **Key assessment findings for gastrocnemius strain (tennis leg)**
>
> - History of sudden acceleration from stationary position or uphill running in a cold environment; client 30–50 years old
> - Functional tests:
>   - AROM: painful ankle plantarflexion
>   - PROM: painful dorsiflexion (passive stretch of gastrocnemius)
>   - RROM: positive plantarflexion
>   - Resisted and length tests: positive for gastrocnemius
> - Palpation: tender in belly ~5 cm superior and medial to musculotendinous junction; muscle defect may be palpable

position, climbing a slope or suddenly changing direction. It is often associated with a cold environment.

Assessment

HISTORY

The client is usually an older athlete (30–50 years old). Sudden onset of pain in the medial head of gastrocnemius is characteristic. The client sometimes reports a sudden stinging or popping sensation in the calf.

FUNCTIONAL TESTS

Lumbar AROM tests do not reproduce symptoms.
Hip AROM tests do not reproduce symptoms.
Knee AROM tests do not reproduce symptoms.

Ankle tests

AROM: painful plantarflexion
PROM: painful dorsiflexion (passive stretch of gastrocnemius)
RROM: positive plantarflexion
Resisted and length tests: positive for gastrocnemius
Special tests: negative

PALPATION

The client usually reports tenderness in the muscle belly approximately 5 cm superior and medial to musculotendinous junction. In severe cases muscle defects may be palpable.

Overview of treatment and management

In the acute phase ice application may provide pain relief. Crutches may be necessary. A heel raise may be used on both legs to limit full muscle lengthening. Gentle stretching to pain tolerance may be commenced soon after injury.

A typical remedial massage treatment for a subacute/chronic mild or moderate gastrocnemius tear includes:

- Swedish massage therapy to the lower limb, lumbar spine and pelvis.
- Remedial massage techniques including (see Table 20.3 on p 410):
  - deep gliding frictions along the muscle fibres
  - cross-fibre frictions
  - soft tissue releasing techniques
  - deep transverse friction applied directly to the injury site to help stimulate collagen production
  - trigger point therapy
  - muscle stretching.

Table 20.3 Remedial massage techniques for muscles of the leg and foot[6,7]

Muscle	Soft tissue release	Trigger point	Deep transverse friction	Stretch	Corrective action[12]	Home exercises
Gastrocnemius	Client: prone, leg extended and abducted so that the foot is off the side of the table. Practitioner: stands at the foot of the table, facing cephalad. The practitioner applies pressure to the injury site or performs a deep longitudinal glide with fingers, thumbs or knuckles as the client slowly plantarflexes and dorsiflexes their ankle. 			Client: supine, knee extended and heel overhanging the end of the table. Practitioner: standing or kneeling at the foot of the table. The practitioner holds the ankle with both hands and dorsiflexes the client's foot as far as possible. The client tries to plantarflex their ankle for 6–8 seconds against the practitioner's resistance. Next the practitioner dorsiflexes the client's ankle as far as possible. This whole procedure is repeated three times. Alternatively, the client's foot can be placed on the practitioner's anterior thigh and the ankle passively dorsiflexed as the practitioner transfers their weight to their front foot. 	Avoid high-heeled shoes. Change running shoes regularly. Use a footrest if heels do not reach the floor when seated.	Stretch: 1. Stand with one foot in front of the other and bend the front knee. Keep the heel of the back foot on the ground to stretch gastrocnemius. 2. Stand on the end of a step with both feet and lower the heel of one foot off the step while keeping the other foot on the step. Strengthen: Calf raise (standing heel raise) Leg curls.

Continued

Table 20.3 Remedial massage techniques for muscles of the leg and foot—cont'd

Muscle	Soft tissue release	Trigger point	Deep transverse friction	Stretch	Corrective action[12]	Home exercises
Soleus	Client: prone, knee flexed and bolster placed under leg proximal to the ankle. Practitioner: stands at side of the table, facing cephalad. The practitioner applies pressure to the injury site or performs a deep longitudinal glide with thumbs, knuckles or elbow as the client slowly plantarflexes and dorsiflexes their ankle.			Client: prone, knee flexed to 90°. Practitioner: stands at the side of the table facing across the client. The practitioner holds the calcaneus with the caudal hand and places their forearm on the sole of the client's foot. The other hand holds the leg just proximal to the ankle. The practitioner dorsiflexes the ankle as far as comfortable with the caudal hand. The client tries to plantarflex their ankle for 6–8 seconds against the practitioner's resistance. Next the practitioner dorsiflexes the client's ankle as far as possible again. This whole procedure is repeated three times.	Modify activities that overload or maintain a fixed shortened position (e.g. use a footrest, avoid high-heeled shoes). Change running technique and surface. Correct leg length inequality	Stretch: Stand with one foot in front of the other. Bend both knees. 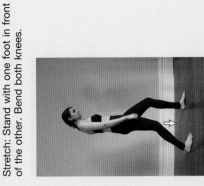 Strengthen: Calf raise (standing heel raise) Leg curls.

Table 20.3 Remedial massage techniques for muscles of the leg and foot—cont'd

Muscle	Soft tissue release	Trigger point	Deep transverse friction	Stretch	Corrective action[12]	Home exercises
Tibialis anterior	Client: supine. Practitioner: stands at the side of the table facing caudad. The practitioner applies pressure to the injury site or performs a deep longitudinal glide with fingers, thumbs or knuckles as the client slowly plantarflexes and dorsiflexes their ankle.			Client: supine. Practitioner: at foot of table. The practitioner plantarflexes (± everts) the client's foot and holds the stretch for up to 30 seconds. Repeat three times.	Eliminate prolonged shortening of the muscle (e.g. avoid long car trips (use of pedal)). Avoid prolonged walking on sloping surfaces.	Stretch: 1. Kneel and sit on your heels. Lift one knee. Hold 6–8 seconds and repeat three times. 2. Sit in a chair and flex the knee so that the dorsum of the toes touch the ground. Strengthen: Foot flat, raise the toes and forefoot leaving heel on the ground.

Table 20.3 Remedial massage techniques for muscles of the leg and foot—cont'd

Muscle	Soft tissue release	Trigger point	Deep transverse friction	Stretch	Corrective action[12]	Home exercises
Tibialis posterior	As for gastrocnemius or soleus Or Client: sidelying. Practitioner: standing or sitting, facing towards the client's head. The practitioner applies pressure to the medial border of the tibia as the client plantarflexes and dorsiflexes their ankle.			As for gastrocnemius or soleus.	When running or jogging use a full arch support, run only on smooth flat surfaces. May require referral for orthotics.	As for gastrocnemius or soleus.

Continued

Table 20.3 Remedial massage techniques for muscles of the leg and foot—cont'd

Muscle	Soft tissue release	Trigger point	Deep transverse friction	Stretch	Corrective action[12]	Home exercises
Fibularis longus and brevis	Client: sidelying. Practitioner: Standing behind the client. The practitioner applies pressure to the injury site as the client plantarflexes and dorsiflexes their ankle. Or Client: supine. Practitioner at the side of the table facing cephalad. The practitioner contacts the taut band/lesion in the muscle as the client plantarflexes/everts and dorsiflexes/inverts. The practitioner can perform a deep glide from behind the lateral malleolus to the fibular head as the muscle lengthens (i.e. dorsiflexes/inverts the ankle).	Peroneus longus / Peroneus brevis / Peroneus tertius		Client: supine. Practitioner: stands at foot of table. The practitioner passively dorsiflexes and inverts the client's ankle as far as comfortable for the client. The client then tries to plantarflex and evert their foot against the practitioner's resistance for 6–8 seconds. When the resistance is released, the practitioner passively dorsiflexes and inverts the foot as far as comfortable for the client. Repeat the procedure three times.	Avoid high-heeled shoes. Ensure that footwear is appropriate for the foot shape (e.g. Morton's foot). May require referral for orthotics.	Stretch: As for gastrocnemius and soleus. Strengthening: calf raises.

- Myofascial release including cross-arm techniques and the leg pull (see Chapter 8).
- Other remedial techniques such as knee and ankle joint articulation may also be introduced as required (see Chapter 7).
- Correct underlying biomechanical and predisposing factors if possible (e.g. ankle pronation, pes planus, muscle tightness/weakness in the lower limb).

CLIENT EDUCATION

Advise the client to rest from aggravating activities to reduce the stress on the injured muscle. A progressive strengthening and stretching program for the gastrocnemius should be commenced as soon as pain permits. Strengthening exercises can begin with isometric contractions, progressing to concentric bilateral calf raises and to unilateral calf raises, gradually adding weights. Finally add eccentric calf lowering over a step. Stretches should include both gastrocnemius and soleus. The client should also stretch and strengthen hamstrings, quadriceps and tibialis anterior. Refer for osseous manipulation.

SHIN SPLINTS

Shin splints is a term used to describe shin pain due to repetitive overuse such as running or dancing. Long periods of standing on a concrete floor or other hard surface in hardsoled shoes has also been implicated. There are two main types of shin splints:

- Anterior/lateral shin splints: tibialis anterior strain, tendinopathy or periostitis. Anterior shin splints is associated with excessive eccentric dorsiflexion (e.g. downhill walking or running)
- Posterior shin splints: tibialis posterior strain, tendinopathy or periostitis. Flexor digitorum longus and soleus may also be involved. It is associated with overpronation or incorrect running stride.

Assessment

HISTORY

The client describes anterolateral or posteromedial leg pain after exercise (e.g. downhill running or running on uneven surfaces, long-distance running, repeated impacts on a hard surface or with poor footwear). Pain is initially relieved by rest but can progress to constant pain.

FUNCTIONAL TESTS

Lumbar AROM tests do not reproduce symptoms.
Hip AROM tests do not reproduce symptoms.
Knee AROM tests do not reproduce symptoms.

Ankle tests

AROM: painful (e.g. dorsiflexion and inversion for tibialis anterior, plantarflexion and inversion for tibialis posterior).
PROM: painful as the involved muscle is passively stretched.
RROM: positive for involved muscles.
Resisted and length tests: positive for involved muscles (e.g. tibialis anterior and posterior may be weak).

PALPATION

Pain is elicited on palpation of the affected soft tissue and along the medial tibial border. Small nodules are often palpable in the muscle attachments to the medial tibia.

Overview of treatment and management

In the acute phase, ice can be applied for pain relief. Advise the client to rest from aggravating activities such as exercise on hard, uneven surfaces. Gentle stretching should be commenced as soon as possible within pain tolerance. The client may be referred for mobilisation and manipulation of the low back, hip, knee, ankle and foot. Referral for orthotics may also be required.

In chronic presentations, massage therapy is directed towards reducing hypertonicity in affected muscles. A typical remedial massage treatment for subacute or chronic shin splints includes:

- Swedish massage therapy to the lower limb, lumbar spine and pelvis. Avoid all techniques that pull on the tibial attachments of muscles. A useful technique involves compressing muscles back onto the bone (see Figure 20.33).

Key assessment findings for shin splints

- History of anterolateral or posteromedial shin pain related to excessive exercise, repetitive impacts, downhill walking or running (anterior shin splints) or overpronation of the ankle (posterior shin splints)
- Functional tests:
  - AROM: painful
  - PROM: painful due to passive stretch
  - RROM: positive for involved muscles
  - Resisted and length tests: positive for involved muscles (e.g. tibialis anterior, tibialis posterior, flexor digitorum longus, soleus)
  - Special tests: negative
- Palpation: pain on palpation at the site of inflammation; small lumps or nodules may be palpable along muscle attachments to the tibia

Fig. 20.33 Shin splints technique

SHIN SPLINTS TECHNIQUE

The client lies supine with the knee extended. Stand to the side of the foot of the table facing the client and hold the leg, with one hand on either side, just proximal to the ankle. Using both hands draw the leg muscles anteriorly, compressing them onto the tibia with the thenar eminences. This drawing and compressing movement is repeated, progressing from the ankle to just below the knee. Alternatively, the same movement can be performed with the client lying supine with their knee flexed and their foot flat on the table.

- Remedial massage techniques including (see Table 20.3 on p 410):
  - deep gliding frictions along the muscle fibres (including soleus, popliteus)
  - cross-fibre frictions
  - soft tissue releasing techniques – for example, for tibialis posterior and soleus muscles, with the client sidelying, apply pressure to the medial border of the tibia as the client plantarflexes and dorsiflexes their ankle

- deep transverse friction applied directly to the injury site may help stimulate collagen production
  - trigger point therapy
  - muscle stretching.
- Myofascial release including cross-arm techniques and the leg pull (see Chapter 8 and Figure 20.34).
- Heat therapy is usually beneficial.
- Other remedial techniques such as ankle joint articulation may also be introduced as required (see Chapter 7):
  - ankle prone circumduction
  - calcaneus prone circumduction
  - tarsals prone plantarflexion
  - ankle traction
  - metatarsal shearing
  - phalanges mobilisation.
- Correct underlying biomechanical and predisposing factors where possible (e.g. overpronation of ankles, foot flare, externally rotated hips, apparent leg length inequality, tight quadriceps, hamstrings, hip flexors or abductors as indicated).

Fig. 20.34 Myofascial release techniques for the leg

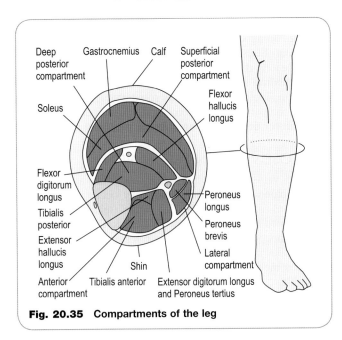

Fig. 20.35 Compartments of the leg

In the figure, the following labels appear:
Deep posterior compartment — Gastrocnemius — Calf — Superficial posterior compartment — Flexor hallucis longus — Soleus — Flexor digitorum longus — Tibialis posterior — Extensor hallucis longus — Peroneus longus — Peroneus brevis — Lateral compartment — Anterior compartment — Tibialis anterior — Shin — Extensor digitorum longus and Peroneus tertius

CLIENT EDUCATION

Approximately 20% of jumping and running athletes have shin splints at some point while engaging in sporting activities. Despite its frequency, best management strategies have not been established. The most logical rehabilitation currently is load management, increasing loading capacity through gradual load exposure and strengthening the calf muscles.[13] Advise the client to rest from aggravating activities such as downhill running or excessive impacts on hard surfaces. Gentle stretching should be introduced as soon as pain permits and continued throughout the rehabilitation. Weakness and/or tightness of tibialis anterior and posterior, gastrocnemius, soleus, quadriceps, hamstrings, hip flexors and hip abductors should be addressed in a progressive strengthening and stretching program. The client may need to change footwear and be referred for orthotics.

Refer for osseous manipulation and for additional physical therapy modalities such as electro-acupuncture if required. If the condition does not improve within two weeks, refer for further assessment for possible stress fracture. Osteosarcoma is another possible serious cause of pain.

CHRONIC COMPARTMENT SYNDROME

The leg has four compartments separated by fascial sheets: anterior, lateral, superficial posterior and deep posterior (see Figure 20.35).

Compartment syndrome occurs most commonly in the anterior compartment which contains tibialis anterior, extensor digitorum longus, extensor hallucis longus, the tibial artery and vein and the deep peroneal nerve.

Note: Compartment syndrome is a collection of symptoms that signal increased pressure in the muscle compartment and results in compromised tissue perfusion. This is a medical emergency and requires immediate referral. Failure to diagnose and treat the condition can result in permanent neurovascular deficit, tissue ischaemia, limb amputation and

rhabdomyolysis[b].[14] Refer any client with persistent pain in the anterior leg with visible swelling or 'stocking' numbness or tingling for immediate surgical decompression.

Lateral compartment syndrome involves the peroneal muscles and may be associated with paraesthesia or a trickling pain on the outer lower border of the leg. This is due to compression of the superficial peroneal nerve usually from increased pressure in both the lateral and the posterior compartments. Refer any client with persistent pain and numbness or tingling in the leg and foot.

Remedial massage therapy may be beneficial for clients with chronic compartment syndrome when symptoms are mild to moderate and transient.

Assessment

HISTORY

Signs and symptoms of chronic compartment syndrome may be difficult to differentiate from shin splints. Clients describe crampy pain after exercise, relieved by rest and transient colour changes in the limb, sensations of coldness in the extremity or feet. Nerve compression produces numbness, tingling or motor loss to the dorsiflexors of the foot. Pain out of proportion to the injury and pain on passive muscle stretch are the most effective clinical observations. Paresis/paralysis, parasthesia and pallor may help in diagnosis but are late signs.[14]

The most significant risk factor for anterior compartment syndrome is fracture of the distal radius. Other factors include calcaneal fractures, male gender, age <35 years, high energy trauma, soft tissue injuries (especially in clients with bleeding disorders), open fracture, limb compression due to traction, padding and casts and surgical management of fractures.

FUNCTIONAL TESTS

Lumbar AROM do not reproduce symptoms.
Hip AROM do not reproduce symptoms.
Knee AROM do not reproduce symptoms.

---

[b]Rhabdomyolysis is a rare condition that occurs when muscle fibres die and release their contents into the bloodstream. It can have serious consequences including kidney failure.

Ankle tests

AROM: painful and limited.
PROM: painful and limited.
RROM: positive for involved muscles (pain or weakness).
Resisted and length tests: positive for involved muscles.
Special tests: negative.

PALPATION

Palpating muscles in the affected compartment elicits pain and muscle tightness is evident.

Overview of treatment and management

Treatment of chronic compartment syndrome requires vigilance for any change in signs or symptoms of neurological and vascular compression that indicate progression from transient symptoms to persistent ones which require immediate referral.

The most important massage therapy techniques for chronic compartment syndrome are myofascial release (Chapter 8) and lymphatic drainage (Chapter 9). Note: massage techniques that increase blood flow to the compartments are contraindicated, as is the application of ice on compromised circulation. Stretching of the whole lower limb kinetic chain may be useful. Discontinue treatment if symptoms are aggravated.

When pain level is reduced, articulation of the ankle, especially the talotibial articulation, can assist in the restoration of proper function of the lower limb (see Chapter 7).

- Ankle prone circumduction
- Calcaneus prone circumduction
- Tarsals prone plantarflexion
- Ankle traction
- Metatarsal shearing
- Phalanges mobilisation.

STRESS FRACTURE OF THE TIBIA

Stress fracture of the tibia is a hairline break that occurs without history of trauma. Chronic shin splints may be a precursor. It usually occurs after prolonged activity such as running, skiing or marching on a hard surface or in a hard-soled boot. Stress fracture can also occur from osteoporosis in female long-distance runners. Stress fractures require referral for medical assessment. They are diagnosed by X-ray or bone scan. Table 20.4 highlights some characteristics of shin splints, compartment syndrome and stress fracture that may be useful for determining appropriate treatment.

VARICOSE VEINS AND SPIDER VEINS

Varicose veins occur when valves in veins are damaged causing blood to pool. They commonly occur in the saphenous veins of the legs. Spider veins (telangiectasia) are small dilated blood vessels that lie close to the surface of the skin or mucous membranes. Their formation is associated with venous hypertension within varicose veins. Common locations include the face (nose, cheeks, chin), upper thigh and ankle.

Pregnancy and prolonged sitting or standing predispose to the formation of varicose veins and spider veins. Note that massage directly on varicose veins or spider veins is contraindicated.

ANKLE

It is important to rule out fracture for any traumatic ankle or foot injury. The Ottawa Ankle Rules are a clinical decision-making tool to determine the need for X-ray in injuries of the mid-foot and ankle. They have been validated in adult populations.[16] Refer any client for radiographic examination of the foot or ankle if there has been a traumatic ankle injury and any of the following are met:

- the client is unable to bear weight for four successive steps (two with each foot)
- localised tenderness along the posterior aspect of lateral or medial malleolus
- localised tenderness over the navicular, cuboid or base of 5th metatarsal

Table 20.4 Characteristics of shin splints, compartment syndrome and tibial stress fracture[15]

Shin splints	Compartment syndrome	Stress fracture
Excessive activity (e.g. running on hard or uneven ground), overtraining, poor shoes, repeated impacts on a hard surface.	Activity induced, repeated episodes, fails to respond to conservative treatment.	Following prolonged activity (e.g. marching, skiing, running), especially in a hard-soled shoe/boot. Common in athletes.
Pain anterolateral or posteromedial border tibia.	Pain out of proportion to the injury, crampy ache, tightness, swelling in the legs. Anterior compartment – pain on dorsiflexion; lateral. Compartment – pain on eversion.	Severe anterior shin pain. Acute, sharp focal pain, unilateral.
Pain decreases as the muscle warms up.	Increases with exercise (can continue to increase for a short time after exercise).	Constant, increasing with exercise. Worse with impact.
Pain worse in morning and after exercise.	Occasionally muscle weakness or sensory symptoms.	Night ache. May be worse in morning.
Palpatory tenderness over a wide region of the tibia and involved muscle.	Tightness evident on palpation.	Palpation elicits localised pain.

Adapted from Brukner P, Khan K. Clinical sports medicine. 4th edn. North Ryde, NSW: McGraw-Hill; 2012.

ACHILLES TENDINOPATHY

The Achilles tendon is commonly injured in running and sports that involve jumping. The client complains of pain and tenderness along the Achilles tendon. An injury to the Achilles tendon may be insertional or non-insertional and a partial or complete (total) rupture, Achilles tedenopathy can be categorised according to the location of the pathology. According to frequency of injury these include:

- Mid-portion Achilles tendinopathy located 2–6 cm above the insertion of the Achilles tendon into the calcaneus where the tendon becomes poorly vascularised
- Insertional Achilles tendinopathy where the tendon degrades at the point of insertion into the calcaneus[17]

Continued sustained overloading of tendons leads to stress relaxation, deformation or 'creep' and eventually tearing occurs.[3] It is associated with shoes with heels that are too low, excessive dorsiflexion on uphill areas, tight calf muscles, shoes with insufficient flexibility in the soles, overpronation of the ankle or excessive activity on hard surfaces. Most of the histological findings in tendinopathy suggest chronic degeneration, regeneration and microtears in the tendon and the absence of evidence of acute inflammation. However, recent work on biopsied tendon tissue provided evidence of an inflammatory process. For example, a marked accumulation of macrophages, stromal fibroblasts primed for inflammation and increased collagen turnover have been identified. Gene expression analysis identified activation of pro-inflammatory pathways that might contribute to the neovascularisation.[18]

Assessment

HISTORY

The client presents with pain in the Achilles tendon above the heel. Pain increases with activity and stretching and decreases with rest. Morning pain is common in chronic cases. There is usually a history of repetitive overuse (e.g. running, jumping).

FUNCTIONAL TESTS

Lumbar AROM tests do not reproduce symptoms.
Hip AROM tests do not reproduce symptoms.
Knee AROM tests do not reproduce symptoms.

Ankle tests

AROM: painful plantarflexion.
PROM: painful dorsiflexion as the muscles are passively stretched.
RROM: positive for plantarflexion.
Resisted and length tests for specific muscles: positive for gastrocnemius and soleus.
Special tests: negative. (Note: squeezing the Achilles from the sides increases pain.)
Thompson test positive in complete Achilles tendon rupture.

PALPATION

Tenderness is elicited in the tendon above the heel.

Overview of treatment and management

If acute, ice application may provide pain relief. Advise the client to avoid any aggravating activities. Using a small heel lift or using higher-heeled shoes is often useful for decreasing pain. Commence range of motion exercises as soon as pain permits.

A typical remedial massage treatment for subacute or chronic Achilles tendinopathy includes:

- Swedish massage therapy to the lower limb, low back and pelvis.
- Remedial massage techniques including (see Table 20.3):
  - deep gliding frictions along the muscle fibres
  - cross-fibre frictions
  - soft tissue releasing techniques (see Figure 20.36)
  - deep transverse friction applied directly to the site of lesion, which may help stimulate collagen production
  - trigger point therapy
  - muscle stretching.
- Focus treatment on agonists and antagonists to restore optimal range of motion (e.g. gastrocnemius, soleus, hip external rotators).
- Myofascial release including cross-arm techniques and the leg pull (see Chapter 8).
- Other remedial techniques such as ankle joint articulation may also be introduced as required (see Chapter 7):
  - ankle prone circumduction
  - calcaneus prone circumduction
  - tarsals prone plantarflexion

Key assessment findings for achilles tendinopathy

- Achilles tendon pain, history of repetitive overuse (e.g. running, jumping)
- Functional tests:
  - AROM: painful plantarflexion
  - PROM: painful dorsiflexion as the muscle is passively stretched
  - RROM: positive for plantarflexion
  - Resisted and length tests tests positive for gastrocnemius ± soleus
  - Special tests: negative
- Palpation: tenderness and pain along the tendon, usually 2–6 cm above calcaneus.

Fig. 20.36 Soft tissue release for Achilles tendinitis

Retrocalcaneal bursa

Subcutaneous bursa
of medial malleolus

Subcutaneous
calcaneal bursa

Fig. 20.37   Calcaneal bursae

- ankle traction
- metatarsal shearing
- phalanges mobilisation.

Correct underlying biomechanical and predisposing factors if possible (e.g. excessive ankle pronation, muscle imbalances).

CLIENT EDUCATION

Advise the client to rest from aggravating activities to reduce the stress on the damaged tendons. Replace low-heeled or worn-out shoes. Adequate warm-up/stretching of the calf muscles is required before exercise. Gradually introduce toe and forefoot raises and eccentric exercises (e.g. standing on edge of a step and dropping the heel below the level of the step). Refer for osseous manipulation if required.

CALCANEAL BURSITIS

The bursa which cushions the insertion of the Achilles tendon at the heel can become inflamed, usually from direct rubbing from shoes in which the upper border heel counter is too tight, too loose or convex (see Figure 20.37). Bursitis can also follow a direct impact on the heel. The client complains of pain at the Achilles insertion which may be swollen.

Treatment

Ice applications are used to provide pain relief. A heel pad may be worn to protect the area from further rubbing. Avoid wearing the offending shoes. In the subacute phase, the remedial massage approach prescribed for Achilles tendinopathy may be applied.

SEVER'S DISEASE

Sever's disease is a common foot problem in active children aged 8 to 15 years. It is a traction apophysitis at the Achilles insertion into the calcaneus that often occurs during rapid growth spurts when bone growth can cause muscles and tendons to become tight.

Assessment

HISTORY

The client is a physically active adolescent (8 to 15 years) who complains of heel pain, which is aggravated by activity and relieved by rest.

Key assessment findings for Sever's disease

- The client is a physically active adolescent (8 to 15 years); history of pain at the Achilles insertion that is aggravated by activity and relieved by rest
- Functional tests:
  - AROM: painful plantarflexion
  - PROM: painful dorsiflexion as the calf muscles are passively stretched
  - RROM: positive for ankle plantarflexion
  - Resisted and length tests: postitive for ankle plantarflexors
  - Special tests: negative
- Palpation: tenderness and swelling at the Achilles insertion

FUNCTIONAL TESTS

Lumbar AROM tests do not reproduce symptoms.
Hip AROM tests do not reproduce symptoms.
Knee AROM tests do not reproduce symptoms.

Ankle tests

AROM: painful plantarflexion.
PROM: painful dorsiflexion as the muscles are passively stretched.
RROM: positive for plantarflexion.
Resisted and length tests for specific muscles: positive for gastrocnemius and soleus.
Special tests: negative.

PALPATION

Palpation at the Achilles insertion elicits tenderness or pain. Swelling may be present. Palpation may reveal tightness in the gastrocnemius and soleus muscles.

Overview of treatment and management

Advise the client to reduce the level of physical activity for one to two weeks. Ice application after exercise may help control pain. Shoes should be replaced when they become too small or if the heel counter is too tight. The condition can become chronic and persist until about 16 years of age. Massage therapy in chronic cases focuses on restoring muscle balance, especially of gastrocnemius, soleus and tibialis anterior.

ANKLE SPRAIN

The ankle is a hinge joint supported by ligament on either side. The medial deltoid ligament is the strongest of the ankle ligaments. Consequently eversion sprains are rare and when they do occur often involve fractures or ligament avulsions. Any client with an eversion sprain should be referred for further investigation. Inversion sprains account for the majority of ankle sprains.[19] The lateral collateral ligaments, from weakest to strongest, are the anterior talofibular ligament, the calcaneofibular ligament and the posterior talofibular ligament (see Figure 20.38 on p 421).

Sprains can occur as a result of improper landing on the foot, muscle tightness/weakness or proprioception deficit. Inversion sprains are likely to be worse if the foot is both inverted and plantar flexed. Bruising will often occur after the injury and is likely to remain for some weeks.

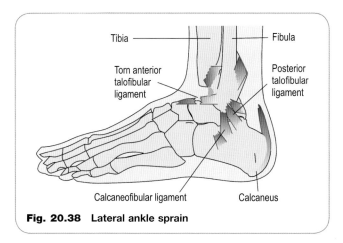

Fig. 20.38 **Lateral ankle sprain**

Key assessment findings for inversion ankle sprain

- History of rolling onto the outside of the ankle; may be accompanied by a popping or tearing sensation; swelling.
- Functional tests:
  - AROM: painful inversion
  - PROM: painful inversion
  - RROM: negative (unless associated muscle strain)
  - Special test: positive (ankle anterior draw, posterior draw and/or lateral ligament stability)
- Palpation: tenderness and swelling at the site of ligament damage

---

Assessment

HISTORY

The client reports rolling onto the lateral side of the ankle. This may be accompanied by a popping or tearing. Swelling occurs over the anterior talofibular ligament. Bruising may follow in the next day or two.

FUNCTIONAL TESTS

Lumbar AROM tests do not reproduce symptoms.
Hip AROM tests do not reproduce symptoms.
Knee AROM tests do not reproduce symptoms.

Ankle tests

AROM: painful inversion.
PROM: painful inversion.
RROM: negative unless the injury is accompanied by muscle strain.
Resisted and length tests for specific muscles: negative (unless associated muscle strain).
Special tests: positive ankle anterior draw (anterior talofibular ligament sprain), posterior draw (posterior talofibular ligament sprain), or lateral ligament stability (calcaneofibular ligament).

PALPATION

Tenderness is elicited anterior to the lateral malleolus in anterior talofibular sprain and inferior to the malleolus in calcaneofibular sprain. Swelling is usually evident. Suspect fracture if tenderness is present posterior or superior to the lateral malleolus.

Overview of treatment and management

The treatment goal immediately after the injury is to decrease pain, increase pain-free range of motion and to protect the ankle from further damage. For acute sprains ice applications may provide pain relief. Ankle splints and taping provide protection for the joint. Reduce weight bearing (crutches may be required). Commence pain-free range of motion exercises as soon as pain permits. A concern for healthcare providers is the potential progression of acute ankle sprains to chronic problems, including arthritic changes in the talocrural joint. Manual joint mobilisation is recommended to diminish pain and increase dorsiflexion range of motion. A 2017 overview of systematic reviews with meta-analysis on ankle sprain found strong evidence for early mobilisation and non-steroidal anti-inflammatory drugs for acute ankle sprains. For pain, swelling and function there is moderate evidence supporting exercise and manual therapy techniques.[20] There was insufficient evidence to support the use of ultrasound and conflicting evidence regarding the efficacy of surgery and acupuncture for the treatment of acute ankle sprains. To prevent recurrence there is strong evidence for bracing and moderate evidence for neuromuscular training.[20]

A typical remedial massage treatment for subacute or chronic ankle inversion sprain includes:

- Swedish massage therapy to the lower limb, low back and pelvis.
- Remedial massage techniques including:
  - light lymphatic drainage to promote reduction of swelling
  - deep transverse friction at the site of lesion to help prevent adhesion formation. This should be performed within the client's pain tolerance. Recommendations vary as to how long to perform deep transverse friction. Good results have been obtained with short applications (20–30 seconds) interspersed with active movement and other massage strokes.
- Massage techniques for associated muscle strains (e.g. peroneal muscles) or tightness include (see Table 20.3 on p 410):
  - deep gliding frictions along the muscle fibres
  - cross-fibre frictions
  - soft tissue releasing techniques
  - trigger point therapy
  - muscle stretching.

Use the client's pain threshold as a guide for when to progress to more vigorous massage techniques.

- Myofascial release including cross-arm techniques (see Chapter 8).
- Ankle joint articulation is introduced when appropriate (see Chapter 7). Note that initially active movement is preferred to passive movements for safety.

Longer-term management involves correcting underlying biomechanical and predisposing factors where possible (e.g. genu varum, weak ankle everters and/or tight ankle inverters).

Client education

Early mobilisation is important to stimulate collagen production. Most ankles regain functional mobility within several weeks. However, full structural recovery takes longer (1–2 months for Grade 1 sprains, 6–12 months for Grade 2 sprains and up to 1 year for Grade 3 sprains).[3,17] Grade 1 injuries are usually managed with RICE for 2 or 3 days before complete weight bearing can commence. Rehabilitation of Grade 2 and 3 sprains is generally divided into three phases:[21]

1. Ice application, compression bandaging, non-weight-bearing according to pain.
2. Rehabilitation of movement, strength and proprioception of the ankle: Rehabilitation begins with isometric exercises of the ankle everters, active pain-free ankle range of motion. Progressively increase walking distance and speed. Resisted theraband/elastic tubing exercises for ankle everters, dorsiflexors and eventually inverters are gradually introduced. Calf muscle strengthening exercises and balance drills can be introduced. Restoring neuromuscular control appears to be vital for functional stability of the joint.[22] To improve proprioception, for example, the client can trace the letters of the alphabet in the air with their big toe.
3. Exercises and retraining of specific skills. In the late rehabilitation phase clients can use wobble boards, hopping and sports-specific drills including running forward and backward, sudden stopping and zig-zagging.

For some clients laxity of ligaments permits recurrent inversion sprain. This is thought to occur because of neuromuscular deficits such as impaired balance, reduced joint position sense, slower firing of peroneal muscles, slower nerve conduction velocity, impaired cutaneous sensation, strength deficits and decreased dorsiflexion range of motion.[22] Rehabilitation should therefore address restoration of neuromuscular function as well as mechanical stability.[20] Encourage clients to continue active proprioceptive training and massage therapy for optimal muscle balance and neuromuscular control. A 2015 study of grade 2 ankle sprain patients compared a massage treatment group to an ankle brace control group.[23] The massage group received 15-minute effleurage and friction massages on their ankles administered by a sport rehabilitation specialist and professional massager. The control group used ankle braces. The 8-week study found that the massage group had significant benefit in range of motion (dorsiflexion, plantarflexion, inversion and eversion), thera-band strength test and balance board test.[23] Another study found that balance training decreased the incidence of ankle sprains and increased dynamic neuromuscular control, postural sway, and the joint position sense in athletes.[24]

ANKLE IMPINGMENT SYNDROME

Impingement refers to entrapment of structures causing pain or restricted range of motion. Ankle impingement syndrome encompasses a range of bone and soft tissue pathologies that can be broadly classified as anterior and posterior.[24] Anterior ankle impingement usually refers to entrapment caused by osteophytes at the anterior tibial margin and the talar neck during dorsiflexion.[26] It is also called 'footballer's ankle' because it is commonly observed in professional soccer players. It is often a consequence of incomplete healing following lateral ankle sprain. Posterior ankle impingement is caused by compression of structures posterior to the tibiotalar and talocalcaneal joints during end-range plantar flexion.[25]

Assessment

HISTORY

Anterior ankle impingement

Ankle pain persisting 6 months after inversion injury sprain; pain at full dorsiflexion; aggravated by climbing stairs, running or walking uphill, climbing ladders, deep squatting; locking sensation or snapping during dorsiflexion and eversion.

Posterior ankle impingement

Pain deep to Achilles tendon; pain at full plantar flexion; aggravated by repetitive push-offs, including downhill running and walking, descending stairs, high-heeled shoes; common in dancers.

FUNCTIONAL TESTS

Lumbar AROM do not reproduce symptoms.
Hip AROM do not reproduce symptoms.
Knee AROM do not reproduce symptoms.

Ankle tests

AROM: painful ± limited (dorsiflexion for anterior ankle impingement/plantarflexion for posterior impingement).
PROM: painful ± limited (dorsiflexion for anterior ankle impingement/plantarflexion for posterior impingement).
RROM usually negative.
Resisted and length tests for specific muscles: usually negative.
Special tests: positive impingement sign.

PALPATION

Anterior and anterolateral tenderness in anterior ankle impingement; posterior impingement more difficult to elicit and localise tenderness.

Overview of treatment and management

For acute symptoms, rest and avoidance of aggravating activities is recommended. Ice and non-steroidal anti-inflammatory drugs are often used. In chronic cases footwear modification, including heel lift orthoses to limit dorsiflexion have been used.

A typical remedial massage treatment for ankle impingement syndrome includes:

- Swedish massage therapy to the lower limb, low back and pelvis.
- Remedial massage techniques including:
  - joint articulation (see Chapter 7)
  - ankle prone circumduction
  - calcaneus prone circumduction
  - tarsals prone plantarflexion
  - ankle traction
  - metatarsal shearing
  - phalanges mobilisation.
- Heat therapy.
- Myofascial release (see Chapter 8).
- Massage techniques for associated muscle strains or imbalances include (see Table 20.3 on p 410):
  - deep gliding frictions along the muscle fibres
  - cross-fibre frictions

- soft tissue releasing techniques
- trigger point therapy
- muscle stretching.

Correct underlying biomechanical and predisposing factors where possible (e.g. leg length inequality).

Client education

Advise the client of the importance of avoiding aggravating activities and of an exercise rehabilitation program to reduce pain and optimise long-term function. Heat packs may be useful for pain relief.

PALPATION

Anterior and anterolateral tenderness in anterior ankle impingement; posterior impingement more difficult to elicit and localise tenderness.

OSTEOARTHRITIS OF THE ANKLE

Osteoarthritis is common in older patients or those with significant previous trauma. Clients complain of limited range of motion and chronic pain which is aggravated by weight-bearing activity.

Assessment

HISTORY

The client is older or has a history of previous significant trauma and complains of limited range of motion and/or chronic pain. Pain is aggravated by weight-bearing activity and slight swelling may be present. The client may complain of morning stiffness.

FUNCTIONAL TESTS

Lumbar AROM do not reproduce symptoms.
Hip AROM do not reproduce symptoms.
Knee AROM do not reproduce symptoms.

Ankle tests

AROM: limited ± painful (plantarflexion/dorsiflexion).
PROM: limited ± painful (plantarflexion/dorsiflexion); hard end-feel and crepitus.

RROM negative unless the injury is accompanied by muscle strain or contracture.
Resisted and length tests for specific muscles: negative (unless associated muscle strain or contracture).
Special tests: negative.

PALPATION

Diffuse tenderness may be elicited on palpation around the joint.

Overview of treatment and management

Treatment of osteoarthritis is based on weight loss, exercise and self-management of acute flare-ups. Episodes of acute inflammation can occur after excessive weight-bearing activity and can be treated with with ice applications and anti-inflammatory medications.

A typical remedial massage treatment for chronic osteoarthritis of the ankle includes:

- Swedish massage therapy to the lower limb, low back and pelvis.
- Remedial massage techniques including:
  - joint articulation (see Chapter 7)
  - ankle prone circumduction
  - calcaneus prone circumduction
  - tarsals prone plantarflexion
  - ankle traction
  - metatarsal shearing
  - phalanges mobilisation.
- Heat therapy.
- Myofascial release (see Chapter 8).
- Massage techniques for associated muscle strains (e.g. peroneal muscles) or tightness include (see Table 20.3 on p 410):
  - deep gliding frictions along the muscle fibres
  - cross-fibre frictions
  - soft tissue releasing techniques
  - trigger point therapy
  - muscle stretching.

Correct underlying biomechanical and predisposing factors where possible (e.g. pes planus, leg length inequality).

Client education

Advise the client of the importance of exercise to manage their condition. Heat packs may be useful for pain relief. Recommend weight loss if clients are overweight and shock-absorbing soles should always be worn. Low-impact exercises like swimming, Tai Chi and paddling should be encouraged.

FOOT

Many remedial massage clients suffer with foot pain, often the result of poor biomechanics from congenital problems (e.g. pes planus or cavus, hallux valgus or ankle pronation) or from many years of poor-fitting shoes. Remedial massage usually consists of Swedish massage, passive joint articulation to the ankles and toes and advice about weight loss and supportive shoes. A common condition encountered in remedial massage practice is plantar fasciitis.

PLANTAR FASCIITIS (HEEL SPUR)

Plantar fasciitis is the most common cause of painful feet and it occurs more often in women than men. The plantar fascia contributes to arch support and shock absorption of the foot. It attaches proximally to the anterior calcaneus and distally to the fascia that crosses the metatarsal heads and extends into the toes. Biomechanical dysfunction in the foot, particularly associated with excessive pronation and lowered longitudinal arch or with pes cavus, places excessive tension on the plantar fascia at the medial tubercle of the anterior calcaneus. Prolonged tensile stress on the periosteum may lead to the development of a bony spur. A spur may also develop in the insertion of the Achilles tendon to the superior part of the calcaneus (dancer's heel).

Assessment

HISTORY

Two types of clients are typical: (1) non-athletic middle-aged women, and (2) distance runners and basketball players. Pain on the sole of the foot at the front of the heel is the main complaint. The pain commonly radiates forward to the middle of the foot. The pain is worse on the first few steps on standing and improves as walking continues but worsens again at the end of the day or the next morning. Plantar fasciitis may be associated with standing for prolonged periods on a hard floor.

FUNCTIONAL TESTS

Lumbar AROM tests do not reproduce symptoms.
Hip AROM tests do not reproduce symptoms.
Knee AROM tests do not reproduce symptoms.

Ankle tests

AROM: painful plantarflexion.
PROM: painful dorsiflexion of ankle, extension of toes.
RROM: may be positive for toe flexion.
Resisted and length tests: may be positive for flexor digitorum brevis.
Special tests: Windlass test positive.

PALPATION

Pain is elicited on palpation at the medial tubercle of the calcaneus.

Overview of treatment and management

In the acute phase, ice application may provide pain relief. A small heel lift or wearing a shoe with a slightly elevated heel helps decrease the pain. Refer for osseous manipulation and acupuncture.

A typical remedial massage treatment for subacute or chronic plantar fasciitis includes:

- Swedish massage therapy to the lower limb, low back and pelvis.
- Remedial massage techniques including:
  - myofascial release (see Chapter 8)
    - gentle myofascial release (see Figure 20.39)
    - deep myofascial release
    For example, longitudinal gliding of the plantar fascia (glide towards the calcaneus to avoid additional stress on the fascia), and cross-fibre frictions on the fascia, avoiding pressure on the medial tubercle (see Figure 20.40 on p 425).
  - passive joint articulation (see Chapter 7)
    - ankle prone circumduction
    - calcaneus prone circumduction
    - tarsals prone plantarflexion
    - ankle traction

Key assessment findings for plantar fasciitis

- History of overuse (e.g. distance running) in athletes: non-athletic middle-aged women. Client complains of pain at the front of the heel on the sole of the foot on the first few steps after rising
- Functional tests:
  - AROM: painful plantarflexion
  - PROM: painful dorsiflexion, extension of toes
  - RROM: may be positive for toe flexors (flexor digitorum brevis)
  - Resisted and length tests may be positive for affected muscles
  - Special tests: Windlass test positive
- Palpation: tenderness or pain at the medial tubercle of the calcaneus

Fig. 20.39 Myofascial release for the foot

Fig. 20.40 Deep myofascial release for plantar fasciitis

- metatarsal shearing
- phalanges mobilisation.
- Techniques for associated muscle tightness (especially flexor digitorum brevis, gastrocnemius, soleus and tibial muscles) include (see Table 20.3 on p 410):
  - deep gliding frictions along the muscle fibres
  - cross-fibre frictions
  - soft tissue releasing techniques
  - trigger point therapy
  - muscle stretching.

Correct underlying biomechanical and predisposing factors (e.g. pes planus, leg length inequality) where possible.

Client education

Advise the client of the importance of restoring normal biomechanics of the foot. Stretching the fascia by standing on a step and dropping the heels below the level of the step or rolling the foot over a tennis or golf ball may be useful. Progressively introduce a program of stretching and strengthening exercises to promote optimal function of muscles of the lower limb. Recommend weight loss if clients are overweight. Shock-absorbing soles should always be worn. Refer clients for orthotics if required. Kinesiotaping could also be considered. A 2016 systematic review on the effectiveness of soft tissue therapy for the management of musculoskeletal disorders and injuries of the upper and lower extremities found that myofascial release to the gastrocnemius,

and soleus was effective in the treatment of plantar fasciitis.[27] However, trigger point therapy, when combined with self-stretching, provided limited or no additional benefit. Another study on the effectiveness of multimodal care for soft tissue injuries of the lower limb found that mobilisation and stretching exercise may be beneficial for persistent plantar heel pain.[28]

FOREFOOT

METATARSALGIA

Metatarsalgia refers to tenderness under the 2nd and 3rd (occasionally 3rd and 4th) metatarsal heads following collapse of the transverse metatarsal arch. Often a callus develops under the foot. Chronic foot biomechanical dysfunction causes changes in weight bearing from the heel and 1st metatarsal to the 2nd to 4th metatarsals. Metatarsalgia is associated with prolonged standing on a hard surface, pes planus, pregnancy, hallux valgus, high heels, pes cavus, short gastrocnemius and poor footwear. Often a change of shoes, especially to a higher heel, triggers the condition.

Treatment

The purpose of remedial massage is to improve the biomechanics of the foot. Massage therapy includes Swedish massage and a range of remedial massage techniques designed to optimise muscle function and to mobilise the ankle and foot, such as passive joint articulation (see Chapter 7), myofascial release, deep gliding, cross-fibre frictions, soft-tissue release techniques, trigger point therapy and muscle stretching. Correct underlying biomechanical and predisposing factors where possible.

CLIENT EDUCATION

Advise the client to wear supportive shoes and to avoid high-heeled shoes. A metatarsal bar (transverse arch support) may be worn under the metatarsal heads. Exercises to strengthen intrinsic foot muscles and stretches for gastrocnemius and hamstrings are recommended. Referral to a podiatrist, chiropractor, osteopath or physiotherapist may be required.

MORTON'S NEUROMA (INTERDIGITAL NEUROMA)

A fusiform swelling develops on the interdigital nerve following chronic compression by the metatarsal heads, most commonly between the 3rd and 4th metatarsal heads. The client complains of tenderness at the site and may report numbness in the interdigital space distal to the neuroma. Symptoms are relieved by removing the shoe.

Treatment

Advise the client to wear shoes that are wide enough to avoid compressing the metatarsal heads. Remedial massage treatment focuses on improving the biomechanics of the foot using such techniques as myofascial release, passive joint articulation (see Chapter 7) and muscle techniques for reducing muscle tightness (see Table 20.3 on p 410).

KEY MESSAGES

- Assessment of clients with conditions of the leg, ankle and foot involves history, outcome measures, postural analysis, gait analysis, functional tests and palpation.
- Assessment findings may indicate the type of tissue involved (contractile or inert, muscle, joint, fascia, ligament), duration of condition (acute or chronic), and severity (grade).
- Assessment findings may indicate a common presenting condition such as ankle sprains, shin splints and plantar fasciitis.
- Assessment findings also indicate client perception of injury and preferences for treatment.
- Consider Clinical Guidelines, available evidence and client preferences when planning therapy.

- Although serious conditions of the lower limb, ankle and foot are rare, be vigilant for red flags during assessment.
- The selection of remedial massage techniques depends on assessment results. Swedish massage to the lower limb, low back and pelvis may be followed by muscle techniques (e.g. deep gliding, cross-fibre frictions, soft tissue releasing techniques, trigger point therapy, deep transverse friction and muscle stretching), passive joint articulation, myofascial release and thermotherapy as indicated.
- Educating clients about likely causal and predisposing factors and exercise rehabilitation are essential parts of remedial massage therapy.
- Prioritise the client self-help component of treatment wherever possible to reduce likelihood of recurrence and/or to promote health maintenance and illness prevention.

Review questions

1. The symptoms of anterior compartment syndrome include:
   a) a dull ache along the anteromedial border of the tibia which is aggravated by activity
   b) weakness of the dorsiflexors of the foot
   c) night ache
   d) pain and paraesthesia in the sole of the foot
2. Which test is likely to reproduce symptoms in a client with tennis leg?
   a) resisted ankle plantarflexion
   b) posterior draw test
   c) passive ankle plantarflexion
   d) resisted ankle dorsiflexion
3. Which statement does not apply to plantar fasciitis?
   a) Pain is increased with dorsiflexion of the foot.
   b) Tenderness is felt at the posteromedial aspect of the calcaneus.
   c) Pain is worse with the first few steps on rising.
   d) Tenderness is felt on the sole of the foot between the 3rd and 4th metatarsal heads.
4. The most commonly sprained ankle ligament is:
   a) anterior talofibular ligament
   b) calcaneofibular ligament

   c) talofibular ligament
   d) deltoid ligament
5. Heel pain in a very active 10-year-old boy is most likely to be:
   a) Osgood-Schlatter's disease
   b) Sever's disease
   c) Achilles tendinitis
   d) Retrocalcaneal bursitis
6. i) What are shin splints?
   ii) How would you differentiate shin splints from a stress fracture of the tibia?
   iii) What treatment (including advice) would you give a client with shin splints?
7. Where would you palpate the anterior talotibial ligament?
8. Describe your treatment for lateral ankle sprain:
   i) in the acute phase
   ii) in the chronic phase
9. Name some common predisposing or causative factors of plantar fasciitis.
10. A client presents with calf pain. List three signs or symptoms that would make you suspect deep venous thrombosis.

REFERENCES

1. Hill CL, Menz HB, Taylor A. Prevalence and correlates of foot pain in a population-based study: the North West Adelaide health study. J Foot Ankle Res 2008;1:2. https://doi.org/10.1186/1757-1146-1-2.
2. Thomas MJ, Ruddy E, Zhang W, et al. The population prevalence of foot and ankle pain in middle and old age: a systematic review. Pain 2011;152(12):2870–80.
3. Bleecker G. Achilles tendon injury: incidence, etiologies, treatments, and outcomes. Parkway: ProQuest Dissertations and Theses; 2017.
4. Cleland J, Koppenhaver S, Su J. Netter's orthopaedic clinical examination: an evidence-based approach. 3rd edn. Philadelphia: Saunders; 2015.
5. Shane AM, Reeves CL, Vazales R, et al. Soft tissue impingement of the ankle: pathophysiology, evaluation, and arthroscopic treatment. Clin Podiatr Med Sur 2016;33(4):503–20.
6. American College of Occupational and Environmental Medicine. Ankle and foot disorders

guideline. Online. Available: https://www.dir.ca.gov/dwc/MTUS/ACOEM_Guidelines/Ankle-and-Foot-Disorders-Guideline.pdf; 2015.
7. Klingman R, Godges J. Red flags for potentially serious conditions in patients with knee, leg, ankle and foot problems. Online. Available: xnet.kp.org/socal_rehabspecialists/ptr_library/09FootRegion/01MedicalScreening-KneeLegAnkleandFootRegions.pdf; 2009.
8. Carnes M, Vizniak N. Quick reference evidence-based conditions manual. 3rd edn. Burnaby, BC: Professional Health Systems; 2009.
9. Murat E, Tahsin A, Nurettin T, et al. Factors affecting insole usage in patients with pes planus. Sanamed 2018;13(2):139–43.
10. Pita-Fernandez S, Gonzalez-Martin C, Alonso-Tajes F, et al. Flat foot in a random population and its impact on quality of life and functionality. J Clin Diagn Res 2017;11(4):LC22–LC27.

11. Reese N, Bandy WD, Yates C. Joint range of motion and muscle length testing. 2nd edn. St. Louis, MO: Saunders/Elsevier; 2010.
12. Simons D, Travell J, Simons L. Myofascial pain and dysfunction: the trigger point manual. Volume 1 Upper half of body. 2nd edn. Philadelphia: Williams & Wilkins; 1999.
13. Winters M. Medial tibial stress syndrome: diagnosis, treatment and outcome assessment. Br J Sports Med 2018;52(18):1213–14.
14. Ali P, Santy-Tomlinson J, Watson R. Assessment and diagnosis of acute limb compartment syndrome: a literature review. J Orthop and Trauma Nurs 2014; 18(4):180–90.
15. Brukner P, Khan K. Clinical sports medicine. 4th edn. North Ryde, NSW: McGraw-Hill; 2012.
16. Clark J. The role of Ottawa Ankle Rules and expansion of nurse-initiated X-ray of lower limbs in a paediatric emergency department. Neonatal,

Paediatric and Child Health Nursing 2015;
18(2):16–21.

17. Bleecker GA. Achilles tendon injury: incidence,
etiologies, treatments, and outcomes. ProQuest
Number: 10606473. Ann Arbor, MI: ProQuest
Dissertations and Theses; 2015.

18. Mendias C. Inflammation in tendinopathy: the
pendulum swings. Translational Sports Med
2018;1(3):103.

19. Gribble A, Bleakley CM, Caulfield BM, et al. 2016
consensus statement of the International Ankle
Consortium: prevalence, impact and long-term
consequences of lateral ankle sprains. Br J Sports
Med 2016:50:1493–5.

20. Doherty C, Bleakley C, Delahunt E, et al. Treatment
and prevention of acute and recurrent ankle
sprain: an overview of systematic reviews with
meta-analysis. Br J Sports Med 2017;51(2):113–25.

21. Czajka CM, Tran E, Cai AN, et al. Ankle sprains
and instability. Med Clin N Am 2014;98(2):
313–29.

22. Ju S, Park G. Effects of the application of ankle
functional rehabilitation exercise on the ankle joint
functional movement screen and isokinetic muscular
function in patients with chronic ankle sprain.
J Phys Ther Sci 2017;29(2):278–81.

23. Mehdi. Effect of friction technique on ankle sprain
grade II treatment. Biomed Pharmacol J 2015;
8(2):523–8.

24. De Vasconcelos G, Cini A, Sbruzzi G, et al. Effects
of proprioceptive training on the incidence of
ankle sprain in athletes: systematic review and
meta-analysis. Clin Rehabil 2018; 32(12):
1581–90.

25. Lavery KP, McHale KJ, Rossy WH, et al. Ankle
impingement. J Ortho Sur Res 2016;11(1):97.

26. Molinier F, Benoist J, Colin F, et al. Does
antero-lateral ankle impingement exist? Orthop
Traumatol-Sur 2017;103:S249–S252.

27. Piper S, Shearer H, Cote P, et al. The effectiveness
of soft-tissue therapy for the management of
musculoskeletal disorders and injuries of the upper
and lower extremities: a systematic review by the
Ontario Protocol for Traffic Injury Management
(OPTIMa) collaboration. Manual Ther 2016;21:
18–34.

28. Sutton DA, Nordin M, Côté P, et al. The
effectiveness of multimodal care for soft tissue
injuries of the lower extremity: a systematic
review by the Ontario Protocol for Traffic
Injury Management (OPTIMa) collaboration.
J Manipulative Physiol Ther 2016;39(2):95–109.e2.

21 Specific client groups

Learning Outcomes

- Assess suitability of clients from specific client groups (children and adolescents, women, men, geriatric clients, clients with a mental illness and sports people) for remedial massage.
- Describe the current evidence for the effectiveness of massage for these clients.
- Manage specialised remedial massage treatments, including obtaining informed consent and selecting appropriate techniques and duration of treatment, for these clients.
- Provide specialised remedial massage treatment for these clients.

INTRODUCTION

Contraindications and precautions for the remedial massage techniques described in this book have been discussed in each chapter. This chapter brings together special considerations for the following remedial massage clients:

- children and adolescents
- women
- men
- geriatric clients
- clients with a mental illness
- sports people.

In the following sections special considerations for both assessing and treating these specific client groups are discussed.

CHILDREN AND ADOLESCENTS

Childhood is the period of life between infancy and the onset of puberty. The importance of cultivating a practice of paediatric clients lies in the long-term benefits of prevention and early intervention of many musculoskeletal conditions. Any trauma has the potential to disrupt normal musculoskeletal development, and the longer excessive stresses and strains persist in the body, the greater the potential disturbance to a developing skeleton. Physical therapy interventions should be commenced as soon as possible following major trauma. Children often respond well to treatment and can make sustained recoveries. Left untreated, compensations to musculoskeletal

distortions can become entrenched and more difficult to treat over time. Remedial massage therapy may also be beneficial in management of such conditions as Osgood-Schlatter's disease, adolescent idiopathic scoliosis and slipped capital femoral epiphysis, often when used to support chiropractic, osteopathy and physiotherapy care.

IMPORTANT CONSIDERATIONS FOR ASSESSING AND TREATING CHILDREN

- A parent or guardian is required to give informed consent for all children under 18 years of age and must be present throughout the consultation. However, it is generally accepted that most young people over 16 are capable of giving their own informed consent. The mature minor principle has been confirmed in Australian common law: minors (< 18 years) may be able to give informed consent if they have sufficient understanding and intelligence to enable full understanding of what is proposed.
- It is every practitioner's responsibility to report any suspected case of child abuse to the statutory child protection service in their jurisdiction. For example, in New South Wales it is mandatory for 'a person who in the course of his or her professional work or other paid employment delivers health care, welfare, education, children's services, residential services or law enforcement, wholly or partly to children' to report suspected cases of child abuse and neglect.[1]
- Be vigilant during assessment for musculoskeletal conditions affecting children that require referral to a medical practitioner, chiropractor, osteopath or physiotherapist. Such conditions include congenital foot problems, congenital hip dysplasia, Osgood-Schlatter's disease, Perthes' disease, capital femoral slipped epiphysis, adolescent idiopathic scoliosis (see Table 21.1 on p 429), and trauma to growth plates and other vulnerable areas (e.g. condylar process of the temporomandibular joint which consists of thin cartilage).
- Modify treatment to suit the age, size and personality of the child. Keep consultations short for young children. A parent or guardian may be recruited to distract the child or assist by holding them during the treatment. Apply techniques lightly and slowly. A reward system (e.g. balloons and stickers) may be useful for establishing a child-friendly practice.
- Adolescence is the period between childhood and adulthood. It is a period of growing autonomy marked by the onset of puberty and involves both biological and psychosocial changes. Adolescents develop physically, cognitively

Table 21.1 Common musculoskeletal conditions affecting children

Congenital foot problems	Check the borders of the foot. Many foot problems arise from in utero positioning and will be self-limiting. A guideline for deciding when to refer a client with congenital foot problems is to determine if the deviation is passively over-correctable (i.e. can the foot be passively moved slightly beyond the correcting position?). Refer all conditions that are not passively over-correctable, such as: ■ metatarsus adductus (lateral border of foot is convex and the medial border concave). If the adducted forefoot is not passively over-correctable refer for further investigation; ■ metatarsus primus varus (adduction of hallux, i.e. the hallux points inwards and there is a large space between the first and second metatarsals). Avoid narrow shoes to prevent the development of bunions; ■ clubfoot (congenital talipes equinovarus).
Pronated foot (flat foot)	An infant's foot looks flat because of a fat pad under the longitudinal arch. Flexible pronated feet (flat feet) are common and usually do not require treatment in children up to 5 years of age. If the foot is inflexible (i.e. unable to be passively over-corrected) refer for further examination. Pronation observed when the child begins to take weight on their lower limbs could be the result of a short Achilles tendon (refer for further examination if the foot cannot be passively dorsiflexed past neutral), an in-toeing gait (refer for further examination if the foot does not assume the normal position when non-weight bearing) or rigid flat foot (refer for further examination if the pronation does not disappear when non-weight bearing and cannot be passively over-corrected). Pronating feet in children over 5 years of age suggests ligament laxity. Refer for a corrective exercise program. Pronated feet due to wide-based gait will usually correct after the first year of weight bearing.
Achilles tendon pain	If obvious causes like pressure from shoes have been ruled out, Achilles tendon pain in adolescents and pre-adolescents suggests Sever's disease which is an uncommon traction-type injury. There may be fragmentation at the calcaneal apophysis. Treatment usually involves modifying activity and teaching young people how to manage flare-ups (e.g. by decreasing or modifying load for a short period, avoiding stretches and eccentric exercises, foot taping, exercises to improve neuromuscular control around the foot and ice packs). Symptoms usually disappear when the apophysis closes.
Genu valgus	Common in young children (up to 75% of 3–5-year-olds) and usually corrects itself by the time they are 7 or 8 years old. Refer if severe, unilateral or not resolving by 7 years of age.
Genu varum	Genu varum is normal until about 18 months of age. Refer if severe, unilateral or not decreasing by 2 years of age.
Genu recurvatum	Congenital genu recurvaturm may be due to intrauterine positioning. It is also associated with connective tissue disorders. Mild genu recurvatum may be due to weak gastrocnemius or popliteus or leg length discrepancy.
Tibial torsion	Tibial torsion is evaluated by measuring the thigh–foot angle (client prone, knee flexed to 90°, measure the angle between the longitudinal axis of the foot and the midline of the thigh). The thigh–foot angle is usually 0° at birth and 20° by the time the child is walking. The child should avoid sitting and sleeping positions which perpetuate the torsion. It is common in babies and may persist for a few years but in most cases gradually disappears as the child grows.
Osgood-Schlatter's disease	Symptoms include pain and tenderness, often bilateral, over the tibial tubercule in a rapidly growing adolescent, especially in athletic boys. The child is often limping. This is a traction-type injury of the apophysis of the tibial tuberosity. Treatment involves a period of activity modification (e.g. avoiding painful activities, stretching and strengthening exercises, pain relief and ice (see Chapter 19). Symptoms usually resolve when the apophysis closes.
Recurrent patella subluxation	This is characterised by episodes of knee collapse associated with lateral displacement of the patella due to a number of conditions including a congenitally flat femoral condyle, shallow patellar ridge, tibial torsion or previous acute patella dislocation. Refer for taping and a quadriceps strengthening program (see Chapter 19). Treatment includes pain relief, limiting activities that excessively load the patellofemoral joint, ice and patella taping.
In-toeing gait (excessive femoral anteversion)	Femoral anteversion is the angle between the femoral neck and a line between the distal femoral condyles. Normally children have 40° of femoral anteversion at birth which decreases to 10° by about 8 years of age. The normal course of excessive femoral anteversion is to decrease over time. Referral is not required unless femoral anterversion is severe by 8 years of age. Discourage children from sitting in the 'W' position.
Developmental hip dysplasia	Developmental hip dysplasia occurs if the hip joint is very shallow and the femoral head is not held tightly in place. It can occur in both hips but is more common in the left. Ortolani's test assesses abduction of the flexed hip. It is performed on newborns and repeated at 6 weeks and 3 months. A child with limited hip abduction at any time must be referred for further investigation (see Chapter 18).

Continued

Table 21.1 Common musculoskeletal conditions affecting children—cont'd

Transient synovitis of the hip	Pain and limp of sudden onset or developing gradually over 1 to 2 weeks. The probable cause is trauma or viral infection. The child is usually 3 to 8 years of age but can be up to 12 years old. The child has a toe-walking gait and holds the hip in flexion. Hip range of motion is limited and painful. Symptoms usually resolve in several days. Nevertheless, the child should be referred to rule out Perthes' disease.
Perthes' disease (avascular necrosis of the femoral head)	Perthes' disease affects children 3–12 years, boys more than girls. It occurs when part or all of the femoral head loses its blood supply and may become misshapen. Groin pain and limp may begin abruptly or develop over months. Symptoms are aggravated by activity and relieved by rest. Examination reveals a flexion contraction of the hip, painful and limited range of motion and causes pain. Refer for further examination (see Chapter 18).
Slipped capital femoral epiphysis	This hip condition occurs in 10–17-year-old children, especially tall thin boys and obese boys. One in four cases is bilateral. Symptoms include groin pain, often referred to the knee, and a limp. Note that hip pain sometimes presents as knee, abdomen or back pain instead of the expected groin pain or limp. Onset may be sudden after trauma or gradual over weeks to months. Examination reveals a flexion contraction and marked restriction of internal rotation of the hip. Hormonal factors are thought to weaken and fracture the epiphyseal plate, allowing the head of the femur to slip posteriorly and inferiorly. Refer for surgical intervention (see Chapter 18).
Scheuermann's disease	This condition affects adolescents 10–15 years of age, boys more than girls. Symptoms include tiredness or pain in the back from an idiopathic breakdown of the developing vertebral endplate (see Chapter 11). Sometimes increased kyphosis is observed. Refer for postural advice, osseous manipulation and extension exercises.
Structural scoliosis	Scoliosis or lateral curvature of the spine is observed on postural observation (see Chapter 11). Adolescent idiopathic scoliosis appears in early adolescence, much more commonly in girls than boys. Adam's test is positive (i.e. lateral curvature persists on forward flexion of the trunk). Refer for further investigation if moderate or severe.
Torticollis	Sudden onset of unilateral neck pain. Torticollis can be brought on by sleeping in a new or uncomfortable position, by swollen neck glands, trauma and a range of other causes. It is managed as for adults (see Chapter 12).
Radial head subluxation (pulled elbow in a toddler)	The head of the radius subluxes through the annular ligament, which normally holds it in place. Refer for reduction.
Little league elbow	This is an uncommon condition that results from excessive throwing. Elbow pain results from traction apophysitis of the medical epicondyle. Treatment includes avoiding throwing activities until the symptoms resolve.
Juvenile rheumatoid arthritis	Polyarticular joint pain and stiffness for more than 6 weeks in a child aged 16 years or less. It can be associated with systemic illness (e.g. fever, rash, lymphadenopathy). Refer promptly for further examination.
Rheumatic fever	This is a rare condition following untreated Streptococcus bacterial infection. Symptoms include migratory arthritis involving several joints. It is rare in Australia except for remote parts of northern Australia. Refer for further examination.

and psychosocially at different rates and adolescents of the same age can vary considerably. Most adolescents are healthy but psychosocial issues and risk-taking behaviour are prominent causes of morbidity and mortality. Physical complaints are commonly connected to psychosocial issues. Practitioners need to gain their client's trust but always remain vigilant of professional boundaries. A respectful and non-judgmental approach should be used. Be explicit with adolescents about confidentiality requirements and encourage young people to talk to parents about important issues.

In this period of rapid transition from childhood to physical and sexual maturity, many adolescents are very shy about their bodies and remedial massage therapists need to be particularly respectful of their clients' modesty. Some adolescents become stressed and anxious as they deal with their physical and emotional changes. Stress is further compounded when students are preparing for important school exams. Remedial massage may be part of a range of treatment strategies for adolescents dealing with stress and more serious mental health issues such as depression and eating disorders. Liaise with the client's medical or other health practitioner. Permission should always be obtained from a young person before talking to their family, school or health practitioners.

EVIDENCE FOR THE EFFECTIVENESS OF MASSAGE FOR CHILDREN

Research into the effectiveness of massage therapy for children and pregnancy is dominated by the work of Tiffany Field.

Her studies have investigated the benefits of massage for infants, children and pregnant women over a range of conditions including childhood leukaemia, asthma, depression and anxiety. According to the Touch Research Institute (established by Tiffany Field in 1992) massage therapy has been shown to 'enhance growth (e.g. in preterm infants), diminish pain (e.g. fibromyalgia), decrease autoimmune problems (e.g. increased pulmonary function in asthma and decreased glucose levels in diabetes), enhance immune function (e.g. increased natural killer cells in HIV and cancer), and enhance alertness and performance (e.g. EEG pattern of alertness and better performance on math computations)'.[2] Decreased stress hormones appear to be responsible for many of these effects. A Cochrane review[3] examined infant massage using 14 randomised controlled trials where babies were stroked for about 15 minutes, three or four times a day, usually for 5 or 10 days. On average, the studies found that when compared to babies who were not touched, babies receiving massage gained more weight each day (about 5 grams), spent less time in hospital, had slightly better scores on developmental tests and slightly fewer postnatal complications, although there were problems with the reliability of the findings. The studies did not show any negative effects of massage. The authors concluded that the evidence for the use of massage to promote growth and development of preterm and low birth weight infants was weak and suggested that wider use of preterm infant massage was unwarranted. Another Cochrane review[4] of trials investigating the effectiveness of infant massage with low-risk groups of parents and infants also found low-quality trials that did not support the use of infant massage. The authors recommended that the focus of future research should be in high-risk groups (e.g. demographically and socially deprived parent–infant dyads) where there may be more potential for change.

Massage therapy has shown promising results in the treatment of childhood asthma. In one study parents of children with asthma were trained to administer a daily 20-minute massage for 30 days.[5] Results for the 6–8-year-olds showed reduced behaviour anxiety and cortisol levels directly after massage but these were not maintained after the series of treatments. Lung function tests had significantly improved after 30 days of regular massage. However, the 9–16-year-olds experienced considerably less benefit.[5] A systematic review in 2005[6] found insufficient evidence from trials to show that a range of manual therapies, including chiropractic, osteopathy and massage could improve asthma and that more research is needed.

Poland et al's[7] study included people from 16 years and older. The study set out to determine whether Swedish massage therapy reduced depression in subjects with human immunodeficiency virus (HIV) disease. The authors found that massage significantly reduced the severity of depression beginning at week 4 (p ≤ 0.04) and continuing at weeks 6 (p ≤ 0.03) and 8 (p ≤ 0.005) compared to no intervention and/or touch.

A number of studies have also examined the effect of massage on children with cancer. Field et al[8] reported increases in white blood cell and neutrophil counts in 20 children with leukaemia following daily massage by their parents for one month. Massage is well known for its positive effect on reducing stress and anxiety. A pilot study by Post-White et al[9] found that massage was more effective than quiet time for reducing heart rate and anxiety in children with cancer under 14 years of age. There were no significant changes in blood pressure, cortisol, pain, nausea or fatigue.

WOMEN

Health issues specifically related to women are largely concerned with the physical and emotional responses to the hormonal changes that occur from the onset of puberty, throughout the monthly menstrual cycle, during pregnancy and childbirth, to menopause and the post-menopausal period. Social changes associated with child rearing (women still outnumber men in this role), including pressures on relationships and balancing child rearing and work, may also affect women's health.

IMPORTANT CONSIDERATIONS FOR ASSESSING AND TREATING WOMEN

- Always consider the influence of hormone fluctuations during assessment. For example, headaches may be associated with pre-menstrual syndrome and menopause.
- Breast cancer is the most common cancer affecting Australian women and accounts for 25% of all cancers diagnosed. Its incidence rose over 35% from 2004 to 2014.[10] Risk factors for developing breast cancer include older age and family history of breast cancer. A common site of metastasis is bone. One of the first symptoms of cancer in the bone is a constant ache or pain in the bone which is aggravated by movement and interferes with sleep.
- Ovarian cancer was the sixth most common cause of cancer-related death among Australian women in 2006.[11] It is mainly a disease of post-menopausal women, with 60% of cases diagnosed in women 60 years and over. Risk factors include older age and family history of ovarian cancer. Metastases may be found in the peritoneal cavity or in the liver, lungs or other organs. The prognosis for women with ovarian cancer is often poorer than for those with other common cancers. This may be attributable partly to the non-specific nature of symptoms, which often leads to diagnosis at a relatively advanced stage of the disease.
- Normal menstruation is associated with a range of symptoms such as bloating, breast tenderness, irritability, anxiety, insomnia, headache, fatigue, mood swings, abdominal cramps, constipation and occasionally joint or muscle pain. For most women these symptoms are mild but for about 25% of menstruating women they can be severe. Pre-menstrual syndrome (PMS) refers to those symptoms occurring during the luteal phase of the cycle (10 days before the menstrual period) that interfere with daily life. PMS symptoms disappear when menses begins. Women with PMS are hypersensitive to progesterone and progestogens that are part of their normal cycle. It appears that oestrogen-related genes and the neurotransmitters serotonin and gamma butyric acid are involved.[12]
- Dysmenorrhoea refers to painful or difficult menstruation. In primary dysmenorrhoea, pain is most severe on the first 2 days of bleeding; in congestive dysmenorrhoea pain commences a few days before bleeding and is relieved by the onset of bleeding; in endometriosis pain commences a few days before bleeding and increases to a maximum within

3 days of onset of bleeding. Refer patients who have menstrual cramps that disrupt their life every month, if symptoms get progressively worse, or the onset of severe menstrual cramps occurred after age 25.[13]

- Many pregnant women seek massage for relaxation, muscle soreness, insomnia and back pain. Special considerations for massage during pregnancy include:
  - First trimester: Many women may not know they are pregnant in the first few weeks. Early symptoms of pregnancy include nausea, vomiting, taste and smell sensitivities, exhaustion, constipation and mood swings. In the first few months of pregnancy massage clients may be comfortable lying prone with pillows under the chest and pelvis. Relaxin, which increases ligament laxity, peaks during the first trimester and at delivery.
  - Second trimester: Later in pregnancy sidelying or seated positions are preferred. In the second trimester, clients may experience shortness of breath, heartburn, frequent urination and backache, and may develop varicose veins and haemorrhoids.[14] Oedema can occur from the pressure of the growing fetus on the large lymphatic vessels of the abdomen and pelvis. In the second trimester fluid retention can cause carpal tunnel syndrome. Although oedema is common during pregnancy, generalised oedema associated with high blood pressure suggests pre-eclampsia and requires medical referral.
  - Third trimester: Massage only in the seated or sidelying position. Oedema may be present in the lower limbs, forearms and hands. Some women experience muscle cramps, incontinence, sacroiliac joint pain, indigestion, frequent urination and sleeplessness throughout their pregnancy and these can continue in the third trimester.
- In addition to the usual contraindications for massage, those for massage during pregnancy include presence of cramping, bleeding or pelvic pain. Abdominal massage, deep remedial techniques for the lumbar spine, acupuncture and reflexology are contraindicated during pregnancy. Vigorous techniques and over-stretching should be avoided.[15] Essential oils that should not be used at all, regardless of whether the client is pregnant or not, include sassafras, wormwood, cassia, pennyroyal, mustard and elecampane.[15] Care should also be taken with oregano, thyme, savoury, clove, cinnamon, cumin, aniseed, anise star, sweet birch and wintergreen. Sage and hyssop should not be used for lengthy periods.[16]
- Women are at risk of injury to the lower back in the weeks and months following childbirth. Their abdominal and pelvic floor muscles have not yet returned to their pre-pregnancy condition and they are required to undertake many unaccustomed lifting and bending tasks to care for their baby. As children grow so do physical demands on new parents (e.g. carrying infants, chasing toddlers, bathing children). Advise new mothers of the importance of muscle-strengthening exercises and of postures for breastfeeding, bathing, lifting and carrying their babies that minimise the risk of injury. Relaxation massage is a good remedy for sleep-deprived and physically exhausted mothers.
- Women may bring their young children with them when they are having remedial massage. In the interest of safety, keep children in the consultation room during their mother's treatment.

- Hormone fluctuations during the normal menstrual cycle may affect ligament laxity.[17] For example, anterior cruciate ligaments may become increasingly lax throughout the menstrual cycle. Changes in knee joint laxity during the menstrual cycle in response to 17β-estradiol fluctuations have been shown to alter neuromuscular control around the knee during running.[18]
- Declining oestrogen levels in menopause increase visceral fat mass and decrease bone mass density, muscle mass and strength.[19] Oestrogen is thought to have a protective effect: (i) it acts as an antioxidant, (ii) it is a membrane stabiliser, and (iii) it binds to oestrogen receptors, thereby regulating the expression of a number of genes. Declining oestrogen has important consequences for the musculoskeletal system, such as an increased risk of osteoporosis and fracture. Weight gain after menopause increases the load on the low back and lower limbs and aggravates many pre-existing conditions including osteoarthritis. Muscle and joint pain is also associated with menopause, along with an increased incidence of muscle injury and slower recovery times.[20, 21]

EVIDENCE FOR THE EFFECTIVENESS OF MASSAGE FOR WOMEN'S HEALTH

Several studies have examined the effects of massage therapy for breast cancer patients. For example, a qualitative study of the experience of massage for 10 breast cancer patients found that massage offered a retreat from uneasy, unwanted, negative feelings connected with chemotherapy treatment. The authors suggested that massage can be added to the treatment choices available to oncology staff.[22] Another study examining the effect of massage on 39 breast cancer patients undergoing chemotherapy found that massage treatment significantly reduced nausea compared with control treatment when improvement was measured as a percentage of the five treatment periods.[23] The results of a systematic review that examined randomised controlled trials providing support for the highest graded therapy recommendations for breast cancer and for treatment-related side effects found that massage improved mood.[24] The authors recommended that massage, along with other integrative therapies like yoga, mindfulness and acupuncture, be incorporated as an option for cancer patients, given the high level of evidence of benefit and the relative low level of risk. Cho et al[25] conducted a prospective randomised trial with 41 breast cancer patients and found that physical exercise combined with manual lymphatic drainage significantly improved quality of life including improved shoulder function and shoulder flexor strength after the 4-week intervention. Another treatment that combined acupuncture and reflexology was found to have the potential to improve symptoms of breast cancer patients with chemotherapy-induced peripheral neuropathy.[26]

A number of studies has examined the effectiveness of massage during pregnancy and childbirth. Field et al[27] compared two groups of women diagnosed with prenatal depression. One group received one session of interpersonal psychotherapy per week for 6 weeks and the other received a combination of interpersonal psychotherapy and massage therapy once a week for the same period. The authors concluded that interpersonal psychotherapy was particularly effective when combined with massage therapy in reducing prenatal depression. There is strong evidence supporting the use of perineal massage to reduce the incidence of perineal trauma although such massage is outside the scope of remedial massage practice.[28–30]

Studies of the effect of aromatherapy and reflexology on the symptoms of menopause, particularly psychological symptoms, have found encouraging results.[31, 32]

MEN

Chronic conditions like obesity, cancer, diabetes and cardiovascular disease are more common in men than women and yet for many men visiting the doctor for a health check-up is a last resort. As a result many health conditions among men go untreated until they become serious, more difficult to treat and/or life-threatening. A report in 2013[33] on Australian males aged 25 years and over found that coronary heart disease was the leading cause of death followed by lung cancer. In 2011–2012, 44% of males aged 25 and over were overweight; 31% were obese. One in 10 males aged 50–59 (11%) and 60–69 (10%) were at risk of injury resulting from excessive alcohol consumption. The prevalence rate for treated psychotic disorders was 5.8 cases per 1000 males aged 25–64, higher than the rate among males aged 18–24 years. Nearly 1 in 5 males aged 25 years and over were estimated to have activity limitation and need help, have difficulty with or use aids or equipment to assist with mobility, self-care or communication. Married males have lower mortality rates compared with males who have never married.

Remedial massage therapists are primary contact practitioners and have a responsibility for promoting healthy lifestyles for their clients. This includes encouraging healthy diets, reduced consumption of alcohol and smoking, and promoting physical fitness. The Australian Bureau of Statistics National Health Survey 2017–2018 showed that the same health risks for men's health had continued since 2012:[34] men continued to be more likely than women to smoke daily; a greater proportion of men aged 18 years and over were overweight or obese compared to women; and men were more likely than women to exceed the guidelines for alcohol consumption (although the proportion of men exceeding the guideline had declined since 2014–15). Only just over half the Australian population (men and women) met the guidelines for fruit and vegetable consumption and only a minority met recommendations for physical activity.

IMPORTANT CONSIDERATIONS FOR ASSESSING AND TREATING MEN

- Men are less likely than women to use health services. Encourage male clients to see their doctors and other healthcare practitioners when required.
- Approximately 18,700 new cases of prostate cancer are diagnosed in Australia every year and approximately 3000 Australian men die from the disease each year. When assessing older males, be mindful that 50% of males over 50 years have a carcinomatous change in their prostate. Most of these changes are benign (e.g. benign prostatic hypertrophy); nevertheless, it is important to refer all males over 50 years who report urinary symptoms (such as

frequency, urgency, nocturia or hesitancy) associated with back, hip or rib pain. Risk factors for prostate cancer include age and family history of prostate, breast or ovarian cancer, and a diet high in processed meat or fat.[35] Be vigilant for young men with a family history of prostate cancer and older men with urinary symptoms.
- Refer clients who are demonstrating signs of mental illnesses like depression or substance abuse to their medical practitioners. Depression in men may manifest as fatigue, irritability, difficulty sleeping and loss of interest in work and hobbies. In some cases signs of depression include anger, aggression, violence, reckless behaviour and substance abuse. Look out for men with physical pain associated with anger, and reckless behaviour. Men, especially older men, are at a higher suicide risk than women.[36]

EVIDENCE FOR THE EFFECTIVENESS OF MASSAGE FOR MEN'S HEALTH

Only a limited number of studies have focused specifically on men's health issues. One Cochrane review investigated non-pharmacological interventions for treating chronic prostatitis/chronic pelvic pain syndrome. These interventions included myofascial trigger point therapy, acupuncture, thermotherapy and lifestyle interventions. Only one myofascial trigger point study could be found but the authors were unable to draw any conclusions based on the quality of the trial.[37] Newby's study[38] found one massage study (Reiki) that reduced depression symptoms in men diagnosed with prostate cancer.

GERIATRIC CLIENTS

Projections for Australia's population place the proportion of people aged over 65 at between 21% and 22% by 2031. This raises particular concerns about the projected health care needs of this ageing population, concerns which include the treatment and management of chronic conditions and the costs required to meet these needs.[39] Remedial massage therapists are likely to be called upon to treat an increasing number of geriatric clients in their clinics, in aged care facilities and in clients' homes.

IMPORTANT CONSIDERATIONS FOR ASSESSING AND TREATING GERIATRIC CLIENTS

- Extra time may be needed for older clients to complete administration requirements, to complete case histories and other assessments, to dress and undress and to get on and off the treatment table. Speak slowly and allow time for the client to respond.
- Many older clients have more than one pathology occurring simultaneously. For example, in the Netherlands comorbidity is present in over 25% of adults, with four or more co-morbidities present in 55% of patients over the age of 75 years; in Canada two or more distinct conditions are present in over 90% of the population aged over 65 years.[40] Co-morbidities could include cardiovascular disease, diabetes, osteoporosis or arthritic joints.
- Many older clients are taking prescription medication. Always consider side effects of medication when assessing clients and negotiating treatment plans.

- Clients may have hearing problems. Speak slowly and clearly. Minimise background noise.
- Adjust techniques to suit the individual client's needs. In general, techniques are applied lightly because of skin fragility, the risk of fracture in osteoporotic clients and the risk of bruising in clients taking blood-thinning medication.
- Treatments are often short, at least initially, until the client's response to treatment has been assessed.
- Clients may require assistance getting on and off the treatment table.
- Clients with cardiovascular or respiratory conditions, or clients who are obese, require extra pillows to elevate their head when lying supine.
- Frail aged clients are often treated in chairs or beds. Massage may be confined to hands and feet.
- Do not cover hearing aids with hands during face, neck and head massage.
- Massage may be performed without oils or creams because of skin sensitivities and allergies. If lubricant can be tolerated, use easily absorbed creams.
- Psychosocial factors like isolation, loneliness or the impact of living on a limited income may have particular relevance when treating older clients. Psychosocial benefits may outweigh physical benefits of massage therapy for this population, including the benefits of touch, the social encounter and the element of caring associated with remedial massage therapy.
- Many older clients have chronic health conditions, including chronic pain and limited mobility associated with osteoarthritis. Reassure clients by educating them about the nature of their condition, the influence of lifestyle on their condition, and ways to self-manage their pain. For example, for chronic low back pain advising clients to stay active and to undertake an exercise program are first line treatments.[41] Weight loss, exercise and self-managing acute flare-ups are evidence-based recommendations for people with osteoarthritis.[42]

EVIDENCE FOR THE EFFECTIVENESS OF MASSAGE FOR GERIATRIC CLIENTS

Several studies have examined the benefits of massage therapy for elderly clients. For example, in one study self-reported health outcomes in older adults suggest improved emotional wellbeing.[43] The effect of massage on cognition has been evaluated by several researchers. Fang et al[44] found that acupoint massage was an effective intervention for maintaining cognitive functions in older adults. Moyle et al[45] commented on the severe paucity of research examining the effects of massage on agitated behaviour in older people with dementia. Only one study could be located but it did provide evidence to support the use of massage as a non-pharmacological approach to managing agitation in older people with dementia. In another study Wu et al[46] reviewed 11 studies on the effectiveness of massage on the behavioural and psychosocial problems of older people with dementia and reported that physical aggressive behaviour, physical non-aggressive behaviour, verbal aggressive behaviour and verbal non-aggressive behaviour decreased significantly after receiving massage or touch, while scores of anxiety, sadness and anger did not decrease significantly. Physical benefits have also been reported. A systematic review by de Luca et al[47] on the safety and effectiveness of massage for older people with chronic low back pain found four articles of good methodological quality. These studies provided moderate evidence supporting the use of manual therapy to reduce pain levels and alleviate disability. Researchers in Japan examined the effect of Anma massage on shoulder range of motion in six elderly patients with Parkinson's disease.[48] This small study involved Anma massage to the cervical spine, the back and the lower extremities for a total of 30 to 40 minutes once per week for 7 weeks. The immediate effect of the intervention was significant improvement in range of motion ($P = .013$).

CLIENTS WITH A MENTAL ILLNESS

One in five Australians aged between 16 and 85 years experience a mental illness each year.[49] Mental illnesses can come and go and most can be effectively treated. Stress can trigger some mental illnesses or may prolong episodes. Through its capacity to reduce stress and enhance feelings of wellbeing, massage therapy may have a considerable role to play in management or prevention of some mental health conditions. Mental illnesses can be divided into psychotic and non-psychotic.[50]

1. Psychotic illnesses — a psychosis (e.g. schizophrenia, bipolar mood disorder) belong to a group of illnesses that affect the ability to make sense of thoughts, feelings and external information. People with psychoses may develop delusions or become depressed or overly elated. Medication and support from medical health professionals can be effective treatments.
2. Non-psychotic illnesses — a non-psychotic illness involves feelings of depression, sadness, tension or fear that become so overwhelming that they interfere with normal activities like going to work and maintaining relationships. Such illnesses include phobias, anxiety, some forms of depression, eating disorders and obsessive compulsive disorder. Most non-psychotic illnesses can be effectively treated with medication and therapy.

IMPORTANT CONSIDERATIONS FOR ASSESSING AND TREATING CLIENTS WITH A MENTAL ILLNESS

- If a client is unable to give informed consent, it may be given by a guardian who must be present throughout the consultation.
- Remedial massage can be used as an adjunct to support primary treatments for mental illness. Effective communication among practitioners is required.
- Practitioners should be vigilant for indications of mental illness and refer clients to medical practitioners when required. People with mental disorders often consult general practitioners with a range of physical complaints and psychological complaints like feeling tired all the time, sleeping badly or not coping with day-to-day events. Emotional symptoms are common but do not necessarily mean that the sufferer has a mental disorder. Signs and symptoms suggesting an underlying mental health problem include:
  - seemingly inappropriate requests for urgent attention
  - increased frequency of consultation or requests for tests

- unexpected or disproportionate outbursts during consultation (tears, anger)
- excessive anxiety about another family member or presenting a relative as the patient
- unstable relationships or frequent breakdowns in relationships
- distressing or deteriorating social circumstances (eviction, redundancy, squalor).

- When assessing clients with a mental illness, consider side effects of medication for common conditions such as depression and bipolar disease.
- Massage may be particularly beneficial for stress management and for treating clients with anxiety and depression.

EVIDENCE FOR THE EFFECTIVENESS OF MASSAGE FOR CLIENTS WITH A MENTAL ILLNESS

An increasing number of studies support the effectiveness of massage in reducing stress and anxiety. One meta-analysis has suggested that the most significant effects of massage are reducing anxiety and helping patients with depression.[51] A review by Field[52] found that moderate pressure massage 'reduced depression, anxiety and heart rate, and it altered EEG patterns, as in a relaxation response'. Moderate pressure massage has also led to increased vagal activity and decreased cortisol levels. Using functional magnetic resonance imaging moderate pressure massage was represented in several brain regions including the amygdala, the hypothalamus and the anterior cingulate cortex, all areas involved in stress and emotion regulation.

In a study of 48 stable intensive care unit patients, patients' anxiety status was evaluated by the State-Trait Anxiety Inventory for Adults.[53] Assessments pre- and post-massage showed that 30 minutes of Swedish massage reduced anxiety immediately and 30 minutes after the massage. Vital signs were also reduced immediately after the massage. Stress reduction was also demonstrated by Ruotsalainen et al[54] who found low-quality evidence that CBT and mental and physical relaxation (i.e. massage) reduced stress more than no intervention but not more than alternative interventions.

A lack of high-quality evidence is a perennial problem. Hillier et al[55] found some evidence for the use of massage therapy to 'improve quality of life for people living with HIV/AIDS (PLWHA), particularly in combination with other stress-management modalities, and that massage therapy may have a positive effect on immunological function'. However, the trials were small and at moderate risk of bias. Similarly, Shin et al[56] were unable to assess the effect of adding aromatherapy to massage on the relief of pain, psychological symptoms including anxiety and depression, physical symptom distress, or quality of life.

A number of studies have been conducted into the use of massage therapy in autism. It is relevant to include autism in discussions of mental health as clients with this complex developmental disability have many behaviours and states in common with clients with mental health conditions. One study found that 13 children with autism aged between 3 and 6 years who received daily massage treatments for 5 months showed significant improvement of sensory impairments and demonstrated increased social skills and basic living skills on standardised measures compared with untreated children.[57] Another randomised controlled trial examined the effects of Thai traditional massage on 60 autistic children and found that Thai traditional massage over an 8-week period had a positive effect on stereotypical behaviours in autistic children.[58] In a preliminary study into the use of alternative healthcare practices by people with serious mental illnesses, 31% of participants reported benefit from massage therapy.[59]

ATHLETES/SPORTS PEOPLE

Sports massage has grown significantly in popularity over the past 30 years and is now incorporated into the regular training regimens of many sports. Its popularity with many elite athletes is well known; many travel with a personal massage therapist as part of their support team. Its popularity is largely based on clinical experience and high-quality evidence is needed to supporting its use.[60] Claims about its effectiveness include increased blood flow, reduced muscle soreness, increased range of motion, increased sense of wellbeing and neurological excitability (both increased before exercise and decreased after exercise).

IMPORTANT CONSIDERATIONS FOR MASSAGING SPORTS PEOPLE

- Sports massage therapists are often one of a team working with sports people to maintain fitness, improve performance and rehabilitate injuries. Team members can include coaches, managers, physiotherapists, chiropractors, medical practitioners and trainers. Effective communication with other members of the team will promote optimal outcomes for clients.
- Sports people are often highly psychologically motivated to improve performance and to return to sport after injury. They are usually keen to comply with recommendations, although they may be reluctant to miss sporting events. The therapist should provide accurate and evidence-based information about injury prevention and recovery and clear instructions for self-directed activities, including exercise rehabilitation.
- The nature of sports massage varies with the level of the athlete and the training schedule. For example, mechanical pressure on muscles can be varied to either increase or decrease neural excitability (measured by the Hoffman reflex). Massage can promote changes in parasympathetic activity (measured by heart rate, blood pressure and heart rate variability) and hormonal levels (measured by cortisol levels) resulting in a relaxation response (physiological mechanisms).[60]

Pre-exercise massage

This style of massage is designed to prepare the body physically and psychologically for sport. It can form part of a warm-up routine.

Massage therapy during exercise

Some sports massage therapists work on the sideline or in the dressing room providing first aid massage during breaks in play.

Post-exercise massage

Sport massage can be part of the cool-down routine to promote immediate recovery from sport (e.g. after fun runs).

Massage between events

Massage for athletes and sports people between events usually takes place in the therapist's clinic as part of routine maintenance, prehabilitation or rehabilitation between events.

■ Given the importance of lifestyle on many health conditions, including cardiovascular disease, diabetes, overweight and obesity, low back pain and osteoarthritis, prioritise physical activity, good nutrition and mental health in all clients.

EVIDENCE FOR THE EFFECTIVENESS OF MASSAGE FOR SPORTS PEOPLE

Sports massage is widely popular despite the paucity of evidence supporting its practice. The effects of different types of massage and the influence that the timing of massage (pre-exercise, post-exercise, between exercise) has on performance, injury recovery or injury prevention remain to be confirmed by further high-quality research.

Pre-exercise massage

A systematic review by Weerapong[60] found limited research investigating the effects of pre-exercise massage on performance and injury prevention. Most of the research on psychological effects of massage concluded that massage produces positive effects on recovery (via psychological mechanisms).

Post-exercise massage

Post-exercise massage is one of the most popular interventions used to enhance recovery after exercise. One systematic review and meta-analysis evaluated the effects of massage on delayedonset muscle soreness and muscle performance after strenuous exercise.[61] Muscle soreness was measured using self-reported rating scales and performance measures included muscle maximal isometric force and peak torque and creatine kinase. Eleven articles involving a total of 504 participants were included. The review found that muscle soreness rating decreased significantly when the participants received massage at 24 hours, 48 hours and 72 hours after intense exercise compared with no intervention. Maximal isometric force and peak torque as total effects also improved. Serum creatine kinase levels reduced after massage. The authors concluded that current evidence suggests that massage therapy after strenuous exercise could be effective for alleviating delayed onset muscle soreness and improving muscle performance.

Another study investigated the effectiveness of different types and duration of massage on performance. Poppendiek et al[62] conducted a systematic review and meta-analysis of the literature on massage for performance recovery. In this review 22 randomised controlled trials met the study inclusion criteria. Five of the 22 studies used automated massage (e.g. vibration); the other 17 used manual massage. Findings showed a tendency for shorter massages of 5–12 minutes to have larger effects (+6.6%, g = 0.34) than massages of more than 12 minutes duration (+1.0%, g = 0.06). Massage therapy appeared to be more effective for short-term recovery of up to 10 minutes than for recovery periods of more than 20 minutes. Effects were 'medium positive' (+14.4%,

g = 0.61) after high-intensity mixed exercise; smaller effects were found after strength exercise (+3.9%, g = 0.18) and endurance exercise (+1.3%, g = 0.12). The effectiveness of massage therapy on performance also appeared to be more beneficial for untrained sports people (+6.5%, g = 0.23) than for trained athletes (+2.3%, g = 0.17). Overall the effects of massage on performance recovery were small but may be useful for short-term recovery after intensive mixed training. Ntshangase and Peters-Futre[63] found that manual massage was no more effective than light automated vibration therapy in controlling functional decline following physiological response to exercise-induced muscle damage. However, the study was based on a small number of randomised controlled studies (28), many of which were methodologically flawed.

Intense physical activity is thought to produce a decrease in immune function as demonstrated by reduced salivary IgA and peripheral blood neutrophil levels after physical activity. High-quality but preliminary evidence supports the possibility that massage has immunological effects. A review of five studies found that post-exercise massage could modulate immune parameters after high-intensity exercise, facilitating the recovery of immunoglobulin A and reducing the presence of exercise-induced pro-inflammatory mediators.[64] If this were confirmed massage therapy could be useful after high-intensity exercise for avoiding performance loss mediated by immunosuppression. The timing of massage after physical activity may also be important. Massage at 2 hours after exercise was shown to increase circulating neutrophils. Immune function effects of massage performed immediately after exercise may be greater than after a 2-hour delay although such comparisons need to be confirmed.

Massage between events

Massage between events is widely used to enhance recovery and prepare athletes for the next event. However, there is insufficient research to date to support this claim.[60]

KEY MESSAGES

■ Informed consent must be obtained from the client, a parent or guardian (in the case of a child under 18 years of age or a client with a mental illness who is unable to provide their own informed consent). The parent or guardian is required to remain with the client throughout the consultation.

■ Managing the consultation requires time management, effective communication skills and modification of techniques to suit the needs of individual clients.

■ When assessing children and adolescents, consider common conditions that occur at specific ages. Treat all musculoskeletal pain as serious until proven otherwise.

■ Adolescents are often particularly sensitive to their developing bodies. Careful attention is required to maintain their modesty and comfort.

■ Always consider the influence of hormones on symptoms in female clients.

■ Be aware that men are often reluctant to discuss health issues with their healthcare practitioners.

- When treating older males, be mindful that 50% of males over 50 years of age have a carcinomatous change in the prostate. Refer all clients with urinary symptoms (frequency, urgency, hesitancy and nocturia) for further investigation.
- Treating older clients requires time and patience. They often have several pathologies at the same time, take prescribed medication and suffer from chronic conditions. Psychological benefits of remedial massage treatment are important.
- Massage appears to be particularly beneficial in the treatment of anxiety and depression.

Review questions

1. i) What effect does excessive femoral anteversion have on gait?
   ii) What is the normal degree of femoral anterversion in neonates and in adults?
2. Briefly describe the pathogenesis of slipped capital femoral epiphysis. What symptoms can it produce?
3. What symptoms could be used to differentiate primary dysmenorrhoea, congestive dysmenorrhoea and endometriosis?
4. What effects can declining oestrogen levels have on the musculoskeletal system?
5. List three common chronic health conditions that males are more likely to experience than females.
6. What common condition affecting older males should be considered when assessing a 60-year-old male with low back pain?
7. How is a remedial massage consultation modified for a frail aged client?
8. List four signs or symptoms that could indicate a client has a mental health problem.

Research activity

Review recent research articles (published in the past 5 years) on the effectiveness of massage for one of the specific client groups discussed in this chapter.

For example, the effect of massage on:
- childhood asthma
- adolescent idiopathic scoliosis
- depression.

Sources of information include:
- Freely available journals such as
  - *BMC complementary and alternative medicine* (peer-reviewed)
  - *Massage Australia* magazine
  - *Massage and Bodywork*
  - *Massage Today*
  - *Sport Health* (Australia)
- Freely available databases such as
  - Cochrane reviews http://www2.cochrane.org/reviews/
  - Pubmed (Medline) http://www.ncbi.nlm.nih.gov/sites/entrez

Other databases are available through libraries including EBSCOhost, AMED (Allied and Complementary Medicine), CINAHL.
- Professional association websites
- Government websites
  - Australian Institute of Health and Welfare
  - Dept of Health and Ageing, Therapeutic Goods Administration
  - NSW Health
  - WorkCover authorities in each state

The quality of research is highly variable. To guide selection of readings, choose a reputable source (e.g. a peer-reviewed journal). Systematic reviews or meta-analyses are regarded as the highest form of evidence. Prioritise the use of these when they are available.

REFERENCES

1. Australian Institute of Family Studies. Mandatory reporting of child abuse. Online. Available: https://aifs.gov.au/cfca/publications/mandatory-reporting-child-abuse-and-neglect; 2018
2. Touch Research Institute. About us. Miami, FL: Touch Research Institute. Online. Available: https://www6.miami.edu/touch-research/Research.html; 2019.
3. Vickers A, Ohlsson A, Lacy JB, et al. Massage for promoting growth and development of preterm and/or low birth-weight infants. Cochrane Database Syst Rev 2004;2:CD000390.
4. Bennett C, Underdown A, Barlow J. Massage for promoting mental and physical health in typically developing infants under the age of six months. Cochrane Database Sys Rev 2013, Issue 4. Art. No.: CD005038. Doi: 10.1002/14651858.CD005038.pub3.
5. Ernst E. Massage therapy is promising for childhood asthma. Focus on Alternative and Complementary Therapies 1999;4(1):30–1.
6. Hondras MA, Linde K, Jones AP. Manual therapy for asthma. Cochrane Database Syst Rev 2005, Issue 2. Art. No.: CD001002. Doi: 10.1002/14651858.CD001002.pub2.
7. Poland R, Gertsik L, Favreau J, et al. Open-label, randomized, parallel-group controlled clinical trial of massage for treatment of depression in HIV-infected subjects. J Altern Complement Med 2013;19(4):334–40.
8. Field T, Cullen C, Diego M, et al. Leukemia immune changes following massage therapy. J Bodyw Mov Ther 2001;5(4):271–4.
9. Post-White J, Fitzgerald M, Savik K, et al. Massage therapy for children with cancer. J Pediatr Oncol Nurs 2009;26(1):16–28.
10. Breast Cancer Australia. Statistics. Online. Available: https://www.breastcanceraustralia.org/about-breast-cancer.html; 2019.
11. Australian Institute of Health and Welfare. Ovarian cancer in Australia: an overview. Canberra: Australian Institute of Health and Welfare; 2010.
   Online. Available: http://www.aihw.gov.au/publications/index.cfm/title/11158.
12. The Better Health Channel. Menstrual cramps overview. Melbourne: Victoria Department of Health. Online. Available: https://www.mayoclinic.org/diseases-conditions/menstrual-cramps/symptoms-causes/syc-20374938; 2019.
13. Mayo Clinic. Menstrual cramps. Online. Available: https://www.mayoclinic.org/diseases-conditions/menstrual-cramps/symptoms-causes/syc-20374938; 2018.
14. Braun M, Simonson S. Introduction to massage therapy. 3rd edn. Baltimore, MD: Lippincott Williams and Wilkins; 2013.
15. Fritz S. Mosby's essential sciences for therapeutic massage. Anatomy, physiology, biomechanics, and pathology. 5th edn. St Louis, MO: Mosby Elsevier; 2017.
16. International Federation of Professional Aromatherapists (IFPA). Pregnancy Guidelines. IFPA: Leicestershire; 2013.

17. Bell DR, Blackburn JT, Hackney AC, et al. Jump-landing biomechanics and knee-laxity change across the menstrual cycle in women with anterior cruciate ligament reconstruction. J Athlet Train 2014;49(2):154–62.

18. Khowailed IA, Petrofsky J, Lohman E, et al. 17beta-estradiol induced effects on anterior cruciate ligament laxness and neuromuscular activation patterns in female runners. J Women's Health (2002). 2015;24(8):670–80.

19. Maltais ML, Desroches J, Dionne IJ. Changes in muscle mass and strength after menopause. J Musculoskelet Neuronal Interact [Research Support, Non-U.S. Gov't Review] 2009;9(4): 186–97.

20. Faria A, Gabriel R, Abrantes J, et al. Ankle stiffness in postmenopausal women: influence of hormone therapy and menopause nature. Climacteric [Research Support, Non-U.S. Gov't] 2009;13(3): 265–70.

21. Enns DL, Tiidus PM, Enns DL, et al. The influence of estrogen on skeletal muscle: sex matters. Sports Med 2010;40(1):41–58.

22. Billhult A, Stener-Victorin E, Bergbom I. The experience of massage during chemotherapy treatment in breast cancer patients. Clin Nurs Res 2007;16(2):85–9.

23. Billhult A, Bergbom I, Stener-Victorin E. Massage relieves nausea in women with breast cancer who are undergoing chemotherapy. J Altern Complement Med – New York 2007;13(1):53–7.

24. Greenlee H, DuPont-Reyes MJ, Balneaves LG, et al. Clinical practice guidelines on the evidence-based use of integrative therapies during and after breast cancer treatment. Cancer J Clin 2017;67(3):194–232.

25. Cho Y, Do J, Jung S, et al. Effects of a physical therapy program combined with manual lymphatic drainage on shoulder function, quality of life, lymphedema incidence, and pain in breast cancer patients with axillary web syndrome following axillary dissection. Support Care Cancer 2016;24(5): 2047–57.

26. Ben-Horin I, Kahan P, Ryvo L, et al. Acupuncture and reflexology for chemotherapy-induced peripheral neuropathy in breast cancer. Integr Cancer Ther 2017;16(3):258–62.

27. Field T, Deeds O, Diego M, et al. Benefits of combining massage therapy with group interpersonal psychotherapy in prenatally depressed women. J Bodyw Mov Ther 2009;13(4):297–303.

28. Beckmann MM, Garrett AJ. Antenatal perineal massage for reducing perineal trauma. Cochrane Database Syst Rev 2006;1:CD005123.

29. Eason E, Labrecque M, Wells G, et al. Preventing perineal trauma during childbirth: a systematic review. Obstet Gynecol 2000;95(3):464–71.

30. Demirel G, Golbasi Z. Effect of perineal massage on the rate of episiotomy and perineal tearing. Int J of Gynaecol 2015;131(2):183–6.

31. Murakami S, Shirota T, Hayashi S, et al. Aromatherapy for outpatients with menopausal symptoms in obstetrics and gynecology. J Altern Complement Med – New York 2005;11(3):491–4.

32. Babakhanian M, Ghazanfarpour M, Kargarfard L, et al. Effect of aromatherapy on the treatment of psychological symptoms in postmenopausal and elderly women: a Systematic review and meta-analysis. J Menopausal Med 2018;24(2): 127–32.

33. Australian Institute of Health and Welfare. The health of Australia's males 25 years and over. Canberra: Australian Institute of Health and Welfare; 2013.

34. Australian Bureau of Statistics. National Health Survey First Results 2017-2018. Online. Available: http://www.abs.gov.au/ausstats/abs@.nsf/mf/4364 .0.55.001; 2018.

35. Prostate Cancer Foundation of Australia. What you need to know about prostate cancer: Prostate Cancer Foundation of Australia. Online. Available: http:// www.prostate.org.au/awareness/general-information/ what-you-need-to-know-about-prostate-cancer/; 2017.

36. Helpguide.org. Depression in men.Online. Available: https://www.helpguide.org/articles/depression/ depression-in-men.htm; 2019.

37. Franco JVA, Turk T, Jung JH, et al. Non-pharmacological interventions for treating chronic prostatitis/chronic pelvic pain syndrome: a Cochrane systematic review. BJU International 2018.

38. Newby TA, Graff JN, Ganzini LK, et al. Interventions that may reduce depressive symptoms among prostate cancer patients: a systematic review and meta-analysis. Psycho-oncology 2015;24(12): 1686–93.

39. Jones R. Chronic disease and co-morbidity. Brit J Gen Pract 2010;60:394.

40. Munk N, Zanjani F. Relationship between massage therapy usage and health outcomes in older adults. J Bodywork Mov Ther 2011;15(2):177–85.

41. Foster NE, Anema JR, Cherkin D, et al. Prevention and treatment of low back pain: evidence, challenges, and promising directions. Lancet 2018;391:2368–83.

42. Hunter DJ. Everything you ever wanted to know about osteoarthritis. The Health Report 2017. Online. Available: https://www.abc.net.au/ radionational/programs/healthreport/everything-you -ever-wanted-to-know-about-osteoarthritis/8664218 #transcript; 2017.

43. Munk N, Kruger T, Zanjani F. Massage therapy usage and reported health in older adults experiencing persistent pain. J Altern Complem Med 2011;17(7):609–16.

44. Fang L, Shen C, Yao L, et al. Acupoint massage for managing cognitive alterations in older adults: a systematic review and meta-analysis. J Altern Complem Med 2018;24(6):532–40.

45. Moyle W, Murfield J, O'Dwyer S, et al. The effect of massage on agitated behaviours in older people with dementia: a literature review. J Clin Nurs 2012;22: 601–10.

46. Wu J, Wang Y, Wang Z. The effectiveness of massage and touch on behavioural and psychological symptoms of dementia: a quantitative systematic review and meta-analysis. J Adv Nurs 2017;73: 2283–95.

47. de Luca K, Fang S, Ong J, et al. The effectiveness and safety of manual therapy on pain and disability in older persons with chronic low back pain: a systematic review. J Manipulative Physiol Ther 2017;40(7):527–34.

48. Suoh S, Donoyama N, Ohkoshi N. Anma massage (Japanese massage) therapy for patients with Parkinson's disease in geriatric health services facilities: effectiveness on limited range of motion of the shoulder joint. J Bodyw Mov Ther 2016; 20(2):364–72. Doi:10.1016/j.jbmt.2015.11.008.

49. Black Dog Institute. Facts & figures about mental health. Online. Available: https://www .blackdoginstitute.org.au/docs/default-source/ factsheets/facts_figures.pdf?sfvrsn=8; 2015.

50. Victoria State Department. Better Health Channel. Forensic mental health. Online. Available: https://www.betterhealth.vic.gov.au/health/ ConditionsAndTreatments/forensic-mental-health; 2018.

51. Moyer CA, Rounds J, Hannum JW. A meta-analysis of massage therapy research. Psychol Bull 2004;130(1):3–18.

52. Field T. Massage therapy research review. Complement Ther Clin Pract 2017;20(4): 224–9.

53. da Silva A, Schuimann S, da Silveira Y, et al. Effect of therapeutic Swedish massage on anxiety level and vital signs of Intensive Care Unit patients. J Bodyw Mov Ther 2017; 21(3): 565–8.

54. Ruotsalainen JH, Verbeek JH, Mariné A, et al. Preventing occupational stress in healthcare workers. Cochrane Database Syst Rev 2015, Issue 4. Art. No.: CD002892. Doi: 10.1002/14651858.CD002892. pub5.

55. Hillier SL, Louw Q, Morris L, et al. Massage therapy for people with HIV/AIDS. Cochrane Database Syst Rev 2010, Issue 1. Art. No.: CD007502. Doi: 10.1002/14651858.CD007502. pub2.

56. Shin ES, Seo KH, Lee SH, et al. Massage with or without aromatherapy for symptom relief in people with cancer. Cochrane Database Syst Rev 2016, Issue 6. Art. No.: CD009873. Doi: 10.1002/ 14651858.CD009873.pub3.

57. Silva L, Cignlini A, Warren R, et al. Improvement in Sensory Impairment and Social Interaction in Young Children with Autism Following Treatment with an Original Qigong Massage Methodology. Am J Chin Med 2007;35(3):393–406.

58. Piravej K, Tangtrongchitr P, Chandarasiri P, et al. Effects of Thai traditional massage on autistic children's behavior. J Altern Complement Med – New York 2009;15(12):1355–61.

59. Russinova Z, Wewiorski N, Cash D. Use of alternative health care practices by persons with serious mental illness: perceived benefits. Am J Public Health 2002;92(10):1600–3.

60. Weerapong P, Hume PA, Kolt GS. The mechanisms of massage and effects on performance, muscle recovery and injury prevention. Sports Med (Auckland) 2005;35(3):235–56.

61. Guo J, Li L, Gong Y, et al. Massage allieviates delayed onset muscle soreness after strenuous exercise: a systematic review and meta-analysis. Frontiers in Physiotherapy 2017;8: Article 747. Doi: 10.3389/fphys.2017.00747.

62. Poppendieck W, Wegmann M, Farrauti A, et al. Massage and performance recovery: a meta-analytical review. Sports Med 2016;46(2): 183–204.

63. Ntshangase S, Peters-Futre. The efficacy of manual versus local vibratory massage in promoting recovery from post-exercise muscle damage: a systematic review. J Sci Med Sport 2017; 20(S1):e42.

64. Tejero-Fernandez V, Membrilla-Mesa M, Galiano-Castillo N, et al. Immunological effects of massage after exercise: a systematic review. Phys Ther Sport 2015;16:187–92.

Answers to Review Questions

Chapter 2

1. a) clinical features that may be associated with the presence of a serious physical condition

    b) observed in post-menopausal women and associated with osteoporotic compression fractures and low levels of oestrogen

    c) the integrity of inert tissue (e.g. articulation itself, ligaments, joint capsule, bursae)

    d) an area of skin that provides sensory input to one pair of spinal nerves

    e) Adam's

2. Night sweats are a possible indicator of serious underlying infection. Refer for medical assessment.

3. a) right gluteal fold lower on the right

    b) gluteal cleft deviates to the right

    c) the left PSIS is higher than the right

    d) the right foot is anterior

    e) right knee is slightly flexed

    f) waist curve on the right appears to decrease

4. a) False

    b) True

    c) False (usually dull and hard to localise)

    d) False (should be T7)

5. Contractile tissue (muscles)

6. Inert tissue (joint, ligaments, bursae, joint capsule)

7. Both contractile and inert tissues could be involved. Further testing is required:
- Strength and length tests for specific muscles
- Special functional tests (e.g. Valsalva)
- Palpation

8. The length of the hamstring muscles can be assessed by straight leg raising when the client is supine. Shortness is assessed by comparison to population norms (normal hamstring length permits approximately 65–80° straight leg raising) and by bilateral comparison.

9. a) lymph glands

    b) tendon

    c) peripheral nerves

    d) blood vessels

10. a) weak dorsiflexors

    b) weak hamstrings

    c) weak quadriceps

    d) weak quadriceps

11. A functional test with a sensitivity of 95% or more rules a condition in – that is, suggests that the client has the condition indicated by the test.

12. Lumbar flexion severely restricted, right lateral flexion moderately restricted

Lumbar flexion severely restricted, right lateral flexion moderately restricted and right rotation mildly restricted

Chapter 3

1. Match the following descriptions with their injury grade:

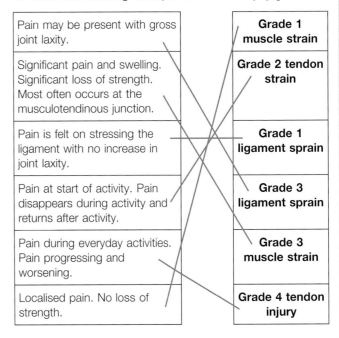

Pain may be present with gross joint laxity.	**Grade 1 muscle strain**
Significant pain and swelling. Significant loss of strength. Most often occurs at the musculotendinous junction.	**Grade 2 tendon strain**
Pain is felt on stressing the ligament with no increase in joint laxity.	**Grade 1 ligament sprain**
Pain at start of activity. Pain disappears during activity and returns after activity.	**Grade 3 ligament sprain**
Pain during everyday activities. Pain progressing and worsening.	**Grade 3 muscle strain**
Localised pain. No loss of strength.	**Grade 4 tendon injury**

2. Never apply cold:

If the client has cold hypersensitivity

To an open wound

Directly to the skin (unless applying ice massage)

If the client is taking analgesics

If the client has circulatory insufficiency (e.g. Raynaud's disease, diabetes mellitus)

3. Contractile tissue

4. a) History – recent (usually within previous 1 or 2 days); redness, heat, pain, swelling and loss of function

    b) The RICE regimen is still widely used in clinical practice. Evidence supports the use of ice for pain relief.

5. As soon as possible after injury but only within the client's pain-free range.

6. Observing active range of motion helps practitioners identify the severity of the client's condition before any passive movements are attempted. This strategy helps ensure the client's safety during assessment and treatment.

7. Sweet basil, peppermint, lemon, lemongrass, tea tree, Virginian cedarwood, juniper berry, sweet orange, clary sage

8. Acute injury management: first aid (e.g. RICE), exercise advice
Subacute injury management: remedial massage therapy, electrophysical therapy, heat therapy, joint mobilisation, exercise rehabilitation

9. permeability
kinins and histamine
monocytes and macrophages
clearing the area of infectious and toxic substances and tissue debris
clotting and anti-clotting factors, and proteins in the complement system
fibrin
granulation (scar) tissue

Chapter 4

1. Functional deficit demonstration (active functional testing)
Postural assessment
Muscle length testing
Muscle strength testing
Palpation

2. Apley's scratch test or standing active ROM tests.
Functional deficit assessments are preferred because they assess multiplanar movements that mimic everyday functions

3. Contracting muscles tend to limit bony approximation

4. When an agonist is contracting its antagonist will be neurally inhibited to allow unopposed joint motion. Relieving the spasm in a shortened muscle may lead to the withdrawal of the neural inhibition of the locked long muscle with an immediate improvement in function testing results.

5. i) Latissimus dorsi
Client standing, sidebend (tests unilateral lat dorsi)
Or client standing, touch toes (tests bilateral lat dorsi)
Other passive versions
ii) Pectoralis major
Sternal division – client supine, abduct extended arm to about 135° (see p 28)
Clavicular division – client supine, abduct extended arm to 90°
iii) Pectoralis minor
Client supine. Observe if back of shoulders touch the table (see p 29)
iv) Quadriceps
Client prone, heel to buttock

6. Postural muscles (e.g. upper trapezius, levator scapulae, quadratus lumborum, rectus femoris, iliopsoas, hamstrings) become hypertonic when overstressed; while phasic muscles (e.g. middle and lower trapezius, serratus anterior, rhomboids, rectus abdominis, gluteals) tend towards hypotonicity when overstressed. Postural muscles require massage, heat, stretching etc. Phasic muscles require strengthening exercises.

7. A muscle or functional group of muscles which become structurally shortened either as a results of spasm or contracture are referred to as *locked short*; a muscle or functional group of muscles, often antagonistic, which are overstretched and usually functionally weak, are referred to as *locked long*.

8. Contracture refers to a muscle which is locked short but is electrically silent; a spasm refers to a muscle which is locked short but is electrically active. Both may test weak during function testing. Contractures will be unlikely to respond to treatment – work on functional balance in surrounding muscles. Spasms are likely to respond well to massage and exercise therapy.

9. Gymnastics – hypermobile lumbar and hip ROM
Water polo – reduced bilateral iliopsoas ROM

10. Compare both sides

11.

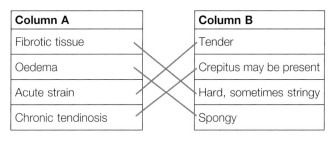

Column A	Column B
Fibrotic tissue	Tender
Oedema	Crepitus may be present
Acute strain	Hard, sometimes stringy
Chronic tendinosis	Spongy

12. i) What was the technique originally thought to achieve? Breakdown of scarring and adhesive conditions in muscles, tendons and ligaments.
ii) Further research is needed to confirm the effects of deep transverse friction.

Chapter 5

1. • Excitability (also called irritability) – the ability to receive and respond to stimuli. The response is contraction of muscle fibres.
• Contractility – muscle can actively shorten its length. This is the unique property of muscle tissues.
• Extensibility – muscle can be stretched beyond its resting length.
• Elasticity – muscle fibre can recoil and resume its resting length after being stretched.

2. In post-isometric relaxation the muscle is passively stretche and minimal resistance applied against isometric contraction.

In CRAC stretching, after the tight muscle is contracted isometrically against the practitioner's resistance, the client concentrically contracts the muscle opposite the tight muscle to actively move the joint through the increased range. A static stretch is then applied at the end of this new range of motion. The process can be repeated several times.

3. Contraindications and precautions for muscle stretching include:
- joint instability
- pain in the region of treatment
- pre-existing injury in muscle or tendon being treated
- active local inflammation of tissues
- geriatric clients – connective tissue begins losing elasticity from around the age of 30 years
- children – according to Appleton,[21] PNF stretching is not recommended for when bones are still growing.
- post surgery
- pre-event and post-event athletics
- recent or unresolved haematoma
- advanced osteoporosis and conditions that weaken bone such as osseous tumour and osteomalacia
- muscle fatigue or weakness

4. Taut muscle that feels like a stretched fibrous rope suggests chronic hypertonicity.

5. Match items in Column A with their function in Column B.

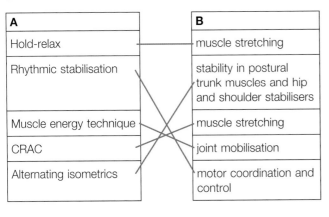

A	B
Hold-relax	muscle stretching
Rhythmic stabilisation	stability in postural trunk muscles and hip and shoulder stabilisers
Muscle energy technique	muscle stretching
CRAC	joint mobilisation
Alternating isometrics	motor coordination and control

6. Give priority to the most at risk tissue that could be affected by the stretch when planning a stretching routine.

Begin with Swedish massage or heat application to the area. Stretches performed during the consultation can be supplemented by a stretching program performed by the client at home.

7. i) an athlete
      sitting and toe touching
   ii) a 35-year-old who plays football once a week, does no other exercise and has a sedentary job
      standing and bending forward towards the toes.
   iii) a 70-year-old
      lying and raising a straight or slightly flexed leg

8. a) Eccentrically

9. c) Stretch reflex

10. b) Reciprocal inhibition

11. c) Ballistic

12. c) PNF

Chapter 6

1.
- Pain referred in a specific pattern that is characteristic of each trigger point
- Occasionally autonomic reactions (e.g. sweating, local vasoconstriction, lacrimation, coryza, salivation, pilomotor activity) and proprioceptive disturbances (e.g. dizziness and tinnitus)
- Pressure on an active trigger point usually elicits a jump sign (i.e. the client quickly pulls away when the trigger point is palpated)
- Snapping palpation (rapid movement across the muscle so that fibres snap back) frequently evokes a local twitch response
- Skin sometimes evinces dermographia (elevations or wheals caused by scratching the skin) or panniculosis (sensitive thickenings or nodules in the subcutaneous tissue) in the area overlying trigger points

2. The main difference between active and latent trigger points is the presence of pain. Active trigger points are always painful and refer pain at rest and/or when the specific muscle containing the trigger point is moved. Active trigger points prevent full lengthening of muscles and weaken the muscle. They can mediate a local twitch response (i.e. a brisk contraction of a taut band of skeletal muscle fibres elicited by snapping palpation of a trigger point[9]) and often produce autonomic phenomena such as local sweating and vasomotor activity, generally in the pain reference zone. Active trigger points are likely to be found in postural muscles of the neck, shoulder and pelvic girdle and the muscles of mastication.

Latent trigger points do not refer pain but are tender on palpation. They may become active through physical or emotional events such as sleeping position, chilling, or viral disease. Latent trigger points are often found incidentally during routine massage.

3.
- Mechanical stresses (e.g. skeletal asymmetry, poor lifting techniques, poor posture, prolonged immobility)
- Nutritional inadequacies (low level of vitamins B1, B6, B12 and C, folic acid, calcium, potassium, iron)
- Metabolic and endocrine inadequacies (thyroid underactivity, hyperuricemia, hypoglycemia) or any impairment to muscle metabolism (anaemia, hypoxia)
- Psychological factors
- Chronic infection
- Allergy, impaired sleep, radiculopathy, chronic visceral disease

Unless due attention is given to addressing perpetuating factors, treatment effect is not likely to be long lasting.

4. Draw an X on the following diagrams to indicate the locations of trigger point(s) in each of the following muscles.

i) Levator scapulae

ii) Upper trapezius

iii) Iliopsoas

iv) Piriformis

5. On the following diagrams, draw in the pain referral patterns for the trigger points indicated.

i) Quadratus lumborum

Deep

ii) Infraspinatus

iii) Rhomboids

iv) Sternocleidomastoid

6. i) Erector spinae muscles
Could be: standing touching toes, sitting legs out straight in front touching toes, or lying supine, pulling both knees to chest

ii) Upper trapezius muscle
Could be: sitting, hold under seat of chair and take head to opposite shoulder (unlitateral) or chin to chest (bilateral)

iii) Piriformis
Could be: lying prone, both knees bent to 90°, let feet drop out to sides. Alternatively, lie supine, knees bent and feet flat on the floor. Place one foot on top of the other knee allowing the knee to drop to the side. Pull the thigh of the bottom leg towards the chest.

7. A trigger point is said to shorten and weaken the muscle.

8. Digital ischaemic pressure is sustained; intermittent takes pressure off and on and is therefore safer and more tolerable.
Intermittent digital pressure: Apply gradually increasing pressure to 7 or 8 out of 10 on the pain scale, maintain the pressure until the client reports 3 or 4 out of 10, then gradually increase the pressure to 7 or 8 again. Repeat the process up to three times.
Intermittent digital pressure is suitable for most clients; digital ischaemic pressure is contraindicated in osteoporotic and hypertensive clients.

9. Snapping palpation (rapid movement across the muscle so that fibres snap back) frequently evokes a local twitch response.

10. Autonomic signs include increased vasomotor activity, changes in skin temperature, erythema of overlying skin, lacrimation, coryza, sweating, goose bumps.

11. Key trigger points are those that when treated can also reduce or eliminate satellite trigger points. Sternocleidomastoid has key trigger points associated with satellite trigger points in temporalis and masseter. See Table 6.1 for other examples.

12. Both piriformis and hamstrings have key trigger points. Treat piriformis first and then if need be, the hamstrings.

13. i) a central trigger point in the upper trapezius
A range of massage techniques can be used to treat central trigger points including:
Intermittent digital pressure, gliding massage techniques from the muscle belly out towards the muscle attachments, mild stretching, thermotherapy, deep stroking or stripping massage over the trigger point area.

ii) an attachment trigger point in the hamstring muscles
Ice massage
Short 20–30-second cold applications
Regardless of the method used to deactivate the trigger point, restoring the normal resting length of the muscle is recommended.

Chapter 7

1. Joint mobilisations use accessory movements but remain within the elastic barrier of the joint. Manipulative techniques are thought to overcome the elastic barrier but remain within the limit of anatomical integrity.

2.

a) Physiological movements can be actively performed by clients. **True**/False

b) Joint play is determined by the laxity of the joint capsule. **True**/False

c) Joint articulation uses physiological and accessory movement. **True**/False

3. When a joint is in the loose-pack position, the articulating surfaces are maximally separated and the joint has the greatest amount of free play. For example, the resting (loose-packed) position of the glenohumeral joint is 55° to 70° abduction and 30° horizontal abduction.

4.

Cervical spine	lateral flexion = rotation, extension
Shoulder joint	external rotation > abduction > flexion > internal rotation
Hip joint	flexion > internal rotation > abduction (order varies)
Knee joint	flexion > extension

That is, cervical lateral flexion is as equally limited as rotation and extension
Also, shoulder – external rotation more limited than abduction, which is more limited than flexion.

5. The usual contraindications of Swedish massage apply to joint articulation as well as
- acutely inflamed joints
- recent fracture
- osteoporosis
- malignancy
- joint instability
- rheumatoid collagen necrosis
- joint ankylosis
- vertebrobasilar insufficiency (for cervical articulation)
- infections
- joint replacement
- severe degenerative joint disease
- history of disc lesions or radiculopathy

6. Begin with Swedish massage to relax the muscles of the lower back, buttocks and right hip. Alternatively, the area may be warmed with a heat pack in preparation for joint articulation. Then apply hip joint articulation.

Guidelines for joint articulation

- Place the joint in mid-range. In general, mid-range positions are loose-packed; that is, the articulating surfaces are maximally separated and the joint has the greatest amount of free play. For example, the resting (loose-packed) position of the glenohumeral joint is 55° to 70° abduction and 30° horizontal abduction.
- Stablise the body part.
- The practitioner's hands should be as close to the joint as possible.
- Usually the proximal bone is stabilised and the distal bone is mobilised.
- Work with gravity where possible.
- Work within the client's pain tolerance.

Finally send the patient home with appropriate instructions (e.g. heat applications, gentle stretches, avoiding walking on hard surfaces in hard soled shoes, weight loss etc).

7. After treatment advise clients to avoid all aggravating conditions. Wearing shoes with good shock absorption and controlling body weight is advisable, especially for clients with low back or lower limb complaints. Range of motion exercises within pain tolerance should be encouraged and heat therapy may provide pain relief. A program of muscle stretching and strengthening can be introduced to address specific muscle imbalances around the joints. Refer clients for osseous manipulation, acupuncture and/or herbal/nutritional support as required.

If joint articulation is carried out after adequate warm-up and within pain tolerance then adverse effects are unlikely. If joint inflammation does occur after treatment, advise the client to use ice and rest the joint for a day or two. If symptoms persist, refer clients for further investigation.

8. History – including elimination of red flags

Functional tests – Active ROM then passive ROM. Observe for capsular pattern

Palpation – including assessment of end-feel of joint ROM

9. Osteoarthritis

Adhesive capsulitis

Other conditions secondary to upper cross syndrome (although directly related to chronic muscle imbalance, joint articulation may be useful)

10. b) Ankylosing spondylitis

Chapter 8

Review Questions

1. b) solid matter suspended in a fluid

2. c) fibroblasts and chondrocytes

3. a) loosen adhesions between connective tissue layers

4. d) cold, dry and tight

5. c) the lower the temperature, the more solid the ground substance

True/False Questions

6. The resistance of a colloid increases in proportion to the pressure applied to it. **True**/False

7. Thoracic inlet release is suitable for clients with breathing problems. **True**/False

8. Myofascial release is performed progressively towards the heart. True/**False**

9. Gentle myofascial release is suitable for most clients. **True**/False

10. When fascia is immobilised the ground substance gradually liquefies. True/**False**

11. Functions of fascia include:
- Maintaining normal shape
- Maintaining vital organs in their correct position
- Resisting mechanical stress (strength, support, elasticity and cushioning)
- Nutritive: loose connective tissue contains fluid that serves as a transport medium for cellular elements of other tissues, blood and lymph
- Providing an additional surface area for muscle attachments (deep fascia)
- Conserving body heat in fat stores (superficial fascia)
- Fighting bacterial infection: histiocyctes offer defence when infectious substances pass through planes in connective tissue
- Healing: fascia deposits collagen fibres (scar tissue) to assist in healing injuries

12. Refer clients to a psychologist, counsellor or medical practitioner when dealing with emotional responses that are beyond the scope of remedial massage therapy.

13. Gentle, sustained techniques are likely to encourage softening and elongation of fascia.

14. Deep myofascial release involves working through superficial layers, slowly applying pressure to a deep myofascial layer, working in time with the client's breathing and using a pain scale; gentle myofascial release involves gentle sustained pressure (3 to 5 minutes).

15. See Table 8.1

MFR initially, augmented by remedial massage techniques

Or

Other remedial techniques initially, augmented by MFR

Both approaches are followed by client education

16. The practitioner feels tissue resistance as a firm barrier.

17. Fascial restrictions often palpate as tight, cold and dry. Trigger points palpate as hyper-irritable painful spots in muscles that refer pain in a predictable pattern.

Chapter 9

1. Three functions of the lymphatic system:
1. remove protein from interstitial fluid
2. produce small lymphocytes which play a key role in cellular immunity: produce large lymphocytes which can synthesise antibiodies
3. drainage system to return interstitial fluid back to the cardiovascular system to be flushed out of the body

2. Complete the following:
a) Lymph is filtered as it passes through <u>lymph nodes</u> as it travels through the body.
b) Contractions of the smooth muscle in the walls of the <u>lymphangions</u> (the functional units of lymphatic vessels) stimulate the flow of lymph towards the thorax.
c) There are approximately <u>500–700</u> lymph nodes in the body.

3. b) right lymphatic duct

4. Mechanical impairment of organ function.

5. Lymphoedema is localised oedema due to lymphatic obstruction. There are many possible causes of oedema including acute nephritic syndrome, heart failure, pregnancy.

6. Surgical intervention and lymph node dissections (e.g. associated with mastectomy).

7.

Primary lymphoedema	Secondary lymphoedema
Mainly affects <u>lower extremity</u>	Occurs in any part of the body
Developmental abnormality. Can be triggered by <u>trauma or simple event like an insect bite</u>	Usually develops after <u>surgical intervention and lymph node dissection</u>

8. Absolute contraindications
- Chronic congestive heart failure, untreated heart failure or cardiac oedema, acute renal insufficiency. A load is placed on the venous system when there is an increase in the volume of lymph arriving at the subclavian veins. Significantly increasing the load could place strain on the heart and kidneys.[2]
- Acute infections and fever.
- Acute deep vein thrombosis (known or suspected).
- Unexplained pain.
- After recent surgery.
- After recent trauma (e.g. whiplash, fractures, sprains or dislocations, or when the extent of the injury is not known).
- Severe unstable hypertension (i.e. elevated blood pressure above the normal range for a prolonged period of time).
- Systemic illness (e.g. fever, diarrhoea, vomiting, unexplained oedema).
- Oedema that contributes to joint stability.

Relative contraindications
- Malignancies. Advise clients who have active cancer or who are recovering from cancer to get clearance from their doctor before commencing lymphatic drainage massage.
- Recent thrombosis. Older clients, clients with veins in poor condition and past history of thrombosis may be a contraindication.
- Varicose veins. Massage above the involved area.
- Bronchial asthma. Treat clients when the condition is receding, omitting sternum and chest massage. Never treat bronchial asthma in an acute phase. Care should always be taken with asthmatics to keep treatments short as overtreatment can bring on a mild attack of asthma.[4]
- Low blood pressure. A full body lymphatic drainage massage may lower blood pressure. Treatment time should be reduced for the first session and increased in subsequent sessions if no problems occur.[4]
- Moles, beauty spots, burns, fresh scars, bruises or skin problems.
- Renal insufficiency or clients receiving haemodialysis. Care should be taken to keep treatments short as such clients tire and bruise easily.
- Gynaecological cysts and other conditions of the uterus. Avoid deep abdominal massage.

Local contraindications
- Varicose veins, thrombosis after inflammation has subsided.
- Local inflammation without fever (e.g. open wound, sprains).
- Sports injuries with oedema or inflammation.

Neck
- Hypersensitivity of the carotid sinus.
- Hyperthyroidism.

Abdomen
- Pregnancy.
- During menstruation.
- After recent abdominal surgery.
- Radiation fibrosis.
- After pelvic deep venous thrombosis.
- Crohn's disease.
- Diverticulosis.

9. c) is always bilateral and pits on pressure

10. Complete the following guidelines for lymphatic drainage massage.
a) The pressure of lymphatic drainage massage is <u>light</u>
b) The rate of lymphatic drainage is <u>slow and rhythmic</u>
c) Begin lymphatic drainage massage at the <u>major proximal lymph nodes in the area</u>
d) Lymphatic drainage massage is always performed in the direction of <u>lymph flow</u>
e) In lymphatic drainage massage each stroke is performed <u>5–7</u> times.
f) Strokes are predominantly <u>circular</u> and performed in a wave-like rhythm.
g) Each stroke has a working phase and a resting phase to create a variation in <u>pressure</u>

11. c) shortness of breath

Chapter 10

1. a) Non-specific low back pain

2. b) Lower crossed syndrome/hyperlordosis

3. c) Sciatica and hamstring tightness

4. d) L5/S1 (closely followed by L4/L5)

5. a) A space-occupying lesion such as a disc prolapse

6. b) Spondylolisthesis

7. Severity of pain, positive Valsalva or compression test, neurological symptoms (e.g. radiating pain into the back of the leg)

8. All clients with spondylolisthesis should be assessed by a medical practitioner, chiropractor, osteopath or physiotherapist. This is potentially a very serious condition. Great attention is required to avoid lumbar extension in all phases of treatment. For example, incorrect pillow placement when the client is prone could increase lumbar lordosis and exert anterior pressure on the displaced vertebra. When the client is supine, ensure that clients lie with their knees flexed or place pillows under their knees to increase lumbar flexion. Posture and exercise advice for managing spondylolisthesis is similar to that for hyperlordotic (lower-crossed posture), including avoiding all activities that extend the spine and cultivating flexion activities such as bringing knees to chest.
AVOID ALL LUMBAR EXTENSION

9. Hip flexors (e.g. iliopsoas, quadriceps)
Back extensors (e.g. erector spinae, quadratus lumborum)

10. a) The sciatic nerve exits the sciatic notch and runs underneath the piriformis muscle. In 15% of the population the sciatic nerve passes through the muscle and muscle spasm or contracture can press on the nerve and cause sciatic neuritis (piriformis syndrome). If straight leg raising has produced pain, numbness or tingling in the low back, posterior thigh and/or lower leg, straight leg raising is performed a second time with the hip externally rotated (i.e. foot turned out). If the posterior thigh and leg pain is relieved in the second test, piriformis syndrome is suggested. Although not a common cause of posterior thigh and leg pain compared with nerve compression originating from the lumbosacral spine, piriformis syndrome can usually be simply and effectively treated when identified.
b) The client lies prone, knees flexed to 90° and lets their feet drop out to sides. The side on which the foot drops least is the side of the tighter piriformis.

11. a) iliopsoas
Lunges
b) quadratus lumborum
Sidebends
c) quadriceps femoris
Heel to buttock (see Table 10.4)

12. Red flags for acute lumbar pain:

Symptoms and signs of infection (e.g. fever) Risk factors for infection (e.g. underlying disease, immunosuppression, penetrating wound)	Infection
History of trauma Minor trauma (if >50 years, history of osteoporosis, taking corticosteroids)	Fracture
Past history of malignancy Age >50 years Failure to improve with treatment Unexplained weight loss Pain at multiple sites Pain at rest	Cancer
Absence of aggravating factors	Aortic aneurysm Other serious condition
Widespread neurological symptoms and signs in the lower limb (e.g. gait abnormality, saddle area numbness) +/− urinary retention, faecal incontinence	Cauda equine syndrome (a medical emergency and requires urgent hospital referral)
Morning stiffness in the lower back that improves with exercise and worsens with rest	Axial spondyloarthropathy (anklyosing spondylitis)

Chapter 11

1. c) unknown cause

2. a) an increased kyphosis at the level of C7 to T3

3. b) fractured rib

4. b) referral to a medical practitioner for further assessment

5. a) Scheuermann's disease

6. Adam's test. In functional scoliosis the spinal curvature straightens on forward bending of the trunk; in structural scoliosis the curvature persists.

7. a) Scheuermann's disease is a disorder of the vertebral epiphysis characterised by anterior vertebral wedging, irregular endplates and loss of vertebral disc height. It is usually limited to several vertebrae, most often in the lower thoracic spine. It is a self-limiting condition. The cause of the condition is unclear although a hereditary component appears to be involved.
b) The active phase occurs in the teenage years (13–17 years). Its ratio of males to females is 2:1.
c) Hyperkyphosis usually in the mid or low thoracic spine
AROM: limited especially in extension
PROM: limited especially in extension
Special tests: springing over affected vertebrae reveals limited mobility
d) Advise clients to be vigilant with posture (avoid slouching in flexion). Practise thoracic extension activities (e.g. the doorway stretch, backstroke swimming) as much as possible. Advise clients about correct lifting techniques. Clients should be referred for spinal manipulation.

Home exercise program
Place a rolled towel along the entire length of the thoracic spine. Lie on the towel for at least 10 minutes per day in order to oppose the increased kyphosis.
Daily extension exercises of the thoracic spine are recommended to increase the mobility of the affected area and to strengthen the back extensor muscles (see Figure 11.13).

8. Describe or draw a resisted muscle test for each of the following muscles:
a) pectoralis major – The client lies supine, arm extended and pointing towards the ceiling. Apply resistance as the client tries to adduct their arm across their chest
b) rhomboid muscles – Stand behind the client. The client takes their flexed elbow behind their back and adducts it as far as possible. Instruct the client to hold this position. Apply downward pressure with one hand on the client's shoulder. At the same time, with the other hand, try to push the elbow into flexion and abduction
c) serratus anterior – The client lies supine and raises their straight arm vertically in front of them (so that the shoulder is flexed to 90°) and thrusts their arm upward to lift their scapula off the table. The client resists as you apply downward pressure to the client's fist.
d) middle trapezius – The client is prone and instructed to abduct their straight arm to 90°, thumbs pointed up to the ceiling. Place one hand on the client's forearm and the other on the client's back over the trapezius muscle. Instruct the client to hold this position as you apply pressure towards the floor.

9. b) thoracic outlet syndrome

10. a) osteophytic lipping
c) muscle spasm

11. A rib fracture may be differentiated from an intercostal muscle spasm through:
History of trauma or likely to be osteoporotic
Severity of pain
Sharp pain
Inability to take a deep breath without pain
Reflex muscle guarding may be apparent on palpation

12. b) pectoralis major

Chapter 12

Review Questions

1. c) Acute torticollis

2. b) a ligament has been sprained

3. d) All of the above

4. c) C5/C6

5. Weak neck flexors – applying resistance with palm across forehead, as the client tries to flex their neck
Weak rhomboids, serratus anterior – wall push-ups keeping shoulder blades back and down

6. See Table 12.4

a) Upper trapezius – Sit and hold under the seat of the chair. Laterally flex neck to the opposite shoulder.

b) Levator scapulae – Reach behind back towards the opposite hip, laterally flex and rotate neck to the opposite side, and then flex neck to comfortable limit.

c) Scalene muscles – Laterally flex neck to comfortable limit and maintaining that position, look up and then down.

7. See Table 12.2

Symptoms and signs of infection (e.g. fever, night sweats)

History of trauma (minor trauma if older or taking corticosteroids), Down's syndrome, rheumatoid arthritis, osteoporosis

Past history of malignancy, age over 50, unexplained weight loss etc

Neurological symptoms in the limbs

Cerebrovascular symptoms or signs, anticoagulant therapy

Cardiovascular risk factors, stroke

8. a) a space-occupying lesion such as a disc prolapse

9. a) osteoarthritis

10. Usually over 50 years or have a history of previous significant trauma, recurrent dull ache in the neck that developed slowly or after a period of increased activity; pain increased by repetitive use and relieved by rest; morning stiffness.

Chapter 13

1. See Table 13.1

Red flags for serious causes of headache include:

- Abrupt onset of headache
- New onset or headache pattern especially when <5 y old or >50 y old
- Neurologic signs or symptoms
- Head or neck trauma
- Fever
- Weight loss
- Systemic disease
- Pregnancy
- Headaches triggered by exertion, sexual activity, cough, or Valsalva
- Postural headaches

2. Migraine headaches – usually one side of the head, often severe pain, pulsating, last 4–72 hours, with or without aura)

3. 20%

Symptoms include:

fully reversible visual symptoms including flickering lights, spots or lines, loss of vision

fully reversible sensory symptoms including pins and needles and numbness

fully reversible dysphasic speech disturbance

4. See Table 13.2

Vascular – 10–40 years onset, more common in females, rapid onset, temporal or frontal, throbbing/pulsing, moderate to severe, episodic, 4–72 hours, neurological signs symptoms common, triggered by foods, drugs, stress

Cervicogenic – 20–60 years, more common in females, slow onset, occipital, behind the eyes, temporal, unilateral, mild to moderate, dull ache, constant, lasts days, triggered by trauma, posture

5. Muscle and joint-specific techniques, heat therapy, myofascial release, posture and exercise rehabilitation; stress management including Swedish massage

6.

a) The most common type of headache is cervicogenic. **True**/False

b) Migraines often strike in the middle of the night. True/**False**

c) Tension-type headaches last no more than 1 or 2 days. True/**False**

d) Rhinosinusitis headache is aggravated by bending forward. True/**False**

e) Cervicogenic headaches typically start at the back of the neck and radiate over the head to the forehead. **True**/False

7. Questions based on red flags include:

How severe is the headache? (e.g. can you continue working?, does the headache wake you in the middle of the night?)

How long does the headache take to peak?

Is this a new or unaccustomed headache?

Are the headaches getting progressively worse?

Does the headache wake you from sleep?

How frequent are the headaches?

Sinusitis

1. The paranasal sinuses are located around the nasal cavity in the maxillary, sphenoid, ethmoid and frontal bones.

2. Infection of the frontal sinuses

Allergic reaction

3. To help reduce sinus congestion and thereby bring about symptom relief

4. Prone: Avoid long effleurage, kneading or friction strokes from the shoulders to the occiput. These strokes should be performed in the reverse direction.

Do not leave patient in prone position for long (pressure on the sinuses) and if you do use the prone position make sure the patient's head is level with their trunk (not lower).

Supine: Use a pillow to elevate the head slightly above the level of the trunk. Stroke only from face down the neck towards the clavicles.

(Use essential oils to aid in decongestion.)

5. The client needs to address the cause of the sinusitis (e.g. pharmaceutical treatment for bacterial infections, allergy testing if required, avoiding known allergens). Increase daily water intake, use steam inhalations. Refer to Quit Smoking programs as required.

Temporomandibular Joint Disorder

1. The two heads of lateral pterygoid act asynchronously – upper head pivots the head of the mandible, the lower head glides the mandible forward. The pattern of pivot and glide is repeated many times to open the jaw.

2. Headache
Clicking jaw
Difficulty chewing
Ear symptoms – pain, impaired hearing, tinnitus
Neuralgia

3. A client with normal range of motion of the TMJ should be able to:
a) Open their mouth wide enough <u>to put three fingers vertically in their mouth</u>
b) Protrude their jaw far enough to put <u>their bottom teeth in front of their top teeth</u>

4. Draw the pain referral patterns for the following trigger points.
See Table 13.6
a) Temporalis

b) Masseter

c) Lateral pterygoid

d) Medial pterygoid

5. Avoid hard foods, cut food into small pieces, chew using molars on both sides and avoid chewing gum.
Symptoms usually resolve with simple conservative treatment.
Heat for sub-acute/chronic pain, ice for acute inflammation.
Correcting forward head carriage.
Stress management – refer as indicated.

Chapter 14

1. b) a fractured rib

2. i) Observe the client lying supine. The back of the client's shoulder would normaly lie flat on the table.
ii) With the client supine, shoulder level with the edge of the table, the client abducts their arm to 135° and lets their arm drop down towards the floor. Shortness of the pectoralis major (sternal part) prevents the arm from dropping to the level of the table.
iii) Visceral pain may have associated symptoms like palpitations, shortness of breath, sweating, productive cough or pain relieved with antacid medication.

3. a) cardiovascular disease

4. c) inflammatory bowel disease

5. a) benign (e.g. referred from the thoracic spine)

6. b) childhood asthma

7. Rib subluxations may be difficult to distinguish from fractures. The rib cage is highly innervated to enable normal co-ordinated breathing. Consequently, rib subluxations are initially intensely painful. The severity of the trauma or the presence of underlying pathology suggests fracture. Severe pain that does not decrease over days and the presence of involuntary muscle guarding also suggest fracture. An X-ray of the region is required in order to make a definitive diagnosis.

8.
- Angina, headache, arm/neck pain, palpitations; cardiovascular risk factors
- Sharp/stabbing chest pain which may refer to lateral neck or shoulder, increased by sidelying, relieved by bending forward
- Tearing sensation, pain radiates to back/abdomen, most severe at onset
- Acute onset dyspnea, sharp chest pain aggravated by inspiration
- Acute onset dyspnea, chest, shoulder, or upper abdominal pain aggravated by deep breathing, haemoptysis, risk factors for deep venous thrombosis
- Pleuritic pain associated with productive cough, pain may refer to shoulder, fever, chills, headaches, malaise, nausea, dyspnea
- History of malignancy, night sweats, older age, tobacco use, weight loss
- History of trauma, osteoporosis, prolonged steroid use, age >70

9. Musculoskeletal chest pain has been defined as chest pain that is aggravated by movement; pain is reproduced by anterior pressure over the costochondral junctions. Thoracic spinal pain is reproduced on movement or on compression.

10. Remedial massage can assist in the management of the condition. Techniques include:

- Swedish massage to the back, including T3 (nerve supply to lungs, bronchial tubes, pleura, chest), neck (the phrenic nerve which supplies the diaphragm, originates mainly from C4), and chest (focus on intercostal muscles). Tapotement is useful in loosening mucus.
- Remedial massage techniques include:
    - Specific muscle techniques particularly for muscles of respiration (pectoralis minor, external intercostals, subclavius, scalene and sternocleidomastoid muscles). Techniques include (see Table 14.5)
        - deep gliding frictions
        - cross-fibre frictions
        - soft tissue releasing techniques
        - trigger point therapy
        - muscle stretching
- Acupressure points can be incorporated into Swedish massage.
- Gentle mobilisations of the thoracic spine including (see Chapter 7):
- Further mobilisations including diaphragm release, cat walk etc (see text)
- Reflexology
- Aromatherapy

Client education: Steam inhalations and humidifiers using essential oils (e.g. eucalyptus and pine) have traditionally been used. Breathing exercises, swimming, yoga, Buteyko and hydrotherapy may be recommended.

It is imperative that clients continue their usual medication. Clients can be referred to a naturopath, homoeopath, acupuncturist, and/or manipulative therapist for further treatment. Allergy testing may also be required.

11. Primary – diaphragm, external intercostal
Accessory – internal intercostals, sternocleidomastoid, scalenes, serratus anterior, pectoralis major and minor, upper trapezius, latissimus dorsi, erector spinae (thoracic), iliocostalis lumborum, quadratus lumborum, serratus posterior superior and inferior, levatores costarum, transversus thoracis, and subclavius.

12. a) In paradoxical breathing the rib cage deflates as the client inhales and inflates as they exhale.
   b) If there is no underlying pathology, clients can correct paradoxical breathing by placing one hand on the upper ribs and one on the abdomen and practising breathing in such a way that the hand on the rib cage rises as they inhale and falls as they exhale.

Chapter 15

1.

Column A		Column B
Elastic and firm		Horizontal adduction
Empty		Adhesive capsulitis
Hard and capsular		Horizontal abduction
Soft tissue		Severe instability

2. c) resisted shoulder internal rotation

3. d) bursa

4. c) history of anterior glenohumeral dislocation

5. b) lateral rotation

6. c) AC joint separation

7. i) supraspinatus – reaching arm behind back towards opposite elbow
   ii) teres major – lying supine, hand behind head, elbow to table
   iii) biceps brachii – extend shoulder, extend elbow and pronate forearm

8. i) stretching for general flexibility (e.g. pendulum exercises)
   ii) strengthening for shoulder stabilisers and rotator cuff muscles (e.g. wall push-ups, overhead work, ball throwing)

9. i) Infraspinatus
   ii) DTF is designed to break down adhesions.

10. Biceps brachii tendon

11.
- Deep gliding frictions along the muscle fibres
- Cross-fibre frictions
- Soft tissue releasing techniques
- Deep transverse friction
- Trigger point therapy

12.
- Advise clients to avoid all overhead or painful activities
- Posture correction especially for the cervical spine and pectoral girdle
- Review aggravating sporting techniques or work activities and correct if possible
- A rehabilitation exercise program should be started as soon as tolerated by the client. The goal of the program is to restore normal shoulder biomechanics. This usually involves strengthening the shoulder stabilisers and rotator cuff muscles. Restoration of normal scapular rotation about a medial to lateral axis and serratus anterior muscle function are particularly important in the rehabilitation of clients whose symptoms are related to occupational overhead work.
- Refer for spinal and shoulder manipulation.

Chapter 16

1. c) 10–15°

2. Flexor carpi radialis, palmaris longus, flexor carpi ulnaris, flexor digitorum superficialis

3. Both are tested by pronating the forearm, asking the client to hold the position while the practitioner tries to supinate the forearm. Pronator quadratus is tested with the elbow fully flexed; pronator teres tested with only slight elbow flexion.

4. c) C7
   d) C8

5. a) joint effusion

6. Biceps brachii – resisted elbow flexion with forearm
   supinated
Brachialis – resisted elbow flexion with forearm pronated
Brachioradialis – resisted elbow flexion with forearm
   semi-supinated (thumb facing towards ceiling)

7. Avoid wrist extension movements (e.g. perform long
effleurage and friction strokes with wrists in neutral, use
forearms etc).

8. c) extensor carpi radialis brevis

9. Repetition strain injuries, especially extensor tendinosis.
Less commonly flexor tendinosis.

10. i) In the acute phase
      Apply ice and firm compression. Advise clients to
      eliminate the responsible activity. This may involve
      avoiding resting the elbow on a hard surface,
      modifying the work environment or wearing an
      elbow pad.
   ii) In the sub-acute phase
      If the etiology is associated with a tight triceps brachii
      or forearm extensor muscles, include specific remedial
      massage techniques (including deep gliding,
      cross-fibre frictions, soft tissue release, trigger point
      therapy and muscle stretches) to restore full muscle
      length in the sub-acute or chronic phase. Myofascial
      release might be beneficial. Refer clients for osseous
      manipulation if required.

11. • Deep gliding frictions along the muscle fibres
    • Cross-fibre frictions
    • Soft tissue releasing techniques
    • Deep transverse friction applied directly to the
      damaged tendon may help stimulate collagen
      production
    • Trigger point therapy for wrist extensor muscles
    • Muscle stretches
    • Myofascial release including cross-arm techniques and
      the arm pull

12. c) golfer's elbow

Chapter 17

1. Extensor digiti minimi, extensor carpi ulnaris, externsor
carpi radialis brevis, extensor carpi radialis longus, extensor
pollicis brevis, abductor pollicis longus, extensor pollicis
longus, extensor pollicis longus, extensor indicis (see
Figure 17.29)

2. Scaphoid bone.
The most useful diagnostic sign for scaphoid fracture is pain
on direct pressure to the floor of the anatomical snuffbox.

3. a) Abductor pollicis longus and brevis

4. Repetition strain injuries include:
lateral epicondylitis, carpal tunnel syndrome, de Quervain's
   disease and tenoysynovitis of the wrist or hand.

5. Lunate dislocation usually occurs as a result of a fall onto
the thenar eminence which forces the lunate anteriorly as the
wrist is forcefully extended.

6. c) wrist extensor tendinopathy/tenosynovitis

7. b) Tinel's sign
   c) Phalen's test

8. Other causes of mechanical compression include
degenerative joint disease, neuroma and ganglia that develop
in the tunnel, subluxation of the lunate bone, constant
vibration (e.g. using jack hammer) and trauma. Carpal tunnel
syndrome may also be caused by fluid retention/metabolic
disease (e.g. diabetes, obesity, fluid retention during
pregnancy).

9. Compression of the median nerve in the carpal tunnel can
alter:
i) sensation in the thumb, index and middle finger
ii) motor activity in the thenar muscles and the rest of the
   muscles on the front of the forearm and hand

10. Osteoarthritis is a common presenting condition in older
   clients or those with previous significant trauma or history
   of overuse; rheumatoid arthritis affects 20–40-year-olds.
In osteoarthritis the distal interphalangeal joints are most
   affected and Heberden's nodes may develop in affected
   joints; rheumatoid arthritis worse in the proximal and
   interphalangeal joints.
Osteoarthritis affects men and women equally; rheumatoid
   arthritis predominantly affects females.
Osteoarthritis affects weight-bearing joints, usually
   asymmetrical; rheumatoid arthritis affects fingers and wrists
   first, symmetrically.

11. • Deep gliding frictions along the muscle fibres
    • Cross-fibre frictions
    • Soft tissue releasing techniques
    • Deep transverse friction applied directly to the
      damaged tendon
    • Trigger point therapy
    • Muscle stretching

12. Swedish massage to the entire upper limb and lower
cervical and upper thoracic spines, local heat applications
(e.g. hot wax treatments), gentle joint articulation, myofascial
release techniques and muscle-focused techniques including
muscle stretches.

Chapter 18

1. c) Femoral capital slipped epiphysis

2. a) Quadriceps muscle strain

3. d) vastus intermedialis

4. b) 5–10 years

5. c) Internal rotation

6. i) gluteus medius and minimus
piriform
internal and external obturator
gemelli muscles

ii) Trochanteric bursitis refers to an inflamed trochanteric bursa which lies directly over the greater trochanter. It is more common in the middle to older age groups and more common in women than men.

iii) The bursa may become inflamed from a direct blow or, more commonly, from chronic compression and friction from the ilitotibial band as it rubs over the greater trochanter during flexion and extension of the hip. The condition is often secondary to biomechanical imbalance such as muscle hypertonicity (e.g. tight gluteus maximus or hip abductor muscles) or from overuse injury (e.g. running on a sloped surface). Describe the mechanism(s) which contribute to the development of trochanteric bursitis – can be inflamed from a direct blow or, more commonly, from chronic compression and friction from the ilitotibial band as it rubs over the greater trochanter during flexion and extension of the hip. Aggravated by climbing stairs and getting in and out of a car. The condition is often secondary to biomechanical imbalance such as muscle hypertonicity (e.g. tight gluteus maximus or hip abductor muscles) or from overuse injury (e.g. running on a sloped surface).

7. The stability of the hip joint is enhanced by the depth of the acetabulum and the presence of the acetabular labrum (cartilaginous ring) and ligamentum teres, which keeps the head of the femur in the socket.
Other ligaments of the hip joint include the pubofemoral ligament, ischiofemoral ligament, zona orbicularis and the transverse ligament of the acetabulum (see Figure 18.1).

8. Pain on resisted hip extension could be due to gluteus maximus or the hamstrings. Gluteus maximus can be tested with the client prone, thigh elevated and the client resisting the practitioner's attempt to take the thigh to the table. Hamstrings can be tested by resisted knee flexion.
+ve resisted hip extension suggests strain of the hip extensor muscles. To discriminate between gluteaus maximum and hamstrings: resist knee flexion. If resisted knee flexion also reproduces the pain, then hamstrings are implicated. If resisted knee flexion does not reproduce the pain, then the gluteus maximus is implicated.

9. Pain reproduced by active range of motion tests of the lumbar spine or the hip region are a good indicator.
History
Functional tests
AROM lumbar will reproduce symptoms; hip AROM will not, if lumbar area implicated
AROM lumbar will not reproduce symptoms; hip AROM will, if hip joint implicated

10. i) Trendelenburg test
gluteus medius
iii) Ober's test:
iliotibial band tightness
iii) Patrick's test
usually indicates hip joint pathology but could be sartorius and other hip adductors.

11. Rarely acute, but if so, treatment could include cryotherapy for analgesia, acupressure, Reiki, reflexology or anti-inflammatory medication. The client should be advised to modify activities to avoid aggravating the condition.
A typical remedial massage treatment for mild or moderate sub-acute or chronic osteoarthritis includes:
- Swedish massage therapy to the low back, pelvis and lower limb
- Remedial massage therapy includes heat therapy, myofascial releasing techniques and joint articulation (see Chapter 7) including:
  - Hip rotation
  - Hip figure-8
  - Hip traction
  - Hip rotation sidelying
- Remedial massage techniques (e.g. deep gliding, cross-fibre frictions, soft tissue release and muscle stretching) for associated muscle contractures.
- Client education
The client should be advised to continue to use heat therapy for pain relief and to modify or avoid all aggravating activities. Range of motion exercises should be commenced as soon as possible within the client's pain tolerance. Stretching and strengthening exercises can be introduced as indicated by assessment findings. Educate clients about the importance of getting the right balance between too little activity (which can lead to capsule and muscle contractures and movement compensations) and too much activity (which can inflame the joint). Non-weight bearing activities such as water aerobics are often beneficial. Use of shock-absorbing soles and weight loss are recommended. Nutritional supplements such as glucosamine may be beneficial.[23] Clients may be referred for other supportive therapies including specialist nutritional advice, acupuncture and osseous mobilisation and manipulation of the pelvis and spine.

12. In the sub-acute or chronic phase, remedial massage techniques for muscle strains include:

- Muscle specific techniques (see Tables 10.5 and 18.7)
- Deep gliding frictions along the muscle fibres
- Cross-fibre frictions
- Soft tissue releasing techniques
- Deep transverse friction at the site of lesion. Deep transverse friction is thought to stimulate collagen production and create mobile scar tissue. Apply the technique for several minutes within the client's pain threshold, alternating with other forms of tissue mobilisation including effleurage, sweeping cross-fibre frictions and stretching.
- Trigger point therapy
- Muscle stretching
- Myofascial release including cross-arm techniques and the leg pull (see Chapter 8)
- Thermotherapy may be beneficial for pain relief

Chapter 19

1.

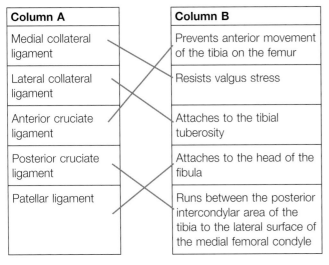

Column A	Column B
Medial collateral ligament	Prevents anterior movement of the tibia on the femur
Lateral collateral ligament	Resists valgus stress
Anterior cruciate ligament	Attaches to the tibial tuberosity
Posterior cruciate ligament	Attaches to the head of the fibula
Patellar ligament	Runs between the posterior intercondylar area of the tibia to the lateral surface of the medial femoral condyle

2. The main function of the popliteus muscle is to unlock the extended (weight-bearing) knee. Popliteus laterally rotates the femur on the tibia and moves the lateral meniscus posteriorly at the beginning of knee flexion. External rotation when the knee is semi-flexed is a function of biceps femoris. Popliteus medially rotates the tibia when the knee is flexed along with sartorius, gracilis and semitendinosus (see Figure 19.4).

3. i) Quadriceps as a group
        Resisted knee extension
     ii) Rectus femoris:
        Resisted hip flexion and resisted knee extension
     iii) Vastus medialis obliquus
        Resisted knee extension in the last 20–30°

4. i) Damage to the medial collateral ligament of the knee
        Valgus stress test
     ii) Rupture to the anterior cruciate ligament of the knee
        Anterior drawer test; Lachman test
     iii) Torn cartilage (meniscus)
        Apley's compression and grind test; Thessaly test

5. Clients complain of knee pain on standing after a prolonged period of sitting. Prolonged sitting with knee flexion maintains the quadriceps in a stretched position and a sudden change in position may elicit knee pain (the movie sign).
Patellofemoral syndrome

6. Tears that occur on the outer third of the meniscus, which has a good vascular supply, have a good chance of healing.

7. The 'unhappy triad' refers to injury to the anterior cruciate ligament, the medial collateral ligament and the medial meniscus.

8. ii) Larger than the medial meniscus

9. i) trunk thrown forward over the centre of gravity
     ii) lifting the hip during swing phase
     iv) manually pushing the knee into extension

10. ii) semimembranosus

11. i) The primary cause of the problem appears to be related to the tracking of the patella during knee extension movements. The patella is embedded in the quadriceps tendon. The patella is pulled superiorly during quadriceps contraction along the line of the pull of the quadriceps. The degree to which this pull deviates from a vertical line is indicated by the Q angle; that is, the angle between a line that connects the tibial tuberosity and the midpoint of the patella, and a line that connects the midpoint of the patella and the anterior superior iliac spine (see Figure 19.5).
     ii) 1. A large Q angle is one of the most common factors that lead to patellar tracking disorders.
        2. Imbalances between the strength of the vastus medialis obliquus, vastus lateralis and ilitotibial band, with its lateral patellar expansion, can contribute to tracking disorders.
        3. Intrinsic factors such as patella alta (a hypermobile and unstable patella that is displaced proximally) and patella baja (in which the patella is displaced distally so that the articular surfaces are incongruent) may also be involved.
     iii) Remedial massage techniques are aimed at addressing the muscle imbalance in the quadriceps and iliotibial band tightness. Techniques especially to vastus lateralis could include:
        - deep gliding frictions along the muscle fibres
        - cross-fibre frictions
        - active and passive soft tissue releasing techniques
        - deep transverse friction
        - trigger point therapy (include all quadriceps muscles)
        - muscle stretches
- Strengthening vastus medialis obliquus may offset the tendency of the other quadriceps to pull the patella laterally.

12. The client should be advised to use heat therapy for pain relief and to modify or avoid all aggravating activities. Weight loss and the use of shock-absorbing soles in shoes may reduce the load on the joint and provide symptom relief. Home exercises should be commenced as soon as pain permits. Non-weight bearing activities such as swimming are often beneficial.

Nutritional supplements may be beneficial. Clients may be referred for other supportive therapies including specialist nutritional advice and acupuncture.

Chapter 20

1. a) A dull ache along the anteromedial border of the tibia which is aggravated by activity
   b) Weakness of the dorsiflexors of the foot

2. a) resisted ankle plantarflexion

3. d) Tenderness is felt on the sole of the foot between the 3rd and 4th metatarsal heads

4. a) Anterior talofibular ligament

5. b) Sever's disease

6. i) Shin splints is a term used to describe shin pain due to repetitive overuse such as running or dancing. Long periods of standing on a concrete floor or other hard surface in hard soled shoes has also been implicated. There are two main types of shin splints:
   a) Anterior/lateral shin splints: tibialis anterior strain, tendinopathy or periostitis. Anterior shin splits is associated with excessive eccentric dorsiflexion (e.g. downhill walking or running)
   Posterior shin splints: tibialis posterior strain, tendinopathy or periostitis. Flexor digitorum longus and soleus may also be involved. It is associated with overpronation or incorrect running stride.

   ii)

Shin splints	Stress fracture
Excessive activity (e.g. running on hard or uneven ground), overtraining, poor shoes, repeated impacts on a hard surface	Following prolonged activity (e.g. marching, skiing, running), especially in a hard-soled shoe/boot
Pain anterolateral or posteromedial border tibia	Severe anterior shin pain. Acute, sharp.
Pain deceases as the muscle warms up	Constant, increasing with exercise. Worse with impact.
Pain worse in morning and after exercise	Night ache. May be worse in morning.
Palpatory tenderness over a wide region of the tibia and involved muscle	Palpation elicits localised pain

iii) In the acute phase, the RICE regime may be beneficial. Advise the client to rest from aggravating activities such as exercise on hard, uneven surfaces. Gentle stretching should be commenced as soon as possible within pain tolerance. The client may be referred for mobilisation and manipulation of the low back, hip, knee, ankle and foot. Referral for orthotics may also be required.

In chronic presentations massage therapy is directed towards reducing hypertonicity in affected muscles. A typical remedial massage treatment for sub-acute or chronic shin splints includes:

- Swedish massage therapy to the lower limb, lumbar spine and pelvis. Avoid all techniques that pull on the tibial attachments of muscles. A useful technique involves compressing muscles back onto the bone (see Figure 20.33).
- Remedial massage techniques including (see Table 20.4):
  - Deep gliding frictions along the muscle fibres (including soleus, popliteus)
  - Cross-fibre frictions
  - Soft tissue releasing techniques
  - Deep transverse friction applied directly to the injury site may help stimulate collagen production
  - Trigger point therapy
  - Muscle stretching
- Myofascial release including cross-arm techniques and the leg pull (see Chapter 8)
- Heat therapy is usually beneficial
- Other remedial techniques such as ankle joint articulation may also be introduced as required (see Chapter 7):
  - Ankle prone circumduction
  - Calcaneus prone circumduction
  - Tarsals prone plantarflexion
  - Ankle traction
  - Metatarsal shearing
  - Phalanges mobilisation
- Correct underlying biomechanical and predisposing factors where possible (e.g. overpronation of ankles, foot flare, externally rotated hips, apparent leg length inequality, tight quadriceps, hamstrings, hip flexors or abductors as indicated)

Client education: Advise the client to rest from aggravating activities such as downhill running or excessive impacts on hard surfaces. Gentle stretching should be introduced as soon as pain permits and continue throughout the rehabilitation. Weakness and/or tightness of tibialis anterior and posterior, gastrocnemius, soleus, quadriceps, hamstrings, hip flexors and hip abductors should be addressed in a progressive strengthening and stretching program. The client may need to change shoes and may need to be referred for orthotics.

7. Sinus tarsi – Anterior talofibular ligament runs from the anterior aspect of the lateral malleolus to the lateral talus. Tenderness and swelling in the sinus tarsi usually indicate a sprain of the anterior talofibular ligament.

8. i) In the acute phase

The treatment goal immediately after the injury is to decrease pain, increase pain-free range of motion and to protect the ankle from further damage. Immediate mobilisation and functional treatment is widely regarded as the best treatment strategy. Ankle splints and taping provide protection for the joint. Reduce weight bearing (crutches may be required). Commence pain-free range of motion exercises as soon as pain permits.

ii) In the chronic phase

A typical remedial massage treatment for sub-acute or chronic ankle inversion sprain includes:

Swedish massage therapy to the lower limb, low back and pelvis

Remedial massage techniques including:

- Light lymphatic drainage to promote reduction of swelling.
- Deep transverse friction at the site of lesion to help prevent adhesion formation.
- Massage techniques for associated muscle strains (e.g. peroneal muscles) or imbalances include (see Table 20.4):
  - Deep gliding frictions along the muscle fibres
  - Cross-fibre frictions
  - Soft tissue releasing techniques
  - Trigger point therapy
  - Muscle stretching
- Myofascial release (see Chapter 8)
- Other remedial techniques such as ankle joint articulation may also be introduced as required (see Chapter 7).
- Longer term management involves correcting underlying biomechanical and predisposing factors where possible (e.g. genu varum, weak ankle everters and/or tight ankle inverters)

Client education: Early mobilisation is important to stimulate collagen production.

9. Biomechanical dysfunction in the foot, particularly associated with excessive pronation and lowered longitudinal arch or with pes cavus, place excessive tension on the plantar fascia at the medial tubercle of the anterior calcaneus. Prolonged tensile stress on the periosteum may lead to the development of a bony spur.

10. In many cases the most significant indicator is history of recent surgery or long plane or bus trip. Suspect deep venous thrombosis when the client has constant pain, tenderness, increased temperature and swelling in the calf. Homan's sign (passive dorsiflexion of the ankle) may reproduce pain (but would also be painful for calf muscle strains).

Chapter 21

1. i) in-toeing gait

ii) 40° in neonates and 10° or less in adults

2. Hormonal factors (associated with the growth spurt in puberty) are thought to weaken the epiphyseal plate allowing the head of the femur to slip posteriorly and inferiorly.

Symptoms include groin pain, often referred to the knee, and a limp. Onset may be sudden after trauma or gradual over weeks to months.

3. Primary dysmenorrhoea – pain is most severe on the first two days of bleeding

Congestive dysmenorrhoea – pain commences a few days before bleeding and is relieved by the onset of bleeding

Endometriosis – pain commences a few days before bleeding and increases to a maximum within 3 days of onset of bleeding

4. Declining oestrogen increases visceral fat mass and decreases bone mass density, muscle mass and strength.

5. Chronic diseases like obesity, cancer, diabetes and cardiovascular disease.

6. Always consider prostate cancer if a male over 50 years presents with low back pain.

7. Allow extra time. In general, techniques are applied lightly because of skin fragility, the risk of fracture in osteoporotic clients and the risk of bruising in clients taking blood-thinning medication. The treatment duration may be short. Clients with cardiovascular or respiratory condition may be uncomfortable lying supine – extra pillows to elevate their head and shoulders may be required.

8. Possible indicators of an underlying mental health condition include:

- seemingly inappropriate requests for urgent attention
- increased frequency of consultation or requests for tests
- unexpected or disproportionate outbursts during consultation (tears, anger)
- excessive anxiety about another family member or presenting a relative as the patient
- unstable relationships or frequent breakdowns in relationships
- distressing or deteriorating social circumstances (eviction, redundancy, squalor).

Index

Page numbers followed by "*f*" indicate figures, "*t*" indicate tables, "*b*" indicate boxes, and "*e*" indicate online content.